Basic Sciences of Nuclear Medicine

Magdy M. Khalil (Ed.)

Basic Sciences of Nuclear Medicine

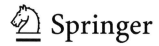 Springer

Magdy M. Khalil
Imperial College London
Hammersmith Campus
Biological Imaging Centre
Du Cane Road
W12 0NN London
United Kingdom
magdy_khalil@hotmail.com

ISBN 978-3-540-85961-1   e-ISBN 978-3-540-85962-8

DOI 10.1007/978-3-540-85962-8

Springer-Verlag Heidelberg Dordrecht London New York

Library of Congress Control Number: 2010937976

Cover design: eStudio calamar, Figures/Berlin

Printed on acid-free paper

Springer is part of Springer Science+Business Media (www.springer.com)

I dedicate this book to my parents

وفوق كل ذي علم عليم.........سورة يوسف (76)

"... and over every lord of knowledge, there is ONE more knowing"
Yousef (12:76)

Acknowledgment

Thanks to my God without him nothing can come into existence. I would like to thank my parents who taught me the patience to achieve what I planned to do. Special thanks also go to my wife, little daughter and son who were a driving force for this project. I am grateful to my colleagues in Department of Nuclear Medicine at Kuwait University for their support and encouragement, namely, Prof. Elgazzar, Prof. Gaber Ziada, Dr. Mohamed Sakr, Dr. A.M. Omar, Dr. Jehan Elshammary, Mrs. Heba Essam, Mr. Junaid and Mr. Ayman Taha. Many thanks also to Prof. Melvyn Meyer for his comments and suggestions, Drs. Willy Gsell, Jordi Lopez Tremoleda and Marzena Wylezinska-Arridge, MRC/CSC, Imperial College London, Hammersmith campus, UK. Last but not least would like to thank Sayed and Moustafa Khalil for their kindness and indispensible brotherhood.

Contents

Basic Physics and Radiation Safety in Nuclear Medicine

1

G. S. Pant

Contents

1.1 Basic Atomic and Nuclear Physics

1.1.1 Atom

All matter is comprised of atoms. An atom is the smallest unit of a chemical element possessing the properties of that element. Atoms rarely exist alone; often, they combine with other atoms to form a molecule, the smallest component of a chemical compound.

G.S. Pant
Consultant Medical Physicist, Nuclear Medicine Section, KFSH, Dammam, KSA
e-mail: gspant2008@hotmail.com

1.1.2 Modern Atomic Theory

1.1.2.1 Wave-Particle Duality

According to classical physics the particle cannot be a wave, and the wave cannot be a particle. However, Einstein, while explaining the photoelectric effect (PEE), postulated that electromagnetic radiation has a dual wave-particle nature. He used the term *photon* to refer to the particle of electromagnetic radiation. He proposed a simple equation to relate the energy of the photon E to the frequency v and wavelength λ of electromagnetic wave.

$$E = hv = h\frac{c}{\lambda} \tag{1.1}$$

In this equation, h is Planck's constant (6.634×10^{-34} J.s) and c is the velocity of light in a vacuum.

De Broglie generalized the idea and postulated that all subatomic particles have a wave-particle nature. In some phenomena, the particle behaves as a particle, and in some phenomena it behaves as a wave; it never behaves as both at the same time. This is called the *wave-particle duality of nature*. He suggested the following equation to relate the momentum of the particle p and wavelength λ:

$$\lambda = \frac{h}{p} \tag{1.2}$$

Only when the particles have extremely small mass (subatomic particles) is the associated wave appreciable. An electron microscope demonstrates the wave-particle duality. In the macroscopic scale, the De Broglie theory is not applicable.

M.M. Khalil (ed.), *Basic Sciences of Nuclear Medicine*, DOI: 10.1007/978-3-540-85962-8_1,
© Springer-Verlag Berlin Heidelberg 2011

1.1.2.2 Electron Configuration

Electrons around a nucleus can be described with wave functions [1]. Wave functions determine the location, energy, and momentum of the particle. The square of a wave function gives the probability distribution of the particle. At a given time, an electron can be anywhere around the nucleus and have different probabilities at different locations. The space around the nucleus in which the probability is highest is called an *orbital*. In quantum mechanics, the orbital is a mathematical concept that suggests the average location of an electron around the nucleus. If the energy of the electron changes, this average also changes. For the single electron of a hydrogen atom, an infinite number of wave functions, and therefore an infinite number of orbitals, may exist.

An orbital can be completely described using the corresponding wave function, but the process is tedious and difficult. In simple terms, an orbital can be described by four quantum numbers.

- The principal quantum number n characterizes the energy and shell size in an atom. It is an integer and can have a value from 1 to ∞, but practically n is always less than 8. The maximum number of electrons in orbital n is $2n^2$. The shells of electrons are labeled alphabetically as $K(n = 1)$, $L(n = 2)$, $M(n = 3)$, and so on based on the principal quantum number.
- The orbital quantum number l relates to the angular momentum of the electron; l can take integer values from 0 to $n - 1$. In a stable atom, its value does not go beyond 3. The orbital quantum number characterizes the configuration of the electron orbital. In the hydrogen atom, the value of l does not appreciably affect the total energy, but in atoms with more than one electron, the energy depends on both n and l. The subshells or orbitals of electrons are labeled as $s(l = 0)$, $p(l = 1)$, $d(l = 2)$ and $f(l = 3)$.
- The azimuthal or magnetic quantum number m_l relates to the direction of the angular momentum of the electron and takes on integer values from $-l$ to $+l$.
- The spin quantum number m_s relates to the electron angular momentum and can have only two values: $-\frac{1}{2}$ or $+\frac{1}{2}$.

Pauli in 1925 added a complementary rule for arrangement of electrons around the nucleus. The postulation is now called *Pauli's exclusion principle* and states that no two electrons can have all quantum numbers the same or exist in identical quantum states.

The filling of electrons in orbitals obeys the so-called Aufbau principle. The Aufbau principle assumes that electrons are added to an atom starting with the lowest-energy orbital until all of the electrons are placed in an appropriate orbital. The sequence of energy states and electron filling in orbitals of a multi-electron atom can be represented as follows:

$$1s - 2s - 2p - 3s - 3p - 4s - 3d - 4p - 5s - 4d$$
$$- 5p - 6s - 4f - 5d - 6p - 7s - 5f - 6d - 7p$$

1.1.2.3 Electron Binding Energies

The bound electrons need some external energy to make them free from the nucleus. It can be assumed that electrons around a nucleus have negative potential energy. The absolute value of the potential energy is called the *binding energy*, the minimum energy required to knock out an electron from the atom.

1.1.2.4 Atomic Emissions

For stability, electrons are required to be in the minimum possible energy level or in the innermost orbitals. However, there is no restriction for an electron to transfer into outer orbitals if it gains sufficient energy. If an electron absorbs external energy that is more than or equal to its binding energy, a pair of ions, the electron and the atom with a positive charge, is created. This process is termed *ionization*. If the external energy is more than the binding energy of the electron, the excess energy is divided between the two in such a way that conservation of momentum is preserved.

If an electron absorbs energy and is elevated to the outer orbitals, the original orbital does not remain vacant. Soon, the vacancy will be filled by electrons from the outer layers. This is a random process, and the occupier may be any electron from the outer orbitals. However, the closer electron has a greater chance to occupy the vacancy. In each individual process of filling, a quantum of energy equal to the difference between the binding energies $E_2 - E_1$ of the two involved orbitals is released, usually in the form of a single photon. The frequency v and wavelength λ of the emitted photon (radiation) are given as follows:

$$E_2 - E_1 = \Delta E = hv = h\frac{c}{\lambda} \qquad (1.3)$$

When an atom has excess energy, it is in an unstable or *excited state*. The excess energy is usually released in the form of electromagnetic radiation (characteristic radiation), and the atom acquires its natural *stable state*. The frequency spectrum of the radiation emitted from an excited atom can be used as the fingerprint of the atom.

1.1.2.5 Nuclear Structure

There are several notations to summarize the nuclear composition of an atom. The most common is $_Z^A X_N$, where X represents the chemical symbol of the element. The chemical symbol and atomic number carry the same information, and the neutron number can be calculated by the difference of A and Z. Hence, for the sake of simplicity the brief notation is $^A X$, which is more comprehensible. For example, for ^{137}Cs, where 137 is the mass number (A + Z), the Cs represents the 55th element (Z = 55) in the periodic table. The neutron number can easily be calculated (A − Z = 82). Table 1.1 shows the mass, charge, and energy of the proton, neutron, and electron.

1.1.2.6 Nuclear Forces

Protons in a nucleus are close to each other ($\approx 10^{-15}m$). This closeness results in an enormously strong repulsive force between protons. They still remain within the nucleus due to a strong attractive force between nucleons that dominates the repulsive force and makes the atom stable. The force is effective in a short range, and neutrons have an essential role in creating such a force. Without neutrons, protons cannot stay close to each other.

In 1935, Yukawa proposed that the short-range *strong force* is due to exchange of particles that he called *mesons*. The strong nuclear force is one of the four fundamental forces in nature created between nucleons by the exchange of mesons. This exchange can be compared to two people constantly hitting a tennis ball back and forth. As long as this meson exchange is happening, the strong force holds the nucleons together. Neutrons also participate in the meson exchange and are even a bigger source of the strong force. Neutrons have no charge, so they approach other nuclei without adding an extra repulsive force; meanwhile, they increase the average distance between protons and help to reduce the repulsion between them within a nucleus.

1.1.2.7 Nuclear Binding Energy and Mass Defect

It has been proved that the mass of a nucleus is always less than the sum of the individual masses of the constituent protons and neutrons (*mass defect*). The strong nuclear force is the result of the mass defect phenomenon. Using Einstein's mass energy relationship, the nuclear *binding energy* can be given as follows:

$$E_b = \Delta m.c^2$$

where Δm is the mass defect, and c is the speed of light in a vacuum.

The *average binding energy* per nucleon is a measure of nuclear stability. The higher the average binding energy is, the more stable the nucleus is.

Table 1.1 Mass and charge of a proton, neutron, and electron

Particle	Symbol	Charge[a]	Mass[b]	Mass (kg)	Energy (MeV)	Relative mass
Proton	p	+1	1.007276	1.6726×10^{-27}	938.272	1,836
Neutron	n	0	1.008665	1.6749×10^{-27}	939.573	1,839
Electron	e^-	−1	0.000548	9.1093×10^{-31}	0.511	1

[a] Unit charge = 1.6×10^{-19} coulombs
[b] Mass expressed in universal mass unit (mass of 1/12 of ^{12}C atom)
Data from Particles and Nuclei (1999)

1.1.3 Radioactivity

For all practical purposes, the nucleus can be regarded as a combination of two fundamental particles: neutrons and protons. These particles are together termed *nucleons.* The stability of a nucleus depends on at least two different forces: the repulsive coulomb force between any two or more protons and the strong attractive force between any two nucleons (nuclear forces). The nuclear forces are strong but effective over short distances, whereas the weaker coulomb forces are effective over longer distances. The stability of a nucleus depends on the arrangement of its nucleons, particularly the ratio of the number of neutrons to the number of protons. An adequate number of neutrons is essential for stability. Among the many possible combinations of protons and neutrons, only around 260 nuclides are stable; the rest are unstable.

It seems that there are favored neutron-to-proton ratios among the stable nuclides. Figure 1.1 shows the function of number of neutron (N) against the number of protons (Z) for all available nuclides. The stable nuclides gather around an imaginary line, which is called the *line of stability.* For light elements (A < 50), this line corresponds to $N = Z$, but with increasing atomic number the neutron-to-proton ratio increases up to 1.5 ($N = 1.5Z$). The line of stability ends at A = 209 (Bi), and all nuclides above that and those that are not close to this line are unstable. Nuclides that lie on the left of the line of stability (area I) have an excess of neutrons, those lying on

the right of the line (area II) are neutron deficient, and those above the line (area III) are too heavy (excess of both neutrons and protons) to be stable.

An unstable nucleus sooner or later (nanoseconds to thousands of years) changes to a more stable proton-neutron combination by emitting particles such as alpha, beta, and gamma. The phenomenon of spontaneous emission of such particles from the nucleus is called *radioactivity,* and the nuclides are called *radionuclides.* The change from the unstable nuclide (parent) to the more stable nuclide (daughter) is called *radioactive decay* or *disintegration.* During disintegration, there is emission of nuclear particles and release of energy. The process is spontaneous, and it is not possible to predict which radioactive atom will disintegrate first.

1.1.3.1 Modes of Decay

The radionuclide, which decays to attain stability, is called the *parent* nuclide, and the stable form so obtained is called the *daughter.* There are situations when the daughter is also unstable. The unstable nuclide may undergo transformation by any of the following modes.

Nuclides with Excess Neutrons

Beta Emission

Nuclides with an excess number of neutrons acquire a stable form by converting a neutron to a proton. In this process, an electron (negatron or beta minus) and an antineutrino are emitted. The nuclear equation is given as follows:

$$n \rightarrow p + e + \bar{v} + Energy$$

where n, p, e, and $\bar{v}$ represent the neutron, the proton, the negatron (beta minus), and the antineutrino, respectively. The proton stays in the nucleus, but the electron and the antineutrino are emitted and carry the released energy as their kinetic energy. In this mode of decay, the atomic number of the daughter nuclide is one more than that of the parent with no change in mass number. The mass of the neutron is more than the sum of masses of the proton, electron, and the antineutrino (the daughter is lighter than the parent). This defect in mass is converted into energy and randomly

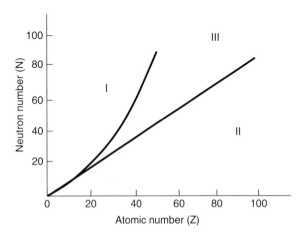

Fig. 1.1 The line of stability and different regions around it. (Reproduced from [3])

shared between the beta particle and the antineutrino. Hence, the beta particle may have energy between zero to a certain maximum level (continuous spectrum). The antineutrino has no mass and charge and has no clinical application.

Radionuclides in which the daughter acquires a stable state by emitting beta particles only are called pure beta emitters, such as ^{3}H, ^{14}C, ^{32}P, and ^{35}S. Those that cannot attain a stable state after beta emission and are still in the excited states of the daughter emit gamma photons, either in a single transition or through cascades emitting more than one photon before attaining a stable state. ^{131}I, ^{132}Xe, and ^{60}Co emit beta particles followed by gamma emissions.

Nuclides that lack Neutrons

There are two alternatives for the nucleus to come to a stable state:

1. Positron emission and subsequent emission of annihilation photons
   In this mode of decay, a proton transforms to a neutron, a positron, and a neutrino.

$$p \rightarrow n + e + v$$

The neutron stays in the nucleus, but a positron and a neutrino are ejected, carrying the emitted energy as their kinetic energy. In this mode of decay, the atomic number of the daughter becomes one less than that of the parent with no change in mass number. The mass of the proton is less than the masses of the neutron, the positron, and the neutrino. The energy for creation of this mass ($E > 1.022$ MeV) is supplied by the whole nucleus. The excess energy is randomly shared by the positron and the neutrino. The energy spectrum of the positron is just like that of the beta particle (from zero to a certain maximum). The neutrino has no mass and charge and is of no clinical relevance. Some of the positron-emitting radionuclides are ^{11}C, ^{13}N, ^{15}O, and ^{18}F.

Just a few nanoseconds after its production, a positron combines with an electron. Their masses are converted into energy in the form of two equal-energy photons (0.511 MeV each), which leave the site of their creation in exactly opposite directions. This phenomenon

is called the *annihilation reaction,* and the photons so created are called *annihilation photons.*

2. Electron captures
   A nucleus with excess protons has an alternative way to acquire a stable configuration by attracting one of its own electrons (usually the k electron) to the nucleus. The electron combines with the proton, producing a neutron and a neutrino in the process.

$$p + e \rightarrow n + v$$

The electron capture creates a vacancy in the inner electron shell, which is filled by an electron from the outer orbit, and characteristic radiation is emitted in the process. These photons may knock out orbital electrons. These electrons are called *Auger electrons* and are extremely useful for therapeutic applications (targeted therapy) due to their short range in the medium.

Electron capture is likely to occur in heavy elements (those with electrons closer to the nucleus), whereas positron emission is likely in lighter elements. Radionuclides such as ^{67}Ga, ^{111}In, ^{123}I, and ^{125}I decay partially or fully by electron capture.

Nuclides with Excess Protons and Neutrons

There are two ways for nuclides with excess protons and neutrons (region III) to become more stable:

1. Alpha decay
   There are some heavy nuclides that get rid of the extra mass by emitting an alpha particle (two neutrons and two protons). The atomic number of the daughter in such decay is reduced by two and mass number is reduced by four. The alpha particle emission may follow with gamma emission to enable the daughter nucleus to come to its ground or stable state. Naturally occurring radionuclides such as ^{238}U and ^{232}Th are alpha emitters.

2. Fission
   It is the spontaneous fragmentation of very heavy nuclei into two lighter nuclei, usually with the emission of two or three neutrons. A large amount of energy (hundreds of million electron volts) is also released in this process. Fission nuclides themselves have no clinical application, but some of their fragments are useful. The fissile nuclides can

be used for the production of carrier free radio-isotopes with high specific activity.

Gamma Radiation and Internal Conversion

When all the energy associated with the decay process is not carried away by the emitted particles, the daughter nuclei do not acquire their ground state. Such nuclei can be in either an excited state or a metastable (isomeric) state. In both situations, the excess energy is often released in the form of one or more gamma photons. The average lifetime of excited states is short, and energy is released within a fraction of a nanosecond. The average lifetime of metastable states is much longer, and emission may vary from a few milliseconds to few days or even longer. During this period, the nucleus behaves as a pure gamma-emitting radionuclide. Some of the metastable states have great clinical application. The transition of a nucleus from a metastable state to a stable state is called an *isomeric transition*. The decay of ^{99m}Tc is the best example of isomeric transition. The decay scheme of ^{99}Mo-^{99m}Tc is shown in Fig. 1.2.

There are situations when the excited nuclei, instead of emitting a gamma photon, utilize the energy in knocking out an orbital electron from its own atom. This process is called *internal conversion,* and the emitted electron is called a *conversion electron.* The probability of K conversion electron is more than L or M conversion electrons, and the phenomenon is more common in heavy atoms. The internal conversion is followed by emission of characteristic x-rays or Auger electrons as the outer shell electrons move to fill the inner shell vacancies.

It should be noted that there is no difference between an x-ray and a gamma ray of equal energy except that the gamma ray originates from the nucleus and has a discrete spectrum of energy, whereas x-ray production is an atomic phenomenon and usually has a continuous spectrum.

Laws of Radioactivity

There is no information available by which one can predict the time of disintegration of an atom; the interest really should not be in an individual atom because even an extremely small mass of any element consists of millions of identical atoms. Radioactive decay has been found to be a spontaneous process

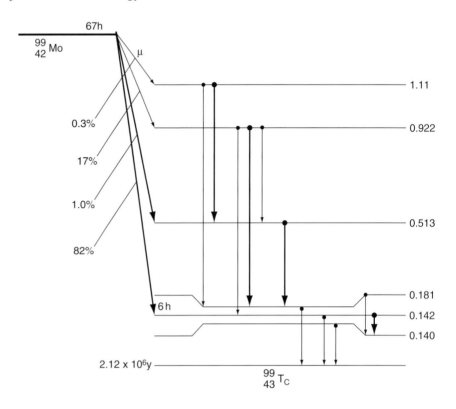

Fig. 1.2 Decay scheme of ^{99}Mo. (Reproduced from [3])

independent of any environmental factor. In other words, nothing can influence the process of radioactive disintegration. Radioactive decay is a random process and can be described in terms of probabilities and average constants.

In a sample containing many identical radioactive atoms, during a short period of time (∂t) the number of decayed atoms (∂N) is proportional to the total number of atoms (N) present at that time. Mathematically, it can be expressed as follows:

$$- \partial N \propto N \partial t$$
$$- \partial N = \lambda N \partial t \qquad (1.4)$$

or

$$\frac{\partial N}{\partial t} = -\lambda N$$

In this equation, the constant λ (known as the *decay constant*) has a characteristic value for each radionuclide. The decay constant is the fraction of atoms undergoing decay per unit time in a large number of atoms. Its unit is the inverse of time.

For simplicity, the decay constant can be defined as the probability of disintegration of a nucleus per unit time. Thus, $\lambda = 0.01$ per second means that the probability of disintegration of each atom is 1% per second. It is important to note that this probability does not change with time.

The exact number of parent atoms in a sample at any time can be calculated by integrating Eq. 1.4, which takes the following form:

$$N = No * \exp(-\lambda t) \qquad (1.5)$$

where No is the initial number of atoms in the sample, and N is the number present at time t.

The term $\frac{\partial N}{\partial t}$ shows the number of disintegrations per unit time and is known as *activity*. The SI unit of activity is the becquerel (Bq; 1 decay per second). The conventional unit of activity is the curie (Ci), which is equal to 3.7×10^{10} disintegrations per second (dps). This number 3.7×10^{10} corresponds to the disintegrations from 1 g ^{226}Ra.

Half-Life

The time after which 50% of the atoms in a sample undergo disintegration is called the *half-life*. The

half-life and decay constant are related by the following equation:

$$T_{1/2} = \frac{0.693}{\lambda} \ or \ \lambda = \frac{0.693}{T_{1/2}} \qquad (1.6)$$

Average Life

The actual lifetimes of individual atoms in a sample are different; some are short, and some are long. The average lifetime characteristic of atoms is related to the half-life by

$$T_{av} = 1.44 \times T_{1/2} \qquad (1.7)$$

The average life is a useful parameter for calculating the cumulated activity in the source organ in internal dosimetry.

Radioactive Equilibrium

In many cases, the daughter element is also radioactive and immediately starts disintegrating after its formation. Although the daughter obeys the general rule of radioactive decay, its activity does not follow the exponential law of decay while mixed with the parent. This is because the daughter is produced (monoexponentially) by disintegration of its parent while it disintegrates (monoexponentially) as a radioactive element. So, the activity of such elements changes biexponentially: First the activity increases, then reaches a maximum, and then starts decreasing. The rate at which the activity changes in such a mixture of radionuclides depends on the decay constant of both the parent and the daughter.

If we start with a pure sample of a parent with a half-life of T_1 and a decay constant λ_1 and it contains $(N_1)_0$ atoms initially, the decay of this parent can be expressed by

$$N_1 = (N_1)_0 e^{-\lambda_1 t} \qquad (1.8)$$

The rate of decay of the parent is the rate of formation of the daughter. Let the daughter decay at the rate $\lambda_2 N_2$, where λ_2 is the decay constant of the daughter and N_2 is the number of atoms of the daughter. The net rate of formation of the daughter can be given by

$$\frac{\partial N_2}{\partial t} = \lambda_1 N_1 - \lambda_2 N_2 \qquad (1.9)$$

The solution of this equation in terms of activity can be given as follows:

$$A_2 = A_1 \frac{T_1}{T_1 - T_2} \left(1 - e^{-0.693\left(\frac{T_1 - T_2}{T_1 T_2}\right)t}\right) \qquad (1.10)$$

where A_1 and A_2 are the activity of the parent and daughter, respectively; T_1 and T_2 are their respective physical half-lives; and t is the elapsed time. This equation is for a simple parent-daughter mixture. In general, three different situations arise from Eq. 1.10.

(a) Secular equilibrium

When the half-life of the parent (T_1) is too long in comparison to that of the daughter (T_2), Eq. 1.10 may be expressed as

$$A_2 = A_1 \left(1 - e^{\frac{-0.693t}{T_2}}\right) \qquad (1.11)$$

After one half-life of the daughter $(t = T_2)$, A_2 will become nearly $A_1/2$; after two half-lives the daughter may grow up to three fourths of the parent, and after four half-lives (of the daughter) this increases to about 94% of the parent activity. Thus, activity of the daughter gradually increases, and after a few half-lives the activity of the parent and daughter become almost equal (Fig. 1.3); they are said to be in *secular equilibrium*.

(b) Transient equilibrium

The half-life of the parent is a few times (~ 10 times or more) longer than that of the daughter, but the difference is not as great as in secular equilibrium. In this case, the activity of the daughter increases and eventually slightly exceeds the activity of the parent to reach a maximum and then decays with the half-life of the parent, as can be seen in Fig. 1.4. For a large value of t, Eq. 1.10 can be written as

$$A_2 = A_1 \frac{T_1}{T_1 - T_2} \quad \text{for } t \gg T_2 \qquad (1.12)$$

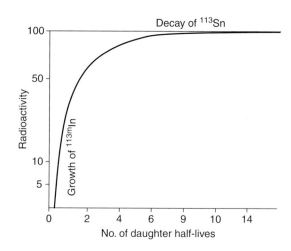

Fig. 1.3 Secular equilibrium

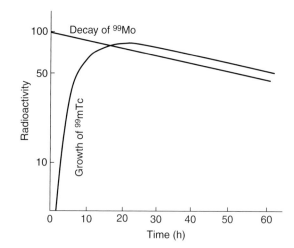

Fig. 1.4 Transient equilibrium

The growth of the daughter for multiples of $T_2 (T_2, 2T_2, 3T_2, 4T_2, etc.)$ will be nearly 50%, 75%, 87.5%, and 94%, respectively of the activity of the parent. It is therefore advisable to elute the activity from the technetium generator after every 24 h (Mo-99 with 67-h half-life and Tc-99m with 6-h half-life).

(c) No Equilibrium

If the half-life of the daughter is longer than the half-life of the parent, then there would be no equilibrium between them.

1.1.4 Interaction of Radiation with Matter

Ionizing radiation transfers its energy in full or part to the medium through which it passes by way of interactions. The significant types of interactions are excitation and ionization of atoms or molecules of the matter by charged particles and electromagnetic radiation (x-rays or gamma rays).

1.1.4.1 Interaction of Charged Particles with Matter

The charged particle loses some of its energy by the following interactions:

1. Ejection of electrons from the target atoms (ionization)
2. Excitation of electrons from a lower to a higher energy state
3. Molecular vibrations along the path (elastic collision) and conversion of energy into heat
4. Emission of electromagnetic radiation

In the energy range of 10 KeV to 10 MeV, ionization predominates over excitation. The probability of absorption of charged particles is so high that even a thin material can stop them completely.

The nature of the interaction of all charged particles in the energy range mentioned is similar. Light particles such as electrons deflect at larger angles than heavier particles, and there is a wide variation in their tortuous path. The path of a heavier particle is more or less a straight line. When electrons are deflected at large angles, they transfer more energy to the target atom and eject electrons from it. These electrons, while passing through the medium, produce secondary electrons along their track (delta rays). The charged particles undergo a large number of interactions before they come to rest. In each interaction, they lose a small amount of energy, and the losses are called *collision losses*.

Energetic electrons can approach the nucleus, where they are decelerated and produce bremsstrahlung radiation (x-rays). The chance of such an interaction increases with an increase in electron energy and the atomic number of the target material. Loss of electron energy by this mode is termed *radiative loss*. The energy lost per unit path length along the track is known as the *linear energy transfer* (LET) and is generally expressed in kilo-electron-volts per micrometer.

1.1.4.2 Range of a Charged Particle

After traveling through a distance in the medium, the charged particle loses all its kinetic energy and comes to rest as it has ample chance to interact with electrons or the positively charged nucleus of the atoms of the medium. The average distance traveled in a given direction by a charged particle is known as its *range* in that medium and is influenced by the following factors:

1. Energy. The higher the energy of the particle is, the larger is the range.
2. Mass. The higher the mass of the charged particle is, the smaller is the range.
3. Charge. The range is inversely proportional to the square of the charge.
4. Density of the medium. The denser the medium is, the shorter is the range of the charged particle.

1.1.4.3 Interaction of Electromagnetic Radiation with Matter

When a beam of x-rays or gamma rays passes through an absorbing medium, some of the photons are completely absorbed, some are scattered, and the rest pass through the medium almost unchanged in energy and direction (transmission). The transferred energy results in excitation and ionization of atoms or molecules of the medium and produces heat. The attenuation of the beam through a given medium is summarized as follows:

– The thicker the absorbing material is, the greater is the attenuation.
– The greater the atomic number of the material is, the greater is the attenuation.
– As the photon energy increases, the attenuation produced by a given thickness of material decreases.

1.1.4.4 Linear Attenuation Coefficient

The linear attenuation coefficient μ is defined as the fractional reduction in the beam per unit thickness as determined by a thin layer of the absorbing material.

$$\mu = \frac{\text{Fractional reduction in a thin layer}}{\text{Thickness of the layers (cm)}}$$

The unit of the μ is cm^{-1}.

1.1.4.5 Exponential Attenuation

The exponential law can explain the attenuation of radiation beam intensity. The mathematical derivation is given next.

Let N_o be the initial number of photons in the beam and N be the number recorded by the detector placed behind the absorber (Fig. 1.5).

The number δN, which gets attenuated, will be proportional to the thickness δx of the absorber and to the number of photons N present in the beam. The number δN will depend on the number of atoms present in the beam and the thickness of the absorber.

Mathematically,

$$\delta N \propto N. \, \delta x$$
$$\text{or } \delta N = -\mu.N.\delta x \tag{1.13}$$

where μ is a constant called the *linear attenuation coefficient* for the radiation used.

The negative sign indicates that as δx increases, the number of photons in the beam decreases. Equation 1.13 can be rearranged as follows:

$$\mu = \frac{\delta N}{N.\delta x} \tag{1.14}$$

The formal definition of attenuation coefficient is derived from the integration of Eq. 1.14, which gives the following relationship:

$$N = No. \, e^{-\mu x} \tag{1.15}$$

Equation 1.15 can also be expressed in terms of beam intensity:

$$I = Io. \, e^{-\mu x} \tag{1.16}$$

where I and I_o are the intensities of the beam as recorded by the detector with and without absorbing material, respectively. The attenuation coefficient may vary for a given material due to nonuniform thickness. This is particularly so if the absorbing material is malleable. It is therefore better to express the mass absorption coefficient, which is independent of thickness of the absorbing material. The mass absorption coefficient is obtained by dividing the linear attenuation coefficient by the density of the material. The unit of the mass attenuation coefficient is square centimeters per gram. The electronic and atomic attenuation coefficients are also defined accordingly. The electronic attenuation coefficient is the fractional reduction in x-ray or gamma ray intensity produced by a layer of thickness 1 electron/cm^2, whereas the

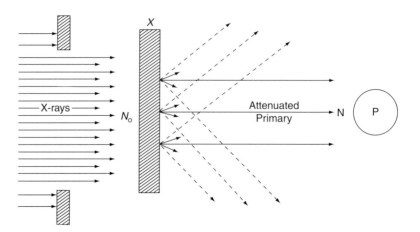

Fig. 1.5 Attenuation of a radiation beam by an absorber. The transmitted beam is measured by detector P. (Reproduced from [4])

atomic attenuation coefficient is the fractional reduction by a layer of thickness 1 atom/cm². Thus, the atomic attenuation coefficient will be Z times the electronic one.

1.1.4.6 Half-Value Layer

From Eq. 1.16, it can be seen that, for a certain thickness ($x = d_{1/2}$) of the absorbing material, the intensity becomes half of its original value, that is, $I = I_o/2$. Substituting these values, Eq. 1.16 can be rearranged as follows:

$$d_{1/2}(HVL) = 0.693/\mu \qquad (1.17)$$

The half-value layer or thickness (HVL or HVT) can be defined as the thickness of an absorbing material that reduces the beam intensity to half of its original value. Depending on the energy of radiation, various materials are used for the measurement of HVL, such as aluminum, copper, lead, brick, and concrete. The HVL for a broad beam is more than that for a narrow beam.

1.1.4.7 Mechanism of Attenuation

There are many modes of interaction between a photon and matter, but only the types discussed next are of importance to us.

Photon Scattering

Photon scattering may or may not result in transfer of energy during the interaction of the photon with an atom of the medium.

Elastic Scattering

In elastic scattering or unmodified scattering, the photons are scattered in different directions without any loss of energy. The process thus attenuates the beam without absorption. In this process, the photon interacts with a tightly bound electron in an atom. The electron later releases the photon in any direction without absorbing energy from it. The contribution of this mode of interaction is relatively insignificant

in medical applications of radiation. However, it has application in x-ray crystallography.

Inelastic (Compton) Scattering

Compton elucidated the mechanism of inelastic (Compton) scattering. In this process, the photon interacts with loosely bound (free) electrons. Part of the energy of the photon is used in ejecting the electron, and the rest is scattered in different directions (Fig. 1.6).

In a so-called head-on collision, the photon turns back along its original track (scattered through 180°), and maximum energy is transferred to the recoil electron. The change in wavelength $\delta\lambda$ of the photon is given by

$$\delta\lambda = 0.024(1 - \cos\varphi)\mathring{A} \qquad (1.18)$$

where φ is the angle of scattering of the gamma photon, and $\mathring{A}$ is the angstrom unit for wavelength. The energy of the scattered photon is expressed as follows:

$$E_1 = E_0/[1 + E_0/m_ec^2\{1 - \cos\varphi\}] \qquad (1.19)$$

where E_0 is the energy of the incident photon and E_1 is that of the scattered photon, m_e is the mass of the electron, and c is the velocity of light in a vacuum. Compton scattering involves interaction between photons and electrons. The probability therefore depends on the number of electrons present and independent of the atomic number. With the exception of hydrogen, all elements contain nearly the same number of electrons per gram (practically the same electron density). Compton scattering, therefore, is

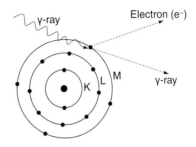

Fig. 1.6 Process of Compton scattering. The incoming photon ejects the electron from outer orbit and is scattered with reduced energy in a different direction. (Reproduced from [4])

independent of atomic number. This is the choice of interaction required in radiation oncology, for which the delivered dose is homogeneous in spite of tissue inhomogeneity within the body.

The total probability σ for the Compton process is given by

$$\sigma = \sigma_s + \sigma_a$$

where σ_s and σ_a are the probabilities for scattering and absorption, respectively.

1.1.4.8 Photoelectric Effect

In the PEE process, the photon disappears when it interacts with the bound electron. The photon energy has to be higher than the binding energy of the electron for this type of interaction to take place.

$$hv = BE + \text{kinetic energy}$$

where hv is the energy of the photon and BE is the binding energy of the electron in the shell (Fig. 1.7). If the photon energy is slightly higher than the binding energy (BE), then the chance of PEE is high. For example, a photon of energy 100 keV has a high probability of undergoing PEE when it interacts with a Pb atom, for which the K shell binding energy is 88 keV. The rest of the (100 to 88) 12-keV energy will be carried away by the ejected electron as its kinetic energy. The ejection of the electron creates a hole in the inner shell, which is filled by an electron from any of the outer shells. Since the electrons in the outer shells possess higher energy than those in the inner shells, the difference in their energy is released as

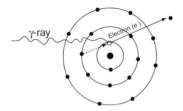

Fig. 1.7 Process of photoelectric absorption. The incoming photon disappears (is absorbed), and the orbital electron is knocked out. An electron from the outer shell falls (*dotted line*) into the inner shell to fill the vacancy. (Reproduced from [4])

x-ray photons. Such photons are characteristic of the atom from which they are emitted. The K, L, M, and so on shells of a given atom have fixed energy, so the difference in their energies is also fixed. The radiation emitted therefore is termed the *characteristic x-rays*.

Three types of possibilities exist during PEE:

1. Radiative transitions
    As explained, during the electron transition from the outer orbit to the inner orbit, a photon is emitted with energy equal to the difference of the binding energies of the orbits involved. The vacancy moves to a higher shell; consequently, a characteristic photon of lower energy follows. The probability of emission of a photon is expressed as the fluorescent yield:

    $$\text{Fluorescent yield}$$
    $$= \frac{\text{Number of x} - \text{ray photons emitted}}{\text{Number of orbital vacancies created}}$$

    Mostly, it is the K shell that is responsible for fluorescent yield.

    $$\text{K shell fluorescent yield } (\omega k)$$
    $$= \frac{\text{Number of K x} - \text{ray photons emitted}}{\text{Number of K shell vacancies}}$$

    The yield increases with an increase in atomic number.

2. Auger electrons
    The characteristic x-ray photon, instead of being emitted, can eject another orbital electron from the atom. These electrons are called Auger electrons (Fig. 1.8). The energy of the Auger electron is equal to the difference of the x-ray photon energy and the binding energy of the shell involved in the process. The process competes with radiative transition. The Auger yield is expressed as the ratio of electrons emitted due to vacancies in subshell i and the total number of atoms with a vacancy in subshell i.

3. Coster–Kronig electrons
    The process for Coster–Kronig electrons is exactly like the Auger transition except that the electron filling the vacancy comes from the subshell of the same principal shell in which the vacancy lies. The kinetic energy of the emitted electrons can be calculated exactly as for Auger electrons. The energy

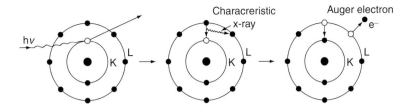

Fig. 1.8 Mechanism of Auger electron emission. (Reproduced from [4])

of Coster–Kronig electrons is so small that they are quickly absorbed in the medium.

1.1.4.9 Pair Production

When a photon with energy in excess of 1.022 MeV passes close to the nucleus of an atom, it may disappear, and in its place two antiparticles (negatron and positron) may be produced as shown in Fig. 1.9. In this process, energy converts into mass in accordance with Einstein's mass energy equivalence ($E = mc^2$). After traversing some distance through the medium, the positron loses its energy, combines with an electron, and annihilates. During combination, both the antiparticles disappear (annihilation) and two 0.511-MeV photons are emitted in the opposite direction.

1.1.4.10 Photonuclear Reaction

When photon energy is too high, either a neutron or a proton may be knocked out (more likely the neutron) from the nucleus. For the majority of atoms, the threshold energy for this effect is more than 10 MeV, and the probability increases with increasing energy until a maximum is reached; above this maximum, the probability falls rapidly.

1.2 Radiation Safety

The applications of radiopharmaceuticals for medical diagnosis and therapy have rapidly increased due to the favorable physical characteristics of artificially produced radionuclides, progress in instrumentation, and computer technology. Efforts are under way to develop newer radiopharmaceuticals in nuclear medicine for both diagnostic and therapeutic procedures.

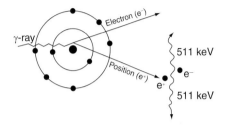

Fig. 1.9 Schematic representation of pair production. (Reproduced from [4])

While such enthusiasm is appreciable, adequate safeguards against radiation exposure are also necessary to minimize the radiation risk to occupational workers, patients, and the public.

1.2.1 Types of Exposure

The following three categories of people are likely to be involved in radiation exposure in medical applications of ionizing radiation:

1. Occupational staff
2. Patients
3. Public

Protection is aimed at achieving a dose as low as reasonably achievable (ALARA) to these categories of people. Spending a minimum of *time* near the radiation sources, keeping a *distance* from them, and using *shielding* devices are the cardinal parameters for radiation safety. The fourth parameter with unsealed sources in nuclear medicine is to avoid or minimize the chance of *contamination*.

For safe use of radionuclides in nuclear medicine, the following basic requirements should be met:

1. The nuclear medicine facility should be well planned with a sufficient number of rooms for intended operations (including the storage and

disposal of radioactive waste) as approved by the competent authority.

2. All the equipment required for safe handling should be available in each room for proposed operations.
3. The staff should be adequate and well trained in handling radioactive material.
4. Radiation monitoring instruments (survey meters, contamination monitors, pocket dosimeters, digital monitors etc.) and decontamination facility should be readily available.

1.2.1.1 Protection of Staff

Nuclear medicine procedures demand preparation of radiopharmaceuticals, their internal movement within the facility, and finally administration to the patient. At each step, there is a possibility of radiation exposure if safety guidelines are ignored. The diagnostic procedures normally do not cause any alarming exposure to the staff and public. However, patients administered radioactive substances for therapeutic purposes become a source of radiation to the staff and their attendants and public. Therapeutic radionuclides are usually beta emitters that do not pose much of a problem from a safety standpoint, and patients treated with them can even be treated as outpatients. However, patients treated with radioiodine (I-131) need hospitalization if treated beyond a certain dose as per national regulatory requirements due to penetrating gamma radiation. These patients stay in a specifically designed isolation room or ward until the body burden decreases to an acceptable level for release from the hospital.

Work Practice

Good work practice is an essential component of radiation safety. This includes observation of all radiation protection rules as applicable to nuclear medicine, use of appropriate safety devices, remote handling of tools/accessories, and maintaining good housekeeping habits in the laboratory.

In addition to the external irradiation, there is a chance of radioactive contamination while handling unsealed sources in nuclear medicine procedures. The radioactive waste generated during preparation, dispensing, and administration of radiopharmaceuticals

shall be handled carefully to minimize exposure to staff and the public.

1.2.1.2 Protection of Patients

Every practice involving ionizing radiation should be justified in terms of net positive benefit. It is particularly important for children, for whom long-term risks of exposure to ionizing radiation are larger. Once clinically justified, each examination involving ionizing radiation should be conducted such that the radiation dose to the patient is the lowest necessary to achieve the clinical aim (optimization). Reference and achievable doses for various radionuclide investigations have been proposed for this purpose by various organizations. The concept of reference doses is recognized as a useful and practical tool for promoting the optimization of patient protection. While reducing the radiation dose to the patient, image quality should not be compromised, which may otherwise lead to repeat investigation. Routine quality control (QC) tests of imaging systems and radiopharmaceuticals have to be done before clinical studies. Another consideration in reducing the patient dose is to avoid misadministration and to provide proper radiation counseling to patients and their family or others involved.

What Is Misadministration?

Error in any part of the procedure starting from patient selection to the interpretation of final results may lead to a repeat study. This in turn leads to an increased radiation dose not only to the patient but also to the staff. A major contributor to increased radiation dose to the patient is misadministration. Misadministration has several components, such as administration of the wrong radiopharmaceutical or the wrong dose or giving the dose to a wrong patient or through a wrong route, which ultimately lead to undesirable exposure to a patient.

The following points should be checked to avoid misadministration:

Identity of the patient: The radiopharmaceutical should be administered to the patient for whom it is prepared. Name, age, and medical record number should be checked before dose administration.

Radionuclide and its physical or chemical form: The physical and chemical form of the radiopharmaceutical should be reconfirmed before administration. Radiopharmaceuticals should go through routine QC procedures to check for any inadequate preparation.

Dose, quantity of radioactivity, QC: The radioactivity should be measured in a dose calibrator before administration. The accuracy and precision of the radionuclide dose calibrator need to be maintained at all times for accuracy in dose estimation. Similarly, imaging equipment should be maintained at its optimum level of performance.

Route: The physician should confirm the route of administration (oral, intravenous) of the radiopharmaceutical.

Pregnancy and breast feeding: Female patient should notify if she is pregnant or breast feeding. This can happen with proper patient education.

Proper counseling is also helpful in reducing exposure to patients and their family members.

1.2.1.3 Protection of the Public or Environment

To ensure that unnecessary exposure to the members of the public is avoided, the following guidelines shall be followed:

1. No member of the public shall be allowed to enter the controlled (hot laboratory and the injection room/area, imaging rooms) and supervised (consoles) areas.
2. Appropriate warning signs and symbols shall be posted on doors to restrict access.
3. Relatives or friends of the patients receiving therapeutic doses of radioactive iodine shall not be allowed to visit the patient without the permission of the radiation safety officer (RSO). The visitors shall not be young children or pregnant women.
4. A nursing mother who has been administered radiopharmaceuticals shall be given instructions to be followed at home after her release from the hospital. The breast-feeding may have to be suspended.
5. An instruction sheet shall be given at the time of release from the hospital to patients administered therapeutic doses of radioiodine; the instructions should be followed at home for a specified period as suggested by the RSO.

6. The storage of radioactive waste shall be done at a location within the hospital premises with adequate shielding to eliminate the public hazard from it.

1.2.2 Control of Contamination

Radioactive contamination can be minimized by carefully designing the laboratory, using proper handling tools, and following correct operating procedures together with strict management and disposal of radioactive waste. In the event of contamination, procedures indicated should be followed to contain the contamination.

1.2.2.1 Management of a Radioactive Spill

1. Perform a radiation and contamination survey to determine the degree and extent of contamination.
2. Isolate the contaminated area to avoid spread of contamination. No person should be allowed to enter the area.
3. Use gloves, shoe covers, lab coat, and other appropriate clothing.
4. Rapidly define the limits of the contaminated area and immediately confine the spill by covering the area with absorbent materials with plastic backing.
5. First remove the "hot spots" and then scrub the area with absorbent materials, working toward the center of the contaminated area. Special decontamination chemicals (Radiacwash) shall be used in the case of a severe spill.
6. All personnel should be surveyed to determine contamination, including their shoes and clothing. If the radioactive material appears to have become airborne, the nostrils and mouth of possible contaminated persons should be swabbed, and the samples shall be evaluated by the RSO.
7. Shut off ventilation if airborne activity is likely to be present (rare situation).
8. A heavily contaminated individual may take a shower in the designated decontamination facility as directed by the RSO. Disposable footwear and gloves should be worn in transit.
9. If significant concentrations of radioiodine have been involved, subsequent thyroid uptake

measurements should be made on potentially exposed individuals after 24 h.

10. Monitor the decontaminated area and all personnel leaving the area after the cleanup. Particular attention should be paid to checking the hands and the soles of shoes.

11. All mops, rags, brushes, and absorbent materials shall be placed in the designated waste container and should be surveyed by the RSO. Proper radioactive disposal should be observed.

12. The RSO should provide the final radiation survey report with necessary recommendations or advice to avoid such an incident in the future.

1.2.2.2 Personnel Decontamination

Contaminated eyes

- If eye contamination is found, the eye should be flushed profusely with isotonic saline or water by covering other parts with a towel to prevent the spread of contamination. An ophthalmologist shall be consulted if there are signs of eye irritation.

Contaminated hair

- If hair is contaminated, try up to three washings with liquid soap and rinse with water.
- Prevent water from running onto the face and shoulders by shielding the area with towels.
- Perform a radiation survey.

Contaminated skin

- Remove any contaminated clothing before determining the level of skin contamination. Levels below 0.1 mR/h (1 μSv/h) are considered minimal hazards.
- If there is gross skin contamination, it shall be given attention first. Wipe with a cotton swab moistened with water and liquid soap using long forceps. Place all swabs in a plastic container for radiation level measurement and storage before disposal.
- If a large skin area is contaminated, the person should have a 10-min shower. Dry the body with a towel in the shower room and monitor the radiation level over the whole body. Do not allow any water to drip on the floor outside the shower room to avoid the spread of contamination.

- Place all the towels and other contaminated clothing in a plastic bag for later monitoring of radiation level for storage and decay.
- Specific hot spots on the skin can be localized with a survey meter or appropriate contamination monitor.
- Clean the specific areas with mild soap and warm water. Avoid using detergents or vigorous scrubbing for they might damage the skin. The use of a soft brush is adequate.
- For stubborn contamination, covering a contaminated area with plastic film or disposable cotton or latex gloves over a skin cream helps remove the contamination through sweating.

1.2.2.3 Internal Contamination

- Simple expedients such as oral and nasopharyngeal irrigation, gastric lavage, or an emetic and use of purgatives may greatly reduce the uptake of a contaminant into the circulation.
- Blocking agents or isotopic dilution techniques can appreciably decrease the uptake of the radionuclides into relatively stable metabolic pools such as bone. These should be administered without delay.

When a contaminated person requires treatment (for wounds) by a physician, the emergency room (ER) should be informed. The following points must be remembered:

- Medical emergencies are the priority and must be attended first. Radiation injuries are rarely life threatening to the victim and the attending physician/staff.
- Clean the wound with mild detergent and flush with isotonic saline or water. If necessary, a topical anesthetic, such as 4% lidocaine, can be used to allow more vigorous cleansing. After a reasonable effort, there is no need to attempt to remove all contamination since it will probably be incorporated into the scab.
- Whenever radionuclides have entered the skin via a needle or sharps, induce the wound to bleed by "milking" it as a cleansing action in addition to the use of running water.
- Perform radiation monitoring at the surface.

1.2.3 Radioiodine Therapy: Safety Considerations

Radioiodine has been effectively used for more than five decades to ablate remnant thyroid tissue following thyroidectomy and for treating distant metastases. Looking at the radiation hazard to staff and the public, national regulatory bodies have established guidelines for the hospitalization and subsequent release of patients administered radioiodine from the hospital. The limit of body burden at which these patients are released from the hospital varies from country to country. Groups who may be critically exposed among the public are fellow travelers during the journey home after release from the hospital and children and pregnant women among other family members at home.

The administered dose of radioiodine is concentrated avidly by thyroidal tissue (thyroid remnant, differentiated thyroid cancer). It rapidly gets excreted via the kidney and urinary bladder and to a lesser extent through perspiration, saliva, exhalation, and the gut. The faster biological excretion of the activity in a thyroid cancer patient actually poses less radiation hazard to the environment than actually expected. Counseling of patients and family members from a radiation safety viewpoint is necessary before therapeutic administration.

1.2.3.1 Radiation Monitoring

Routine monitoring of all work surfaces, overcoats, exposed body parts, and so on is essential before leaving the premises. Both Gieger-Muller (G.M.)-type survey meters and ionization chamber-type survey meters are required for monitoring. All persons involved in a radioiodine procedure should be covered by personnel radiation monitoring badges, and their neck counts should also be measured periodically. It is advisable to carry out periodic air monitoring in these areas to ensure that no airborne activity is present.

1.2.3.2 Use of a Fume Hood

Radioiodine in capsule form poses much less radiation safety problems than in liquid form. When in liquid form, the vials containing I-131 should be opened only inside a fume hood using remote-handling bottle openers. If these vials are opened outside the fume hood, there is every possibility that the worker involved may inhale a fraction of the vaporous activity. All operations using I-131 should be carried out wearing face masks, gloves, and shoe covers and using remote-handling tools. Radioactive iodine uptake measurement for the thyroid of staff involved should be done weekly to check for any internal contamination.

1.2.3.3 Specific Instructions to the Patient

It is the combined responsibility of the physician and the medical physicists or technologists to administer the desired dose to the patient. The patient is normally advised to come with an empty stomach or after a light breakfast and not to eat or drink anything for 1–2 h after therapeutic administration. After this time, they are advised to have as much fluids as possible for fast excretion of radioiodine from the kidneys. They are also advised to void the urinary bladder frequently and to flush the toilet twice after each voiding. This practice not only reduces the radiation dose to the kidneys, bladder, and entire body of the patients but also helps in their fast release from the hospital.

In female patients of reproductive age, two important aspects need to be considered:

1. Possibility of pregnancy: Radionuclide therapy is strictly prohibited during pregnancy.
2. Pregnancy after radionuclide therapy should be avoided for at least 4 months (4–6 months) or as advised by the treating physician.

1.2.3.4 Discharge of the Patient from the Hospital

The regulatory authority of each country decides the maximum limit of activity of I-131 at which the patient may be discharged from the hospital. This can be roughly estimated by measuring the exposure rate from the patient at a 1-m distance with a calibrated survey meter, which should read approximately 50 µSv/h (5 mR/h) for a body burden of 30 mCi or less.

1.2.3.5 Posttreatment

The patient must be provided with an instruction card detailing the type and duration of any radiation protection restrictions that must be followed at home. This should also contain details of therapy and necessary radiation protection procedures.

1.2.3.6 Contact with Spouse or Partner and Others at Home

The patient should make arrangements to sleep apart from his or her partner for some time as suggested by the RSO. The duration of such restriction actually depends on the body burden of the patient at the time of release from the hospital [5–8]. Contact with family and friends at home should not be for prolonged periods for a few initial days after release from the hospital [5, 9]. Close contact with pregnant women and young children on a regular basis should be avoided for such time as suggested by the RSO. It would be ideal if an arrangement could be made for young children to stay with relatives or friends after the treatment, at least for the initial few days or weeks. If such an arrangement is not possible, then prolonged close contact with them should be avoided as per advice of the RSO. Time duration to avoid close contact can only be estimated on an individual basis depending on the radioiodine burden and socioeconomic status of the patient. Mathieu et al. [10] estimated the radiation dose to the spouse and children at home and observed that the dose to the spouse is greater from patients treated for thyrotoxicosis than for those treated for thyroid cancer. Pant et al. [11] reported that the dose to family members of patients treated with radioiodine (I-131) for thyrotoxicosis and cancer thyroid was within 1 mSv in the majority of the cases with proper counseling of the patient and the family members at the time of release from the hospital.

1.2.3.7 Returning to Work

If work involves close contact with small children or pregnant women, then it should not be resumed by treated patients for a few weeks; otherwise, routine work can be assumed by avoiding close contact with fellow colleagues for a prolonged period. The Luster et al. [12] published the relevant guidelines for radio-iodine therapy for consultation.

1.2.3.8 Personal Hygiene and Laundering Instructions for the First Week After Therapy

A normal toilet should be used in preference to a urinal for voiding urine. The sitting posture is preferred to standing. Spilled urine should be wiped with a tissue and flushed. Hands should always be washed after using the toilet. Any linen or clothes that become stained with urine should be immediately washed separately from other clothes.

1.2.3.9 Records

A proper logbook should be maintained with details of storage and disposal of radionuclides. The record of dose administration to the patients, their routine monitoring, transient storage of waste for physical decay, and the level of activity at the time of disposal should be properly recorded. Decontamination procedures and routine surveys should also be recorded in the radiation safety logbook. The name of the authorized person who supervised the procedure should also be recorded.

1.2.4 Management of Radioactive Waste

Radioactive waste is generated as a result of handling unsealed sources in the laboratory, leftover radioactive material from routine preparations, dose dispensing to patients, contaminated items in routine use, and so on. The waste arises in a large variety of forms depending on the physical, physiochemical, and biological properties of the material. In radionuclide therapy, the waste may also consist of excreta.

1.2.4.1 Storage of Radioactive Waste

The solid waste generated in the working area should be collected in polythene bags and transferred to suitable containers in the storage room. The liquid waste has to be collected in either glass or preferably plastic containers. The waste containing short-lived and long-lived radionuclides should be collected in separate bags and stored in separate containers. If the laboratory is used for preparation of short-lived radiopharmaceuticals, then it is advisable not to collect the waste until the next preparation. This will avoid unnecessary exposure to the staff handling radioactive waste. The storage room should have proper ventilation and an exhaust system. The shielding around the waste storage room should be adequate to prevent any leakage of radiation. The waste must be stored for at least ten half-lives for decay or until such a time disposal is conveniently possible.

1.2.4.2 Disposal of Solid Waste

1. Low-activity waste
    The solid waste comprised of paper tissues, swabs, glassware, and similar materials that are of low activity (only a few becquerels) can be disposed with ordinary refuse provided no single item contains concentrated activity and

    (a) They do not contain alpha or beta emitters or radionuclides with a long half-life.
    (b) The waste does not go through a recycling procedure.
    (c) The radionuclide labels are intact (to guard against misinterpretation).

2. High-activity wastes
    Contaminated clothing and those items that need to be reused are segregated and stored for physical decay of radioactivity or decontaminated separately. A derived working limit (DWL) of 3.7 Bq/cm^2 is indicated for personal clothing and hospital bedding. Disposal methods for solid waste consist of decaying and disposal or ground burial. The method chosen depends on the quantity of radioactive material present in the wastes. From each work area, the wastes are collected in suitable disposable containers. Extra care for radiation protection is necessary during the accumulation, collection, and disposal of radioactive wastes. Containers should be marked with the radiation symbol and suitable designation for segregation [13].
    Solid waste (e.g., animal carcasses, animal excreta, specimens, biologically toxic material) can be

conveniently dealt with by burial or incineration, depending on the national or international guidelines. Incineration of refuse containing nonvolatile radionuclides concentrates the activity in the ash. If the ash contains undesirable high activity, special disposal methods should be adopted. The ash can be diluted and disposed without exceeding the specified limits or buried. The design of the incinerator for handling the radioactive waste should be considered at the planning stage.

1.2.4.3 Management of Cadavers Containing Radionuclides

An unfortunate situation arises if a patient dies after administration of a high amount of radioactivity and the radiation limits are more than the threshold level for releasing the body from the hospital. If the activity is concentrated in a few organs (as can be seen by scanning the cadaver under the gamma camera), then those organs should be removed, and the body released after ensuring that the limits recommended by the competent authority are not exceeded. In case of widespread disease for which organ removal is no solution, the body may be put into an impermeable plastic bag and stored in a mortuary (cold room) for physical decay until the radiation level returns to an acceptable limit. In any compelling social circumstances, the advice of a regulatory body may be sought. Autopsy, management of removed organs or a part of the body, handing over the body, and burial or cremation should be done under the direct supervision of the RSO. Removal of organs from the cadaver is socially not permitted in some countries, the regulatory requirement of that country shall be followed by the RSO.

1.2.4.4 Disposal of Liquid Waste

While disposal of liquid wastes through the sanitary sewage system, the limits of dilution and disposal should not exceed the prescribed limits recommended by the competent authority (normally 22.2 MBq/m^3). If the activity in the waste is too low, then it may be disposed with proper dilution (dilute and dispose). If the activity level is moderate to high and the half-life or lives of the radionuclides is relatively short, then the waste should be stored for physical decay for a period of about ten half-lives (delay and decay).

The quantity of liquid radioactive waste generated due to nuclear medicine investigations hardly poses any problem of storage or disposal. However, it is not the same for therapeutic nuclear medicine, for which a large amount of radioactive waste is generated in the form of effluent from the isolation room or ward of thyroid cancer patients. The large doses of radioiodine used for the treatment of thyroid cancer calls for planned storage and release of waste by sewage disposal. Amounts of ^{131}I as high as 7.4–11.1 GBq (200–300 mCi) are administered to patients with distant metastases. Approximately 80–90% of administered radioactivity is excreted through urine [5]. Therefore, management of radioactive urine poses a radiation safety problem.

Various methods have been recommended for the disposal of high-level radioactive liquid wastes. The widely used technique is the storage delay tank system. Storage of all effluent from the isolation room or ward, or urine alone, in a storage delay tank system is the recommended method and is more feasible in hospitals with tanks of appropriate volumes. The system allows collection of effluent from the isolation room or ward in the first tank. The tank is closed after it is completely filled, and collection takes place in the second tank. Until the second tank is completely filled, the effluent in the first tank gets enough time to decay, which may make its release possible to the sewage system. It will even be better if effluent in each tank is allowed to decay for a given length of time and then released into a big dilution tank before its final release into the sewage line. A large number of small tanks is advisable for allowing decay of radioiodine for at least ten half-lives. Provision of access to the dilution tank is useful for monitoring the activity concentration at any time before its final release to the main sewer system.

1.2.4.5 Disposal of Gaseous Waste

Gaseous wastes originate from exhausts of stores, fume cupboards, and wards and emission from incinerators. Points of release into the atmosphere should be carefully checked, and filters (including charcoal) may be used wherever possible. The concentration of radioactive materials in the air leaving the ventilation system should not exceed the maximum permissible concentrations for breathing unless regular and adequate monitoring or environmental surveys are carried out to prove the adequacy of the disposal system. When large quantities of radionuclides are routinely discharged to the environment, it is advisable to make environmental surveys in the vicinity since many radionuclides will be concentrated on surfaces.

In installations where large amounts of airborne activity are involved, it may be necessary to use suitable air filtration (through charcoal filter) systems and to discharge the filtered effluent through a tall stack. The height of the stack can be chosen to ensure that the radioactivity is sufficiently diluted before it reaches ground level. Combustible low-level radioactive waste may be incinerated with adequate precautions to reduce bulk.

Security: The waste has to be protected from fire, insects, and extreme temperatures.

References

1. Pant GS, Rajabi H (2008) Basic atomic and nuclear physics. In: Basic physics and radiation safety in nuclear medicine. Himalaya Publishing House, Mumbai
2. Povh B, Rith K, Scholz C, Zetche F, Lavell M, Particles and Nuclei: An introduction to the physical concept (2nd ed), Springer 1999
3. Pant GS, Shukla AK (2008) Radioactivity. In: Basic physics and radiation safety in nuclear medicine. Himalaya Publishing House, Mumbai
4. Pant GS (2008) Basic interaction of radiation with matter. In: Basic physics and radiation safety in nuclear medicine. Himalaya Publishing House, Mumbai
5. Barrington SF, Kettle AG, O'Doherty MJ, Wells CP, Somer EJ, Coakley AJ (1996) Radiation dose rates from patients receiving iodine-131 therapy for carcinoma of the thyroid. Eur J Nucl Med 23(2):123–130
6. Ibis E, Wilson CR, Collier BD, Akansel G, Isitman AT and Yoss RG (1992) Iodine-131 contamination from thyroid cancer patients. J Nucl Med 33(12):2110–2115
7. Beierwalts WH, Widman J (1992) How harmful to others are iodine-131 treated patients. J Nucl Med 33:2116–2117
8. de Klerk JMH (2000) 131I therapy: inpatient or outpatient? J Nucl Med 41:1876–1878
9. O'Dogherty MJ, Kettle AG, Eustance CNP et al. (1993) Radiation dose rates from adult patients receiving ^{131}I therapy for thyrotoxicosis, Nucl Med Commun 14:160–168
10. Mathieu I, Caussin J, Smeesters P et al. (1999) Recommended restrictions after ^{131}I therapy: Measured doses in family members. Health Phys 76(2):129–136
11. Pant GS, Sharma SK, Bal CS, Kumar R, Rath GK (2006) Radiation dose to family members of hyperthyroidism and thyroid cancer patients treated with [131]I. Radiat Prot Dosim 118(1):22–27
12. Luster M, Clarke SE, Dietlein M et al. (2008) Guidelines for radioiodine therapy of differentiated thyroid cancer. Eur J Nucl Med Mol Biol 35(10):1941–1959

13. International Atomic Energy Agency (2000) Management of radioactive waste from the use of radionuclides in medicine IAEA publication TECDOC-1183, Vienna, 2000

Further Reading

Cherry SR, Sorenson JA, Phelps ME (2003) Physics in nuclear medicine, 3rd edn. Saunders, Philadelphia

Chandra R (1992) Introductory physics of nuclear medicine. Lea & Febiger, Philadelphia

Meredith WJ, Massey JB (1974) Fundamental physics of radiology. Wright, Bristol

Johns HE, Cunningham JR (1969) The physics of radiology. Thomas, Springfield

Henkin R (ed) (1996) Nuclear medicine. Mosby, Philadelphia

Clarke SM (1994) Radioiodine therapy of the thyroid, Nuclear Medicine in Clinical Diagnosis and Treatment. (Murray, Ell, Strauss, Eds.), Churchill Livingstone, New York, 1833–1845

Radiopharmacy: Basics

2

Tamer B. Saleh

Contents

2.1 Introduction

A *radiopharmaceutical* is a radioactive compound that has two components, a radionuclide and a pharmaceutical; it is used for the diagnosis and treatment of human diseases. All radiopharmaceuticals are legend drugs and are subject to all regulations that apply to other drugs. The difference between a radiochemical and a radiopharmaceutical is that the former is not administered to humans due to the possible lack of sterility and nonpyrogenicity; any material administered to humans must be sterile and nonpyrogenic. A radiopharmaceutical may be a radioactive element like ^{133}Xe or a labeled compound such as ^{99m}Tc-labeled compounds [1].

In nuclear medicine, about 95% of the radiopharmaceuticals are used for medical diagnosis; only about 5% are used for therapeutic purposes. In designing a radiopharmaceutical, a suitable pharmaceutical is chosen on the basis of its preferential localization in a given organ or its participation in the physiological function of the organ. Then, a suitable radionuclide is tagged onto the chosen pharmaceutical and administered to the patient [2]. The radiation emitted from the organ can be detected by an external radiation detector for assessment of the morphological structure and the physiological function of that organ. Radiopharmaceuticals in most cases have no pharmacological effect as they are mainly administered in tracer amounts. So, they mainly do not show any dose–response relationship. For the therapeutic radiopharmaceuticals, however, the observed biological effect is from the radiation itself and not from the pharmaceutical [3].

Nuclear medicine procedures generally have two classifications; the first is those that depend on single-photon emitters, for which planar and tomographic imaging (single-photon emission computed tomography or SPECT) are the options of image acquisition. The other type is positron emission tomography (PET), for which the detection process relies on positron-electron annihilation and the release of two opposing photons (180° apart). The key component that distinguishes these techniques among other modalities is the diversity and ability of their contrast agents to

T.B. Saleh
King Fahed Specialist Hospital, Dammam, KSA
e-mail: tamirbayomy@yahoo.com

M.M. Khalil (ed.), *Basic Sciences of Nuclear Medicine*, DOI: 10.1007/978-3-540-85962-8_2,
© Springer-Verlag Berlin Heidelberg 2011

answer a clinical question. The contrast agents in nuclear medicine are radiolabeled compounds or radiopharmaceuticals that, when localized in the region of interest, emit important information about the pathophysiologic status of the tissue involved. Both imaging techniques have high sensitivity in detecting molecular concentrations in the pico or nano range, and their role in functional or molecular imaging is well addressed. SPECT and PET radiopharmaceuticals have a wide acceptance in molecular imaging, biomedical research disciplines, and drug development. However, many SPECT tracers are approved by the U.S. Food and Drug Administration (FDA), widely available, well reviewed in the literature, and relatively cheaper and perform for a significant patient population on a daily basis, whereas this situation is not true for the use of PET compounds.

SPECT radiotracers have a particular position in the matrix of molecular imaging due to their ability to image endogenous ligands such as peptides and antibodies and their ability to measure relatively slow kinetic processes due to the relatively long half-life of the commonly used isotopes (in comparison to PET). In addition, the capability to measure two different photon energies allows SPECT systems to depict two molecular pathways simultaneously by measuring their corresponding photon emissions [4]. In this chapter, we discuss some basic concepts about properties of radiopharmaceuticals, production, and generator systems used in clinical practice.

2.2 An Ideal Radiopharmaceutical

The definition of an ideal radiopharmaceutical in nuclear medicine procedures varies according to its use. The aim of a diagnostic radiopharmaceutical is to provide detectable photons with minimal biological effect to the cells or organ, whereas it is desired to produce a cytotoxic effect in a therapeutic procedure [5]. Generally, an ideal radiopharmaceutical for diagnostic procedures should meet the following characteristics:

Short half-life: Radiopharmaceuticals should have a relatively short effective half-life, which should not exceed the time assigned to complete the study. It provides a smaller radiation dose to the organ and ambient structures together with reduced exposure to workers, family members, and others. However,

radiotracers with short lifetimes mandate an injection of a high-activity concentration using fast imaging systems and may also compromise image quality. Thus, an optimal half-life satisfies imaging requirements while maintaining the quality of the scan. Protein synthesis and peptide formation involve a slow kinetic process; thus, single-photon emitters provide an opportunity to study the underlying functional disorders while the tracer still is able to emit a signal [1].

Suitable radionuclide emission: Radiopharmaceuticals emitting γ-radiation by electron capture or isomeric transition (energy between 30 and 300 keV) are commonly used in nuclear medicine diagnostic procedures. For therapeutic purposes, α-, β-, and Auger electron emitters are used because of their high linear energy transfer, which leads to maximum exposure and damage of the target cells. The α-particles and Auger electron emitters are mostly monoenergetic, whereas the β-particles have a continuous energy spectrum up to their maximum energy E_{max}.

High target-to-nontarget ratio: In all diagnostic procedures, it is well known that the agent with better target uptake is a superior imaging agent since the activity from the nontarget areas can interfere with the structural details of the organ imaged. Therefore, the target-to-nontarget activity ratio should be as large as possible.

Target uptake rate: The rate at which an organ takes up the administered radiopharmaceutical is also considered a key characteristic of an ideal radiopharmaceutical because it influences the period after which imaging acquisition is done. It is preferable to get images as early as possible for patient convenience. For example, ^{99m}Tc-pertechnetate is preferable to ^{123}I-NaI because the thyroid-imaging procedure can be performed after 20 min of dose administration, while with ^{123}I-NaI it takes 4–6 h to launch the imaging session.

Tracer excretion: The most common excretion route is renal clearance, which is rapid and can reduce exposure to the blood, whole body, and marrow. In contrast, the gastrointestinal tract (GIT) and hepatobiliary excretion is slow and leads to higher GIT and whole-body exposures. With GIT excretion, reabsorption into the blood also occurs. Since organ visualization is better when the background tissues have less uptake than the target organ, the radiopharmaceutical must be cleared from the blood and background tissue to achieve better image contrast.

Availability: The ideal radiopharmaceutical should be cost effective, inexpensive, and readily available in any nuclear medicine facility. This feature also characterizes the spread and diffusion of gamma emitters compared to PET-based compounds.

2.3 Production of Radionuclides

Naturally occurring radionuclides cannot be employed for medical diagnosis because of their long half-lives, which warrant the need for production of other radionuclides that can be safely used for medical applications. Most of the radionuclides for medical use are produced in nuclear reactors or cyclotrons. Some of the radionuclides are eluted from the generators in which the parent radionuclide is produced from a reactor or a cyclotron [2].

The process of all radionuclide production can be described by the general equation

$$X(``BP", ``EP")Y$$

where

X is the target element.
Y is the product element.
BP is the bombarding particle (projectile).
EP is the emitted product.

Pure metals are the best targets to use because of their high ability to sustain the high temperature in cyclotron and reactor systems.

2.3.1 Reactor-Produced Radionuclides

The two major principles of a nuclear reactor are that the neutrons induce fission in the fissile material constructing the fuel rods (e.g., U^{235}, P^{239}) of the reactor and the number of neutrons released in that fission reaction is about two or three neutrons with a mean energy of 1.5 MeV.

$$U^{235} + n \rightarrow \text{fission products} + \upsilon n$$

These new neutrons are used to produce fission in other nuclei, resulting in the release of new neutrons

that initiate the chain reaction. This chain reaction must be controlled to avoid the possible *meltdown* situation in the reactor using special neutron moderators (low molecular weight materials such as water, heavy water, and graphite, which are distributed in the spaces between the fuel rods), and neutron absorbers (e.g., cadmium rods placed in the fuel core) are used to thermalize and reduce the energy of the emitted neutrons to 0.025 eV to maintain equilibrium [1].

From the medical usefulness point of view, there are two types of nuclear reactions used to produce radioisotopes of interest 2 types: thermal neutron reactions and fission (n, f) reactions.

2.3.1.1 Thermal Neutron Reactions

The thermal neutrons around the core of the nuclear reactor can induce the following types of nuclear reactions:

$$A_Z^Y + n \rightarrow A_Z^{Y+1} + \gamma$$

$$A_Z^Y + n \rightarrow A_{Z-1}^Y + p$$

In the first type of reaction, the target atom A captures a neutron and emits gamma rays (γ), also written as an (n, γ) reaction.

For example:

$$^{98}\text{Mo (n,}\gamma\text{) }^{99}\text{Mo}$$

$$^{50}\text{Cr (n,}\gamma\text{) }^{51}\text{Cr}$$

In the second type of reactions, a proton is emitted after absorption of the neutron, resulting in a new element with different atomic number (Z).

For example:

$$^{14}\text{N(n, p) }^{14}\text{C}$$

$$^{3}\text{He(n, p) }^{3}\text{H}$$

Although the (n, γ) reaction produces a radioisotope from a stable one with a low specific activity product that are not carrier free, no sophisticated chemical separation procedures are required.

The (n, p) reaction produces an isotope with a different atomic number (element), enabling the production of high specific activity and carrier-free radioisotopes. *Specific activity* can be defined as the amount of activity per unit mass of a radionuclide or a labeled compound.

Products of (n, γ) reactions include parent isotopes, which are commonly used in nuclear generators to produce daughter radionuclides, which are the isotopes of interest; these are usually separated from their parents by column chromatography procedures.

For example:

$$^{98}Mo(n, \gamma) \, ^{99}Mo \xrightarrow{\, t1/2=67\,h \,} \, ^{99m}Tc$$

$$^{124}Xe(n, \gamma) \, ^{125}Xe \xrightarrow{\, t1/2=67\,h \,} \, ^{125}I$$

2.3.1.2 Fission or (n, f) Reactions

Fission is a process of breaking up a heavy nucleus (e.g., ^{235}U, ^{239}Pu, ^{232}Th) and any other material with an atomic number greater than 90 into two fragments (by-products).

For example:

$$U_{92}^{235} + n \rightarrow U_{92}^{236} \rightarrow Kr_{36}^{89} + Ba_{56}^{144} + 3n$$

$$U_{92}^{235} + n \rightarrow U_{92}^{236} \rightarrow I_{53}^{131} + Y_{39}^{102} + 3n$$

$$U_{92}^{235} + n \rightarrow U_{92}^{236} \rightarrow Mo_{42}^{99} + Sn_{50}^{135} + 2n$$

The neutron interacts with the ^{235}U nucleus to form unstable uranium atom ^{236}U, which breaks into two different smaller atoms and a number of neutrons. The isotopes produced may be employed in nuclear medicine (^{99}M, ^{131}I, ^{133}Xe); the greatest portion of these radioisotopes is not useful in nuclear medicine as they tend to decay by β⁻ emission. Unlike the radioisotopes formed from (n, γ) reactions, fission products can be chemically treated to produce carrier-free radionuclides. But, the major problem is how to separate them from the other products to obtain the highest level of radiochemical purity of the end product. The radioisotopes are mainly separated by appropriate chemical procedures that may involve precipitation, solvent extraction, ion exchange, distillation, and chromatography. Two of the most common isotopes are discussed as examples:

Molybdenum-99: For ^{99}Mo separation, the irradiated uranium target is dissolved in nitric acid, and the solution is adsorbed on an alumina (Al_2O_3) column. The column is then washed with nitric acid to remove uranium and other fission products.

Iodine-131: For chemical separation of ^{131}I from ^{235}U, the latter is dissolved in 18% sodium hydroxide (NaOH) by heating, and hydroxides of many metal ions are then precipitated by cooling. The supernatant containing sodium iodide is acidified with sulfuric acid. Iodide is oxidized to iodine by the effect of the acid, and iodine is collected in a NaOH by distillation.

2.3.2 Cyclotron-Produced Radionuclides

Cyclotron systems, which were invented in 1930, have an obvious role in the production of a wide range of nuclear medicine radiopharmaceuticals, especially those with short half-lives.

The basic principle of their operation is the acceleration of charged particles such as protons, deuterons, and α-particles in a spiral path inside two semicircular, flat, evacuated metallic cylinders called "dees." The dees are placed between the two poles of a magnet (see Fig. 2.1) so that the ion beam is constrained within a circular path inside the dees. At the gap between the dees, the ions experience acceleration due to the imposition of the potential difference. The beam particles originate at the ion source at the center of the cyclotron, and as they spiral outward in the dees, they acquire increasing energy for each passage across the gap of the dees. Eventually, the high-energy particles reach the periphery of the dees, where they are directed toward a target for bombardment [6].

Fixed-frequency cyclotrons can accelerate positively charged ions up to only 50 MeV for protons due to the relativistic increase in the mass of the accelerated particle, while for linear accelerators, particle acceleration can occur up to several hundreds of mega-electron-volts because of the ability of the accelerator to compensate for the increase in mass of high-energy particles. Advanced techniques have been developed to use cyclotrons to accelerate particles to much higher energies [7].

The majority of cyclotrons built prior to 1980 accelerated positively charged ions (i.e., H⁺); medical

Fig. 2.1 Layout of cyclotron

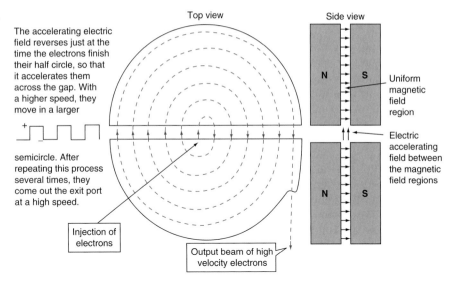

The accelerating electric field reverses just at the time the electrons finish their half circle, so that it accelerates them across the gap. With a higher speed, they move in a larger

semicircle. After repeating this process several times, they come out the exit port at a high speed.

Injection of electrons

Top view

Side view

Uniform magnetic field region

Electric accelerating field between the magnetic field regions

Output beam of high velocity electrons

cyclotrons accelerate negative ions (H⁻). This design allows for a simple deflection system in which the beam is intercepted by a thin carbon foil that extracts the negative ions at the end of the trajectory, resulting in the formation of a positively charged H⁺ beam. The beam then changes the direction without a deflector due to the magnetic field. The H⁺ bombards the target in a manner similar to that in a positively charged ion cyclotron. It is also possible to extract the beam at two different points in the machine, allowing use of a negative-ion cyclotron for production of two different radioisotopes simultaneously [8]. Generally, when the target nuclei are irradiated by the accelerated particles, a nuclear reaction takes place. The incident particle, after interaction, may leave some of its energy in the nucleus or be completely absorbed by it, depending on its incident energy. In either case, the nucleus is excited, resulting in the emission of nucleons (protons and neutrons) followed by γ-ray emission.

Depending on the energy deposited by the incident particle, a number of nucleons may be emitted randomly from the irradiated nucleus, leading to the formation of different nuclides. As the energy of the irradiating particle is increased, more nucleons are emitted and therefore a greater variety of nuclides may be produced.

An example of a simple cyclotron-produced radionuclide is the production of ^{111}In by irradiation of ^{111}Cd with 12-MeV protons. The nuclear reaction can be expressed as follows:

$$^{111}\text{Cd (p, n)}^{111}\text{In}$$

In this case, a second nucleon may not be emitted because there is not enough energy left after the emission of the first neutron. The excitation energy insufficient to emit any more nucleons will be dissipated by γ-ray emission.

The target material must be pure and preferably monoisotopic or at least enriched in the desired isotope to avoid the production of extraneous radioisotopes. In addition, the energy and type of the irradiating particle must be chosen to avoid the presence of undesired radionuclides.

Table 2.1 represents the most common commercial cyclotrons presented by the International Atomic Energy Authority (IAEA) report for cyclotron distribution in member states in 2006 [9].

2.3.3 Generator-Produced Radionuclides

The first commercial radionuclide generator was produced in the United States in the early 1960s (Brookhaven National Laboratories); since then, a number of different types of generators have been developed for various purposes in nuclear medicine. Generators are "parent–daughter systems involving a long-lived parent radionuclide that decays to short half-life daughter" and is called a generator because of its ability to generate continuously a relatively short-lived daughter radionuclide. The parent and its daughter nuclides are not isotopes; therefore, chemical separation is possible. Table 2.2 represents the most commonly used generators in nuclear medicine applications.

Radionuclide generators are formed by a glass or plastic column fitted at the bottom with a filtered disk. The column is fitted with absorbent material such as alumina, on which the parent nuclide is absorbed. Daughter radionuclides are generated by the decay of the parent radionuclide until either a *transient* or *secular* equilibrium is reached; after that, the daughter appears to decay with the half-life of the parent. The daughter is eluted in a carrier-free state (because it is not an isotope of the parent radionuclide) with a sterile and pyrogen-free appropriate solvent; then, the activity of the daughter starts to increase again up to equilibrium, so the elution can be made multiple times. Figure 2.2 shows a typical generator system.

Several methods can be adopted to obtain a sterilized eluted radionuclide:

- The entire column of the generator is autoclaved.
- Column preparation occurs under general aseptic conditions.
- Bacteriostatic agents are added to the generator column.
- A membrane filter unit is attached to the end of the column.
- Elution procedures are carried out under aseptic conditions.

2.3.3.1 Daughter Yield Equations

Assuming that there is initially no daughter activity in the generator, the daughter activity at any given time t is given by

$$A_2 = \frac{\lambda_2}{\lambda_2 - \lambda_1} A_1^0 (e^{-\lambda_1 t} - e^{-\lambda_2 t})$$

where

A_2 is the daughter activity at time t.
A_1^0 is the parent activity at time zero.
λ_1 and λ_2 are decay constants for the parent and daughter, respectively.

In case of transient equilibrium, as time t becomes sufficiently long, $e^{-\lambda_2 t}$ is negligible compared with $e^{-\lambda_1 t}$, and the equation becomes

$$A_2 = \frac{\lambda_2}{\lambda_2 - \lambda_1} A_1^0 (e^{-\lambda_1 t})$$

Table 2.1 Common commercial cyclotrons for cyclotron distribution

Company	Model	Description
CTI, Inc./ Siemens	RDS 111 RDS 112	11 MeV H−, 40,60 µA 11 MeV H−, 40 µA
GE	PETrace	16.5 MeV H−, 8.6 MeV D−, 80 µA
Ion Beam Applications (IBA)	Cyclone 18/9 Cyclone 30+	18 MeV H−, 9 MeV D−, 80 µA 30 MeV H−, 15 MeV D−, 60 µA
Sumitomo Heavy Industries	CYPRIS 370 AVF 930+	16 MeV H+, 10 MeV D+, 60 µA 90 MeV H+, 60 µA
Scanditronix Medical AB	MC40+	10–40 MeV H+, 5–20 MeV D+, 60 µA

Table 2.2 Some generator systems used in nuclear medicine applications

Parent	Parent ($T_{1/2}$)	Nuclear reaction	Daughter	Daughter ($T_{1/2}$)	Mode of daughter decay	Principal keV (% abundance)	Column	Eluant
^{99}Mo	66 h	Fission	^{99m}Tc	6 h	IT	140(90)	Al2O3	0.9% NaCl
^{87}Y	80 h	^{88}Sr(p,2n)	^{87m}Sr	2.8 h	IT	388(82)	Dowex 1 × 8	0.15M NaHCO3
^{68}Ge	271 days	^{69}Ga69 (p,2n)	^{68}Ga	68 min	B+	511(178)	Al$_2$O$_3$	0.005M EDTA
^{62}Zn	9.3 h	^{63}Cu(p,2n)	^{62}Cu	9.7 min	B+	511(194)	Dowex 1 × 8	2N HCL
^{82}Sr	25.5 days	^{85}Rb(p,4n)	^{82}Rb	75 s	B+	511(190)	SnO$_2$	0.9% NaCl

Adapted from [2].

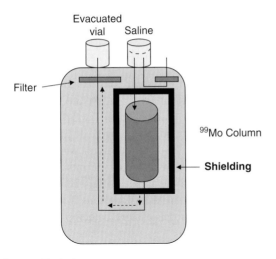

Evacuated
vial   Saline

Filter

^{99}Mo Column

Shielding

Fig. 2.2 Typical generator system

Since $A_1^0(e^{-\lambda_1 t})$ is the parent activity at time t, we can express it by A_1, and the equation can be rewritten as

$$A_2 = \frac{\lambda_2}{\lambda_2 - \lambda_1} A_1$$

In case of secular equilibrium, the parent activity does not decrease dramatically even after many daughter half-lives. As such, the decay constant of the parent λ_1 is much smaller than that of the daughter. So, we can make an approximation and assume that $\lambda_2 - \lambda_1 \approx \lambda_2$ and $A_1 = A_2$; thus, the daughter activity is equal to the parent activity.

2.3.3.2 ^{99}Mo-^{99m}Tc Generator

The ^{99}Mo-^{99m}Tc generator has been the most commonly used radionuclide generator in nuclear medicine practice worldwide since its first commercial introduction in 1965. It has several characteristics and attractive properties, which are summarized as follows [10]:

- Cost effective and simple to use
- Sterile and pyrogen free
- High radionuclide and radiochemical purity
- Used to produce many ^{99m}Tc-labeled radiopharmaceuticals frequently used in nuclear medicine departments
- Ideal half-life of the daughter nuclide (6 h) and optimum energy (140 keV, ~90% abundance)

- ^{99}Mo produced by the (n, f) fission reaction instead of the (n, γ) reaction (to have a carrier-free ^{99}Mo radionuclide) has a half-life of 66 h and decays by β-emission (87%) to metastable state technetium (^{99m}Tc) and in 13% to ground state (^{99}Tc), while ^{99m}Tc has a half-life of 6 h and decays to ^{99}Tc by an isomeric transition with the emission of 140-keV gamma photons [11].

2.3.3.3 Liquid Column (Solvent Extraction) Generator

The basic principle of the liquid column (solvent extraction) generator involves placing a 20% NaOH solution of ^{99}Mo in a glass column and then letting methyl ethyl ketone (MEK) flow through that column to extract ^{99m}TcO$_4$, leaving ^{99}Mo in an aqueous solution. The advantage of this generator is that it is extremely cost effective, but it needs many manipulations in the overall method and causes more radiation exposure to staff involved. Its use in nuclear medicine is diminishing.

2.3.3.4 Solid Column Generator

A solid column ^{99}Mo-^{99m}Tc generator is made initially with alumina (Al$_2$O$_3$) loaded in a plastic or glass column where the ^{99}Mo radionuclide is adsorbed on alumina in the chemical form ^{99}MoO$_4$ (molybdate). The column is washed with isotonic saline to remove any undesirable activity. The amount of alumina used is about 5–10 g, depending on the total ^{99}Mo activity used. ^{99m}Tc radionuclide is eluted as a product of ^{99}Mo decay in the form of sodium pertechnetate (Na^{99m}TcO$_4$) with a 0.9% NaCl solution. After elution, the ^{99m}Tc activity starts to grow again up to equilibrium [12]. Elution may be carried out even before equilibrium if needed, and the amount of activity obtained depends on the time elapsed between the previous and the present elution.

For radiation protection purposes, the generator columns are shielded with lead or depleted uranium in generators with high ^{99}Mo activity because ^{238}U has a higher Z number and therefore attenuates γ-rays more efficiently.

There are two types of solid column ^{99}Mo-^{99m}Tc generators: wet and dry column. Dry column generators are preferable due to the repeated withdrawal of saline from the column after routine generator usage by an evacuated tube, which prevents the formation of hydrogen peroxide (H_2O_2) and perhydroxyl free radical (HO_2), which if present in the ^{99m}Tc eluate can interfere with the ^{99m}Tc labeling procedures because they can act as oxidants. In addition, in wet column generators, saline in the tubing may possibly freeze in extremely cold weather, thus preventing elution until thawed.

2.3.3.5 ^{99m}Tc Yield in the ^{99}Mo-^{99m}Tc Generator

Since ^{99}Mo and ^{99m}Tc radionuclides decay to ^{99}Tc, the generator eluate contains both ^{99m}Tc and ^{99}Tc in various concentrations. The fraction of ^{99m}Tc decreases due to the rapid decay of ^{99m}Tc, especially when the time between elutions increases. ^{99m}Tc and ^{99}Tc have the same chemical structure, so ^{99}Tc can interfere with the preparation of ^{99m}Tc radiopharmaceuticals, especially with kits containing small amounts of stannous ions. This situation becomes critical when the generators are left without elution for several days [13].

The ^{99m}Tc content in the generator eluate can be expressed by the following equation:

$$F = N_A/(N_A + N_B)$$

where F is the ^{99m}Tc mole fraction. N_A and N_B are the number of ^{99m}Tc and ^{99}Tc, respectively.

The mole fraction of ^{99m}Tc (F) at any time t can be calculated as

$$F = 0.87\lambda_1(e^{-\lambda_1 t} - e^{-\lambda_2 t})/(\lambda_2 - \lambda_1)(1 - e^{-\lambda_1 t})$$

where λ_1 and λ_2 are decay constants for the ^{99}Mo and ^{99m}Tc, respectively. The factor 0.87 indicates that 87% of ^{99}Mo decays to ^{99m}Tc.

2.3.3.6 Other Generator Systems

^{113}Sn-^{113}In Generator

Indium-113 can be used to prepare a number of radiopharmaceuticals used for imaging of lungs, liver, brain, and kidneys. ^{113}Sn has a half-life of 117 days,

while the daughter ^{113}In has a half-life of 100 min and energy of 393 keV [14]. The generator is made up of hydrous zirconium oxide contained in a plastic or glass column. Sn-113 produced in a reactor by neutron irradiation and in the stannic form is adsorbed on the column, and the daughter ^{113}In is eluted with 0.05N HCl [15].

Due to the relatively long half-life of ^{113}Sn (117 days), the ^{113}Sn-^{113}In generator can be used for 6–12 months, making it one of the most economical generators. The disadvantage of this generator is the improper energy of 393-keV photons from ^{113}In with routinely used gamma camera detectors. ^{113}Sn-^{113}In generators generally have been replaced by moly generators; however, they are still useful in some developing countries and isolated regions of the world [3].

^{81}Rb-^{81}Kr Generator

^{81}Kr is a gamma-ray-emitting radionuclide with a photon energy of 190 keV (192% abundance). It is commonly used as a lung and myocardial perfusion imaging agent [16]. The generator is formed of a column containing a cation exchange resin (Bio-Rad AGMP-50), where the cyclotron-produced ^{81}Rb ($t_{1/2} = 47$ h) is loaded. The noble gas ^{81}Kr ($t_{1/2} = 13$ s) is eluted by passing humidified oxygen over the generator column [17]. The ^{81}Kr and O_2 are delivered to the patient through a nonbreathing face mask. The major disadvantages of the ^{81}Rb-^{81}Kr generator are the high cost and the 12-h expiration time of the nuclide of the generator [3].

^{82}Sr-^{82}Rb Generator

Rubidium-82 is a positron-emitting radionuclide and is used primarily as a myocardial perfusion agent for PET imaging. It serves as an alternative to the accepted oxygen-15 and nitrogen-13 with an increasing trend for use in research and clinical practice [18]. Its importance also lies in the fact that the production process does not require a cyclotron system and its associated complexities.

^{82}Sr ($t_{1/2} = 25$ days) decays by electron capture to ^{82}Rb ($t_{1/2} = 75$ s), which decays by β^+ emission. To make the generator, the cyclotron-produced ^{82}Sr is loaded on a SnO_2 column, and ^{82}Rb is eluted with

0.9% NaCl solution to obtain it in the form of rubidium chloride. Because of its short half-life, [82]Rb elution can be repeated every 10–15 min with maximum yield [19]. The disadvantage of this generator is the short half-life of the [82]Rb daughter radionuclide. In an effort to overcome the short half-life, a calibrated continuous infusion system has been developed, allowing elution of the generator directly into an intravenous catheter [20].

The activity of [82]Rb produced from a [82]Sr-[82]Rb generator is dependent on elution conditions (volume and eluent flow rate) and sampling conditions (time and position of collection). There is a characteristic curve for the elution of Rb-82 from the generator that depends on the flow rate and the Sr-82 activity within the generator. This results in a variation of the infusion profile, thus altering the amount of tracer injected [21].

[68]Ge-[68]Ga Generator

[68]Ga is primarily used for brain tumor imaging, but with the availability of positron systems and its emission of 2.92-MeV positrons in 89% abundance, its use has increased in PET applications [22]. This generator is made up of alumina loaded in a plastic or glass column. Carrier-free [68]Ge ($t_{1/2} = 271$ days) in concentrated HCl is neutralized in EDTA (ethylenediaminetetraacetic acid) solution and adsorbed on the column. Then, [68]Ga ($t_{1/2} = 68$ min) is eluted with $0.005M$ EDTA solution. Alternatively, [68]Ge is adsorbed on a stannous dioxide column, and ^{68}Ga is eluted with $1.0N$ HCl. This generator can be eluted frequently with a maximum yield in a few hours [23].

[62]Zn-[62]Cu Generator

Copper-62 is also a positron-emitting radionuclide (98% abundance) and is used widely for PET imaging. [62]Zn ($t_{1/2} = 9.3$ h) decays to [62]Cu ($t_{1/2} = 9.7$ min) by electron capture (92%) and β^+ emission (8%). [62]Cu decays by β^+ emission (97%) and electron capture (3%). [62]Zn in $2N$ HCl is adsorbed on a Dowe 1×8 column, and [62]Cu is converted to [62]Cu-PTSM, copper-62 (II) pyruvaldehyde bis-(N-4-methyl)thiosemicarbazone which is used for myocardial and brain perfusion imaging [24]. The biggest disadvantage of this generator is the short half-life of the daughter radionuclide, limiting its use only to the day of delivery [25].

Most nuclear medicine procedures that use single-photon emitters are based on Tc-99m or Tc-99m-labeled compounds, and the recent shortage of this radionuclide (2010 international moly crisis) demonstrated the wide and extensive importance of its clinical utility. However, there are other radiopharmaceuticals that are of particular interest in many diagnostic applications.

2.4 Common Radiopharmaceuticals

2.4.1 Thallium-201

Thallium-201 is a frequently used radiopharmaceutical in cardiac imaging in addition to its role in scanning of tumors and parathyroid adenomas [26].

[201]Tl, which is commercially available as thallium chloride, is produced by exposing pure natural [203]Tl to a high-energy proton beam, resulting in production of Pb-201:

$$^{203}Tl\,[p, 3n]\,Pb\text{-}201$$

Pb-201 is then chemically separated from the target Tl-203 and allowed to decay to Tl-201.

Tl-201 decays to mercury (Hg-201) by Electron Capture with a half-life of 73 h and gives off a mercury-characteristic x-ray (69–80 keV) with 95% abundance and two gamma rays of 135 and 167 keV with a combined abundance of 12%. The commercially produced thalous chloride should contain 95% of its content in the form of Tl-201 [1]. The maximum concentration of thallium in the heart is obtained approximately 10–30 min after injection in the resting state and 5 min after stress induced either physically or pharmacologically. Uptake of Tl-201 into the myocardium is dependent on tissue oxygenation, which governs the blood flow as oxygen is essential in supporting Tl-201 uptake through the Na-K-ATPase (adenosine triphosphatase) concentration mechanism (Tl-201 and K$^+$ are similarly involved in the Na-K-ATPase pump) [27]. Tl-201 has been extensively used as a myocardial perfusion imaging agent in evaluating patients with coronary artery disease and in viability assessment. In addition, its role in tumor imaging has been recognized.

2.4.2 Gallium-67

Gallium-67 is a cyclotron-produced radiopharmaceutical; it can be produced by one of the following nuclear reactions:

Zn-67[p, n]Ga-67

Zn-68[p, 2n]Ga-67

Ga-67 decays by EC with a half-life of 78 h with the following gamma-ray energy and abundances: 93 keV (40%), 184 keV (24%), 296 keV (22%), and 388 keV (7%).

Ga-67 is delivered from the manufacturer as gallium citrate with radiochemical purity greater than 85%. Gallium is presented as Ga^{+3} in aqueous solutions, making radiopharmaceutical production easier than that with ^{99m}Tc because reduction does not have to be performed.

It is considered the master radiopharmaceutical for tumor imaging and detection of inflammatory sites. Its role is highly affected after the introduction of FDG-PET, fluorodeoxyglucose applications. On injection of gallium citrate, more than 90% of gallium becomes bound to plasma proteins, mainly *transferrin*, resulting in slow clearance from plasma. The Ga-transferrin binding procedure can be affected when transferrin is saturated with stable gallium or iron before gallium injection. Under these conditions, gallium distribution is shifted from soft tissue to bones with no change in the tumor uptake, while increasing Ga-transferrin binding causes an increase in soft tissue activity and decreased tumor activity [28].

2.4.3 Iodine Radiopharmaceuticals

Radioisotopes of iodine are widely used in nuclear medicine for diagnostic and therapeutic purposes. Radioiodine can substitute into many iodine radiopharmaceuticals (e.g., ^{131}I-MIBG, ^{123}I-MIBG, meta-iodobenzylguanidine and orthoiodohippurate [OIH]), and when oxidized for iodination (by chloramine T or chloroglycoluril), it can attach itself to aromatic rings to make different radiopharmaceuticals. The most common iodine isotopes are I-131, I-125, I-123, and ^{123}I-ioflupane.

- Iodine-131

Iodine-131 is produced as a by-product of uranium fission. I-131 decays by β emission with a half-life of 8.05 days to X-133. As a result of that decay, four γ-rays are emitted with the following energies and abundances: 364 keV (82%), 637 keV (7%), 284 keV (6%), and 723 keV (2%). The 364-keV energy photons are mainly used diagnostically. The accepted radiochemical purity from the manufacturer for I-131 as NaI is 95%, as MIBG or Norcholesterol is 95%, and as OIH is 97%. I-131 is used as NaI in thyroid therapy and diagnosis in addition to imaging of the adrenal gland (as iodo-methyl-norcholestrol or MIBG) and renal tubular system (as ^{131}I-OIH). Due to the high thyroid radiation uptake (1 rad/µCi), it has been replaced by I-123 for thyroid imaging and ^{99m}Tc-MAG$_3$, Mercaptoacetyltriglycine for renal tubular scan. Recently, I-131 was applied for radioimmunotherapy of non-Hodgkin lymphoma (NHL) when labeled with anti-CD20 monoclonal antibody (^{131}I-tositumobab) in a therapeutic regimen called BEXXAR [29].

- Iodine-125

Iodine-125 is produced from Xe-124 through the following reaction:

Xe-124[n, γ] Xe-125

Then, Xe-125 decays by EC to I-125. I-125 decays by EC with a half-life of 60 days and 35-keV gamma rays. I-125, when labeled with albumin-producing radioiodinated serum albumin (RISA), is frequently used for plasma volume and GFR, Glomerular filtration rate determination. I-125-labeled antibodies are used widely for radioimmunoassay.

- Iodine-123

Iodine-123 is a cyclotron-produced radiopharmaceutical. Different methods have been used for I-123 production, although the current method of production uses the following reactions with 31-MeV protons from the cyclotrons:

1. Xe-124[p, 2n]Cs-123. Cs-123 then decays by EC and β$^+$ emission to Xe-123, which decays to the target radiopharmaceutical (I-123), also by EC and β$^+$ emission.

Xe-124[p, pn] Xe-123

2. Then, Xe-123 decays to I-123 by electron capture. I-125 is present as the only contaminant

with the previous methods at a concentration of less than 0.1%. I-123 decays by EC with a 13-h half-life and emits 159-keV photons with 83% abundance (ideal for imaging). Radiochemical purity of I-123 preparations from the manufacturer must exceed 95%.

I-123 is the preferred thyroid imaging agent, imparting 1% of the thyroid dose per microcurie when compared with I-131. ^{123}I-labeled compounds are commonly used as ^{123}I-MIBG for an adrenal scan, ^{123}I-OIH for a tubular renal scan, and ^{123}I-iodoamphetamine (^{123}I-IMP) for a cerebral perfusion scan [2].

- ^{123}I-Ioflupane (DaTSCAN)
  DaTSCAN is a widely used ^{123}I derivative for detection of the loss of nerve cells that release dopamine in an area of the brain called the striatum; dopamine is a chemical messenger, and therefore it will be useful in diagnosis of the following:

  1. *Movement disorders*: DaTSCAN is used to help distinguish between Parkinson disease and essential tremor (tremors of unknown cause) with a sensitivity of 96.5% [30].
  2. *Dementia*: DaTSCAN is also used to help distinguish between "dementia with Lewy bodies" and Alzheimer disease with 75.0–80.25% sensitivity [31].

Dopamine transporter (DAT) imaging with tropane derivatives such as FP-CIT Fluoropropyl-Carbomethoxy-Iodophenyl-Tropane (^{123}I-Ioflupane) and β-CIT, Beta Carbomethoxy-Iodophenyl-Tropane has been developed to directly measure degeneration of dopamine presynaptic terminal and may be used to quantify changes in DAT density. Ioflupane binds specifically to certain structures of the nerve cells ending in the brain striatum that are responsible for the transport of dopamine. This binding can be detected using tomographic imaging [32].

2.4.4 Indium-111 Radiopharmaceuticals

In-111 is produced in a cyclotron through the following reaction:

$$Cd\text{-}111\ [p, n]\ In\text{-}111$$

Indium-111 decays with a 67-h half-life by EC as a pure gamma emitter with 173-keV (89%) abundance and 247-keV (94% abundance) photons. The gamma energies of In-111 are in the optimum range of detectability for the commercially available gamma cameras. Like Ga-67, In-111 in aqueous solutions exists only as In^{3+} and behaves chemically like iron, forming strong complexes with the plasma protein transferrin.

Because of the great stability of In-111 with transferrin, only strong chelates can be used in vivo to direct the localization of the radiopharmaceuticals to other sites. Strong chelators like DTPA, Diethlenetriaminepentaacetate or EDTA can be easily used with indium using citrates or acetates as a transfer ligand. ^{111}In-DTPA has been used for renal and brain imaging and is currently used for cisternography. ^{111}In-colloids can be used as liver/spleen imaging agents, and larger colloidal particles are commonly used for lung imaging.

The most common applications of In-111 are in labeling blood cells (white blood cells and platelets) for imaging inflammatory processes, thrombi, and proteins [33]. In protein labeling, by which proteins are primarily labeled to DTPA, choosing proper the In-111-specific concentration is of greater importance. In blood cell labeling, the plasma transferrin competes for the In-111 and reduces the labeling efficiency because In-111 binds with higher efficiency to transferrin than blood cells; therefore, isolation of the desired blood component from plasma permits easy labeling of either platelets or white blood cells.

[111]In has been conjugated to octreotide as an agent for the scintigraphic localization of primary and metastatic somatostatin receptor-positive neuroendocrine tumors. A labeled form of octreotide is commercially available as the DTPA chelated compound ^{111}In-DTPA-octriotide (^{111}In-pentetreotide, Octreoscan) [34].

[111]In contributes also in labeling of monoclonal antibodies (MAbs) using bifunctional chelates. The chelating agent (mainly DTPA) is first conjugated to the antibody, and then ^{111}In binds to the conjugated MAb via the chelating agent [35]. The commercially available kit is called Oncoscint. Indium In-111 satumomab pendetide (Oncoscint) is indicated for use in immunoscintigraphy in patients with known colorectal or ovarian cancer. It helps determine the extent and location of extrahepatic foci of disease and can be helpful in the preoperative determination of the resectability of malignant lesions in these patients [36].

A murine monoclonal antibody produced against prostate carcinoma and prostate hypertrophy is chelated to GYK-DTPA, glycyl-tyrosyl-(N,epsilon-diethylenetriaminepentaacetic acid) and lypophilized to give capromab pendetide. After ^{111}In labeling, a ^{111}In-capromab pendetide (ProstaScint) kit is produced for detecting primary and metastatic prostate cancer [37].

2.4.5 Xenon-133

Xenon-133 is an inert gas used mainly for lung ventilation scans and for the assessment of cerebral blood flow. It is a by-product of uranium fission with a 5.3-day half-life and 35% abundance for 81-keV photons. This photon energy requires starting lung scans with ventilation followed by the ^{99m}Tc-MAA (macroaggregated albumin) perfusion scan [1].

2.4.6 Chromium-51

Chromium-51 has a half-life of 27.7 days and has long been used for labeling red blood cells as a method for determination of red cell mass and red cell survival [38].

2.4.7 Phosphorus-32

Phosphorus-32, which is delivered commercially as ^{32}P-sodium phosphate, is produced by irradiating sulfur with neutrons in a reactor. P-32 decays by β^- emission with a half-life of 14.3 days. ^{32}P-sodium phosphate is indicated for therapeutic treatment of polycythemia vera, chronic myelocytic leukemia, and chronic lymphocytic leukemia and for palliation of metastatic bone pain. Chromic ^{32}P-phosphate is used for treatment of peritoneal or pleural effusions caused by metastatic disease [39, 40].

2.4.8 Strontium-89

Strontium-89 (pure β^- emitter) is produced in the reactor and decays with a half-life of 50.6 days [41].

[89]Sr-chloride (Metastron) is used for relief of bone pain since the compound behaves biologically as calcium does and localizes at the sites of active osteogenesis [42].

2.4.9 Rhenium-186

Rhenium-186 is a reactor-produced radiopharmaceutical that decays by β^- emission and has a half-life of 3.8 days. Re-186 is complexed with hydroxyethylene diphosphonate (HEDP) after reduction with stannous ions like Tc-99m. [186]Re-HEDP with radiochemical purity over 97% is useful for bone pain palliative therapy [43]. A whole-body scan can also be obtained using its 137-keV energy photons [44].

2.4.10 Samarium-153

Samarium-153 is a reactor-produced radionuclide that decays by β^- emission and has a half-life of 46.3 h. Sm-153 is complexed with a bone-seeking agent, ethylenediaminetetramethylene phosphonic acid (EDTMP), which localizes in bone metastases by chemisorption. [153]Sm-EDTMP is approved by FDA for relief of metastatic bone pain. Its duration of response is 1–12 months. In addition, its 103-keV photons allow scintigraphic imaging of the whole body [45]46.

2.4.11 [111]In- and ^{90}Y-Ibritumomab Tiuxetan (Zevalin)

Zevalin ([111]In- and ^{90}Y-ibritumomab tiuxetan) consists of a murine monoclonal anti-CD20 antibody covalently conjugated to the metal chelator DTPA, which forms a stable complex with ^{111}In for imaging and with ^{90}Y for therapy. ^{90}Y-ibritumomab tiuxetan is used for the treatment of some forms of B-cell NHL, a myeloproliferative disorder of the lymphatic system, while its ^{111}In derivative is used to scan the predicted distribution of a therapeutic dosage of ^{90}Y-ibritumomab in the body [47].

The antibody binds to the CD20 antigen found on the surface of normal and malignant B cells (but not B-cell precursors), allowing radiation from the attached isotope (yttrium-90) to kill it and some nearby cells. In addition, the antibody itself may trigger cell death via antibody-dependent cell-mediated cytotoxicity, complement-dependent cytotoxicity, and apoptosis. Together, these actions eliminate B cells from the body, allowing a new population of healthy B cells to develop from lymphoid stem cells [48].

An earlier version of anti-CD20 antibody, Rituximab, has also been approved under the brand name Rituxan for the treatment of NHL. Ibritumomab tiuxetan was the first radioimmunotherapy drug approved by the FDA in 2002 to treat cancer. It was approved for the treatment of patients with relapsed or refractory, low-grade or follicular B-cell NHL, including patients with rituximab-refractory follicular NHL. In September 2009, ibritumomab received approval from the FDA for an expanded label for the treatment of patients with previously untreated follicular NHL, who achieve a partial or complete response to first-line chemotherapy.

2.4.12 ^{90}Y-Labeled Microspheres

Treatment of hepatic carcinomas and metastasis have experienced many trials [49] of the use of ceramic or resin microspheres with certain types of beta-emitting radiation to enhance their response rate. However, many side effects observed can contraindicate their usage for this purpose (e.g., secondary medullary toxicity with the release of ^{90}Y from the microspheres). Accordingly, modification of these methods was applied to develop new microspheres containing yttrium-90 in a stable form, preventing the release of the radioactive material in the surrounding matrix. Two products have been presented: SIR-Spheres with a 35-μm diameter (Medical Sirtec Ltd., Australia) and TheraSphere with a 20- to 30-μm diameter (MDS Nordion, Ottawa, Canada) [50]. This therapeutic module should be initiated with a diagnostic estimation of the possibility of locating and quantifying a possible pulmonary shunt. This is achievable by injection of ^{99m}Tc-MAA into the hepatic artery [51]. When yttrium-90 is incorporated into the tiny glass beds, it can be injected through the blood vessels supplying the liver through a long and flexible plastic tube (catheter) with guided fluoroscopy. This procedure allows a large local dose of radiation to be delivered to the tumor with less risk of toxicity to other parts of the body or the healthy liver tissues. The radiation from the induced ^{90}Y activity is contained within the body and becomes minimally active within 7 days after treatment due to physical decay [52].

2.4.13 Lutetium-177 Compounds

Lutium-177 ($T_{1/2} = 6.71$ days) is a radionuclide of exciting potential. It is used in a manner similar to yttrium-90; however, it has slightly different advantages:

1. It has both beta particle emissions ($E_{max} = 497$, 384 and 176 keV) for therapeutic effect and gamma emissions (113 and 208 keV) for imaging purposes.
2. It has a shorter radius of penetration than Y-90, which makes it an ideal candidate for radioimmunotherapy for smaller and soft tumors.

Many Lu-177 derivatives have been developed for many therapeutic purposes, such as

1. Lu-177 labeled EDTMP and 1,4,7,10-tetraazacyclododecane-1,4,7,10-tetraaminomethylenephosphonate (DOTMP) for bone pain palliation [53]
2. Lu-177 labeled radioimmunoconjugates (Lu-177 monoclonal antibody, 7E11) constructs for radioimmunotherapy of prostate cancer [54]
3. Lu-177-DOTA, tetra-azacyclododecanetetra-acetic acid octreotate for targeted radiotherapy of endocrine tumors [55].

References

1. Wilson MA (1998) Textbook on nuclear medicine. Lippincott-Raven, Philadelphia
2. Saha GB (2004) Fundamentals of radiopharmacy, 5th edn. Springer, Berlin
3. Bernier D, Christian P, Langan LJ (1998) Nuclear medicine – technology and techniques, 3rd edn. Mosby, St. Louis
4. Meikle S, Kench P, Kassiou M, Banati R (2005) Small animal SPECT and its place in the matrix of molecular imaging technologies. Phys Med Biol 50(22):R45–R61

5. Karesh S (1996) Radiopharmaceuticals – a tutorial. Loyola University Medical Education Network, Chicago

6. Saha GB, MacIntyre WJ, Go RT (1992) Cyclotrons and positron emission tomography for clinical imaging. Semin Nucl Med 22:150

7. Lewis DM (1995) Isotope production and the future potential of accelerators. In: Proceedings of the.14th international conference on cyclotrons and their applications, Cape Town

8. Grey-Morgan T, Hubbard RE (1992) The operation of cyclotrons used for radiopharmaceutical production. In: Proceedings of the 13th international conference on cyclotrons and their applications, Vancouver

9. IAEA (2006) Directory of cyclotrons used for radionuclide production in member states. IAEA-DCRP, Vienna

10. Eckelman WC, Coursey BM (eds) (1982) Technetium-99m: generators, chemistry and preparation of radiopharmaceuticals. Int J Appl Radiat Isot 33:793

11. Marengo M, Apriele C, Bagnara C, Bolzati C, Bonada C, Candini G, Casati R, Civollani S, Colompo FR, Compagnone G, Del Dottore F, DI Gugliemo E, Ferretti PP, Lazzari S, Minoia C, Pancaldi D, Ronchi A, Di Toppi GS, Saponaro R, Torregionai T, Uccelli L, Vecchi F, Piffanelli A (1999) Quality control of Mo99/Tc99m generators: results of a survey of the radiopharmacy working group of the Italian Association of Nuclear Medicine (AIMN). Nucl Med Commun 20:1077–1084

12. Zolle I (2007) Technetium-99m pharmaceuticals. Springer, Berlin

13. Holland ME, Deutsch E, Heinemann HR (1986) Studies on commercially available 99Mo/99mTc generators. II. Operating characteristics and behavior of 99M/99mTc radionuclide generators. Appl Radiat Isotopes 37:173

14. Sampson C (1995) Textbook of radiopharmacy, theory and practice, 2nd edn. Taylor & Francis, London

15. Teranishi K, Yamaashi Y, Maruyama Y (2002) 113Sn-113mIn generator with a glass beads column. J Radioanal Nucl Chem 254(2):369–371

16. Kleynhans PH, Lötter MG, van Aswegen A, Herbst CP, Marx JD, Minnaar PC (1982) The imaging of myocardial perfusion with 81mKr during coronary arteriography. Eur J Nucl Med 7(9):405–409

17. Johansson L, Stroak A (2006) Kr-81m calibration factor for the npl ionisation chamber. Appl Radiat Isotopes 64(10–11):1360–1364

18. Klein R (2007) Precision-controlled elution of a 82Sr/82Rb generator for cardiac perfusion imaging with positron emission tomography. Phys Med Biol 52:659–673

19. Aardaneh K, van der Walt TN, Davids C (2006) Radiochemical separation of 82Sr and the preparation of a sterile 82Sr/82Rb generator column. J Radioanal Nucl Chem 270 (2):385–390

20. Saha GB, Go RT, MacIntyre WJ et al (1990) Use of the 82Sr/82Rb generator in clinical PET studies. Nucl Med Biol 17:763

21. Gennaro GP, Bergner BC, Haney PS, Kramer RH, Loberg MD (1987) Radioanalysis of 82Rb generator eluates. Int J Rad Appl Instrum A 38(3):219–225

22. Breeman WAP, Verbruggen AM (2007) The 68Ge/68Ga generator has high potential, but when can we use 68Ga-labelled tracers in clinical routine. Eur J Nucl Med Mol Imaging 34(7):978–981

23. Asti M, De Pietri G, Fraternali A, Grassi E, Sghedoni R, Fioroni F, Roesch F, Versari A, Salvo D (2008) Validation of (68)Ge/(68)Ga generator processing by chemical purification for routine clinical application of (68)Ga-DOTA-TOC. Nucl Med Biol 35(6):721–724

24. Haynes NG, Lacy JL, Nayak N, Martin CS, Dai D, Mathias CJ, Green MA (2000) Performance of a 62Zn/62Cu generator in clinical trials of PET perfusion agent 62Cu-PTSM. J Nucl Med 41(2):309–314

25. Guillaume M, Brihaye C (1986) Generators for short-lived gamma and positron emitting radionuclides: current status and prospects. Nucl Med Biol 13:89

26. Vasken D, Pasquale P-F, Arrighi JA, Bacharach SL, Quyyumi AA, Freedman NMT, Bonow RO (1993) Coronary blood flow/perfusion and metabolic imaging: concordance and discordance between stress-redistribution-reinjection and rest-redistribution thallium imaging for assessing viable myocardium: comparison with metabolic activity by positron emission tomography. Circulation 88 (3):941–952

27. Fieno DS, Shea SM, Li Y, Harris KR, Finn JP, Li D (2004) Myocardial perfusion imaging based on the blood oxygen level-dependent effect using T2-prepared steady-state free-precession magnetic resonance imaging. Circulation 110 (10):1284–1290

28. Yutaka N, Akira F, Taiji T, Yukiya H, Susumu M (2004) Ga-67 citrate scintigraphy in the diagnosis of primary hepatic lymphoma. Clin Nucl Med 29(1):53–54

29. Capizzi R (2004) Targeted radio-immunotherapy with Bexxar produces durable remissions in patients with late stage low grade Non-Hodgkin's lymphomas. Trans Am Clin Climatol Assoc 115:255–272

30. Booij J (2001) The clinical benefit of imaging striatal dopamine transporters with [123I] FP-CIT SPET in differentiating patients with presynaptic parkinsonism from other forms of parkinsonism. Eur J Nucl Med 28:266–272

31. Lorberboym M (2004) 123I-FP-CIT SPECT imaging of dopamine transporters in patients with cerebrovascular disease and clinical diagnosis of vascular parkinsonism. J Nucl Med 45:1688–1693

32. Lavalaye J (2000) Effect of age and gender on dopamine transporter imaging with 123-I-FP-CIT SPECT in healthy volunteers. Eur J Nucl Med 27:867–869

33. Thomas P, Mullan B (1995) Avid In-111 labeled WBC accumulation in a patient with active osteoarthritis of both knees. Clin Nucl Med 20(11):973–975

34. Ha L, Mansberg R, Nguyen D (2008) Increased activity on In-111 octreotide imaging due to radiation fibrosis. Clin Nucl Med 33:46–48

35. Paul BJ, George SC, Jack JE, Darlene F-B, Freeman W, Conrad N, Howard DJ (1995) Indium-111 oncoscint CR/OV and F-18 FDG in colorectal and ovarian carcinoma recurrences early observations. Clin Nucl Med 20(3):230–236

36. Bray D, Mills AP, Notghi A (1994) Imaging for recurrent/residual colorectal carcinoma using 111In-oncoscint. Nucl Med Commun 15(4):248

37. Kimura M, Sivian T, Mouraviev V, Mayes J, Price M, Bannister M, Madden J, Wong T, Polascik T (2009) Utilization of 111In-capromab pendetide SPECT-CT for detecting seminal vesicle invasion with recurrent prostate cancer after primary in situ therapy. Int J Urol 16(12):971–975

38. Dworkin HJ, Premo M, Dees S (2007) Comparison of red cell and whole blood volume as performed using both chromium-51-tagged red cells and iodine-125-tagged albumin and using I-131-tagged albumin and extrapolated red cell volume. Am J Med Sci 334(1):37–40

39. Kaplan E, Fels IG, Kotlowski BR (1960) Therapy of carcinoma of the prostate metastatic to bone with P-32 labeled condensed phosphate. J Nucl Med 1:1–13

40. Lewington VJ (1993) Targeted radionuclide therapy for bone metastases. Eur J Nucl Med 20:66–74

41. Blake GM, Wood JF, Wood PJ, Zivanovic MA, Lewington VJ (1989) 89Sr therapy: strontium plasma clearance in disseminated prostatic carcinoma. Eur J Nucl Med 15:49–54

42. Poner A, Mertens W (1991) Strontium 89 in the treatment of metastatic prostate cancer. Can J Oncol 1:11–18

43. Ketring AR (1987) 153Sm-EDTMP and 186Re-HEDP as bone therapeutic radiopharmaceuticals. Nucl Med Biol 14:223–232

44. de Klerk JMH, van Dijk A, van het Schip AD, Zonnenberg BA, van Rijk PP (1992) Pharmacokinetics of rhenium-186 after administration of rhenium-186-HEDP to patients with bone metastases. J Nucl Med 33:646–651

45. Holmes RA (1992) [153Sm] EDTMP: a potential therapy for bone cancer pain. Semin Nucl Med 22:41–45

46. Singh A, Holmes RA, Farhangi M (1989) Human pharmacokinetics of samarium-153 EDTMP in metastatic cancer. J Med 30:1814–1818

47. Otte A (2006) 90Y-ibritumomab tiuxetan: new drug, interesting concept, and encouraging in practice. Nucl Med Commun 27(7):595–596

48. Han S, Iagaru AH, Zhu HJ, Goris ML (2006) Experience with 90y-ibritumomab (Zevalin) in the management of refractory non-Hodgkin's lymphoma. Nucl Med Commun 27(12):1022–1023

49. Gray BN et al (1989) Selective internal radiation (SIR) therapy for treatment of liver metastases: measurement of response rate. J Surg Oncol 42:192–196

50. Biersack HJ, Freeman LM (eds) (2007) Clinical nuclear medicine. Springer, Berlin

51. Ho S, Lau WY, Leung WT, Chan M, Chan KW, Johnson PJ, Li AK (1997) Arteriovenous shunts in patients with hepatic tumors. J Nucl Med 38:1201–1205

52. Gray BN et al (2001) Randomized trial of SIR-spheres plus chemotherapy vs. chemotherapy alone for treating patients with liver metastases from primary large bowel cancer. Ann Oncol 12:1711–1720

53. Chang Y, Jeong J, Lee YS, Kim Y, Lee D, Key Chung J, Lee M (2008) Comparison of potential bone pain palliation agents – Lu-177-EDTMP and Lu-177-DOTMP. J Nucl Med 49(Supplement 1):93

54. Tedesco J, Goeckeler W, Becker M, Frank K, Gulyas G, Young S (2005) Development of optimal Lu-177 labeled monoclonal antibody (7E11) constructs for radioimmunotherapy of prostate cancer. J Clin Oncol 23(June 1 Supplement):4765

55. Ezziddin S, Attassi M, Guhlke S, Ezziddin K, Palmedo H, Reichmann K, Ahmadzadehfar H, Biermann K, Krenning E, Biersack HJ (2007) Targeted radiotherapy of neuroendocrine tumors using Lu-177-DOTA octreotate with prolonged intervals. J Nucl Med 48(Suppl 2):394

Technetium-99m Radiopharmaceuticals

3

Tamer B. Saleh

Contents

Technetium-99m is a transient metal, exists in many oxidation states, and can combine with a variety of electron-rich compounds. ^{99m}Tc-labeled radiopharmaceuticals are partners of 85% of all nuclear medicine procedures because of the unique properties of ^{99m}Tc, which is considered ideal for the following reasons:

1. It is a gamma emitter with an ideal energy of 140 keV for scintigraphy.
2. The half-life of 6.02 h is suitable for preparations and clinical applications.
3. Radiation burden to the patient is considerably reduced because of the absence of particulate radiation and short half-life.
4. When labeled with a specific chemical substrate, the labeled radiopharmaceutical provides a high ratio of target to nontarget.
5. It is readily available through a weekly delivery of ^{99}Mo-^{99m}Tc generators.
6. Quality control of its radiopharmaceuticals can be achieved rapidly and by routinely available tools in any nuclear medicine department [1].

3.1 Technetium Chemistry

3.1.1 Technetium-99m

The name *technetium* was derived by the scientist Mendeleyev from the Greek word *technetos*, meaning "artificial." Technetium-99m was discovered in 1937 by Perrier and Segre in a sample of naturally occurring ^{98}Mo irradiated by neutrons and deuterons. The first generator as a source for Tc-99m was introduced in 1957 at the *Brookhaven National laboratory*, and the first commercially available ^{99}Mo-^{99m}Tc generator was made available in 1965. Use of Tc-99m really revolutionized nuclear medicine procedures, particularly with the modern gamma cameras coupled to advanced electronics and computing systems. This revolution was not completed until 1970, when the stannous ion reduction method of ^{99m}Tc-diethylene-triaminepentaacetate (DTPA) production as an "instant kit" was described, that simple and convenient "shake-and-bake" preparations for a large number of ^{99m}Tc-labeled radiopharmaceuticals were possible.

Technetium can exist in eight oxidation states (i.e., 1− to 7+); the stability of these oxidation states depends on the type of the labeled ligand and the chemical environment. The 7+ and 4+ oxidation states are the most stable. Tc-99 is presented at any ^{99}Mo-^{99m}Tc generator elution due to the decay of Mo^{99} to Tc^{99m}. It represents about 70% of the total technetium concentration in an eluate; however, this percentage may be increased to about 90% for the first eluate and after weekend elutions of generator. Tc-99m and Tc-99 are chemically identical, so they compete for all chemical reactions. In preparations containing only limited Sn^{2+} as a reducing agent (e.g., ^{99m}Tc-HMPAO [hexamethylpropylene amine

T.B. Saleh
King Fahed Specialist Hospital, Dammam, KSA
e-mail: tamirbayomy@yahoo.com

M.M. Khalil (ed.), *Basic Sciences of Nuclear Medicine*, DOI: 10.1007/978-3-540-85962-8_3,
© Springer-Verlag Berlin Heidelberg 2011

oxime] preparation), only freshly prepared Tc-99m elution is used for obtaining maximum labeling yield [2, 3].

3.1.1.1 ^{99m}Tc Reduction

Generator-produced Tc-99m is available in the form of sodium pertechnetate (^{99m}Tc-NaTcO$_4^-$), which has an oxidation state of 7+ for ^{99m}Tc. TcO$_4^-$ has a configuration of a pyramidal tetrahedron with Tc^{7+} at the center and four oxygen atoms at the apex and corners of the pyramid. TcO$_4^-$ is chemically nonreactive and has no ability to label any compound by direct addition; therefore, reduction of Tc^{7+} to a lower oxidation state is required. The reduction process is obtained using a number of reducing agents (e.g., stannous chloride, stannous citrate, stannous tartarate, etc.), with stannous chloride preferred [4].

The TcO$_4^-$/stannous chloride (SnCl$_2$.2H$_2$O) reduction method is described as follows:

$$3\ Sn^{2+} - 6e \rightarrow 3Sn^{4+}$$
$$2TcO_{4^-} + 16H^+ + 6e \rightarrow 2\ TcO_{4^-} + 8H_2O$$
$$\text{Overall, } 3\ Sn^{2+} + 2\ TcO_{4^-} + 16H^+ \rightarrow 3Sn4^+$$
$$+2\ TcO_{4^-} + 8H_2O$$

Since the amount of ^{99m}Tc in the ^{99m}Tc eluant is very small, only a little Sn^{2+} is required for reduction. However, a 10^6:1 ratio of Sn^{2+} ions to ^{99m}Tc atoms is applied for all ^{99m}Tc-labeled radiopharmaceutical kits to ensure complete reduction of all ^{99m}Tc atoms.

The Tc^{4+} is now in the appropriate chemical form to react with an anion like PYP, Pyrophosphate methylene diphosphonate (MDP), or DTPA. The complex formed is known as a *chelate*; the generic equation is shown as follows:

$$Tc^{4+} + \text{chelating agent}^{n-} \rightarrow Tc - \text{chelate}$$

For example,

$$Tc^{4+} + \text{pyrophosphate}^{4-} \rightarrow Tc - \text{pyrophosphate}$$

Generally, for any ^{99m}Tc-labeled preparation, there are three species that may be present:

- Bound ^{99m}Tc-labeled compound, which is the desired product, and its percentage reflects the yield of preparation

- Free pertechnetate (TcO$_4^-$), which has not been reduced by tin or produced by the action of oxygen
- Hydrolyzed technetium that did not react with the chelating agent or that was bound to hydrolyzed Sn^{2+}

3.1.1.2 ^{99m}Tc Reduction Problems

Presence of oxygen: The commercially available ^{99m}Tc labeling kits are flushed with N$_2$ gas to maintain an inert gas atmosphere in it in addition to the implementation of antioxidants (e.g., ascorbic acid). These arrangements are used to prevent the action of oxygen if sneaked into the preparation vial. Oxygen can cause oxidation of the stannous ions present, preventing the reduction to Tc^{7+} and thus increasing the percentage of free TcO$_4^-$ in ^{99m}Tc-labeled radiopharmaceuticals. This problem can also be avoided by using a relatively large quantity of stannous ions.

Further, the high activity of ^{99m}Tc in the presence of oxygen can cause radiolysis of water-producing hydroxyl (OH), alkoxy (RO), and peroxy (RO$_2$) free radicals, which can interact with ^{99m}Tc chelates, producing more TcO$_4^-$ in the preparation [5].

Hydrolysis of reduced technetium and tin: In aqueous solutions, ^{99m}Tc may undergo hydrolysis to form many hydrolyzed species of ^{99m}TcO$_2$ complexes [6]. Hydrolysis competes with the chelation process of the desired compound, reducing the radiopharmaceutical preparation yield. In addition, these compounds can interfere with the diagnostic test when present in relatively high proportion. Hydrolysis of stannous compounds can also occur in aqueous solutions at pH 6–7, producing insoluble colloids that have the ability to bind to the reduced ^{99m}Tc, resulting in a low labeling yield. An acid is added to the kit to change the pH value of the solution and hence prevent hydrolysis of Sn^{2+} ions. Hydrolysis of reduced technetium and Sn^{2+} can be recovered by adding an excess amount of the chelating agent [7].

3.1.1.3 Technitium-99m Labeling Kit Designation

The kit designation is optimized to ensure that the desired ^{99m}Tc-labeled complex is obtained in its higher yield [8]. Several factors influence the preparation process; they are primarily the nature and amounts of reducing agents and ligands, pH, and temperature.

An ideal Tc-99m labeling kit should contain the following:

Ligand: For targeting ^{99m}Tc to its desired location (e.g., DTPA, MDP, 2,6-dimethylphenylcarbamoyl-methyl iminodiacetic acid [HIDA], and macroaggregated albumin [MAA])

Reductant: For reduction of free pertechnetate (TcO_4^-) (e.g., stannous chloride)

Buffer: To provide a suitable pH environment for the formation of a specific ^{99m}Tc-labeled complex

Antioxidant: To prevent reoxidation of the labeled compounds and hence increase the stability of the radiopharmaceutical (e.g., ascorbic acid, gentisic acid, and p-aminobenzoic acid)

Catalyst: Might be a ligand introduced to form an intermediary coordination complex when the formation of the desired complex is slow relative to formation of hydrolyzed-reduced technetium (e.g., DTPA, gluconate, and citrate)

Accelerators: To increase the radiochemical purity and the rate of complex formation

Surfactants (optional): Required to solubilize lipophilic ^{99m}Tc-labeled complexes (methoxyisobutyl isonitrile, MIBI) and particulate preparations (MAA and microspheres)

Inert fillers: To achieve rapid solubilization of the vial content through the control of particle size during the lyophilization process

3.1.2 Technetium and Technetium-Labeled Compounds

3.1.2.1 ^{99m}Tc-Sodium Pertechnetate

^{99m}Tc-sodium pertechnetate (TcO_4^-) is eluted from the ^{99m}Tc-^{99}Mo generator with sterile isotonic saline. Aseptic conditions should be maintained during the elution and dispensing processes, and the resultant ^{99m}Tc activity concentration depends on the elution volume [9]. Figure 3.1 shows the pertechnetate anion.

^{99m}Tc-sodium pertechnetate is used clinically in the following applications:

- Labeling with different chemical ligands to form ^{99m}Tc-labeled complexes

Fig. 3.1 Pertechnetate anion

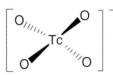

- Thyroid scintigraphy
- Salivary gland scintigraphy
- Lachrymal duct scintigraphy
- Meckle's diverticulum scintigraphy

In blood, 70–80% of ^{99m}Tc-pertechnetate is bound to proteins. The unbound fraction is preferentially concentrated in the thyroid gland and other related structures, such as salivary glands, gastric mucosa, choroid plexus, and mammary tissue. ^{99m}Tc-pertechnetate is excreted mainly by the kidneys, but other pathways may be relevant in certain circumstances, such as saliva, sweat, gastric juice, milk, etc [10]. Lactating women secrete 10% of pertechnetate in milk. Pertechnetate can also cross the placental barrier [11].

3.1.2.2 ^{99m}Tc-Labeled Skeletal Imaging Agents

Since phosphonate and phosphate compounds are localized with high concentrations to bony structures, phosphate derivatives were initially labeled with ^{99m}Tc for skeletal imaging in 1972. However, phosphonate compounds are preferable because they are more stable in vivo than phosphate compounds due to the week P–O–P bond of phosphates, which can be easily broken down by phosphatase enzymes, whereas the P–C–P bond in diphosphonate is not affected [12] (Fig. 3.2).

Three commonly used diphosphonate compounds are MDP, hydroxymethylene diphosphonate (HDP), and 1-hydroxyethylidene diphosphonate (HEDP). The first two are shown in Fig. 3.3. ^{99m}Tc-diphosphonate agents are weak chelates and tend to degrade with time in the presence of oxygen and free radicals. Excess tin in the labeling kit can prevent these oxidative reactions while maintaining the optimal value of the tin/chelating agent ratio to avoid the presence of undesired ^{99m}Tc-Sn-colloid.

^{99m}Tc-diphosphonate complexes are used for multipurpose bone imaging, whereas ^{99m}Tc-pyrophosphate

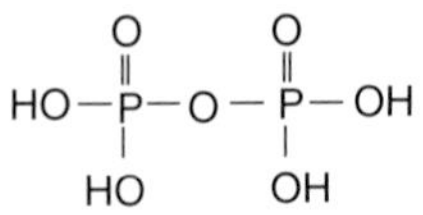

Fig. 3.2 Diphosphonic acid

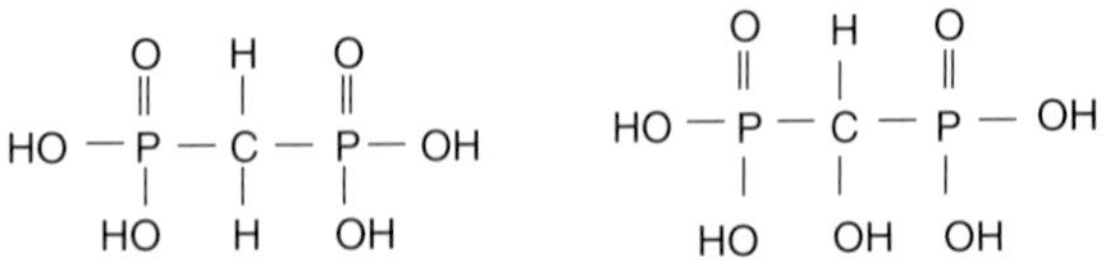

$$HO-\overset{\overset{\displaystyle O}{\|}}{\underset{\underset{\displaystyle HO}{|}}{P}}-O-\overset{\overset{\displaystyle O}{\|}}{\underset{\underset{\displaystyle OH}{|}}{P}}-OH$$

Diphosphoric acid

$$HO-\overset{\overset{\displaystyle O}{\|}}{\underset{\underset{\displaystyle HO}{|}}{P}}-\overset{\overset{\displaystyle H}{|}}{\underset{\underset{\displaystyle H}{|}}{C}}-\overset{\overset{\displaystyle O}{\|}}{\underset{\underset{\displaystyle OH}{|}}{P}}-OH$$

Methlene
diphosphonic acid

$$HO-\overset{\overset{\displaystyle O}{\|}}{\underset{\underset{\displaystyle HO}{|}}{P}}-\overset{\overset{\displaystyle H}{|}}{\underset{\underset{\displaystyle OH}{|}}{C}}-\overset{\overset{\displaystyle O}{\|}}{\underset{\underset{\displaystyle OH}{|}}{P}}-OH$$

Hydroxymethylene
diphosphonic acid

Fig. 3.3 MDP and HDP

compounds are used in red blood cell (RBC) labeling for gated blood pool and gastrointestinal tract (GIT) bleeding procedures.

Many mechanisms of tracer uptake by the skeleton have been proposed, and many factors play a role. The most common and applicable principle states that the calcium and phosphate on mature bone are presented as hydroxyapatite (HAB; sheets of calcium and hydroxyl ions with phosphate bridges linking them), which constructs any bony structure. In immature HAB, in which the calcium-to-phosphorus molar ratio is low, phosphate groups of the tracer can be obtained in this reactive new bone formulation phase. This idea has been evidenced by the higher uptake of these tracers in the joint and active areas of bone formulation in children. It is not well known if the technetium molecule can liberate itself from this bony structure or if it remains [13].

About 40–50% of ^{99m}Tc-HDPs accumulate in the skeleton following intravenous injection, while the rest is excreted mostly with urine.

Maximum bone accumulation occurs after 1 h and remains constant for 72 h. Cumulative activity excretion percentage varies according to the diphosphonate agent; however, it has been observed that about 75–80% of the activity is excreted through urine in the first 24 h.

^{99m}Tc-MDP, ^{99m}Tc-HDP, and ^{99m}Tc-HEDP have almost the same diagnostic efficiency, especially in detection of bone metastasis, trauma, infection, and vascular and metabolic diseases [14, 15].

3.1.2.3 ^{99m}Tc-Labeled Renal Imaging Agents

Diethylenetriaminepentaacetate (DTPA)

DTPA is produced commercially as a pentasodium or calcium salts in the presence of an appropriate amount of stannous chloride for reduction of the added free technetium [16]. The structural formula is shown in Fig. 3.4. The exact oxidation state of the ^{99m}Tc-DTPA complex is not known, although several valency states have been suggested (III–V).

The ^{99m}Tc-DTPA complex is used successfully in

• Renal studies and glomerular filtration rate (GFR) determination
• Cerebral scintigraphy when a blood-brain barrier (BBB) leak is expected
• Lung ventilation studies when used as an aerosol
• Localization of inflammatory bowel disease

The ^{99m}Tc-DTPA complex should undergo extensive quality control testing when used for GFR determination and pyrogenicity testing when used as a cerebral imaging agent since the brain is sensitive to pyrogens. After intravenous injection, ^{99m}Tc-DTPA penetrates the capillary walls to enter the extravascular space within 4 min. Because of its hydrophilicity and negative charge, it is eliminated from cells to the extracellular space. ^{99m}Tc-DTPA is removed from the circulation exclusively by the kidneys. ^{99m}Tc-DTPA cannot pass through the BBB unless there is a structural defect that permits diffusion of the tracer and hence is used for detection of vascular and neoplastic brain lesions. As an aerosol, diffusion of 0.5-μm diameter particles is to the lung periphery and alveolar retention, whereas larger particles (≥1 μm) tend to diffuse to the trachea and upper bronchial tree [17].

Dimercaptosuccinic Acid (DMSA)

The kit contains an isomeric mixture of dimercaptosuccinic acid (DMSA) as a mesoisomer (>90%) in addition to D- and L-isomers (<10%). The structural formula of DMSA is shown in Fig. 3.5. Precaution should be taken with The ^{99m}Tc-DMSA labeling procedure because of the high sensitivity of the formulated complex to oxygen and light. In an acidic medium, the ^{99m}Tc(III)-DMSA complex (renal agent)

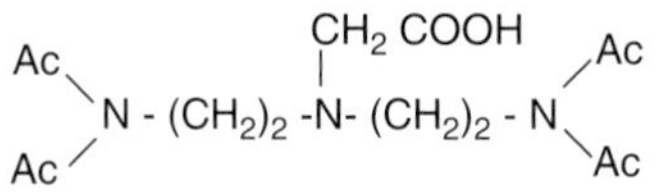

Fig. 3.4 Pentetate

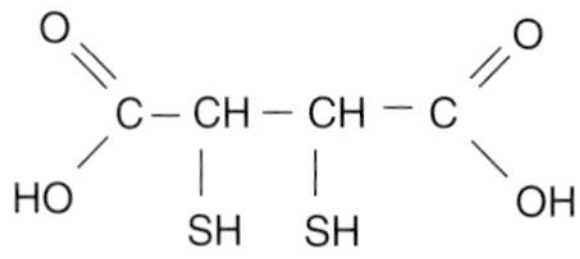

Fig. 3.5 Dimercaptosuccinic acid

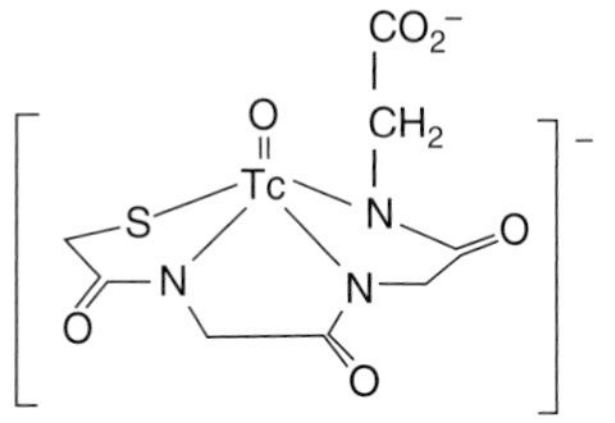

Fig. 3.6 ^{99m}Tc(V)-MAG$_3$ (mercaptoacetyltriglycine) complex

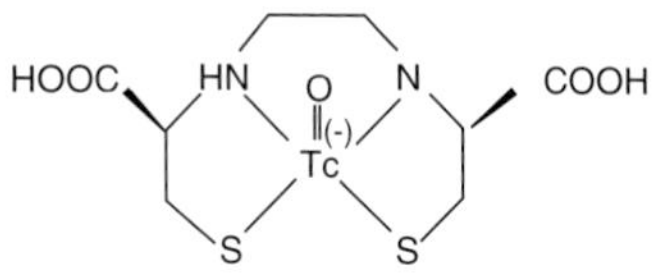

Tc(V)oxo-L,L-EC

Fig. 3.7 Tc-99m-labeled ethylene dicysteine

is formed with high yield (95%). On the other hand, with elevated pH up to 7.5–8.0, the pentavalent ^{99m}Tc (V)-DMSA complex is produced.

After intravenous injection, the ^{99m}Tc(III)-DMSA complex is taken up in the renal parenchyma [18]. After 1 h, approximately 25% of the injected dose is found in the proximal tubules, 30% in the plasma, and 10% in the urine. The main uses of ^{99m}Tc-DMSA are to diagnose renal infection in children and in morphological studies of the renal cortex. Pentavalent ^{99m}Tc (V)-DMSA is used to detect medullary thyroid cancer cells and their soft tissue and bone metastases [19].

Mercaptoacetyltriglycine (DMSA)

The ^{99m}Tc-labeled mercaptoacetyltriglycine (MAG$_3$), ^{99m}Tc-MAG$_3$ (^{99m}Tc-Mertiatide) (Fig. 3.6), is the radiopharmaceutical of choice for renal tubular function assessment, particularly in renal transplants, replacing ^{123}I- and ^{131}I-hippuran (orthoiodohippurate, OIH) because of the unique characteristics of ^{99m}Tc for diagnostic purposes.

^{99m}Tc-Mertiatide is obtained by adding ^{99m}TcO$_4$ to the kit vial and heating in a water bath (100°C for 10 min) followed by cooling for 15 min [20, 21]. Heating is required because at room temperature, formation of the ^{99m}Tc-MAG$_3$ is slow (52% in 2 h).

Generally, labeling should be performed with the highest possible specific concentration, although there are two recommended methods:

1. Use 3 ml of fresh eluate with an activity up to 30 mCi and dilute to 10 ml, then add ^{99m}TcO$_4$ to the vial and heat for 10 min in a water bath. The 10 ml of complex volume is stable for 4 h.

2. Use 1 ml fresh eluate with maximum activity of 25 mCi and dilute to 4 ml to obtain a higher activity concentration. A complex stable for only 1 h will be obtained.

After intravenous injection, ^{99m}Tc-MAG$_3$ is rapidly distributed in the extracellular fluid and excreted by the renal system. The maximum renal accumulation occurs after 3–4 min injection. ^{99m}Tc-MAG$_3$ is used to evaluate renal dynamic function in obstructive uropathy, renovascular hypertension, and complications of transplant. It is also used to evaluate renal function as a presurgical assessment for donors admitted for kidney transplant [22].

Ethylene Dicysteine (EC)

The ethylene dicysteine (EC) kit consists of three vials: A, B, and C. The labeling procedure is achieved by adding ^{99m}TcO$_4$ to vial A containing the EC active ingredient. Then, the dissolved contents of vial B (stannous chloride as a reducing agent) are added to vial A to react for 15 min. Finally, the contents of vial C (ascorbic acid in a buffer solution as a stabilizer) are dissolved and injected in vial A [23].

The ^{99m}Tc-EC complex (Fig. 3.7) has been used successfully since 1992 as a renal agent for the determination of the tubular extraction rate and examination of renal function in patients with transplanted kidneys, but it is not widely used because of its long and complicated preparation procedure in comparison to MAG$_3$. It has similar clinical applications as MAG$_3$ [24].

Many other radiopharmaceuticals have been introduced for renal scan purposes, as ^{99m}Tc-p-aminohippuric acid (^{99m}Tc-PAH) and ^{99m}Tc-DACH, diaminocyclohexane but they have possessed inferior diagnostic and biokinetic features [25].

3.1.2.4 ^{99m}Tc-Labeled Myocardial Perfusion Agents

Methoxyisobutyl Isonitrile

^{99m}Tc-sestamibi was introduced initially under the brand name Cardiolite as a technetium-based radiopharmaceutical to replace Tl-201 in myocardial perfusion imaging.

The Cardiolite kit contains a lyophilized mixture of the MIBI chelating agent in the form of copper salt to facilitate labeling with ligand exchange at elevated temperature [26].

Labeling is achieved by addition of 1–3 ml of ^{99m}Tc-pertechnetate (25–150 mCi) to the reaction vial and shaking vigorously. Figure 3.8 shows the Tc-99m-labeled sestamibi complex. As with all other types of preparations that need heat, vial pressure normalization is essential in ^{99m}Tc-sestamibi preparation procedures. Heating in a water bath (100°C for 10 min) or in a microwave oven for 10 s is required to complete the formulation procedure [27].

^{99m}Tc-sestamibi is used for

1. Myocardial perfusion studies; diagnosis of ischemic heart disease, diagnosis and localization of myocardial infarctions, and assessment of global ventricular function
2. Diagnosis of parathyroid hyperfunctioning adenoma
3. Tumor (breast, bone and soft tissue, lymphoma, and brain) imaging

^{99m}Tc-sestamibi accumulates in the viable myocardial tissue according to blood flow like thallous chloride but is not dependent on the functional capability of the Na/K pump. Elimination of the complex from blood is fast, and the hepatobiliary tract is the main clearance pathway of the complex [28].

Tc-99m-Labeled Tetrofosmin

With the brand name Myoview, tetrofosmin was introduced as a myocardial imaging agent with the advantage that heating is not required. The ^{99m}Tc-tetrofosmin complex (Fig. 3.9) is formulated by adding up to 240 mCi of free technetium in a 4- to 8-ml volume with a specific concentration not greater than 30 mCi/ml to the reaction vial and shaking gently. Although the complex formation could be enhanced by heating, it is formed rapidly at room temperature in high yield. Tetrofosmin is sensitive to the preparation variables, especially the age of the eluate (less than 6 h) and the time interval from the last elution [29]. ^{99m}Tc-tetrofosmin is used in the diagnosis of myocardial perfusion abnormalities in patients with coronary artery

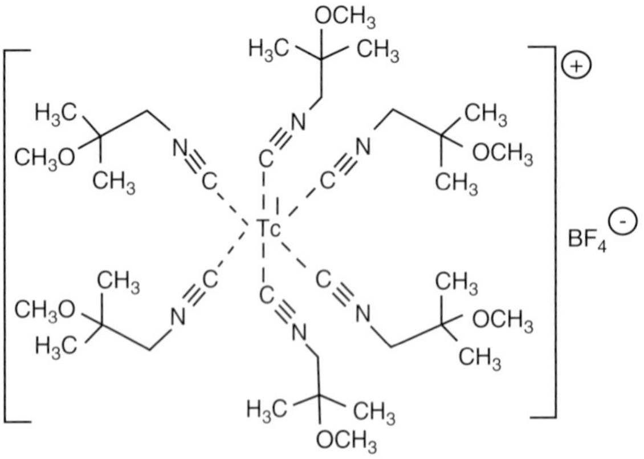

Fig. 3.8 ^{99m}Tc(I) sestamibi complex

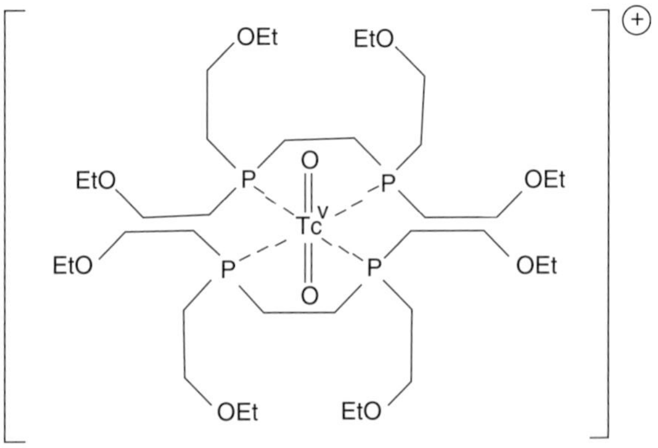

Fig. 3.9 ^{99m}Tc(V)-tetrofosmin complex

disease [30–32]. ^{99m}Tc-tetrofosmin is diffused to the viable myocardial tissue proportional to blood flow. After 5 min of intravenous injection, myocardial uptake is 1.2% at rest and 1.3% during stress and remains constant for at least 4 h. Elimination from blood is fast, and the major pathway of tetrofosmin clearance is the hepatobiliary tract.

3.1.2.5 ^{99m}Tc-Labeled Brain Perfusion Agents

Hexamethylpropylene Amine Oxime (HMPAO)

Use of ^{99m}Tc-HMPAO (exametazime) (Fig. 3.10) as a brain perfusion agent is based on its ability to cross the BBB as a lipophilic complex. The complex is obtained by adding up to 30 mCi of ^{99m}TcO$_4$ to the reaction vial and inverting gently for 10 s. The ^{99m}Tc-HMPAO complex (primary complex) is initially unstable and tends with time to convert to a less-lipophilic form (secondary complex) that has less ability to cross the BBB [33]. Hence, it should be used within 30 min postpreparation after labeling to obtain radiochemical purity more than 85%. Instability of the complex has been attributed to the following three main factors:

1. High (9–9.8) pH
2. Radiolysis by hydroxy free radicals
3. Excess stannous ions

Stabilization of the ^{99m}Tc-HMPAO primary complex for up to 6 h could be achieved by adding stabilizers like methylene blue in phosphate buffer or cobalt (II)-Chloride to the reaction vials [34].

As mentioned, ^{99m}Tc-HMPAO is primarily used in brain perfusion imaging, although it is used for leukocyte labeling substituting ^{111}In-oxine. Methylene blue and phosphate buffer should not be used when the complex formulation is designed for labeling of leukocytes.

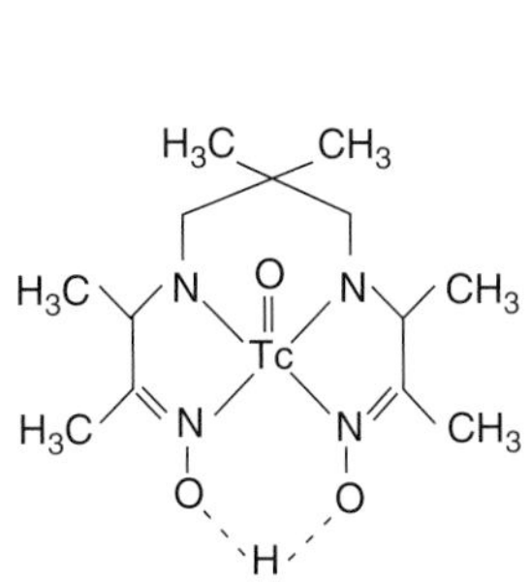

Neutral lipophilic molecules may cross the BBB by diffusion or active transport depending on the molecular size and structural configuration. The lipophilic ^{99m}Tc-HMPAO complex can cross the BBB and be extracted from blood with high efficiency. Cerebral extraction is about 5% of the total injected radioactivity. In vivo, the primary complex decomposes rapidly to a charged, less-lipophilic complex and then is trapped in the brain [35, 36].

After injection, 50% of the radioactivity is eliminated from blood within 2–3 min. After 5 min when the lipophilic complex has disappeared from blood and brain, the persisting image of the brain due to the trapped activity will be stable for 24 h.

Ethyl Cysteinate Dimer (ECD)

Ethyl cysteinate dimer (ECD) is also called Neurolite and contains two vials, A and B. The ^{99m}Tc-ECD (bicisate) complex (Fig. 3.11) is obtained as follows:

1. Add 3 ml saline to vial A, which contains the active ingredients, and then invert the vial to dissolve the kit contents.
2. Add 2 ml of ^{99m}TcO$_4$ (25–100 mCi) aseptically to vial B, which contains 1 ml phosphate buffer.
3. Withdraw 1 ml of vial A contents, add to vial B, and allow the reaction to take place for 30 min at room temperature. The produced ^{99m}Tc-bicisate complex shows high in vitro stability.

^{99m}Tc-ECD is indicated for brain scintigraphy for diagnosis of acute cerebral ischemia, epilepsy, head trauma, and dementia [37]. After intravenous injection, ^{99m}Tc-ECD is distributed in the normal brain proportional to blood flow. The lipophilic complex crosses the BBB with a percentage of 6.5% of the total injected activity after 5 min. After 1 h, less than 5% of the radioactivity is present, mainly as the non-lipophilic complex. Excretion of ^{99m}Tc-ECD from the body is primarily by the kidneys, approximately 50% during the first 2 h [38].

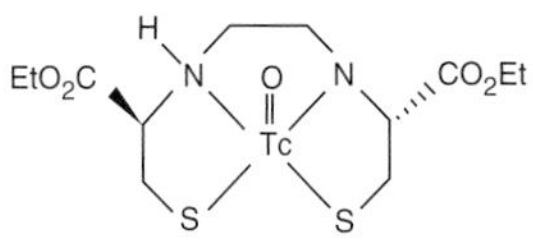

Fig. 3.10 ^{99m}Tc(V)-D,L-HMPAO (hexamethylpropylene amine oxime) complex

Fig. 3.11 ^{99m}Tc(V)O-L,L-ECD (ethyl cysteinate dimer)

3.1.2.6 ^{99m}Tc-Labeled Hepatobiliary Agents

Iminodiacetic Acid Derivatives (IDA)

Since the first iminodiacetic acid (IDA) derivative, HIDA, was developed, several N-substituted IDA derivatives have been prepared: 2,6-diethyl (DIDA or etilfenin), paraisopropyl (PIPIDA or iprofenin), para-butyl (BIDA or butilfenin), diisopropyl (DISIDA or disofenin), and bromotrimethyl (mebrofenin) (Fig. 3.12) [39].

^{99m}Tc-IDA complexes are formed by mixing 1–5 ml of ^{99m}TcO$_4$ (8–40 mCi) with the vial contents and allowing the reaction to be completed in 15 min. ^{99m}Tc-IDA complexes are formed easily with reduced technetium at room temperature. Yield, radiochemical purity, and stability are not affected by the size of the substituents attached to the phenyl ring [40].

^{99m}Tc-IDA derivatives are used to

- Evaluate hepatocyte function
- Rule out or prove acute cholecystitis
- Demonstrate common bile duct partial or complete obstruction
- Verify hepatic bile duct atresia in infants

After intravenous injection, the ^{99m}Tc-IDA complex is bound to the plasma protein (mainly albumin) and carried to the liver; maximum liver uptake is

measured at 10 min. Whole activity is seen in biliary trees and the gall bladder in 15–25 min and in the intestines in 45–60 min. Hepatobiliary excretion of ^{99m}Tc-IDA complexes is governed by molecular size and affected by the type of the substituents attached to the phenyl ring.

3.1.2.7 ^{99m}Tc-Labeled Human Serum Albumin

Human Serum Albumin (HSA)

^{99m}Tc-labeled albumin is a product derived from human serum albumin (HSA), which is a natural constituent of human blood. The labeling of a kit containing HSA and Sn^{+2} is carried out by adding up to 60 mCi of ^{99m}TcO$_4$ in a volume of 1–8 ml to the kit vial; labeling efficiency should be greater than 90%. The contents of the vial should be thoroughly mixed before drawing the patient dosage. The oxidation state of technetium in ^{99m}Tc-HSA is not known but has been postulated to be 5$^+$ [41]. ^{99m}Tc-HSA is used for cardiac blood pool imaging and first-pass and gated equilibrium ventriculography [42].

Macroaggregated Human Serum Albumin

MAA is obtained by aggregation of HSA at acidic pH. The number of particles varies from 1 to 12 million particles per milligram of aggregated albumin. The shape of the particles is irregular, and the size ranges between 10 and 90 μm, with no particles larger than 150 μm.

Preparation of ^{99m}Tc-MAA is carried out by adding 2–10 ml of ^{99m}Tc-pertechnetate with activity up to 100 mCi aseptically to the reaction vial; the complete reaction time is from 5 to 20 min. Prior to injection and dosage administration, the contents of the vial should be agitated gently to make a homogeneous suspension. Similarly, the contents of the syringe also should be thoroughly mixed before administration [43].

Following intravenous injection, more than 90% of the ^{99m}Tc-MAA is localized in lung capillaries and arterioles. Organ selectivity is directly related to particle size, small particles (<8 μm) pass the capillaries and retained in the reticuloendothelial system while relatively larger particles (>15 μm) accumulate in the lung capillaries [44]. ^{99m}Tc-MAA is the

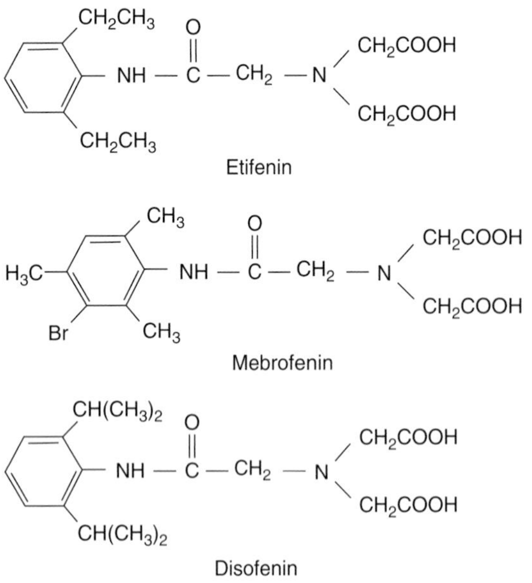

Fig. 3.12 Iminodiacetic derivatives

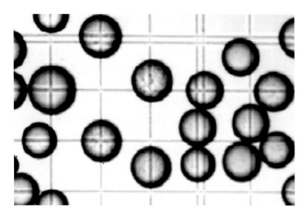

Fig. 3.13 Albumin microspheres (40 μm) (small square 50 × 50 μm, 150 fold), From [7] with permission from Springer+Business Media.

radiopharmaceutical of choice for lung perfusion scan with ventilation scan to exclude pulmonary embolism. In addition it is also used for radionuclide venography for detection of deep vein thrombosis (DVT).

Human Serum Albumin Microspheres (HSAM)

Human serum albumin microspheres (HSAM; Fig. 3.13) are produced by heat denaturation of HSA in vegetable oil [45]. A particle size between 12 and 45 μm is regularly obtained from the commercial kit. The commercial kit may contain 10 mg of microspheres, corresponding to 800,000–1,600,000 microspheres per vial. Complex preparation is obtained when 5–150 mCi of ^{99m}Tc-pertechnetate in 2–10 ml is added to the reaction vial followed by labeling time at room temperature for 15 min. Clinically, ^{99m}Tc-HSAM is used for pulmonary perfusion scintigraphy and determination of right-to-left shunts [46].

3.1.2.8 ^{99m}Tc-Labeled Colloids

Sulfur Colloid (SC)

^{99m}Tc-sulfur colloid (SC) complex is obtained by mixing ^{99m}TcO$_4$ and the kit contents of sodium thiosulfate in an acidic medium and then heating at 95-100°C in a water bath for 5–10 min. The pH of the mixture is adjusted from 6 to 7 with a suitable buffer. Kits of ^{99m}Tc-SC available from commercial manufacturers,

in addition to the basic ingredients of thiosulfate and an acid, may contain gelatin as a protective colloid and ethylenediaminetetraacetic acid (EDTA) to remove by chelation any aluminum ion present in the $_{99m}$Tc-eluate [47]. The particle size ranges from 0.1 to 1 μm, with a mean size of 0.3 μm, and the size distribution can vary from preparation to preparation and from kit to kit.

The ^{99m}Tc-SC complex formation procedure is a two-step procedure:

Step 1: The acid reacts with sodium thiosulfate in the presence of ^{99m}TcO$_4$ and forms colloidal ^{99m}Tc$_2$S$_7$:

$$2Na^{99m}TcO_4 + 7Na_2S_2O_3 + 2HCl \rightarrow {}^{99m}Tc_2S_7 + 7Na_2SO_4 + H_2O + 2NaCl$$

Step 2: Colloidal sulfur is precipitated as

$$Na_2S_2O_3 + 2HCl \rightarrow H_2SO_3 + S + 2NaCl$$

Certain precautions should be taken to eliminate large colloidal particles and to avoid usage of ^{99m}Tc-pertechnetate with eluate containing an alumina concentration above 10 μg aluminum/ml [48].

^{99m}Tc-SC may be useful for the following diagnostic applications:

- Determination of GIT bleeding sites
- Gastric-emptying scan
- Bone marrow imaging
- Liver-spleen scintigraphy

Tin Colloid (TC)

^{99m}Tc-tin colloid (TC) is now considered the agent of choice for liver-spleen scintigraphy since it does not need special labeling conditions (heating or pH adjustment). The complex is formed simply by adding up to 100 mCi of ^{99m}Tc-pertechnetate to the reaction vial. Labeling occurs with high efficiency after 20 min at room temperature. ^{99m}Tc-tin colloid shows a particle size distribution between 0.2 and 0.8 μm [49]. Biodistribution of colloids is typically dependent on the particle size. With a particle size of 0.3–0.6 μm, 80–90% of the radioactivity accumulates in the liver, with 5–10% in the spleen and 5–9% in the bone marrow [50]. Larger particles tend to localize in the spleen and smaller ones in the bone marrow. Colloids are rapidly removed from blood by phagocytosis, mainly in the liver. It has similar application as those of sulfur colloid and is more commonly used because of its easier preparation, which avoids the need for boiling.

Albumin Nanocolloid

The commercial nanocolloid kit contains the HSA colloid and stannous dihydrate and is characterized by small size particles (almost 95% of the particles are less than 0.08 mm with a mean size of 0.03 mm). Complex labeling is obtained when proper $^{99m}TcO_4$ activity (up to 150 mCi) in a small volume is added aseptically to the vial and the reaction is continued for 10 min at room temperature [51]. Because of the smaller size of the particles, more nanocolloid localizes in the bone marrow ($\approx$15%) relative to ^{99m}Tc-SC (2–5%).

^{99m}Tc-albumin nanocolloid is used in

- Sentinel lymph node (SLN) scintigraphy [52]
- Lymphoscintigraphy
- Bone marrow scintigraphy
- Inflammation scintigraphy

Biodistribution of ^{99m}Tc-albumin nanocolloid was discussed in regard to a small size colloidal particle.

3.1.2.9 ^{99m}Tc-Labeled Monoclonal Antibodies

Arcitumomab (CEA Scan)

Carcinoembryonic antigen (CEA) (CEA Scan kit introduced by Mallinckrodt Medical) as a single-dosage kit contains the active ingredient Fab$^-$ fragment of arcitumomab, a murine monoclonal antibody IMMU-4. ^{99m}Tc-CEA labeling is carried out by adding 1 ml of ^{99m}TcO$_4$ (20–30 mCi) to the reaction vial and incubating the mixture for 5 min at room temperature. The labeling yield should be more than 90%. The complex is stable for 4 h after labeling. CEA is expressed in a variety of carcinomas, particularly of the GIT, and can be detected in the serum. IMMU-4 is specific for the classical 200,000-Da CEA, which is found predominantly on the cell membrane. ^{99m}Tc-CEA Scan complexes the circulating CEA and binds to CEA on the cell surface. The Fab$^-$ fragment of arcitumomab is

cleared rapidly by the urinary tract and plasma clearance due to its small particle size [53].

The IMMU-4 antibody is targeted against the CEAs of colorectal tumors; therefore, ^{99m}Tc-CEA Scan is used for the detection of recurrence or metastatic carcinomas of the colon or rectum, particularly when high levels of CEA are detected [54]. However, it is an uncommon procedure following positron emission tomographic/computed tomographic (PET/CT) scan.

Sulesomab (LeukoScan)

The kit vial for LeukoScan contains the active ingredient Fab$^-$ fragment, called sulesomab, obtained from the murine monoclonal antigranulocyte antibody IMMU-MN3. It is a single-dose kit introduced by Immunomedics Europe in 1997. Labeling is carried out by adding 0.5 ml of isotonic saline and swirling the content for 30 s; immediately after dissolution, 1 ml of ^{99m}TcO$_4$, corresponding to an activity of 30 mCi, is added to the vial. The reaction is allowed for 10 min, and the labeling yield should be more than 90%. After intravenous injection, elimination of ^{99m}Tc-LeukoScan from the blood is indicated by 34% of the baseline activity after 1 h. The route of excretion is essentially renal, with 41% of the activity excreted in urine over the first 24 h [55]. ^{99m}Tc-sulesomab targets the granulocytes and therefore is primarily used to detect infection and inflammation, particularly in patients with osteomyelitis, joint infection involving implants, inflammatory bowel disease, and foot ulcers of diabetics [56].

3.1.2.10 ^{99m}Tc-Labeled Peptides and proteins

Depreotide (NeoSpect)

The depreotide (NeoSpect) kit vial contains a lyophilized mixture of depreotide, sodium glucoheptonate, stannous chloride, and sodium EDTA. Labeling of the depreotide (cyclic decapeptide) with ^{99m}Tc is performed by ligand exchange of intermediary ^{99m}Tc-glucoheptonate. The ^{99m}Tc-NeoSpect complex is obtained by aseptically adding up to 50 mCi ^{99m}Tc-pertechnetate in a volume of 1 ml to the vial. After normalizing the pressure, the vial should be agitated carefully for 10 s and then placed in a water bath for

10 min; when the labeling procedure is completed, the vial should be left for cooling at room temperature for 15 min (running water should not be used for cooling) [57]. Depreotide is a synthetic peptide that binds with high affinity to somatostatin receptors (SSTRs) in normal as well as abnormal tissues. This agent is used to detect SSTR-bearing pulmonary masses in patients proven or suspected to have pulmonary lesions by CT or chest x-ray. Negative results with ^{99m}Tc-depreotide can exclude regional lymph node metastasis with a high degree of probability [58].

Some reports showed that ^{99m}Tc-depreotide was accumulated in pulmonary nodules 1.5–2 h following the intravenous injection [58, 59]. ^{99m}Tc-depreotide can be also seen in the spine, sternum, and rib ends [60]. The main route of elimination of the compound is the renal system. This is an uncommon procedure when PET/CT is available that can show lesions as small as 5 mm.

Apcitide (AcuTect)

[99m]Tc-apcitide was introduced under the brand name of AcuTect as a single-dosage kit. The kit vial contains bibapcitide, which consists of two apcitide monomers, stannous chloride and sodium glucoheptonate. Labeling is performed by adding up to 50 mCi of [99m]TcO_4 to the kit vial and heating for 15 min in a boiling water bath. The labeling yield should be greater than 90%. ^{99m}Tc-apticide binds to the GP glycoprotein IIb/IIIa receptors on activated platelets that are responsible for aggregation in forming the thrombi and therefore is used for the detection of acute DVT in lower extremities [40].

Annexin V (Apomate)

Annexin V (Apomate) is a human protein with a molecular weight of 36 kDa, has a high affinity for cell membranes with bound phosphatidyl serine (PS) [61]. In vitro assays have been developed that use annexin V to detect apoptosis in hematopoietic cells, neurons, fibroblasts, endothelial cells, smooth muscle cells, carcinomas, and lymphomas. ^{99m}Tc-annexin V has also been suggested as an imaging agent to detect thrombi in vivo because activated platelets express large amounts of PS on their surface [62]. The radiopharmaceutical is prepared by adding about 1,000 MBq ^{99m}Tc-pertechnetate to 1 mg freeze-dried (n-1-imino-4-mercaptobutyl)-annexin V (Mallinckrodt, Petten, The Netherlands). This mixture is incubated for 2 h at room temperature [63].

[99m]Tc-Annexin strongly accumulates, with a biological half-life of 62 h, in the kidneys (21%) and the liver (12.8%) after 4 h of injection. Accumulation in myocardium and colon is limited, and excretion is obtained exclusively by urine (75%) and feces (25%) [63].

References

1. Murray IPC, Ell PJ (1998) Nuclear medicine in clinical diagnosis and treatment. Churchill Livingstone, Edinburgh
2. Dewanjee MK (1990) The chemistry of 99mTc-labeled radiopharmaceuticals. Semin Nucl Med 20:5
3. Fleming WK, Jay M, Ryo UY (1990) Reconstitution and fractionation of radiopharmaceutical kits. J Nucl Med 31:127–128
4. Kowalsky RJ, Falen SW (2004) Radiopharmaceuticals in nuclear pharmacy and nuclear medicine, 2nd edn. American Pharmacists Association, Washington
5. Hung JC, Iverson BC, Toulouse KA, Mahoney DW (2002) Effect of methylene blue stabilizer on in vitro viability and chemotaxis of Tc-99m-exametazime-labeled leukocytes. J Nucl Med 43(7):928–932
6. Bogsrud TV, Herold TJ, Mahoney DW, Hung JC (1999) Comparison of three cold kit reconstitution techniques for the reduction of hand radiation dose. Nucl Med Commun 20 (8):761–767
7. Zolle I (2007) Technetium-99m pharmaceuticals. Springer, Berlin
8. Eckelman WC, Steigman J, Paik CH (1996) Radiopharmaceutical chemistry. In: Harpert J, Eckelman WC, Neumann RD (eds) Nuclear medicine: diagnosis and therapy. Thieme Medical, New York, p 213
9. European Pharmacopoeia (Ph. Eur.) ver. (5.0). Council of Europe, Maisonneuve, Sainte-Ruffine, 2005
10. Oldendorf WH, Sisson WB, Lisaka Y (1970) Compartmental redistribution of 99mTc-pertechnetate in the presence of perchlorate ion and its relation to plasma protein binding. J Nucl Med 11:85–88
11. Ahlgren L, Ivarsson S, Johansson L, Mattsson S, Nosslin B (1985) Excretion of radionuclides in human breast milk after administration of radiopharmaceuticals. J Nucl Med 26:1085–1090
12. Tofe AJ, Bevan JA, Fawzi MB, Francis MD, Silberstein EB, Alexander GA, Gunderson DE, Blair K (1980) Gentisic acid: a new stabilizer for low tin skeletal imaging agents: concise communication. J Nucl Med 21:366–370
13. Wilson MA (1998) Textbook on nuclear medicine. Lippincott-Raven, Philadelphia
14. Francis MD, Ferguson DL, Tofe AJ, Bevan JA, Michaels SE (1980) Comparative evaluation of three diphosphonates: in vitro adsorption (C14-labeled) and in vivo osteogenic uptake (Tc-99m complexed). J Nucl Med 21:1185–1189

15. Fogelman I, Pearson DW, Bessent RG, Tofe AJ, Francis MD (1981) A comparison of skeletal uptakes of three diphosphonates by whole-body retention: concise communication. J Nucl Med 22:880–883

16. Carlsen JE, Moller MH, Lund JO, Trap-Jensen J (1988) Comparison of four commercial Tc-99m-(Sn)-DTPA preparations used for the measurement of glomerular filtration rate. J Nucl Med 21:126–129

17. Agnew JE (1991) Characterizing lung aerosol penetration (abstract). J Aerosol Med 4:237–250

18. de Lange MJ, Piers DA, Kosterink JGW, van Luijk WHJ, Meijer S, de Zeeuw D, Van-der Hem GJ (1989) Renal handling of technetium-99m-DMSA: evidence for glomerular filtration and peri-tubular uptake. J Nucl Med 30:1219–1223

19. Ramamoorthy N, Shetye SV, Pandey PM, Mani RS, Patel MC, Patel RB, Ramanathan P, Krishna BA, Sharma SM (1987) Preparation and evaluation of ^{99m}Tc(V)-DMSA complex: studies in medullary carcinoma of thyroid. Eur J Nucl Med 12:623–628

20. Murray T, Mckellar K, Owens J, Watson WS, Hilditch TE, Elliott AT (2000) Tc-99m – MAG3: problems with radiochemical purity testing (letter). Nucl Med Commun 21:71–75

21. Van Hemert FJ, Lenthe H, Schimmel KJM, van Eck-smit BLF (2005) Preparation, radiochemical purity control and stability of Tc-99m mertiatide (Mag-3). Ann Nucl Med 19(4):345–349

22. Oriuchi N, Miymoto K, Hoshino K, Imai J, Takahashi Y, Sakai S, Shimada A, Endo K (1997) Tc-99m-MAG3: a sensitive indicator for evaluating perfusion and rejection of renal transplants. Nucl Med Commun 18:400–404

23. Gupta NK, Bomanji JB, Waddington W, Lui D, Costa DC, Verbruggen AM, Ell PJ (1995) Technetium-99m-1,1-ethylenedicysteine scintigraphy in patients with renal disorders. Eur J Nucl Med 22:617–624

24. Kabasakal L, Turoğlu HT, Onsel C, Ozker K, Uslu I, Atay S, Cansiz T, Sönmezoğlu K, Altiok E, Isitman AT et al (1995) Clinical comparison of technetium-99m-EC, technetium-99m-MAG3 and iodine-131-OIH in renal disorders. J Nucl Med 36:224–228

25. Jaksic E, Artikoa V, Beatovic S, Djokic D, Jankovic D, Saranovic D, Hana R, Obradovic V (2009) Clinical investigations of 99mTc-p-aminohippuric acid as a new renal agent. Nucl Med Commun 30:76–81

26. Cooper M, Duston K, Rotureau L (2006) The effect on radiochemical purity of modifications to the method of preparation and dilution of Tc-99m sestamibi. Nucl Med Commun 27:455–460

27. Varelis P, Parkes SL, Poot MT (1998) The influence of generator eluate on the radiochemical purity of Tc-99m-sestamibi prepared using fractionated Cardiolite kits. Nucl Med Commun 19(7):615–623

28. Millar AM, Murray T (2006) Preparation of Tc-99m sestamibi for parathyroid imaging. Nucl Med Commun 27(5):473

29. Patel M, Owunwanne A, Tuli M, al-Za'abi K, al-Mohannadi S, Sa'ad M, Jahan S, Jacob A, Al-Bunny A (1998) Modified preparation and rapid quality control test for technetium-99m-tetrofosmin. J Nucl Med Technol 26(4):269–273

30. Graham D, Millar AM (1999) Artifacts in the thin-layer chromatographic analysis of Tc-99m-tetrafosmin Injections. Nucl Med Commun 20:439–444

31. Ramírez A, Arroyo T, Díaz-Alarcón JP, García-Mendoza A, Muros MA, Martinez del Valle MD, Rodríguez-Fernández A, Acosta-Gómez MJ, Llamas-Elvira JM (2000) An alternative to the reference method for testing the radiochemical purity of Tc-99m-tetrofosmin. Nucl Med Commun 21(2):199–203

32. Hammes R, Joas LA, Kirschling TE, Ledford JR, Knox TL, Nybo MR et al (2004) A better method of quality control for Tc-99m-tetrafosmin. J Nucl Med Technol 32:72–78

33. Webber DI, Zimmer AM, Geyer MC, Spies SM (1992) Use of a single-strip chromatography system to assess the lipophilic component in technetium-99m exametazime preparations. J Nucl Med Technol 20:29–32

34. Solanki C, LI D, Wong A, Barber R, Wraight E, Sampson C (1994) Stabilization and multidose use of exametazime for cerebral perfusion studies. Nucl Med Commun 15(9):718–722

35. Catafau A (2001) Brain SPECT in clinical practice. Part I: perfusion. J Nucl Med 42:259–271

36. Pi-lien H, Shu-hua H, Chao-ching H, Song-chei H, Ying-chao C (2008) Tc-99m HMPAO brain SPECT imaging in children with acute cerebellar ataxia. Clin Nucl Med 33(12):841–844

37. Dormehl IC, Oliver DW, Langen K-J, Hugo N, Croft SA (1997) Technetium-99m-HMPAO, technetium-99m-ECD and iodine-123-IMP cerebral blood flow measurements with pharmacological interventions in primates. J Nucl Med 38:1897–1901

38. Holman BL, Hellman RS, Goldsmith SJ, Mean IG, Leveille J, Gherardi PG, Moretti JL, Bischof-Dela-loye A, Hill TC, Rigo PM, Van Heertum RL, Ell PJ, Bçll U, DeRoo MC, Morgan RA (1989) Bio-distribution, dosimetry and clinical evaluation of Tc-99m ethyl cysteinate dimer (ECD) in normal subjects and in patients with chronic cerebral infarction. J Nucl Med 30:1018–1024

39. Myron LL, Anthony RB, John DS (1985) Failure of quality control to detect errors in the preparation of Tc-99m disofenin (DISIDA). Clin Nucl Med 10(7):468–474

40. Saha GB (2004) Fundamentals of radiopharmacy, 5th edn. Springer, Berlin

41. Zolle I, Oniciu L, Hofer R (1973) Contribution to the study of the mechanism of labelling human serum albumin (HSA) with technetium-99m. Int J Appl Radiat Isotopes 24:621–626

42. Strauss HW, Zaret BL, Hurley PJ, Natarajan TK, Pitt P (1971) A scintiphotographic method for measuring left ventricular ejection fraction in man without cardiac catheterization. Am J Cardiol 28:575–580

43. Chandra R, Shannon J, Braunstein P, Durlov OL (1973) Clinical evaluation of an instant kit for preparation of 99m Tc-MAA for lung scanning. J Nucl Med 14:702–705

44. Wagner HN, Sabiston DC, Iio M, McAfee JG, Langan JK (1964) Regional pulmonary blood flow in man by radioisotope scanning. JAMA 187:601–603

45. Zolle I, Rhodes BA, Wagner HN Jr (1970) Preparation of metabolizable radioactive human serum albumin microspheres for studies of the circulation. Int J Appl Radiat Isotopes 21:155–167

46. Rhodes BA, Stern HS, Buchanan JW, Zolle I, Wagner HN Jr (1971) Lung scanning with Tc-99m-microspheres (abstract). Radiology 99:613–621

47. Stern HS, McAfee JG, Subramanian G (1966) Preparation, distribution and utilization of technetium-99m-sulfur colloid. J Nucl Med 7:665–675

48. Ponto JA, Swanson DP, Freitas JE (1987) Clinical manifestations of radiopharmaceutical formulation problems. In: Hladik WB III, Saha GB, Study KT (eds) Essentials of nuclear medicine science. Williams & Wilkins, Baltimore, pp 271–274

49. Whateley TL, Steele G (1985) Particle size and surface charge studies of a tin colloid radiopharmaceutical for liver scintigraphy. Eur J Nucl Med 19:353–357

50. Schuind F, Schoutens A, Verhas M, Verschaeren A (1984) Uptake of colloids by bone is dependent on bone blood flow. Eur J Nucl Med 9:461–463

51. SolcoNanocoll Product monograph of the kit for the preparation of Tc-99m nanocolloid, issued by Sorin Biomedica, Italy (1992)

52. Alazraki N, Eshima D, Eshima LA, Herda SC, Murray DR, Vansant JP, Taylor AT (1997) Lymphoscintigraphy, the sentinel node concept, and the intraoperative gamma probe in melanoma, breast cancer and other potential cancers. Semin Nucl Med 27:55–67

53. Immunomedics Europe product monograph for the CEA-Scan (arcitumomab) kit for the preparation of Tc-99m CEA-Scan. Immunomedics Europe, Darmstadt, Germany (2000)

54. Moffat FL Jr, Pinsky CM, Hammershaimb L, Petrelli NJ, Patt YZ, Whaley FS, Goldenberg DM (1996) Immunomedics study group clinical utility of external immunoscintigraphy with the IMMU-4 technetium-99m Fab' antibody fragment in patients undergoing surgery for carcinoma of the colon and rectum: results of a pivotal, phase III trial. J Clin Oncol 14:2295–2305

55. Immunomedics Europe product monograph for LeukoScan (sulesomab). Issued by Immunomedics Europe, Darmstadt, Germany (1997)

56. Gratz S, Schipper ML, Dorner J, Hoffken H, Becker W, Kaiser JW, Behe M, Behr TM (2003) LeukoScan for imaging infection in different clinical settings: a retrospective evaluation and extended review of the literature. Clin Nucl Med 28(4):267–276

57. Berlex laboratories product monograph for the neotect kit for the preparation of Tc-99m depreotide. Berlex Laboratories, Wayne, NJ (2001) (Diatide, NDA No. 21-012)

58. Danielsson R, Bââth M, Svensson L, Forslæv U, Kælbeck K-G (2005) Imaging of regional lymph node metastases with 99m Tc-depreotide in patients with lung cancer. Eur J Nucl Med Mol Imaging 32:925–931

59. Kahn D, Menda Y, Kernstine K, Bushnell DL, McLaughlin K, Miller S, Berbaum K (2004) The utility of 99mTc-depreotide compared with F-18 fluorodeoxyglucose positron emission tomography and surgical staging in patients with suspected non-small cell lung cancer. Chest 125:494–501

60. Menda Y, Kahn D, Bushnell DL, Thomas M, Miller S, McLaughlin K, Kernstine KH (2001) Nonspecific mediastinal uptake of 99m Tc-depreotide (NeoTect). J Nucl Med 42 (Suppl):304P

61. Blankenberg FG, Katsikis PD, Tait JF et al (1999) Imaging of apoptosis (programmed cell death) with ^{99m}Tc annexin V. J Nucl Med 40:184–191

62. Tait JF, Cerqueira MD, Dewhurst TA (1994) Evaluation of annexin V as platelet directed thrombus targeting agent. Thromb Res 75:491–501

63. Kemerink D, Liem IN, Hofstra L, Boersma HH, Buijs W, Reutelingsperger C, Heidendal G (2001) Patient dosimetry of intravenously administered 99mTc-annexin V. J Nucl Med 42:382–387

Radiopharmaceutical Quality Control

4

Tamer B. Saleh

Contents

4.1 Introduction

Like all other drugs intended for human administration, radiopharmaceuticals should undergo strict and routine quality testing procedures in addition to their own specific tests for radionuclidic and radiochemical purity. Radiopharmaceutical quality control tests can be simply classified as *Physiochemical* and *Biological* tests [1–3].

T.B. Saleh
Senior Medical Physicist, RSO, King Fahed Specialist Hospital, Dammam, Kingdom of Saudi Arabia
e-mail: tamirbayomy@yahoo.com

4.2 Physiochemical Tests

4.2.1 Physical Tests

Physical characteristics should be observed for any radiopharmaceutical for the first and frequent use. Color alterations should be identified for both true solution and colloidal preparations. True solutions should also be checked for turbidity and presence of any particulate matter; in colloidal preparations, determination of particle size is of most interest.

4.2.2 pH and Ionic Strength

The administered radiopharmaceutical should have a proper pH (hydrogen ion concentration) with an ideal value of 7.4 (pH of blood), but it can vary between 2 and 9 because of the high buffer capacity of the blood. The pH of any radiopharmaceutical preparation can be measured by a pH meter [4].

Ionic strength, isotonicity, and osmolality should be observed properly in any radiopharmaceutical preparation so it is suitable for human administration.

Note: Since pH and ionic strength are important factors for the stability of a radiopharmaceutical, the preparation diluent is preferred to be the same solvent used in the original preparation.

4.2.3 Radionuclidic Purity

The term *radionuclidic* purity refers to the presence of radionuclides other than the one of interest and is defined as the proportion of the total radioactivity

M.M. Khalil (ed.), *Basic Sciences of Nuclear Medicine*, DOI: 10.1007/978-3-540-85962-8_4,
© Springer-Verlag Berlin Heidelberg 2011

present as the stated radionuclide. Measurement of radionuclide purity requires determination of the identity and amounts of all radionuclides that are present. The radionuclide impurities which, vary according to the method of radionuclide production, can affect dramatically the obtained image quality in addition to the overall patient radiation dose.

Radionuclidic impurities may belong to the same element of the desired radionuclide or to a different element. Examples of radionuclidic impurities are ^{99}Mo in ^{99m}Tc-labeled preparations and iodide isotopes in ^{131}I-labeled preparations [5]. Radionuclidic purity is determined by measuring the half-lives and characteristic radiations emitted by each radionuclide. The γ-emitters can be differentiated by identification of their energies on the spectra obtained by an NaI(Tl) crystal or a lithium-drifted germanium [Ge(Li)] detector coupled to a multichannel analyzer (MCA). The β-emitters can be tested by a β-spectrometer or a liquid scintillation counter. Since a given radiation energy may belong to a number of radionuclides, half-life must be established to identify each radionuclide.

4.2.4 Radiochemical Purity

Radiochemical purity is defined as the proportion of the stated radionuclide that is present in the stated chemical form. Image quality (as a function of the radiopharmaceutical biological distribution) and the radiation absorbed dose are directly related to the radiochemical purity. Radiochemical impurities are produced from decomposition due to the *action of solvent, change in temperature or pH, light, presence of oxidation or reducing agents, and radiolysis.*

Free and hydrolyzed ^{99m}Tc forms in many ^{99m}Tc-labeled preparations; secondary hexamethyl-propylene amine oxime (HMPAO) complex in ^{99m}Tc-HMPAO preparations and free ^{131}I-iodide in ^{131}I-labeled proteins are good examples of the radiochemical impurities [6].

The stability of a compound is time dependent on exposure to light, change in temperature, and radiolysis, and the longer the time of exposure is, the higher the probability of decomposition will be. Sodium ascorbate, ascorbic acid, and sodium sulfite are normally used for maintaining the stability of a radiopharmaceutical. Several analytical methods are used to determine the radiochemical purity of a given radiopharmaceutical, and these methods are discussed next.

4.2.4.1 Thin-Layer Chromatography

Thin-layer chromatography (TLC), which was developed by Hoye in 1967 is considered the most commonly used method for determination of radiochemical purity in nuclear medicine. The main principle of a TLC chromatography system is that a mobile phase (solvent) migrates along a stationary phase (adsorbent) by the action of the capillary forces [7]. Depending on the distribution of components between the stationary and the mobile phases, a radiopharmaceutical sample spotted onto an adsorbent will migrate with different velocities, and thus impurities are separated.

In TLC, each component in a given sample is identified by an R_f value, which is defined as "the ratio of the distance traveled by the sample component to the distance the solvent front has advanced from the original point of starting the chromatography test in the stationary phase."

$$R_f = \text{Distance traveled by the component/distance of the solvent front}$$

The R_f values range from 0 to1. If a component migrates with the solvent front, the R_f is [1], while the R_f for the component remaining at the origin is [0]. R_f values are established with known components and may vary under different experimental conditions. The main principles of separation are adsorption (electrostatic forces), partition (solubility), and ion exchange (charge), and the movement of the mobile phase may take either ascending or descending modes. When the solvent front moves to the desired distance, the strip is removed from the testing container, dried, and measured in an appropriate radiation detection system; histograms are obtained for the activity of all sample components [8].

Stationary Phases

Standard TLC materials: Standard TLC plates are available as glass plates, as plastic or aluminum foils covered with the stationary phase. A wide range of stationary phases are commercially available, including silica gel, reversed-phase silica, aluminum oxide, synthetic resins, and cellulose. The main advantage of standard TLC materials is that they have the ability to provide relatively high-resolution tests, while the relatively long developing time of the mobile phase (mainly >30 min) through the high-particle-size adsorbent material (20 μm) is considered its main disadvantage [9].

High-performance TLC (HPTLC): HPTLC provides a good solution to the long chromatographic developing time by use of materials with a smaller particle size.

Instant TLC (ITLC): ITLC plates are made of fiberglass sheets integrated with an adsorbent, usually silica gel, and can be cut to any size, developing an economic chromatographic solution. Due to the fine mesh material, the migration properties are increased manyfold compared to the standard TLC materials, reducing the chromatographic time to less than 5 min without affecting the separation of radiochemical impurities. Because of the advantages mentioned, ITLC materials are the most frequently used for the stationary phase in nuclear medicine since they fulfill the need for a rapid and accurate method for testing the radiochemical purity of a radiopharmaceutical sample. Silica stationary phases have been produced for ITLC as silica gel (ITLC-SG) and silicic acid (ITLC-SA). ITLC-SG is the most widely used adsorbent for routine radiochemical purity determination [10].

Paper: Papers (e.g., Whatman no. 1 and Whatman 3MM) were commonly used in the early days of chromatography, although they are still used and recommended for many chromatographic procedures.

The main disadvantage of paper chromatography is the poor resolution it provides for radiochemical purity tests; however, Whatman 3MM is the material of choice for partition chromatography procedures.

Aluminum oxide: Aluminum-coated plates are commonly used for separation of some radiopharmaceuticals (e.g., Sesta-MIBI[methoxyisobutyl isonitrile]) depending on the aluminum oxide (Al_2O_3) polar properties.

Cellulose: Cellulose can interact with water and serve as a stationary phase for separation of polar substances by paper chromatography; also, it can be used in the powder form as an adsorbent for TLC.

Mobile Phases

Saline, Water, Acetone, Methyl Ethyl Ketone (MEK), Ethanol, Acetic Acid, Chloroform, and *Acetonitrile* represent the most common group of mobile phases used as the mobile partner in most TLC chromatographic procedures.

4.2.4.2 TLC Chromatography Procedure

To determine the radiochemical purity by ITLC or paper chromatography for a radiopharmaceutical sample, the following steps should be applied [11]:

- Fill a small beaker with about 10 ml (3–5 mm high) with the proper solvent and then cover the beaker with a glass plate or with a foil sheet.
- Prepare the chromatography strip (5–10 cm long) and mark the solvent front ($R_f = 0$) with a colored pen and the start point ($R_f = 1$) with a pencil.
- Using a 1-ml syringe with a fine needle (25 gauge), put one small drop of the sample onto the starting point on the strip.
- Immediately, insert the strip into the beaker so the spot sample does not dry, observing that initially the solvent level is below the starting point.
- When the solvent has reached the front, the strip should be removed and dried.
- Quantify the regional distribution of radioactivity on the strip using any of the radiation detection methods discussed next.

Figure 4.1 shows a sample procedure for determination of radiochemical purity of a radiopharmaceutical by ITLC using two different solvents.

4.2.4.3 Methods for Regional Radioactivity Measurement in TLC Chromatography

Many analytical methods were developed for determination of the radioactivity percentage of the different radiochemical species along the TLC chromatography strip, starting with the *autoradiography* method by which a chromatogram is placed on an x-ray film and exposed in the dark for about 1 h. However, the most popular methods in nuclear medicine were achieved using one of the following systems [9]:

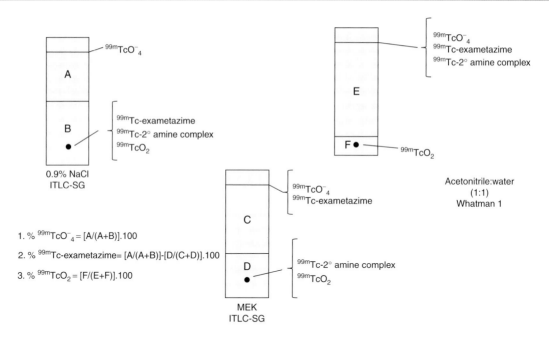

Fig. 4.1 Chromatographic system for determination of radiochemical purity of Tc-99m labeled HMPAO. (Adapted from [7])

- *Gamma camera*: A dried strip is placed close to the detector head of the camera, and an image is obtained. The region of interest (ROI) is drawn for each radioactive area. The radiochemical purity is expressed as a fraction of the total recovered activity.
- *Ionization chamber*: The dried strip is cut into two segments and measured in the chamber. This method is frequently used for simple separation techniques (compounds of $R_f = 0$ or 1) but is not applicable in multisegmental strips or samples with low radioactive concentration [12].
- *NaI(Tl) scintillation counter*: Chromatographic plates are cut in segments (up to ten) and counted in the scintillation counter. This method is preferrede to the ionization chamber because it provides more sensitive results, giving the chance to determine the radiochemical purity of a sample at different and close R_f values.
- *Chromatography scanner*: A slit-collimated radiation detector [mainly NaI(Tl) scintillation counter] is moved along the thin-layer plate, and the radioactivity distribution between the start and the solvent front points is recorded and plotted as radioactive peaks [13]. This method is considered the most accurate one because it provides values with high sensitivity and resolution .

- *Linear analyzer*: This device operates as a position-sensing proportional counter, measuring a fixed number of channels along the length of the chromatographic plate. It gives us the most sensitive results, but resolution is less than that obtained with NaI(Tl) scintillation counters [14].

A comparison of four different methods of quantification is shown in Fig. 4.2, in which a phantom chromatographic plate with increasing amount of radioactivity (0.25, 1.0, 4.0, 16.0, and 64.0 kBq) spotted at exact intervals was measured bythe following:

A:	Linear analyzer
B:	Conventional scanner
C:	Cut-and-measure scintillation counter
D:	Ionization chamber

The highest sensitivity was achieved in A and C, while the best resolution occured with B and C.

The ionization chamber indicated a low detection efficiency of radioactivity below 20 kBq (peaks 1, 2, 3, and 4).

For ^{99m}Tc, the main impurities are the *free pertechnetate* (TcO_4) and the *reduced, hydrolyzed technetium* (TcO_2) (in another words, colloidal ^{99m}Tc).

Fig. 4.2 Phantom chromatography plate analyzed by four different methods of measurement. The highest sensitivity was achieved with a and c, the best resolution with b and c. Using the ionization chamber (d), activities less than 20 kBq (peaks 1, 2, 3, 4) were not resolved accurately. (From [9] with permission from Springer)

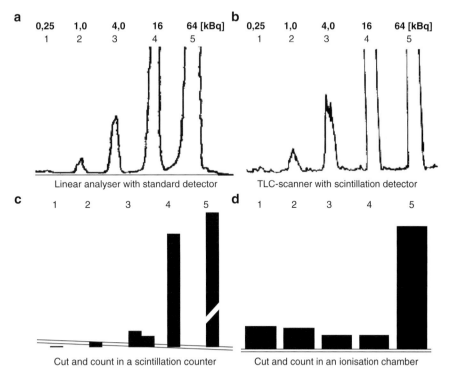

a Linear analyser with standard detector

b TLC-scanner with scintillation detector

c Cut and count in a scintillation counter

d Cut and count in an ionisation chamber

Free pertechnetate migration properties and hence its R_f value are governed by the type of mobile and stationary phases used for the TLC test, while reduced, hydrolyzed technetium is present mainly at the origin ($R_f = 0$) due to its insolubility properties (like all other colloidal components), explaining why reduced, hydrolyzed technetium species cannot be recognized in colloidal and particulate preparations (e.g., macro-aggregated albumin [MAA] preparations).

Tables 4.1 and 4.2 summarize the TLC chromatographic data for Tc-99m and non-Tc-99m radiopharmaceuticals, respectively.

4.2.5 Precipitation

Precipitation is the method of separating a radiochemical form from another with an appropriate chemical reagent. The precipitate is separated by centrifugation. $^{51}Cr^{3+}$ in ^{51}Cr-sodium chromate can be estimated by precipitating chromates as lead chromate and determining the radioactivity of the supernatant.

4.2.6 Distillation

Distillation is a method applicable to compounds with different vapor pressures. The two compounds can be separated by simple distillation at a specific temperature. The compound with higher vapor pressure is distilled off first, leaving the other compound in the distilling container. Iodide impurities can be separated from any iodine-labeled compound by distillation.

4.2.7 Ion Exchange

Ion exchange is performed simply by passing a radiopharmaceutical sample through a column of ionic resin and eluting the column with a suitable solvent. Separation of different chemical forms is dependent on the ability and affinity of exchange of ions from a solution onto the resin. Polymerized and high molecular weight resins are of two kinds: cation exchange and anion exchange resins.

An example of that method is the determination of the presence of $^{99m}TcO_4^-$ in ^{99m}Tc-labeled albumins,

Table 4.1 Chromatographic data for ^{99m}Tc-radiopharmaceuticals

^{99m}Tc-Radiopharmaceutical	Stationary Phase	Solvent	R_f ^{99m}TcO$_4$	^{99m}Tc-Complex	Hydrolyzed ^{99m}Tc
Bone radiopharmaceuticals					
^{99m}Tc-PYP	ITLC-SG	Acetone	1.0	0.0	0.0
	ITLC-SG	Saline	1.0	1.0	0.0
^{99m}Tc-MDP	ITLC-SG	Acetone	1.0	0.0	0.0
	ITLC-SG	Saline	1.0	1.0	0.0
^{99m}Tc-HDP (hydroxymethylene diphosphonate)	ITLC-SG	Acetone	1.0	0.0	0.0
	ITLC-SG	Saline	1.0	1.0	0.0
Renal radiopharmaceuticals					
^{99m}Tc-DTPA	ITLC-SG	Acetone	1.0	0.0	0.0
	ITLC-SG	Saline	1.0	1.0	0.0
^{99m}Tc-MAG$_3$	Whatman 3MM	Acetone	1.0	0.0	0.0
	Whatman 3MM	Water	1.0	1.0	0.0
^{99m}Tc-gluceptate	ITLC-SG	Acetone	1.0	0.0	0.0
	ITLC-SG	Saline	1.0	1.0	0.0
^{99m}Tc(III)-DMSA (dimercaptosuccinic acid)	Whatman 3MM	Acetone	1.0	0.0	0.0
	ITLC-SA	Butanol	0.9	0.5	0.0
^{99m}Tc(V)-DMSA	ITLC-SG	MEK (methyl ethyl ketone)	1.0	0.0	0.0
	ITLC-SG	Saline	1.0	1.0	0.0
^{99m}Tc-IDAs (iminodiacetic acids)	Whatman 3MM	MEK	0.9	0.0	0.0
	ITLC-SG	Water	1.0	1.0	0.0
Cardiac radiopharmaceuticals					
^{99m}Tc-sestamibi	Whatman 3MM	Ethyl acetate	0.0–0.1	0.5–0.8	0.0–0.1
^{99m}Tc-tetrofosmin	ITLC-SG	Acetone-dichloromethane (35:65)	0.9–1.0	0.4–0.7	0.0–0.1
Brain radiopharmaceuticals					
^{99m}Tc-HMPAO	ITLC-SG	MEK	1.0	1.0 (primary)	0.0
	ITLC-SG	Saline	1.0	0.0	0.0
	Whatman 1	50% acetonitrile	1.0	1.0	0.0
^{99m}Tc-bicisate	Whatman 3MM	Ethyl acetate	0.0	1.0	0.0

(continued)

Table 4.1 (continued)

99mTc-Radiopharmaceutical	Stationary Phase	Solvent	R_f		
			$^{99m}TcO_4$	^{99m}Tc-Complex	Hydrolyzed ^{99m}Tc
Miscellaneous					
^{99m}Tc-MAA	ITLC-SG	Acetone	1.0	0.0	0.0
^{99m}Tc-HSA (human serum albumin)	ITLC-SG	Ethanol:NH$_4$OH:H$_2$O (2:1:5)	1.0	1.0	0.0
^{99m}Tc-SC (sulfur colloid)	ITLC-SG	Acetone	1.0	0.0	0.0
^{99m}Tc-nanocolloid	Whatman ET-31	Saline	0.8	0.0	0.0
^{99m}Tc-architumomab	ITLC-SG	Acetone	1.0	0.0	0.0
^{99m}Tc-nofetumomab	ITLC-SG	12% TCA in H$_2$O	1.0	0.0	0.0

Data adapted from [9, 21] and UKRG Handbook (Bev Ellis, United Kingdom Radiopharmaceutical Group, London, 2002)
Adapted from [2].
ITLC-SA instant thin-layer chromatography silicic acid, *ITLC-SG* instant thin-layer chromatography silica gel

Table 4.2 Chromatographic data of radiopharmaceuticals other than 99mTc-complexes

Radiopharmaceutical	Stationary phase	Solvent	R_f values	
			Labeled product	Impurities
125I-RISA (radioiodinated serum albumin)	ITLC-SG	85% methanol	0.0	1.0(I$^-$)
131I-hippuran	ITLC-SG	CHCl$_3$:acetic acid (9:1)	1.0	1.0(I$^-$)
131I-NP-59	ITLC-SG	Chloroform	1.0	1.0(I$^-$)
131I-MIBG	Silica gel plated plastic	Ethyl acetate:ethanol (1:1)	0.0	0.6(I$^-$)
131I-NaI	ITLC-SG	85% methanol	1.0	0.2(IO^{-3})
51Cr-sodium chromate	ITLC-SG	n-Butanol saturated with 1N HCl	0.9	0.2(Cr3+)
67Ga-citrate	ITLC-SG	CHCl$_3$:acetic acid(9:1)	0.1	1.0
111In-DTPA (diethylenetriaminepentaacetate)	ITLC-SG	10% ammonium acetate: methanol (1:1)	1.0	0.1(In3+)
111In-capromab pendetide	ITLC-SG	Saline	0.0	1.0(In3+)
18F-FDGh	ITLC-SG	CH$_3$CN/H$_2$O (95:5)	0.37	0.0
90Y-,111In-ibritumomab tiuxetan		0.9%NaC1 solution	0.0	1.0

Adapted from [21]
ITLC-SG instant thin-layer chromatography silica gel

by which the $^{99m}TcO_4^-$ is adsorbed to the Dowex-1 resin, leaving the ^{99m}Tc-labeled albumins and the hydrolyzed ^{99m}Tc to go with the elute when using 0.9% NaCl as a solvent to wash the resin column.

4.2.8 Solvent Extraction

When two immiscible solvents are shaken together, any solute present will distribute between the two phases according to its solubility in each phase. Equilibrium is reached and governed by the partition coefficient D:

$$D = \text{Concentration in organic phase/Concentration in aqueous phase}$$

Lipid-soluble molecules may have $D \geq 100$, so it becomes highly concentrated in the organic phase. If the solvent is volatile (e.g., ether or chloroform), the solute can be recovered by distillation or evaporation. An example of this method is the separation of ^{99m}Tc-pertechnetate by dissolving ^{99}Mo in a strongly alkaline solution (e.g., potassium hydroxide) and then extracting with MEK. ^{99m}Tc-pertechnetate dissolved in the organic phase can be recovered by evaporation to dryness; this method has been used initially to prepare ^{99m}Tc-pertechnetate for ^{99m}Tc-labeled radiopharmaceuticals [15].

4.2.9 Electrophoresis

The basic idea of electrophoresis is the property of charged molecules (atoms) to migrate in an electric field. The migration rate is dependent on the charge and size of the molecule. The apparatus used in electrophoresis consists simply of a direct current power supply to provide a potential difference of 400 V or greater, connected through an electrolyte buffer solution (barbitone/barbituric acid) to either end of a strip of support medium, which may be cellulose acetate or filter paper. Since ^{99m}Tc-pertechnetate is considered a small ion, it migrates rapidly and is readily separated from larger negatively charged complexes, such as ^{99m}Tc-DTPA (diethylenetriaminepentaacetate) or insoluble ^{99m}TcO$_2$, which remain at the origin [16].

4.2.10 Gel Filtration

Gel filtration chromatography is a process obtained when a mixture of solutes is passed down a column of suitable medium, such as *cross-linked dextran Sephadex,* and then eluted with a proper solvent, allowing the large molecules to be released first while the smaller ones are selectively retarded due to penetrating the pores of the gel polymeric structure.

Sequential fractions of the eluate are collected by an automated fraction collector, and the radioactivity is measured for each fraction.

Gel chromatography is the method of choice for separating proteins of different molecular weights. In addition, this method is equally important in detecting impurities in ^{99m}Tc-labeled radiopharmaceuticals. To obtain the percentages of free, bound, and unbound hydrolyzed ^{99m}Tc species, a Sephadex gel-saline filtration system is widely used. In this case, ^{99m}Tc-chelate is eluted first, followed by the free ^{99m}TcO$_4^-$, while the hydrolyzed ^{99m}Tc is retained by the column.

It has been observed that some ^{99m}Tc chelates may bind to or dissociate on the column, producing inaccurate results.

4.3 High-Performance Liquid Chromatography

High-performance liquid chromatography (HPLC) is a recent modification of the gel chromatography method; the liquid phase is forced at a high pressure through an adsorbent, densely packed column. When the different species of the sample are eluted from the column, they pass through a radiation detector or any other detector, which records its presence, normally in a graph form. The stationary phase most frequently consists of beads of silica bounding an organic pad containing long-chain (C$_{18}$) carbon groups. A wide range of stationary and mobile phases has been used; by suitable choice, this technique is extremely valuable in the development and evaluation of new radiopharmaceuticals. In addition, HPLC is considered a suitable technique for estimation of short-lived radiopharmaceuticals because of its rapidity [17].

If the components are irreversibly adsorbed on the stationary phase of the HPLC system (e.g., hydrolyzed ^{99m}Tc species), the system required is expensive; therefore, the use of HPLC is not routine in hospital practice. As an example, HPLC has been used for separation of ^{99m}Tc-MDP (methylene diphosphonate) prepared by borohydride reduction into several different components. A schematic diagram of the general components of the radio-HPLC system can be seen in Fig. 4.3.

Fig. 4.3 Components of a
radio-high-performance liquid
chromatographic (HPLC)
system

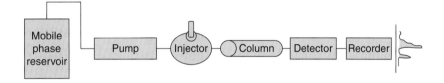

4.3.1 Sep-Pak Analysis

Sep-Pak cartridges (Millipore Water) have been developed for isolation and cleanup of sample components as a modification of the HPLC technology. This method is applicable for radiochemical analysis of ^{99m}Tc-MAG$_3$ (mercaptoacetyltriglycine), ^{99m}Tc-sestaMIBI, and radiolabeled MIBG.

4.4 Biological Tests

The presence of microorganisms (bacteria, fungi, etc.) should be examined for all pharmaceuticals intended for human administration and is defined by the sterility test.

Living organisms also can produce metabolic by-products (endotoxins) that can undesirably affect the radiopharmaceutical preparation, so special testing procedures should be applied (pyrogenicity and toxicity tests).

4.4.1 Sterility

The objective of the sterility test is to ensure that the sterilization processes, mainly by autoclaving for long-lived radiopharmaceuticals and membrane filtration for short-lived ones, are conducted properly [18]. A proper sterility test involves the incubation of the radiopharmaceutical sample for 14 days in

- *Fluid thioglycollate medium* for growth of aerobic and anaerobic bacteria
- *Soybean-casein digest medium* for growth of fungi and molds

The sterility test requires 14 days, so ^{99m}Tc-labeled compounds and other short-lived radiopharmaceuticals could be released prior to the completion of the test [19].

4.4.2 Pyrogenicity

Pyrogens are either *polysaccharides* or *proteins* produced by the metabolism of microorganisms. They are mainly soluble and heat stable, represented primarily as bacterial endotoxins. Pyrogens produce symptoms of fever, chills, malaise, joint pain, sweating, headache, and dilation of the pupils within 30 min to 2 h after administration.

Pyrogenicity testing was developed from the rabbit test (monitoring of the temperature of three healthy rabbits for 3 h after injection of the test sample) to a more sophisticated and rapid method called the *limulus amebocyte lysate* (LAL) method. LAL, which is isolated from the horseshoe crab (*limulus*), reacts with gram-negative bacterial endotoxins in nanogram or greater concentrations, forming an opaque gel. The thicker the gel, the greater the concentration of pyrogens in the sample. Gram-negative endotoxins are known as the most important source of pyrogen contamination, so the LAL test is a rapid and sensitive pyrogenicity test [20].

Generally, manufacturers are required to perform the sterility and pyrogenicity tests prior to release of their products to the end users. However, the short half-lives of ^{99m}Tc radiopharmaceuticals prohibit their testing for sterility and pyrogenicity, emphasizing aseptic labeling techniques by using laminar flow enclosures containing high-efficiency particle air (HEPA) filters improves the environment for radiopharmaceutical formulation.

4.4.3 Toxicity

Toxicity tests should be applied for all radiopharmaceuticals approved for human use. A quantity called $LD_{50/60}$ describes the toxic effect of a radiopharmaceutical by determination of the dose required to produce mortality of 50% of a species in 60 days after administration of a radiopharmaceutical dose [21].

The test should be done for at least two different species of animals. Because of the strict regulations on the use of animals for research and due to the expected differences on reactions from animal species to humans, cell culturing and computer modeling have been used to achieve toxicity tests.

References

1. European Pharmacopoeia (Ph. Eur.) ver. (5.0). Council of Europe, Maisonneuve, Sainte-Ruffine, 2005.
2. United States Pharmacopoeia (USP), Official Monographs, United States Pharmacopeial Convention, 2005.
3. General International Pharmacopoeia Monograph for Radiopharmaceuticals, World Health Organization, Geneva, 2007.
4. Kowalsky RJ, Falen SW. Radiopharmaceuticals in nuclear pharmacy and nuclear medicine. 2nd ed. American Pharmacists Association, 2004.
5. Hammermaier A, Reich E, Bogl W. Chemical, radiochemical, and radionuclidic purity of eluates from different commercial fission ^{99}Mo/^{99m}Tc generators. Eur J Nucl Med. 1986;12:41–6.
6. Eckelman WC, Levenson SM, Johnston GS. Radiochemical purity of ^{99m}Tc-radiopharmaceuticals. Appl Radiol. 1977;6:211.
7. Wilson MA. Textbook on nuclear medicine. Philadelphia: Lippincott-Raven; 1998.
8. Robbins PJ. Chromatography of technetium 99mTc-radiopharmaceuticals – a practical guide. New York: Society of Nuclear Medicine; 1984.
9. Zolle I. Technetium-99m Pharmaceuticals. Berlin: Springer; 2007.
10. Zimmer AM, Pavel DG. Rapid miniaturized chromatographic quality-control procedures for Tc-99m radiopharmaceuticals. J Nucl Med. 1977;18:1230–3.
11. Pauwels EKJ, Feitsma RIJ. Radiochemical quality control of 99mTc-labeled radiopharmaceuticals. Eur J Nucl Med. 1977;2:97.
12. Robbins PJ. Chromatography of technetium-99m radiopharmaceuticals. A practical guide. New York: Society of Nuclear Medicine; 1983.
13. Janshold AL, Krohn KA, Vera DR, Hines HH. Design and validation of a radio-chromatogram scanner with analog and digital output. J Nucl Med Tech. 1980;8:222.
14. Wieland DM, Tobes MC, Mangner TJ, editors. Analytical and chromatographic techniques in radiopharmaceutical chemistry. Berlin: Springer; 1986.
15. IAEA research program report. Alternative technologies for 99mTc generators. IAEA-TECDOC-852. ISSN 1011-4289, 1995.
16. Belkas EP, Archimandritis S. Quality control of colloid and particulate ^{99m}Tc-labelled radiopharmaceuticals. Eur J Nucl Med. 1979;4:375.
17. Mallol J, Bonino C. Comparison of radiochemical purity control methods for Tc-99m radiopharmaceuticals used in hospital radiopharmacies. Nucl Med Commun. 1997;18:419–22.
18. Snowdon GM. Is your technetium generator eluate sterile? J Nucl Med Technol. 2000;28:94–5.
19. Brown S, Baker MH. The sterility testing of dispensed radiopharmaceuticals. Nucl Med Commun. 1986;7:327–36.
20. U.S. Food and Drug Administration. Guideline on validation of the limulus amebocyte lysate test as an end-product endotoxin test for human and animal parenteral drugs, biological products, and medical devices. Rockville, 1987
21. Saha GB. Fundamentals of radiopharmacy. 5th ed. Berlin: Springer; 2004.

PET Chemistry: An Introduction

Tobias L. Roß and Simon M. Ametamey

Contents

5.1 Introduction

One major advantage of radioactivity is its extremely high sensitivity of detection. Regarding the medical applicability of radioactivity, it permits non-invasive in vivo detection of radiolabelled compounds at nano- to picomolar levels. The use of substances at such low concentrations usually precludes a physiological, toxic or immunologic response of the investigated biological system. Consequently, the considered physiological process or system is examined in an unswayed situation. Furthermore, a wide range of substances,

even those which are toxic at higher concentrations, become considerable for the development of radiopharmaceuticals and use in nuclear medicine. In contrast to the wide range of employable bioactive molecules, the range of suitable radioactive nuclides is much more restricted by their nuclear physical and chemical properties. In particular, radionuclides for diagnostic applications should provide appropriate (short) half-lives and radiation properties for detection and imaging, but at the same time the radiation dose of patients and personnel have to be kept to minimum. Nonetheless, to date, a couple of radionuclides have proven suitable for both nuclear medical diagnostic applications, single photon emission computed tomography (SPECT), and positron emission tomography (PET).

As indicated by their names, SPECT is based on photon or γ-ray emitting nuclides while PET is derived from those nuclides which belong to the group of neutron-deficient nuclides and emit positrons (β^+-decay). Large scale production of positron emitting radionuclides became possible for the first time by the invention of the cyclotron by Ernest Orlando Lawrence in 1929 [1]. Since then, many (medical) cyclotrons have been built and have been in use at various nuclear medicine PET facilities. As a result, short-lived positron emitters such as most commonly employed fluorine-18 and carbon-11 are routinely produced at most nuclear medicine centres on a daily basis.

In the β^+-decay of a neutron-deficient nucleus, a positron (β^+) and a neutrino (ν) are synchronously emitted, while in the nucleus, a proton is converted into a neutron. Neutrinos show practically no interaction with matter and thus they are not detectable by PET cameras. In contrast, the emitted positron is able to interact with an electron, its anti-particle. As a result, both particles annihilate and give two γ-rays with a total energy of 1.022 MeV, the sum of the

T.L. Roß (✉)
Radiopharmaceutical Chemistry, Institute of Nuclear Chemistry, Johannes Gutenberg-University Mainz, Fritz-Strassmann-Weg 2, D-55128 Mainz, Germany
e-mail: ross@uni-mainz.de

S.M. Ametamey
Animal Imaging Center-PET, Center for Radiopharmaceutical Sciences of ETH, PSI and USZ, ETH-Hönggerberg, D-CHAB IPW HCI H427, Wolfgang-Pauli-Str. 10, CH-8093, Zurich, Switzerland
e-mail: amsimon@ethz.ch

M.M. Khalil (ed.), *Basic Sciences of Nuclear Medicine*, DOI: 10.1007/978-3-540-85962-8_5,
© Springer-Verlag Berlin Heidelberg 2011

masses of positron and electron, 511 keV each. Both γ-rays show a nearly $180°$ distribution and each carries the characteristic energy of 511 keV. Accordingly, the decay of positron emitters which are used as label for PET radiopharmaceuticals results in two γ-rays and as these are body-penetrating photons, they can be detected by an appropriate PET camera. This physical phenomenon provides the base of PET imaging.

In PET scanners, a circular ring of detector pairs, which record only coincidence events, registers the in vivo generated pairs of γ-rays. An appropriate computer-aided data acquisition provides PET images with information about in vivo distribution and levels of accumulation of the radionuclide and the radiopharmaceutical, respectively. Consequently, biochemical processes can be visualised and a dynamic data acquisition further allows for registration of a temporal component such as pharmacokinetics of a certain drug. In combination with bio-mathematical models and individual corrections of attenuation, transmission and scatter effects, physiological and pharmacological processes can be precisely acquired and quantified [2].

The most important radionuclides for PET imaging are fluorine-18 and carbon-11. Particularly, the ^{18}F-labelled glucose derivative 2-deoxy-2-[^{18}F]fluoro-D-glucose ([^{18}F]FDG) represents the most widely used PET radiopharmaceutical which has contributed most to the worldwide success of clinical PET imaging. The combination of a highly efficient radiochemistry and a high yielding ^{18}O(p,n)^{18}F nuclear reaction makes [^{18}F]FDG available in large amounts and also enables shipment and distribution by commercial producers. Since its development in the 1970s [3], [^{18}F]FDG has been employed in many PET studies in oncology, neuroscience and cardiology [4–7]. However, further substances have followed and to date, several PET radiopharmaceuticals for specific targets have been developed and evaluated for a wide range of applications in clinical nuclear medicine as well as in preclinical research [8–11].

The following chapter deals with the development and the use of PET radiopharmaceuticals. Here a comprehensive overview of basic considerations and possibilities in development of PET radiopharmaceuticals is given. An outline of commonly employed clinically established PET radiopharmaceuticals, their most important production routes and clinical applications follows in the next chapter, in which also aspects of routine production and quality control of PET radiopharmaceuticals as well as their use in drug development are introduced and briefly summarised. Both chapters principally cover literature until the beginning of 2009.

5.2 Choice of the Radionuclide

There is a variety of basic functions and effects which can generally be followed and visualised by PET such as metabolism, pharmacokinetics, (patho)physiological and general biochemical functions; receptor-ligand biochemistry; enzyme functions and inhibition; immune reactions and response; pharmaceutical and toxicological effects. However, a close look into the designated processes and the related biochemistry is necessary to find a positron emitter with appropriate characteristics.

Although fluorine-18 is the most commonly preferred positron emitter for PET radiopharmaceuticals, monoclonal antibodies labelled with fluorine-18 for immuno-PET imaging are normally not useful because the physical half-life of 110 min does not fit to the slow accumulation (normally 2–4 days) of most monoclonal antibodies in solid tumours [12]. In such cases, longer-lived PET nuclides as iodine-124 ($T_{1/2} = 4.18$ days) and zirconium-89 ($T_{1/2} = 3.27$ days) are more suitable for this particular application. On the other hand, longer half-lives increase radiation doses to the patients and thoughtful considerations towards a health/risk–benefit analysis are mandatory.

As a basic principle, short-lived radionuclides should preferably be used if their suitability is similarly good with respect to a certain application. Blood flow tracers are a perfect example for the use of extremely short-lived radionuclides such as oxygen-15 ($T_{1/2} = 2$ min), nitrogen-13 ($T_{1/2} = 10$ min) and rubidium-82 ($T_{1/2} = 1.3$ min). The scanning times of blood flow studies using PET are normally very short and not longer than 2–5 min. Hence, radiolabelled substances such as [^{15}O] water, [^{15}O]butanol, [^{13}N]ammonia and [^{82}Rb]RBCl are particularly suitable. However, the relatively short half-lives of the these radionuclides place some constraints on imaging procedure and execution.

Besides half-lives, there are further physical aspects to be considered. One is the β^+-energy ($E_{\beta+}$) of the emitted positrons. The $E_{\beta+}$ also clearly affects the radiation dose to the patients and thus the lower the $E_{\beta+}$ the better it is for the patients. Since the $E_{\beta+}$ is also responsible for the positron range (travelling distance of the positron) and a short positron range enhances the spatial resolution in PET, a low $E_{\beta+}$ is also very favorable for high resolution PET imaging. However, in human PET scanners, the distance of the detectors to the object is long and the positron range is no longer significant for the absolute spatial resolution as demonstrated in comparable studies using different positron emitters in imaging phantoms [13, 14]. In contrast, high-resolution small animal PET scanners show dramatically degraded image quality by the use of positron emitters with high $E_{\beta+}$ or complex decay schemes [15].

In comparison with most of the available positron emitters for PET, it is already quite evident from the nuclear properties that fluorine-18 is the most preferred radionuclide for PET. The optimal half-life of fluorine-18 offers multi-step radiochemistry, extended PET studies of slower biochemistry as well as the shipment of the ^{18}F-labelled radiopharmaceuticals to clinics without an on-site cyclotron or a radiochemistry facility. Furthermore, it has one of the lowest $E_{\beta+}$ among the PET nuclides and provides high-resolution PET images. An overview of the nuclear data of important positron emitters for PET is given in Table 5.1.

In the same way as the radionuclide must fulfil the physical requirements of the PET imaging, it needs to exhibit suitable chemical properties with respect to available labelling techniques. Thereby, the labelling strategy depends on the initial situation and attendant restrictions. If a certain radionuclide is given by reasons such as availability or imaging characteristics, the target structure often needs to be modified towards its suitability for corresponding labelling methods. In contrast, if the structure of a biomolecule is stipulated, a combination of a radionuclide with an appropriate and efficient labelling procedure needs to be found. However, a restricted number of PET radionuclides and a limited selection of reactions for their introduction into biomolecules generally necessitate the approach of tailored structures. Noteworthy, those structural modifications of the parent biomolecule are mostly accompanied by changes in the pharmacological behaviour and usually a compromise covering pharmacological performance, radiochemistry, dosimetry and PET imaging requirements must be found.

In general, the choice for the right positron emitter for a new PET radiopharmaceutical can be described as the best match between efficient radiochemistry,

Table 5.1 Important positron emitters used for PET and their nuclear data from [16, 17]

Nuclide	Half-life	Decay mode (%)	$E_{\beta+,max}$ [keV]
Organic			
^{11}C	20.4 min	β^+ (99.8) EC (0.2)	960
^{13}N	9.96 min	β^+ (100)	1,190
^{15}O	2.03 min	β^+ (99.9) EC (0.1)	1,720
^{30}P	2.5 min	β^+ (99.8) EC (0.2)	3,250
Analogue			
^{18}F	109.6 min	β^+ (97) EC (3)	635
^{73}Se	7.1 h	β^+ (65) EC (35)	1,320
^{75}Br	98 min	β^+ (75.5) EC (24.5)	1,740
^{76}Br	16.2 h	β^+ (57) EC (43)	3,900
^{77}Br	2.38 days	β^+ (0.7) EC (99.3)	343
^{120}I	81.1 min	β^+ (64) EC (36)	4,100
^{124}I	4.18 days	β^+ (25) EC (75)	2,140
Metallic			
^{38}K	7.6 min	β^+ (100)	2,680
^{45}Ti	3.09 h	β^+ (85) EC (15)	1,040
^{60}Cu	23.7 min	β^+ (93) EC (7)	3,772
^{61}Cu	3.33 h	β^+ (61) EC (39)	1,215
^{62}Cu	9.7 min	β^+ (98) EC (2)	2,930
^{64}Cu	12.7 h	β^+ (18) β^- (37) EC (45)	655
^{68}Ga	68.3 min	β^+ (90) EC (10)	1,900
^{72}As	26 h	β^+ (88) EC (12)	2,515
^{82}Rb	1.3 min	β^+ (96) EC (4)	3,350
^{86}Y	14.7 h	β^+ (34) EC (66)	1,300
^{89}Zr	3.27 days	β^+ (33) EC (77)	902
^{94m}Tc	52 min	β^+ (72) EC (28)	2,470

acceptable dosimetry and favourable pharmacological and PET imaging properties.

5.2.1 Labelling Methods – Introduction of the Radionuclide

Organic positron emitters: The introduction of the radionuclide into a biomolecule or a structure of (patho)physiological interest obviously is one of the essential steps in the development of radiopharmaceuticals. Biomolecules and pharmaceuticals mainly consist of carbon, hydrogen, oxygen, nitrogen, sulphur and phosphorous due to that fact the so-called organic radionuclides (see Table 5.1), carbon-11, oxygen-15, ammonia-13 and phosphorous-30 allow the so-called authentic labelling without any changes in (bio)chemical and physiological behaviour of the radiolabelled molecule. However, these organic radionuclides are extremely short-lived isotopes with half-lives only from 2 to 20 min and that strongly limits their applicability. Only the half-life of 20 min of carbon-11 offers the possibility of radiosyntheses with more than one step and the detection of physiological processes with slower pharmacokinetics. Besides an unchanged pharmacology, the major advantage of such short half-lives is a low radiation dose to the patients and possible repeat studies within a short period.

Analogue positron emitters: Biomolecules and pharmaceuticals are generally relatively complex organic compounds and claim for multi-step radiosyntheses for their radiolabelled counterparts. In addition, many (patho)physiological processes are slower and thus not detectable with the extremely short-lived radionuclides. Alternatively, the so-called analogue radionuclides with longer half-lives from 80 min to 4 days are commonly introduced into biomolecules. The labelling with analogue radionuclides makes use of similarities in steric demand and/or in electronic character of the substituted atom or functional group. The steric demand of an atom or a functional group refers to the amount of space occupied by an atom or a functional group. Accordingly, selenium-73 can be used in the manner of sulphur. Selenium as the next homologue to sulphur has very similar steric and chemical properties. The analogue radiopharmaceuticals L-[^{73}Se]selenomethionine [18] and L-homocysteine[^{73,75}Se]selenolactone [19] are examples for such a selenium-sulphur-analogy. Similarly, ^{75,76,77}Br and ^{120,124}I can be regarded as structural analogues for methyl groups.

In the majority of cases, the analogue radionuclides evoke only small insignificant structural differences, but the arising electronic changes and those of chemical reactivity can be important. In each individual case, the pharmacological behaviour and properties of such analogue radiotracers have to be tested for changes in characteristics. In the last decades, the number of new pharmaceuticals has increased rapidly and more and more compounds have been identified as pharmacologically relevant substances which are originally carrying fluorine, bromine or iodine [20, 21]. Consequently, the advantages of authentic labelling and longer half-lives accrue and simplify the development of a corresponding radiopharmaceutical.

Metallic positron emitters: In a third group, there are also some metallic positron emitters which are suitable for PET imaging (see Table 5.1). The half-lives vary from minutes to days and offer a broad range of applicability. In contrast to organic or analogue PET nuclides, some of the metallic radionuclides are achievable from generator systems (e.g. ^{62}Zn/^{62}Cu, ^{68}Ge/^{68}Ga and ^{82}Sr/^{82}Rb) which make them available in places without an on-site cyclotron. Metallic PET nuclides can be used either directly in their free cationic forms or as complexes. Rubidium-82 has been evaluated as a myocardial perfusion PET tracer [22, 23]. In form of [^{82}Rb] RbCl, it is used as radiopharmaceutical for perfusion PET imaging on the market for almost 20 years (CardioGen-82$^{©}$, approved by the FDA in 1989). The similarities of rubidium to the potassium cation lead to a rapid uptake of rubidium-82 into the myocardium and allow the identification of regions of insufficient perfusion by PET imaging [24, 25]. In complexes, the metallic radionuclides are usually incorporated into biomolecules which carry suitable chelators (i.e. Fig. 5.27 for the somatostatin receptor ligand [^{68}Ga-DOTA, Tyr^3]octreotide [26]).

In addition to differences in chemical, physical and nuclear properties of the radionuclides, the production routes or processes can also influence the labelling approach. The production route as well as the work-up provides the radionuclide in a certain chemical form which requires suitable (radio)chemistry in the following synthetic steps. From the production process, PET radionuclides are obtained only in a nano- to picomolar range while they are still very well detectable by their radioactive decay. As a result, the final PET radiopharmaceuticals are so attractive to medicinal purposes. In the body, they can be detected with non-invasive methods while the quantity of material is extremely small and generally toxic and pharmacological effects are negligible.

Specific activity: Owing to the desired insignificant quantities, a fundamental criterion of the quality of a radionuclide and the final radiopharmaceutical is its specific (radio)activity (SA) which depends on the amount of stable isotopes (carrier) present. Carrier can be divided into:

- *Isotopic carrier*: isotopes of the same element as the radionuclide and
- *Non-isotopic carrier*: isotopes of other elements mostly with very similar chemical and physical properties to the radionuclide

On this account, SA is defined as the mass-related radioactivity:

$$SA = A/m [Bq/g]$$

where A is the radioactivity in Becquerel and m is the mass of the radioactive material including all impurities and carrier, respectively. In (radio)chemistry such a specification related to the mass is inconvenient and thus SA is generally expressed on the molar basis as radioactivity related to the amount of substance:

$$SA = A/n [Bq/mol]$$

where m is replaced by n for the amount of substance in moles. In the absence of impurities or isotopic carrier, the theoretically attainable maximum molar SA equals to:

$$SA = N_A (\ln2/T_{1/2}) [Bq/mol] \quad \text{or}$$
$$SA = 1.16 \times 10^{20}/T_{1/2} [Bq/mol]$$

where N_A is Avogadro's number (6.023×10^{23}) in atoms/mol and $T_{1/2}$ is the half-life of the radionuclide in hours. The general abundance of stable isotopes of the PET radionuclides smaller the theoretically attainable SA and the quantity of material become higher by natural isotopic carrier, but it is normally still at a nano- to picomolar level (6.3×10^4 versus 300–600 GBq/μmol for theoretical and practical SA, respectively, for fluoride-18 produced from $^{18}O(p,n)^{18}F$). Most applications in molecular imaging call for high (molar) specific activities and a lot of effort is put into this issue. Especially for brain receptor PET imaging, high specific activities are essential when receptor systems of low density can be saturated by radioligands with low SA. Besides poor PET imaging results, because of an unfavourable signal-to-noise ratio, pharmacological or toxic effects have also to be considered. In general, for radiochemical practice, the radionuclide situations can be classified as:

- Carrier-free (c.f.)
- No-carrier-added (n.c.a.)
- Carrier-added (c.a.)

Carrier free (c.f): Ideally carrier-free systems are not achievable with PET radionuclides as they all have naturally occurring stable isotopes. For example, carbon is the fourth most abundant element on earth and it is present in almost every kind of material. Thus, especially for carbon-11 high specific activities are an exceptional challenge. However, in radiochemistry of PET radionuclides, traces of stable isotopes are omnipresent and act as isotopic carrier. Sources of isotopic carrier are the air, target and vessel materials, transport lines and tubes, chemicals and solvents.

No carrier added (n.c.a): Contaminations in chemicals and solvents are below normal chemical purification limits, but they are still in the quantity of the radionuclide. Those conditions are referred to as no-carrier-added (n.c.a.) conditions and correspond to a state of practically highest SA attainable.

Carrier added (c.a): On the contrary, some circumstances require the addition of stable isotopes what is termed as carrier-added (c.a.). Predominantly, c.a. conditions are employed to achieve weighable quantities of a product for characterisation by non-radioactive analytical methods or to increase radiochemical yields. As a widely used c.a. procedure the production of electrophilic fluorine-18 is well known. The addition of the isotopic carrier fluorine-19 is necessary to mobilise n.c.a. $[^{18}F]F_2$ which is too reactive and adheres to the walls of targets and tubes.

Labelling reactions and radiosyntheses on the n.c.a. scale mean to work at a subnanomolar level regarding the amount of radioactive substance while all other reactants and solvents are still present at a macroscopic scale. Hence, the course of reaction may differ strongly from that of classical chemical reactions at balanced stoichiometric ratios, where all substrates and reagents are present in amounts in a similar or equal range. Such labelling reactions under non-equilibrium conditions generally proceed according to pseudo-first-order kinetics where the precursor amounts are in extreme excess to the radionuclide and can approximately be set as constant. On the other hand, the radionuclide and the labelled product exist on a n.c.a. scale and thus a consecutive labelling reaction or an interaction of two radioactive species can be statistically excluded.

In labelling procedures and radiosyntheses, obviously, the decay has to be taken into account and thus the half-life of the employed radionuclide. With respect to the PET imaging, the final radiopharmaceutical must be obtained in reasonable amounts sufficient for the following PET procedures. As a rule of thumb, the radiosynthesis including purification, formulation and quality control of a PET radiopharmaceutical should not exceed three half-lives of the radionuclide. Consequently, the extremely short-lived PET radionuclides call for very fast chemistry and preclude multi-step procedures.

The efficacy of radiolabelling reactions is generally quantified by the radiochemical yield (RCY) which corresponds to the decay-corrected yield related to the starting activity. In contrast, the real yield reflects the amount of isolated radioactive material, but is not functional as an appraisal factor of the labelling procedure.

5.2.2 Labelling Methods for Fluorine-18

The indisputable importance of fluorine-18 in PET makes ^{18}F-labelled radiopharmaceuticals the most favoured ones; thus, especially procedures for the introduction of fluorine-18 are of great interest and several methods and strategies have been developed [27–31]. There are many established nuclear production pathways for fluorine-18; the most commonly used are listed in Table 5.2 [32, 33].

The main difference between various nuclear reactions is the target material which is either gas or liquid (water) and determines the final chemical form of fluorine-18. From gas targets, fluorine-18 is achieved as electrophilic c.a. [18]F]fluorine gas (^{18}F]F_2) and from the water targets, nucleophilic n.c.a. [18]F]fluoride in aqueous solution is obtained. As mentioned before, in case of the electrophilic ^{18}F]F_2, adsorption of the produced n.c.a. fluorine-18 on the walls of the target requires the addition of non-radioactive F_2

(isotopic carrier) for an isotopic exchange and removal of the n.c.a. fluorine-18 out of the target. Due to this fact, the procedure dramatically lowers the obtainable specific activity which is one of the major disadvantages of these production routes.

Nonetheless, many compounds of (radio)pharmacological interest call for electrophilic labelling methods and thus necessitate c.a. [18]F]F_2 or its derived secondary labelling agents. The most popular PET radiopharmaceutical which is routinely produced via an electrophilic c.a. ^{18}F-labelling (^{18}F-fluorodestannylation) is 6-^{18}F]fluoro-L-DOPA (^{18}F]F-DOPA) (see Fig. 5.3) [34, 35]. So far, an efficient nucleophilic approach for a n.c.a. ^{18}F-fluorination of ^{18}F]F-DOPA is still lacking.

However, the nucleophilic production route using ^{18}O-enriched water as target material is the most efficient procedure and also provides the n.c.a. [18]F]fluoride in high specific activities. As a result, the [18]O(p,n)[18]F reaction is the most widely used method to produce fluorine-18. The required proton energy of $16 \rightarrow 3$ MeV for the nuclear reaction is achievable without problems from small cyclotron, so-called medical cyclotrons. Normal batches of 50–100 GBq for the production of ^{18}F-labelled clinically utilised PET radiopharmaceuticals can be obtained within 30–60 min depending on the target construction and the corresponding beam current.

Regarding the chemical concepts for the introduction of fluorine-18 into organic molecules, the methods of the macroscopic organic chemistry could be principally transferred. In general chemistry, the commonly used fluorination procedures are based on the Wallach reaction [36] and the Balz–Schiemann reaction [37]. However, in n.c.a. ^{18}F-radiosyntheses, these procedures led only to very low radiochemical yields [38, 39]. Effects of the unusual stoichiometric ratios under n.c.a. conditions as well as principle aspects of

Table 5.2 Most common nuclear reactions for production of fluorine-18

Reaction	[18]O(p,n)[18]F	[16]O([3]He,p)[18]F	[20]Ne(d,α)[18]F	[18]O(p,n)[18]F
Target filling	H_2[18]O	H_2O	Ne (200 μmol F_2)	[18]O_2, Kr (50 μmol F_2)
Particle energy [MeV]	$16 \rightarrow 3$	$36 \rightarrow 0$	$14 \rightarrow 0$	$16 \rightarrow 3$
Chemical product form	[18]F]fluoride (aq)	[18]F]fluoride (aq)	[18]F]F_2	[18]F]F_2
Yield [GBq/μAh]	2.22	0.26	0.37–0.44	~0.35
Specific activity [GBq/μmol]	40×10^3	40×10^3	~0.04–0.40	~0.35–2.00

the reactions' mechanisms and reactants led to these results. Both reaction types revealed inappropriate for fluorine-18 chemistry under n.c.a. conditions.

Generally, radiofluorination methods can be divided into electrophilic and nucleophilic reactions (substitutions) according to the chemical form of fluorine-18 and thus the production route. Both methods represent direct ^{18}F-fluorinations and can be completed by two additionally indirect methods, the ^{18}F-fluorinations via prosthetic groups and the ^{18}F-fluorinations via built-up syntheses. In general, the indirect methods are based on direct methods for the ^{18}F-labelling of the required prosthetic group or synthon. Frequently, the nucleophilic ^{18}F-methods are employed here due to higher specific activities, higher radiochemical yields and a better availability of n.c.a. [^{18}F]fluoride.

5.2.2.1 Electrophilic Substitutions

Fluorine-18 for electrophilic substitution reactions is available as c.a. [^{18}F]F$_2$ directly from targets. ^{20}Ne and enriched [^{18}O]O$_2$ can be used as target materials (cf. Table 5.2). Both alternatives come along with an adsorption of the fluorine-18 on the target walls and entail an addition of [^{19}F]F$_2$ to mobilise the produced fluorine-18 by isotopic exchange. In the ^{18}O(p,n)^{18}F reaction, the enriched [^{18}O]O$_2$ target filling is removed after bombardment and the target is filled with 0.1% [^{19}F]F$_2$ in Kr and repeatedly irradiated for the [^{18}F]F$_2$ formation [40]. In comparison, the ^{20}Ne(d,α)^{18}F reaction is more practical as 0.1% [^{19}F]F$_2$ is directly added with the neon and an additional step for recovery of the enriched material and the consecutive irradiation is saved. Furthermore, the process does not require enriched material and is less expensive. Therefore, the ^{20}Ne(d,α)^{18}F reaction is the commonly employed

process for electrophilic fluorine-18, although its production rates are lower [32, 33]. As all production processes for electrophilic fluorine-18 require carrier addition, c.a. [^{18}F]F$_2$ or milder reagents derived from it cannot be used in preparations of PET radiopharmaceuticals where high specific activities are mandatory [41, 42].

Generally, the methods of electrophilic fluorinations from organic chemistry can be directly transferred into c.a. fluorine-18 chemistry. Due to the fact that carrier is added here, the stoichiometric ratios are more balanced than under n.c.a. conditions and thus closer to macroscopic chemistry. In organic chemistry, elemental fluorine is known for its high reactivity and its poor selectivity. Therefore c.a. [^{18}F]F$_2$ is often transferred into less reactive and more selective electrophilic fluorination agents such as [^{18}F]acetyl hypofluoride ([^{18}F]CH$_3$COOF) [43], [^{18}F]xenon difluoride ([^{18}F]XeF$_2$) [44, 45] or [^{18}F]fluorosulfonamides [46]. The maximum radiochemical yield in electrophilic radiofluorinations is limited to 50% as only one fluorine in [^{18}F]F$_2$ is substituted by a ^{18}F atom. Consequently, that is also the situation for all secondary electrophilic radiofluorination agents derived from c.a. [^{18}F]F$_2$.

The most popular example of electrophilic radiofluorinations using c.a. [^{18}F]F$_2$ is the first method to produce 2-deoxy-2-[^{18}F]fluoro-D-glucose ([^{18}F]FDG) by Ido et al. in 1978 (see Fig. 5.1) [3]. [^{18}F]F$_2$ was used in an electrophilic addition to the double bond of triacetoxyglucal and gave [^{18}F]FDG in a radiochemical yield of 8%. As a radioactive side product 3% of the ^{18}F-labelled mannose derivative (2-deoxy-2-[^{18}F] fluoro-D-mannose, [^{18}F]FDM) was obtained. In 1982, a higher RCY of 20% and an improved product-to-byproduct-ratio of 7:1 were achieved in the approach of Shiue et al. using the milder radiofluorination agent [^{18}F]acetyl hypofluoride [47]. Many other approaches

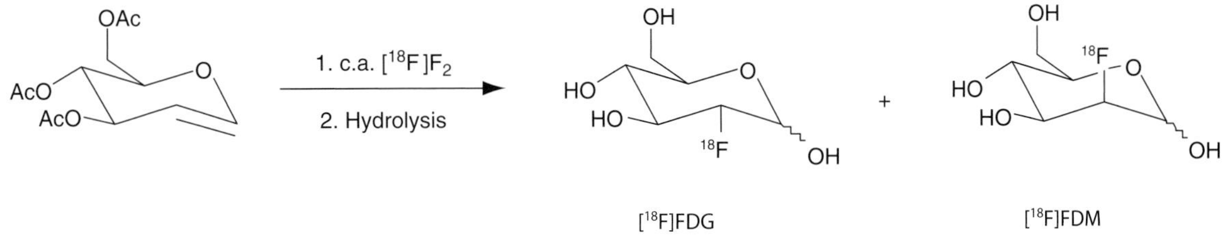

Fig. 5.1 Original radiosynthesis of [^{18}F]FDG (RCY = 8%) by Ido et al. using c.a. [^{18}F]F$_2$. As a side product, the ^{18}F-labelled mannose derivative ([^{18}F]FDM) was obtained in a RCY of 3%

were made to increase radiochemical yields of [^{18}F]
FDG in electrophilic procedures [48–50], including
also attempts with [^{18}F]XeF$_2$ [51–53].

Another example for a direct electrophilic ^{18}F-
fluorination is 5-[^{18}F]fluorouracil which is the ^{18}F-
labelled analogue of 5-fluorouracil. 5-Fluorouracil is
a chemotherapeutic and thus its ^{18}F-labelled analogue
can be used for therapy control, for visualisation of
various tumours and for prediction of therapy response
in liver metastases [54, 55]. 5-[^{18}F]fluorouracil can be
prepared by direct ^{18}F-fluorination of uracil using c.a.
[^{18}F]F$_2$ [56].

The most important PET radiopharmaceutical which
is routinely produced via electrophilic ^{18}F-fluorination
methods is 6-[^{18}F]fluoro-L-DOPA ([^{18}F]F-DOPA).
After [^{18}F]FDG, [^{18}F]F-DOPA ranks second in its
frequency of clinical use. The direct radiofluorination
of 3,4-dihydroxyphenyl-L-alanine using [^{18}F]F$_2$ leads
to three possible ^{18}F-labelled regioisomers namely
2-[^{18}F]F-DOPA (12%), 5-[^{18}F]F-DOPA (1.7%) and
6-[^{18}F]F-DOPA (21%) (see Fig. 5.2) and requires a
complex HPLC purification to obtain the desired
6-[^{18}F]F-DOPA in only 3% RCY [57].

Several attempts have been made to improve radiochemical yields and regioselectivity in the direct
radiofluorination of L-DOPA [58, 59]. So far, the
most efficient procedures for 6-[^{18}F]F-DOPA which
provide adequate RCY of up to 33% for clinical
PET imaging are based on ^{18}F-fluorodemetallation
reactions [60–62]. Among the ^{18}F-demetallation reactions, to date, the ^{18}F-fluorodestannylation is the
most commonly used reaction for routinely produced
6-[^{18}F]F-DOPA (see Fig. 5.3) [34, 63]. An automation
of this radiosynthesis and recently improved precursor
synthesis and quality control allows reliable routine
productions for clinical PET imaging using 6-[^{18}F]
fluoro-L-DOPA [35, 64].

To date, the ^{18}F-fluorodestannylations are generally
the preferred methods for electrophilic ^{18}F-labelling of
complex molecules as they provided satisfactory
radiochemical yields and high regioselectivity.

For higher specific activities in electrophilic ^{18}F-
fluorinations, [^{18}F]F$_2$ can be obtained from n.c.a.
[^{18}F]CH$_3$F via an electric gaseous discharge reaction
in the presence of [^{19}F]F$_2$ (150 nmol) (see Fig. 5.4).
This provides specific activities of up to 55 GBq/µmol

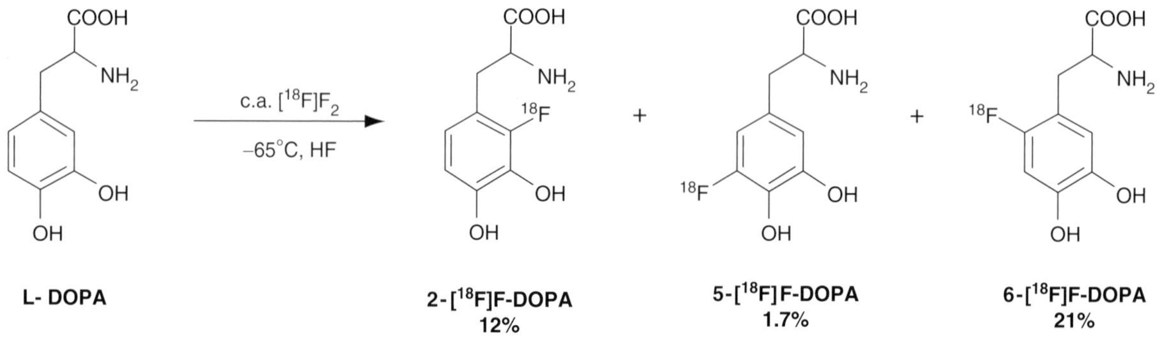

Fig. 5.2 Direct electrophilic radiofluorination of [^{18}F]F-DOPA using c.a. [^{18}F]F$_2$. The product mixture contains 21% of the desired ^{18}F-labelled regioisomer 6-[^{18}F]F-DOPA

Fig. 5.3 Electrophilic radiofluorination of 6-[^{18}F]F-DOPA by regioselective ^{18}F-fluorodestannylation. After 45–50 min 6-[^{18}F]F-DOPA is obtained in RCY of 26–33%

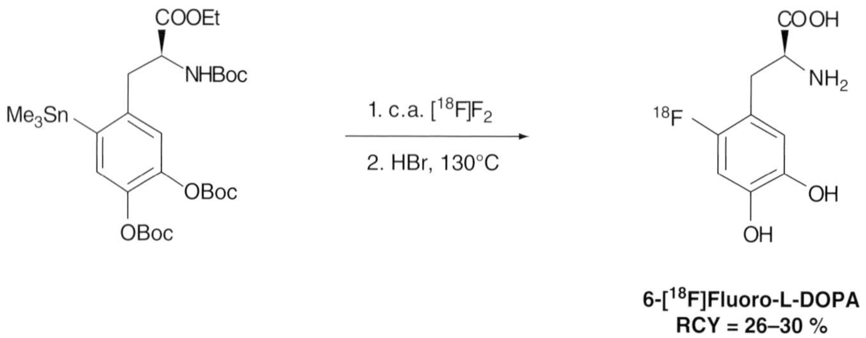

in case of the $[^{18}F]F_2$ which leads to SA of ~15 GBq/μ mol of final ^{18}F-labelled products [65].

However, electrophilic substitution reactions using $[^{18}F]F_2$ and secondary milder fluorination agents derived from it can be used in clinically routine production of PET radiopharmaceuticals where low specific activities and moderate radiochemical yields are not essential. PET imaging of receptor systems and other PET imaging investigations which require high specific activities, still necessitate ^{18}F-radiopharmaceuticals produced under no-carrier-added conditions and thus derive from nucleophilic substitution using n.c.a. $[^{18}F]$fluoride.

5.2.2.2 Nucleophilic Substitutions

As mentioned earlier, the $^{18}O(p,n)^{18}F$ reaction using enriched $[^{18}O]$water as target material is the most efficient and most widely used production route for (nucleophilic) fluorine-18. The required proton energy of 16 MeV can be easily generated by medial cyclotrons and so 50–100 GBq of n.c.a. fluorine-18 can be produced within 30–60 min. The fluorine-18 is obtained directly from the target as nucleophilic n.c.a. $[^{18}F]$fluoride in aqueous solution without any carrier addition.

For saving the costly, enriched material, the first step after the irradiation is the separation of the $[^{18}F]$fluoride from the $[^{18}O]$water. Commonly, $[^{18}F]$fluoride is trapped on an anionic exchange resin (solid phase extraction cartridge systems) while the $[^{18}O]$water is recovered. $[^{18}F]$Fluoride in aqueous solution is strongly hydrated and inactivated for nucleophilic reactions. For an activation of the $[^{18}F]$fluoride, generally, the water is removed by azeotropic distillation with acetonitrile and the remaining dry $[^{18}F]$fluoride is available for nucleophilic substitution reaction as an activated nucleophile.

Due to the strong tendency of fluoride ions to form hydrogen fluoride, the ^{18}F-labelling reactions must be carried out under dry and aprotic conditions. Hence, nucleophilic ^{18}F-labelling is usually performed in dipolar aprotic organic solvents. For further activation and increased nucleophilicity of the $[^{18}F]$fluoride, it is used in combination with weak and soft cations, those of caesium or rubidium. As a result, a so-called 'naked' $[^{18}F]$fluoride of high nucleophilicity is produced. Similarly, phase transfer catalyst such as tetraalkylammonium salts, mainly as their carbonates, hydroxides or hydrogen carbonates, can be used. One of the most efficient and commonly applied system in radiofluorinations is the combination of a cryptand, the aminopolyether Kryptofix©2.2.2, and potassium carbonate (see Figs. 5.5 and 5.6) [66, 67]. In case of base-

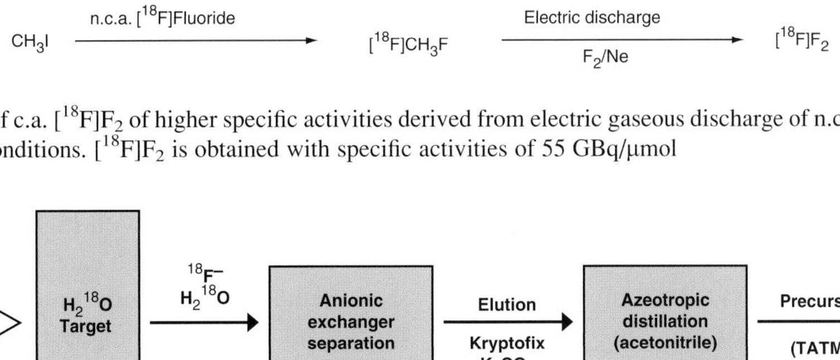

$$CH_3I \xrightarrow{\text{n.c.a. } [^{18}F]\text{Fluoride}} [^{18}F]CH_3F \xrightarrow[\text{F}_2/\text{Ne}]{\text{Electric discharge}} [^{18}F]F_2$$

Fig. 5.4 Production of c.a. $[^{18}F]F_2$ of higher specific activities derived from electric gaseous discharge of n.c.a. $[^{18}F]$fluoromethane under carrier-added conditions. $[^{18}F]F_2$ is obtained with specific activities of 55 GBq/μmol

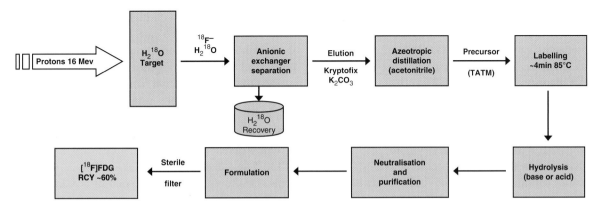

Fig. 5.5 Steps of the $[^{18}F]$FDG routine production. TATM = 1,3,4,6-tetra-O-acetyl-2-O-trifluoro-methanesulfonyl-beta-D-mannopyranose

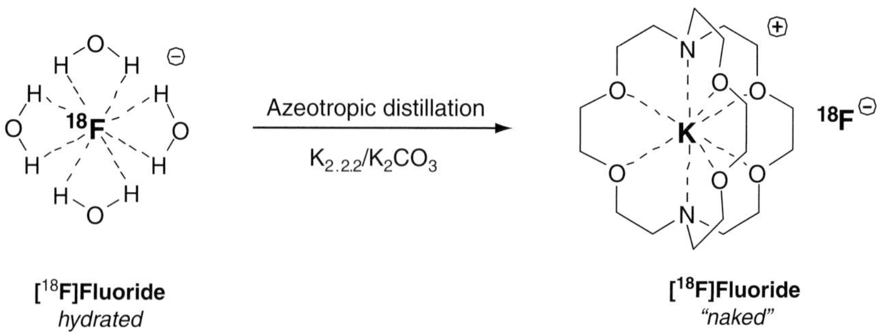

Fig. 5.6 Principle of [^{18}F]fluoride activation by removal of water in combination with the Kryptofix$^©$2.2.2/potassium carbonate system

[^{18}**F**]**Fluoride**
hydrated

Azeotropic distillation
$K_{2.2.2}/K_2CO_3$

[^{18}**F**]**Fluoride**
"naked"

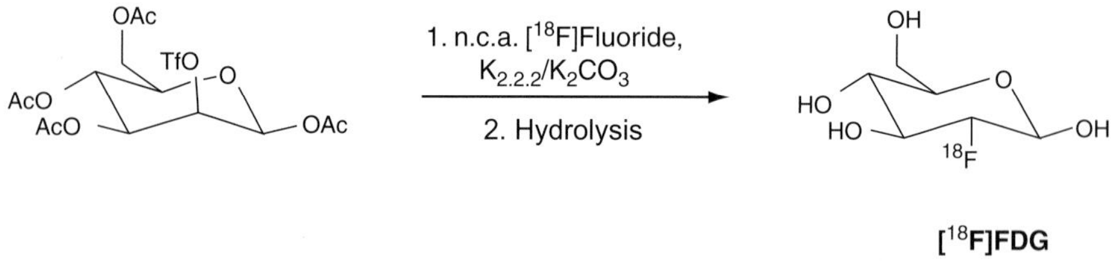

Fig. 5.7 Most commonly used radiosynthesis of n.c.a. [^{18}F]FDG (RCY = 50–70%) by Hamacher et al.

1. n.c.a. [^{18}F]Fluoride, $K_{2.2.2}/K_2CO_3$

2. Hydrolysis

[^{18}**F**]**FDG**

sensitive compounds the carbonate can be exchanged by oxalate which provides less basic conditions. In another method, the [^{18}F]fluoride is separated from [^{18}O]water by an electrochemical anodic adsorption [68]. For drying the cell is flushed two times with acetonitrile or dimethylamide. A polarity change of the electrical field provides a subsequent desorption and release of the [^{18}F]fluoride into a dipolar aprotic solvent containing a phase transfer catalyst system [69]. In recent studies, the use of ionic liquids showed very high ^{18}F-labelling efficiency of up to 90% RCY without previous drying procedures [70]. Small volumes of aqueous ^{18}F-solution are directly added to the reaction mixture containing a base, precursor and ionic liquid. The best results were obtained from the combination of caesium carbonate and the ionic liquid 1-butyl-3-methylimidazolium triflate ([bmim][OTf]). This method was also applied for [^{18}F]FDG productions and showed good RCY of 50–60%, but so far, it has been tested just with small amounts of [^{18}F]fluoride of less than 1 GBq [71].

Generally, the most important procedures to get ^{18}F-labelled radiopharmaceuticals are based on the nucleophilic substitution using n.c.a. [^{18}F]fluoride which is so far also the only way to get ^{18}F-radiopharmaceuticals of high specific activities. Nucleophilic substitution reactions can be divided into aliphatic and aromatic substitutions.

Aliphatic substitution: In case of aliphatic nucleophilic substitutions, the reactions follow the S_N2

mechanism and suitable leaving groups are required. The most efficient leaving groups are sulphonic acid esters such as the methane sulphonic acid ester (mesylate), the trifluoromethane sulphonic acid ester (triflate), the *para*-toluene sulphonic acid ester (tosylate) and the *para*-nitrobenzene sulphonic acid ester (nosylate). Further suitable leaving groups are halogens. The most important and prominent example of such an aliphatic nucleophilic substitution using n.c.a. [^{18}F]fluoride is the synthesis of [^{18}F]FDG using an acetyl-protected mannose precursor (1,3,4,6-tetra-*O*-acetyl-2-*O*-trifluoro-methanesulfonyl-beta-*D*-mannopyranose, TATM) carrying a triflate leaving group which was developed by Hamacher et al. in 1986 (see Fig. 5.7) [67]. This procedure provides [^{18}F]FDG after deprotection and purification in very high radiochemical yields of 50–70% with high specific activities of ~300–500 GBq/μmol. To date, this is the most widely used method for the production of [^{18}F]FDG towards preclinical and clinical applications.

Regarding the reaction conditions for aliphatic nucleophilic substitutions using n.c.a. [^{18}F]fluoride, best results are typically obtained from acetonitrile as solvent and the Kryptofix$^©$2.2.2/potassium carbonate system. Applied reaction temperatures vary from 80°C to 110°C and depend on the individual precursor molecule. Due to the low boiling point of acetonitrile of 82–84°C, temperatures higher than 110°C are not practical. Further suitable solvents are dimethylformamide, dimethylsulfoxide and dimethylacetamide which also allow higher temperatures up to 160–190°C. In recent studies, Kim et al. found increased radiochemical yields in aliphatic nucleophilic ^{18}F-labelling by the use of *tert*-alcohols (frequently *tert*-butanol) as co-solvents to acetonitrile. A beneficial effect was shown for a number of clinically important ^{18}F-labelled PET radiopharmaceuticals [72].

Generally, the aliphatic nucleophilic substitution is high yielding and does not take much longer than 10–15 min for completion. Often, a subsequent deprotection step is necessary, but can also be accomplished within short reaction times of 5–10 min. As a result, aliphatic nucleophilic substitution is widely applied in ^{18}F-labelling chemistry and several routinely produced ^{18}F-labelled PET radiopharmaceuticals are obtained from this reaction type. Besides [^{18}F]FDG, the most popular examples are 3-deoxy-3'-[^{18}F]fluoro-L-thymidine ([^{18}F]FLT) [73], [^{18}F]fluoromisonidazole ([^{18}F]FMISO) [74], O-(2-[^{18}F]fluoroethyl-L-tyrosine) ([^{18}F]FET) [75, 76] and [^{18}F]fluorocholine ([^{18}F]FCH) [77].

Aromatic substitution: The nucleophilic aromatic n.c.a. ^{18}F-fluorinations require an activated aromatic system, an electron deficient system. Otherwise, the desired target ring is not attractive for a nucleophilic attack by n.c.a. [^{18}F]fluoride. Such activation can be reached by strong electron-withdrawing groups (EWG) such as nitro, cyano, carbonyl functionalities

and halogens in *ortho-* or *para*-position to the substitution (see Fig. 5.8).

Suitable leaving groups (LG) are nitro, halogens and especially trimethylammonium salts as their triflate, tosylate, perchlorate or iodide [30, 31, 78]. Generally, dimethylsulfoxide is the solvent of choice for the nucleophilic aromatic substitution, but also dimethylamide and dimethylacetamide or solvent mixtures have been found beneficial. The nucleophilic aromatic substitution usually requires higher energy than its aliphatic variant, especially in case of the fluoro-for-nitro exchange. Therefore, the dipolar aprotic solvents with higher boiling points are preferred and the use of acetonitrile is rare.

An example of a nucleophilic aromatic substitution is the direct ^{18}F-fluorination of the butyrophenone neuroleptic N-methyl-[^{18}F]fluorospiperone using the corresponding nitro-precursor which gave a RCY of ~20% (isolated product) after 70 min synthesis time (see Fig. 5.9) [79]. The aromatic system is activated by the electron-withdrawing effect of the *para*-ketone functionality. However, butyrophenones are base sensitive and the direct ^{18}F-labelling of N-methyl-[^{18}F] fluorospiperone could be realised only with the less basic Kryptofix©2.2.2/potassium carbonate/oxalate buffer system. In the same manner, [^{18}F]haloperidol [79, 80], [^{18}F]altanserin [81] and p-[^{18}F]MPPF (4-[^{18}F]fluoro-N-[2-[4-(2-methoxyphenyl)-1-piperazinyl]

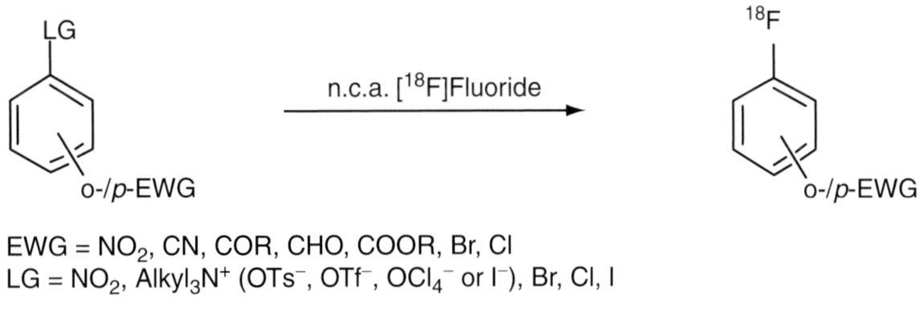

Fig. 5.8 Nucleophilic aromatic substitution using n.c.a. [^{18}F]fluoride

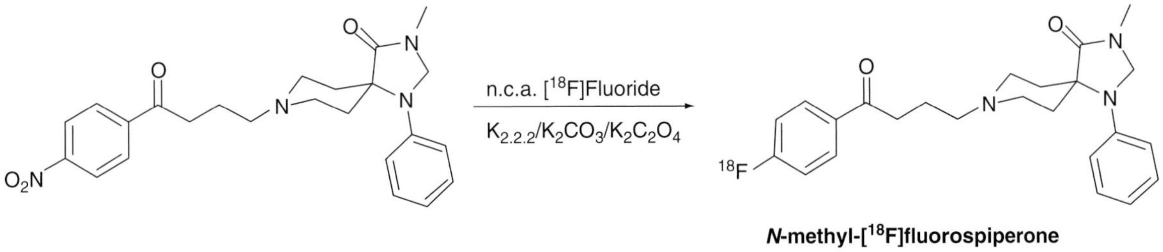

EWG = NO_2, CN, COR, CHO, COOR, Br, Cl
LG = NO_2, $Alkyl_3N^+$ (OTs^-, OTf^-, OCl_4^- or I^-), Br, Cl, I

N-methyl-[^{18}F]fluorospiperone

Fig. 5.9 Nucleophilic aromatic ^{18}F-fluorination of n.c.a. N-methyl-[^{18}F]fluorospiperone

ethyl]-*N*-2-pyridinyl-benzamide) [82, 83] have been successfully labelled with n.c.a. [18F]fluoride by the fluoro-for-nitro exchange.

Another possibility for nucleophilic aromatic substitutions is given by electron-deficient heteroaromatic systems such as pyridines which do not need further activating electron-withdrawing groups [84–86]. 18F-fluoroanalogues of epibatidine have been labelled via a nucleophilic (hetero)aromatic substitution in the *ortho*-position of the pyridinyl group (see Fig. 5.10) and gave radiochemical yields of 55–65% using the trimethylammonium triflate leaving group [87–89]. However, the 18F-labelled epibatidines revealed very toxic [88, 90] and further less toxic 18F-labelled ligands for the nicotine acetylcholine receptor system have been developed, again via the nucleophilic (hetero)aromatic substitution on the *ortho*-position of a pyridinyl group [91, 92]. In case of *meta*-substitutions, the activation of the pyridine is normally not efficient enough and additional activating groups are necessary to obtain sufficient 18F-incorporation [86] as shown by the 18F-labelling of a MAO-B inhibitor in the *meta*-position of the pyridinyl moiety using the fluoro-for-nitro exchange (see Fig. 5.11); 10% RCY after 120 min total synthesis time [93].

Using the direct nucleophilic aromatic substitution, several 18F-labelled PET radiopharmaceuticals have been successfully synthesized including 18F-labelled

butyrophenone neuroleptics [79, 80], [18F]altanserin [81], [18F]methylbenperidol [94], *p*-[18F]MPPF [82, 83], [18F]flumazenil [95], 18F-labelled MAO-B inhibitor [93], 18F-labelled epibatidine analogues [87–89] and further ligands for the nicotine acetylcholine receptor system (nAChR) [91, 92].

In general, radiolabelling chemistry benefits from microwave heating which usually dramatically enhances reaction (labelling) kinetics and provides products within minutes and often with higher (radiochemical)yields [96]. However, the aromatic fluoro-for-nitro exchange, particularly, benefits usually from microwave heating and increased radiochemical yields within markedly reduced reaction times can be obtained [81, 97, 98].

If an aromatic system is somehow non-activated or even deactivated (electron-rich) for nucleophilic 18F-fluorination, a possible strategy is the introduction of auxiliary activating groups transferring the deactivated arene into an activated system. Such supplementary groups or functions need to be removed or modified after the 18F-labelling which implies a multistep radiosynthesis. Aldehydes and ketone functions are particularly suitable as activating groups as they can be removed by reductive decarbonylation [99–101]. This method has been applied for nucleophilic 18F-labelling approaches towards n.c.a. 6-[18F]FDOPA which resulted in only 3–5% RCY

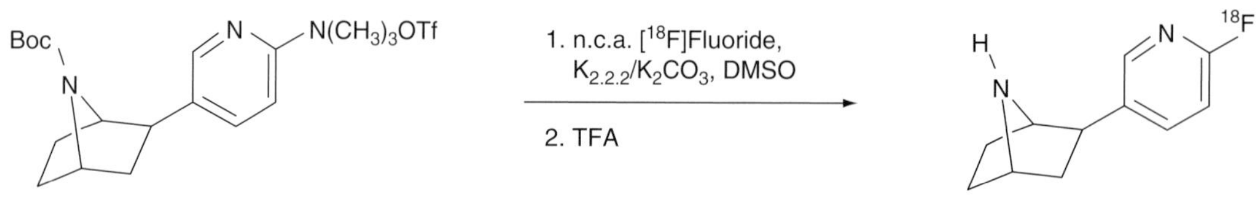

Norchloro-[18F]fluoroepibatidine

Fig. 5.10 18F-Fluoroanalogue of epibatidine. 18F-labelling via nucleophilic (hetero)aromatic substitution

***N*-(2-aminoethyl)-5-[18F]fluoro-pyridine-2-carboxamide**

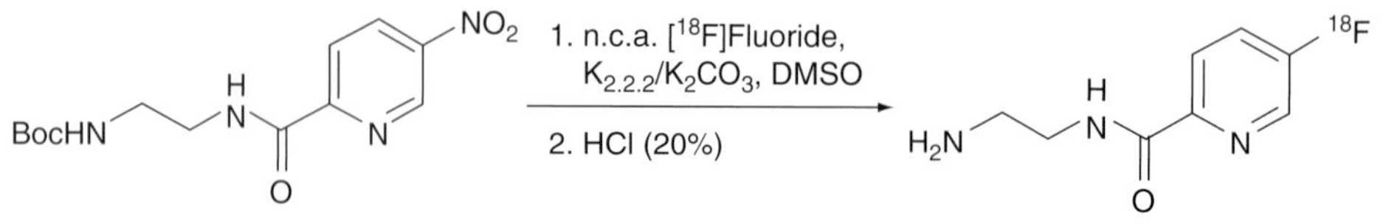

Fig. 5.11 18F-labelling of N-(2-aminoethyl)-5-[18F]fluoropyridine-2-carboxamide, a MAO-B inhibitor, using nucleophilic (hetero) aromatic substitution in pyridine's *meta*-position

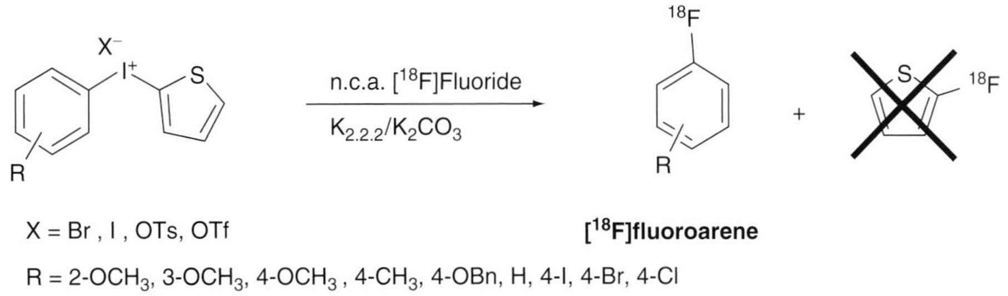

Fig. 5.12 Nucleophilic aromatic ^{18}F-labelling of various arenes including electron-rich systems using aryl(2-thienyl)iodonium salts as precursors

after a three-step radiosynthesis [102] and towards n. c.a. 2-[18F]fluoroestradiol which could be achieved in 10–24% RCY [103].

Another method which allows a direct nucleophilic aromatic ^{18}F-labelling of deactivated systems is the use of diaryliodonium or aryl(heteroaryl)iodonium salts (see Fig. 5.12) [104, 105]. The resulting product distribution after the nucleophilic attack of the n.c.a. [18F] fluoride strongly depends on the electronic and steric character of each aryl ring and its substituents, respectively. Generally, the more electron-deficient ring of the iodonium salt is preferred for the ^{18}F-introduction. Thus, the use of electron-rich heteroaryl systems as one iodonium moiety such as the 2-thienyl group leads to a regioselective ^{18}F-labelling on the counter ring [105]. So far, some attempts of using diaryliodonium salts as precursors for complex structures towards ^{18}F-labelled radiopharmaceuticals have been made, but the ^{18}F-labelling of complex structures via diaryliodonium salts still remains a challenge [103, 106]. One successful example is the PBR ligand [18F]DAA1106 which was recently ^{18}F-labeled in radiochemical yields of 46% from a diaryliodonium precursor [107].

5.2.2.3 ^{18}F-Fluorinations Via Prosthetic Groups

[18]F-labelling via prosthetic groups is based on small molecules which are first ^{18}F-labelled and then introduced into appropriate biomolecules [31, 108–110]. As mentioned before, the direct nucleophilic ^{18}F-labelling methods which usually provide the ^{18}F-labelled PET radiopharmaceutical fast and in high RCY are generally inappropriate for multifunctionalised structures such as peptides, oligonucleotides or antibodies. For that reason, small organic molecules are labelled with fluorine-18 using a direct method and subsequently, they are

conjugated to the target structure forming the final ^{18}F-labelled PET radiopharmaceutical. Principally, both electrophilic and nucleophilic ^{18}F-labelling are suitable for the ^{18}F-introduction into prosthetic groups, but due to high specific activities, higher RCY and better availability of n.c.a. [18F]fluoride, the nucleophilic methods clearly outperform the electrophilic procedures.

The prosthetic group: A variety of prosthetic groups have been developed so far, whereas only limited methods for their introduction into biomolecules are available: acylation [111–122], alkylation [123–125], amidation [126–130], imidation [125], thiol-coupling [131, 132], oxime-formation [133, 134] and photochemical conjugation [122, 135] (see Fig. 5.13).

Most of the procedures for preparation of prosthetic groups are multi-step radiosyntheses and with the final coupling step to bioactive molecules they end as 4–5 – step radiosynthesis. Furthermore, the methods for introduction of certain prosthetic groups require certain functionalities in the target structure and some suffer from low RCY or poor in vivo stability, but prosthetic groups are still indispensable, because of the limitations of direct nucleophilic ^{18}F-labelling.

[18F]SFB: The most commonly applied ^{18}F-labelled prosthetic group is N-succinimidyl-4-[18F]fluorobenzoate ([18F]SFB) which cannot be obtained in a single step [116, 117]. Generally, [18F]SFB derives from n.c.a. ^{18}F-labelling of the triflate salt of 4-trimethylammonium-ethylbenzoate yielding 4-[18F]fluorobenzoic acid ([18F]FBA) after basic hydrolysis; in the next step, [18F]FBA is converted into activated succinimidyl esters using activating agents like N-hydroxysuccinimidine/ 1,3-dicyclohexalcarbodiimide (NHS/DCC) [118], N,N'-disuccinimidyl carbonate (DSC) [119] or O-(N-succinimidyl)-N-N,N',N'-tetramethyluronium tetrafluoroborate (TSTU) [121] to give [18F]SFB. To date, the TSTU-mediated procedure is the fastest and most

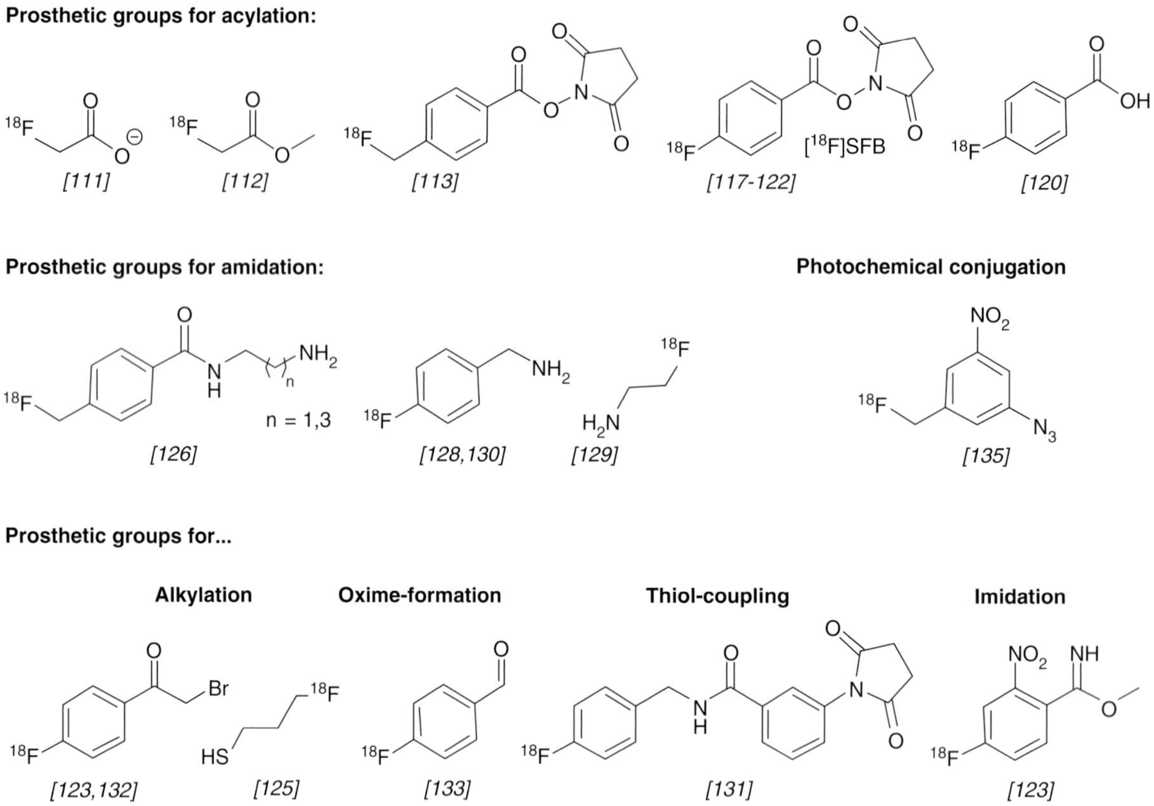

Prosthetic groups for acylation:

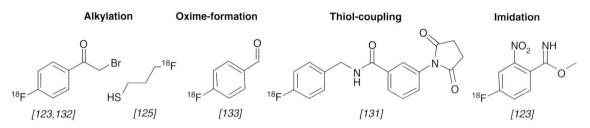

[111] [112] [113] [118]SFB [117-122] [120]

Prosthetic groups for amidation: **Photochemical conjugation**

[126] n = 1,3 [128,130] [129]   [135]

Prosthetic groups for...

Alkylation	Oxime-formation	Thiol-coupling	Imidation

[123,132] [125] [133] [131] [123]

Fig. 5.13 Examples of prosthetic groups and their application in n.c.a. ^{18}F-labelling of biomolecules. References are given in brackets

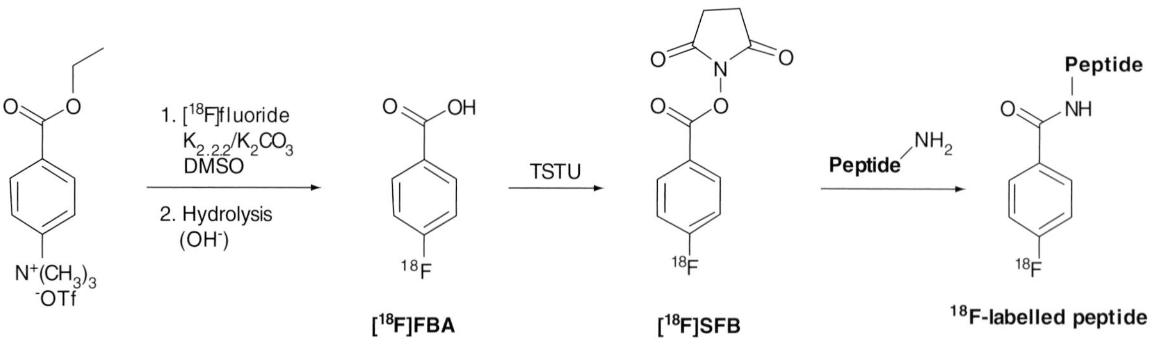

[18]F]FBA ^{18}F]SFB ^{18}F-labelled peptide

1. [18F]fluoride
   K2.2.2/K2CO3
   DMSO

2. Hydrolysis
   (OH−)

TSTU

Peptide

Fig. 5.14 Principle of prosthetic group ^{18}F-labelling of biomolecules using n.c.a. [^{18}F]SFB (TSTU mediated). TSTU: O-(N-succinimidyl)-N-N,N',N'-tetramethyluronium tetrafluoroborate

convenient method to produce [^{18}F]SFB (see Fig. 5.14) [121]. [^{18}F]SFB can then be coupled to an amino function of the target structure.

Recently, the Cu(I)-catalysed 1,3-dipolar cycloaddition between alkynes and azides which is the most prominent representative of the so-called 'click chemistry' [136] has been applied to fluorine-18 chemistry [137–139]. Very mild reaction conditions accompanied by high efficiency, high selectivity and excellent yields make this click reaction particularly suitable for biological applications as well as for the synthesis of PET radiopharmaceuticals.

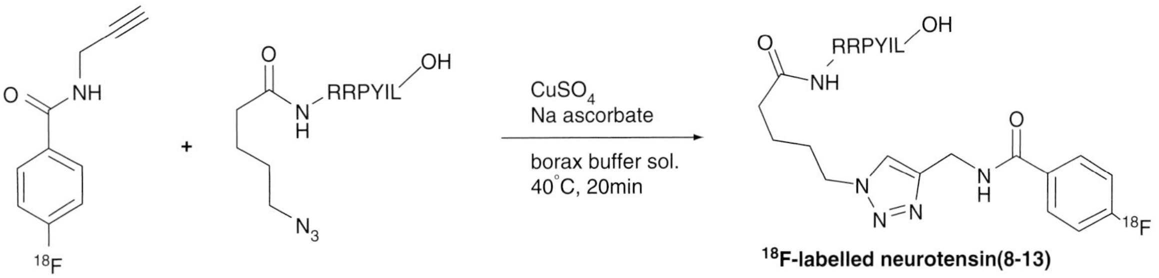

Fig. 5.15 N.c.a. ^{18}F-labelling of neurotensin(8-13) using click chemistry

As an example, the hexapeptide neurotensin(8–13) was successfully n.c.a. ^{18}F-labelled using the click reaction of the ^{18}F-alkyne n.c.a. 4-[^{18}F]fluoro-*N*-(prop-2-ynyl)benzamide and the azide-functionalised $N_3(CH_2)_4CO$-neurotensin(8–13) (see Fig. 5.15) [140]. Under very mild conditions of only 40°C reaction temperature and in borax buffer solution, radiochemical yields of 66% were achieved within 20 min.

In each individual case, the choice of the prosthetic group, and therewith the method of conjugation, depends on the chemical and pharmacological properties of the target structure. Furthermore, the in vivo stability of the prosthetic group and the influence on the pharmacological behaviour of the ^{18}F-labelled compound has to be considered. In terms of the most important requirements for prosthetic group ^{18}F-labelling, to date, the [^{18}F]SFB group seems to be the most suitable prosthetic group. However, the wide scope and the very mild conditions of the ^{18}F-click cycloaddition have added a new and wide flexibility to the ^{18}F-labelling prosthetic groups.

5.2.2.4 Direct ^{18}F-Labelling of Multifunctional Molecules

As mentioned above, the method of choice to introduce the ^{18}F-label into structures like peptides is the use of small ^{18}F-labelled prosthetic groups which are coupled to the biomolecule (see previous paragraph). Recently, the first successful approaches of direct nucleophilic ^{18}F-labelling were reported. Peptides can be selectively functionalised with a highly activated aromatic system bearing a trimethylammonium leaving group which enables a direct one-step nucleophilic aromatic n.c.a. ^{18}F-labelling under very mild conditions [141]. Another new strategy of direct

[18]F-labelling is based on organoboron and organosilicon bioconjugates which can be labelled with n.c.a. [^{18}F]fluoride in one step under aqueous conditions with high RCY [142–144]. In a similar approach, organosilicon building blocks were introduced into a peptide structure and facilitated direct nucleophilic n.c.a. ^{18}F-labelling of peptides in one step under very mild aqueous and even slightly acidic conditions without the need for protection group chemistry (see Fig. 5.16) [145]. Depending on the type of precursor, either 45% RCY or 53% RCY is achieved after 15 min ^{18}F-labelling of the silane precursor or the silanol precursor, respectively.

5.2.2.5 ^{18}F-Labelled Synthons for Built-Up Radiosyntheses

The growing number of complex and multifunctional pharmaceuticals poses a particular challenge to radiolabelling methods. Frequently, the target structure is not suitable for direct ^{18}F-labelling and only an indirect ^{18}F-labelling method can be applied. Besides the prosthetic group ^{18}F-labelling, the ^{18}F-labelling via built-up radiosynthesis offers another indirect alternative [27–31, 86, 146]. Both methods are very similar as they are based on ^{18}F-labelled small organic molecules and indeed the lines between them are often blurred. Generally, the ^{18}F-labelling via built-up radiosyntheses using synthons are used in the direction of small monomeric radiotracers while the ^{18}F-labelled prosthetic groups are mostly applied towards ^{18}F-labelling of macromolecular structures such as peptides or antibody fragments. Obviously, the indirect ^{18}F-labelling methods imply multi-step radiosyntheses of minimum two steps.

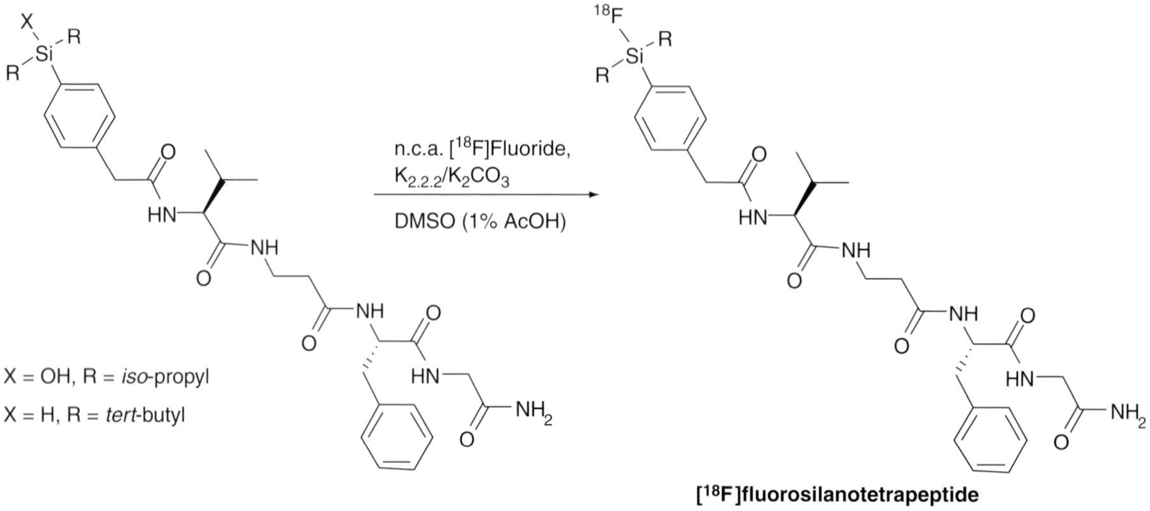

Fig. 5.16 Direct nucleophilic n.c.a. ^{18}F-labelling of a silicon tetrapeptide

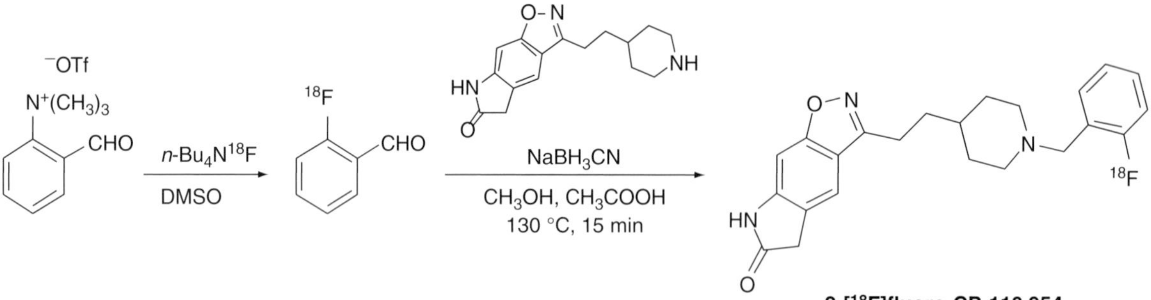

Fig. 5.17 Reductive amination with 2-^{18}F]fluorobenzaldehyde forming the AChE inhibitor 2-^{18}F]fluoro-CP-118,954

The Synthons: The built-up radiosynthesis approach is based on small activated organic molecules which are subsequent to the ^{18}F-fluorination used for a built-up synthesis of the final target compound. Such ^{18}F-labelled synthons are generally derivatives of ^{18}F]fluorobenzene or similar ^{18}F-labelled aryls. Regarding the ^{18}F-introduction they usually bear a leaving group and an activating group. In addition, they need to be functionalised towards further coupling or built-up reactions. Either the activation group is modified or the synthons bear additional substituents which provide further derivatisation and allow coupling reactions. Frequently, the activation group is modified for following coupling or built-up reaction steps.

[18]F]Fluorobenzaldehydes give several possibilities for built-up syntheses and represent the most versatile class of synthons. The aldehyde moiety can be easily transferred into other functionalities. Thus, ^{18}F]fluoro-benzaldehydes can be reduced to their ^{18}F]fluoro-benzamines or –amides and subsequently used in amination reactions towards N-^{18}F]fluorobenzylamines [147–152]. Recently, the AChE inhibitor 5,7-Dihydro-3-[2-[1-(2-^{18}F]fluorobenzyl)-4-piperidinyl]ethyl]-6H-pyrrolo[3,2,f]-1,2-benzisoxazol-6-one (2-^{18}F]fluoro-CP-118,954) has been labelled with fluorine-18 via reductive amination using 2-^{18}F]fluorobenzaldehyde (see Fig. 5.17) [152].

Additional useful derivatives from ^{18}F]fluoroben-zaldehydes are the ^{18}F]fluorobenzyl halides which can be used as alkylation agents for amino [153–155], hydroxyl [156] or thiol [156] functions. 2-^{18}F]fluoro-4,5-dimethoxybenzaldehyde was prepared from its trimethylammonium triflate precursor and used as synthon in a five-step enantioselective radiosynthesis

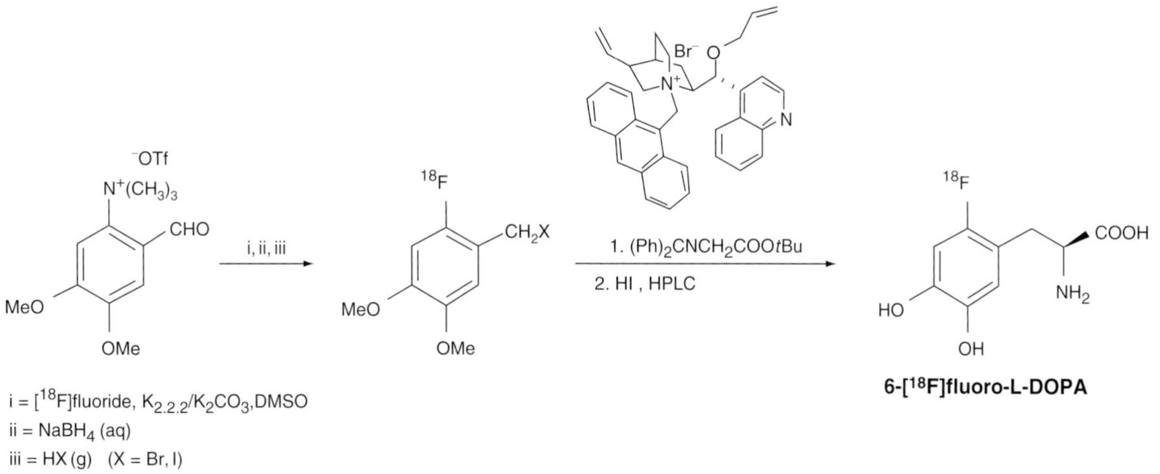

i = [^{18}F]fluoride, K$_{2.2.2}$/K$_2$CO$_3$,DMSO
ii = NaBH$_4$ (aq)
iii = HX (g)   (X = Br, I)

Fig. 5.18 2-[^{18}F]fluoro-4,5-dimethoxybenzyl halides as synthons for n.c.a. radiosynthesis of 6-[^{18}F]fluoro-L-DOPA

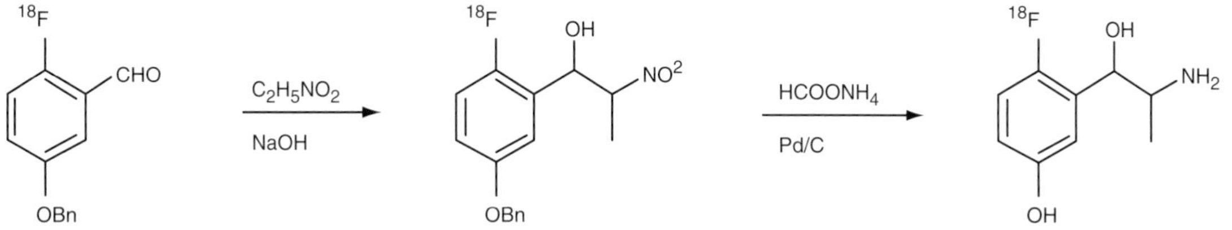

Fig. 5.19 N.c.a. radiosynthesis of 6-[^{18}F]fluorometaraminol via nucleophilic addition of nitroethane to 3-benzyloxy-6-[^{18}F] fluorobenzaldehyde

of n.c.a. 6-[^{18}F]fluoro-L-DOPA (see Fig. 5.18) [157, 158]. After reduction of the aldehyde group with sodium borhydride to the benzylalkohol function, the treatment with the corresponding hydrogen halide leads to the 2-[^{18}F]fluoro-4,5-dimethoxybenzyl halide. N.c.a. 6-[^{18}F]fluoro-L-DOPA was achieved from an enantioselective coupling with *N*-(diphenylmethylene) glycine *tert*-butyl ester, deprotection and semi-preparative HPLC in RCY of 25–30% with an enantiomeric excess of >95%.

Besides the conversion reactions of the aldehyde group, [^{18}F]fluorobenzaldehydes can also function as direct reaction partner according to organic carbonyl chemistry. Prominent representatives of such chemistry which have also been applied to ^{18}F-radiochemistry are the Wittig reaction [159], the Horner–Wadsworth–Emmons reaction [160] and the Knoevenagel condensation [161].

In addition, the electrophilic character of aldehydes also offers the possibility of nucleophilic additions.

[^{18}F]Fluorobenzaldehydes have also been applied in nucleophilic additions [162, 163]. In this way, the nucleophilic addition of nitroethane to n.c.a 3-benzyloxy-6-[^{18}F]fluorobenzaldehyde and following reductive deprotection led to n.c.a. 6-[^{18}F]fluorometaraminol in a diastereomeric mixture from which the stereoisomers could be separately isolated by two subsequent semi-preparative HPLC purifications (see Fig. 5.19) [164]. In the same manner, also the n.c.a 4-[^{18}F]fluorometaraminol was synthesised.

Similar to the carbonyl chemistry of [^{18}F]fluorobenzaldehydes, [^{18}F]fluoroacetophenones offer a broad range of synthetic possibilities [164, 165]. Moreover, secondary derived synthon/prosthetic group 4-[^{18}F] fluorophenacylbromide can be conjugated to peptides and proteins via alkylation reaction or thiol-coupling reactions [125, 134].

Another group of versatile synthons derive from the [^{18}F]fluoro-4-haloarenes which can be used in palladium(0)-catalysed C–C-bond formation reactions

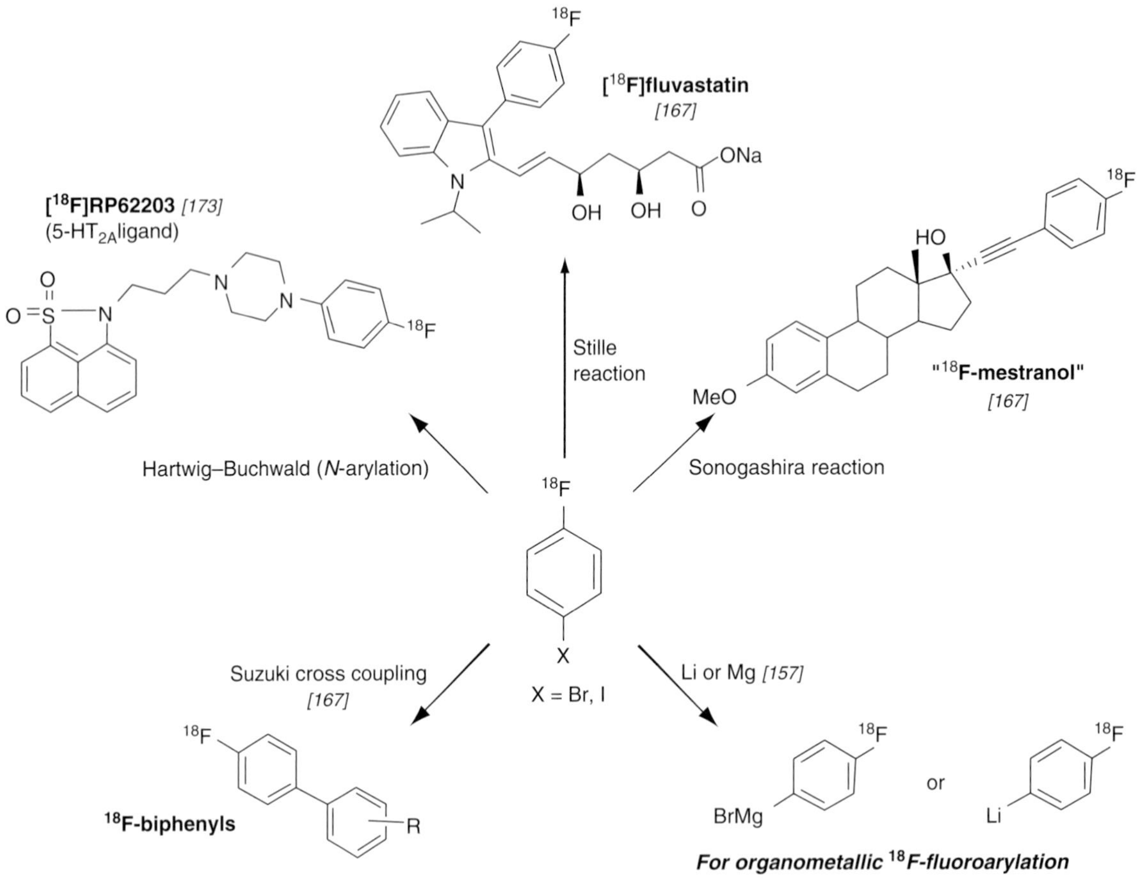

Fig. 5.20 N.c.a. 4-[^{18}F]fluorohalobenzenes as versatile synthons for palladium(0)-catalysed coupling reactions and their transformation into metalorganic reagents for ^{18}F-fluoroarylation reaction

such as the Stille reaction [166–170], the Sonogashira reaction [171] and Suzuki cross-coupling reactions [172] (see Fig. 5.20). Furthermore, 4-bromo and 4-iodo-[^{18}F]fluorobenzenes have been used in palladium-mediated N-arylation reactions, also referred to as Hartwig-Buchwald reactions [173, 174]. In addition, n.c.a. [^{18}F]fluoro-4-haloarenes can also be easily transferred into reactive species such as Grignard reagents or into 4-[^{18}F]fluorophenyl lithium which can be employed in various metalorganic coupling reactions [175].

Due to their broad applicability, [^{18}F]fluorohalobenzenes and their secondary derived ^{18}F-labelling synthons have become more and more attractive. In the past decade, several methods for an efficient preparation of [^{18}F]fluorohaloarenes have been developed and make this class of ^{18}F-labelled synthons readily available [105, 166, 176–179].

In addition to the most widely used ^{18}F-labelling synthons [^{18}F]fluorobenzaldehydes, [^{18}F]fluorobenzyl halides and [^{18}F]fluorohalobenzenes, further primary and secondary ^{18}F-aryls have been developed and proven to be useful for ^{18}F-labelling via built-up radiosynthesis. Accordingly, n.c.a. 4-cyano-1-[^{18}F]fluorobenzene or 4-[^{18}F]fluorobenzonitrile was employed for built-up radiosyntheses of several ^{18}F-butyrophenone neuroleptics [180]. On the other hand, it can also be transferred into the secondary ^{18}F-labelling synthon n.c.a. 4-[^{18}F]fluorobenzyl amine which can be used as prosthetic group [130, 132] or further converted into N-4-[^{18}F]fluorobenzyl-α-bromoacetamide as prosthetic group for the ^{18}F-labelling of oligonucleotides [129]. More in a sense of a prosthetic group n.c.a. 4-[^{18}F]fluorobenzyl amine was recently used for the ^{18}F-labelling of the first ^{18}F-labelled folic acid derivatives [132].

N.c.a. [^{18}F]fluoronitrobenzenes, which is available from high-yielding ^{18}F-labelling of the appropriate dinitrobenzene precursors, can be easily reduced to the corresponding [^{18}F]fluoroanilines by the use of common reducing agents such as NaBH$_4$, SnCl$_2$, N$_2$H$_2$/Pd, H$_2$/Pd-C, BH$_3$ or LiAlH$_4$ [181]. N.c.a. [^{18}F]fluoroanilines have been employed for the ^{18}F-labelling of several anilinoquinazolines as epidermal growth factor receptor (EGFR) ligands [183–185] as well as for fluorophenylureas [183]. A subsequent treatment of the 4-[^{18}F]fluoroaniline with nitrites leads to the 4-[^{18}F]fluorophenyldiazonium derivative which was used for the preparation of ^{18}F-labelled 5-HT$_2$ receptor ligands [182].

Since various biologically active compounds bear a 4-fluorophenoxy moiety [186], the secondary synthon n.c.a. 4-[^{18}F]fluorophenol is of great interest. The first radiosynthesis of this versatile synthon was based on a hydrolysis of the 4-[^{18}F]fluorophenyldiazonium salt [187]. In recent years, new synthetic strategies towards 4-[^{18}F]fluorophenol and several improvements of the radiosyntheses have made 4-[^{18}F]fluorophenol readily available for built-up radiosyntheses [188, 189]. Thus, it was applied for the radiosynthesis of a highly selective dopamine D$_4$ receptor ligand [190] as well as in a catalysed variant of the Ullmann ether coupling to provide 2-(4-[^{18}F]fluorophenoxy)-benzylamines (see Fig. 5.21) [190].

Finding the right ^{18}F-labelling strategies for new radiopharmaceuticals is generally limited by the target structures themselves. Although a variety of ^{18}F-fluorination methods have been developed, many

of them still do not provide the desirable broad applicability and call for very special conditions. Thus, there is still room for improvement and new development of ^{18}F-labelling methods. However, many ^{18}F-labelled PET radiopharmaceuticals from various classes of compounds have been prepared and some are routinely produced and employed in nuclear medicine practice.

5.2.3 Labelling Methods for Carbon-11

Besides fluorine-18, carbon-11 is the most commonly used positron emitter for PET radiopharmaceuticals. Although the short half-life of only 20.4 min of carbon-11 does not allow time-consuming radiosyntheses or the shipment of produced ^{11}C-labelled radiopharmaceuticals, several important ^{11}C-radiopharmaceuticals are routinely employed in the clinics.

Similar to the requirements for fluorine-18 productions, the production of carbon-11 can be facilitated with small medical cyclotrons using protons in an energy range of $15 \rightarrow 7$ MeV. The ^{14}N(p,α)^{11}C nuclear reaction is applied as the general production method [191]. The reaction is carried out with ^{14}N-gas targets. Small portions of oxygen ($\leq 2\%$) added to the target gas cause [^{11}C]CO$_2$ formation and in case of hydrogen (5–10%) addition, [^{11}C]CH$_4$ is the final product form [192, 193].

Several further production routes are known for carbon-11, but generally, they are of much less

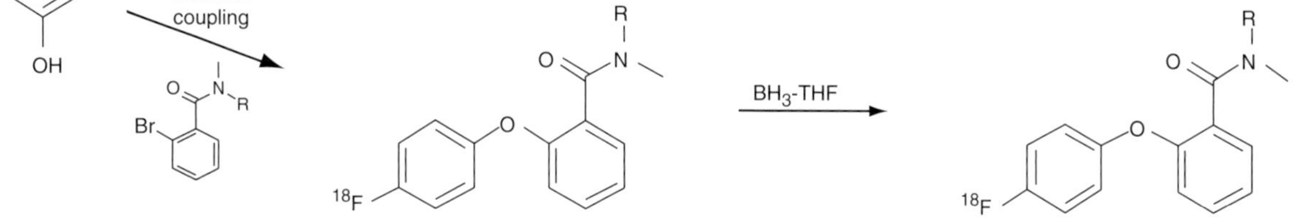

Fig. 5.21 N.c.a. 4-[^{18}F]fluorophenol as versatile synthon in built-up radiosyntheses

Fig. 5.22 Secondary and further ^{11}C-labelling synthons derived from the primary $[^{11}C]CO_2$

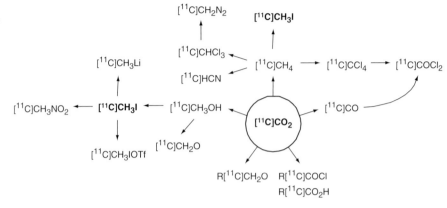

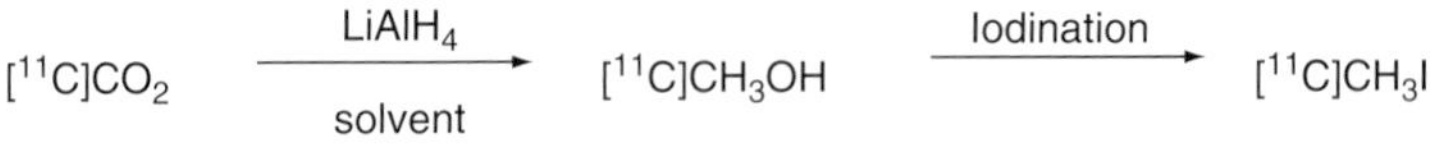

Fig. 5.23 Radiosynthesis of $[^{11}C]CH_3I$ according to the 'wet' method starting from primary $[^{11}C]CO_2$

$$[^{11}C]CO_2 \xrightarrow[\text{solvent}]{\text{LiAlH}_4} [^{11}C]CH_3OH \xrightarrow{\text{Iodination}} [^{11}C]CH_3I$$

importance than the ^{14}N(p,α)^{11}C reaction [16, 32, 194, 195]. Furthermore, using the ^{14}N(p,α)^{11}C nuclear reaction, carbon-11 can be obtained in high radiochemical yields with high specific activities.

^{11}C precursors: Regarding the two product forms and thus the two primary ^{11}C-labelling synthons $[^{11}C]CH_4$ and $[^{11}C]CO_2$, the latter is the most preferred labelling precursor. $[^{11}C]$carbon dioxide offers the possibility of direct ^{11}C-introductions into organic molecules. Accordingly, $[^{11}C]CO_2$ reacts with primary amino functions to form $[^{11}C]$ureas and $[^{11}C]$isocyanates [196]. Another direct ^{11}C-labelling possibility is given by the reaction with organometallic systems. Thus, the treatment of the Grignard reagents CH$_3$MgBr or CH$_3$MGCl with $[^{11}C]CO_2$ gives $[1-^{11}C]$acetate which is the most important ^{11}C-labelled radiopharmaceutical derived from direct ^{11}C-carboxylation [197, 198].

Even though the half-life of 20.4 min of carbon-11 allows only reactions and conversions with fast kinetics, most ^{11}C-labelling methods are based on secondary ^{11}C-labelling synthons derived from $[^{11}C]CO_2$ (see Fig. 5.22) [199]. Along with all the possible pathways, the ones using $[^{11}C]CH_3I$ are the preferred routes for ^{11}C-labelling. However, $[^{11}C]$ HCN and $[^{11}C]CO$ are also important ^{11}C-labelling synthons. Especially, $[^{11}C]CO$ has been proven for its applicability in palladium- or selenium-catalysed reactions [200].

'Wet method': The first efficient radiosynthesis for $[^{11}C]CH_3I$ was developed by Comar et al. in 1973 [201, 202]. This so-called 'wet' method is based on reduction of $[^{11}C]CO_2$ to $[^{11}C]CH_3OH$ by means of lithium aluminium hydride (LiAlH$_4$) in solvents such as ethyleneglycol dimethylether, tetrahydrofuran or diethylether. $[^{11}C]CH_3OH$ is then iodinated using hydroiodic acid or triphenylphosphite ethyliodide (see Fig. 5.23). Diphosphorous tetraiodide [203] and triphenylphosphine diiodide [204] can also be employed as iodination agents. Although the 'wet' method provides reliable and high radiochemical yields, it has one major drawback: the use of LiAlH$_4$. LiAlH$_4$ is a source of non-radioactive carbon dioxide which in turn brings in isotopic carrier carbon-12 and thus dramatically reduces the specific radioactivity of the $[^{11}C]CH_3I$ and the following products.

Dry method: More recently, a new approach to $[^{11}C]CH_3I$, the so-called 'gas phase' or 'dry' method was developed [205, 206]. Starting from $[^{11}C]CO_2$, hydrogen reduction in presence of a nickel catalyst provides $[^{11}C]CH_4$ which is passed through a heated glass tube (~720°C) with iodine vapour for iodination (see Fig. 5.24). The product $[^{11}C]CH_3I$ is trapped on a Porapak column and after completion of the iodination, $[^{11}C]CH_3I$ is released by heating and a stream of helium. The iodination process can be performed in a single pass reaction where the $[^{11}C]CH_4$ slowly passes the heated glass tube for iodination only once

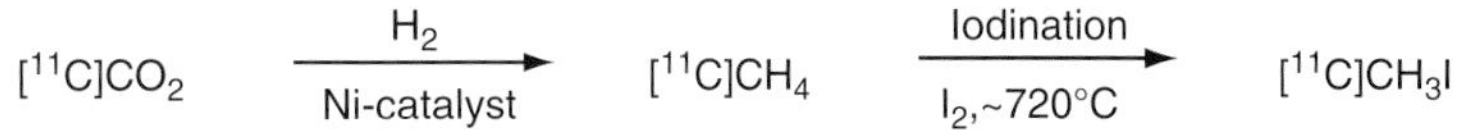

Fig. 5.24 Radiosynthesis of [^{11}C]CH$_3$I according to the 'dry' method starting from primary [^{11}C]CO$_2$

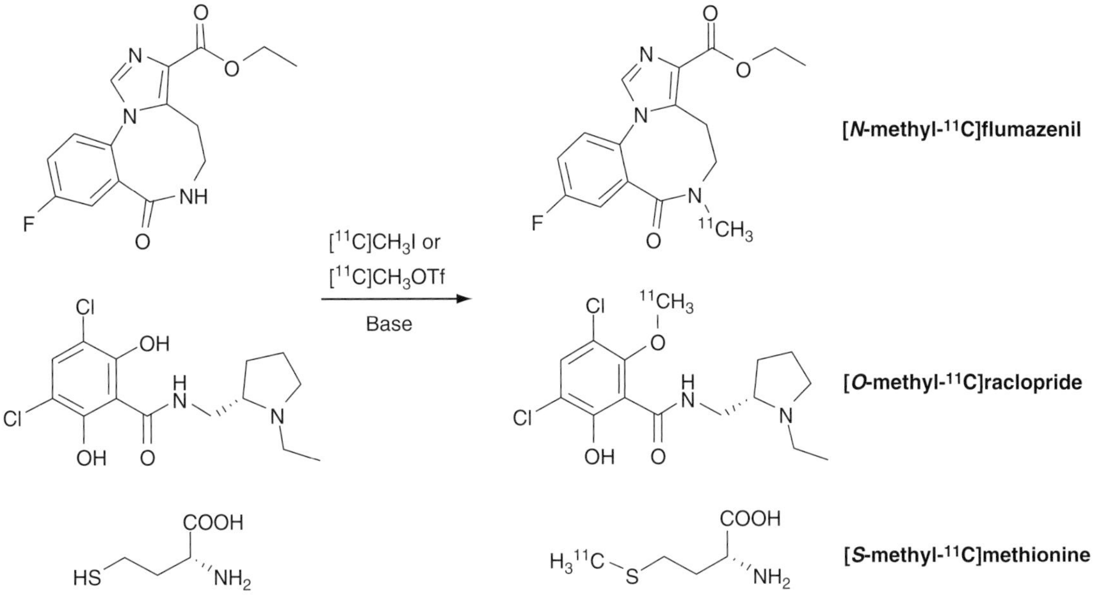

$$[^{11}C]CO_2 \xrightarrow[\text{Ni-catalyst}]{H_2} [^{11}C]CH_4 \xrightarrow[I_2, \sim 720°C]{\text{Iodination}} [^{11}C]CH_3I$$

Fig. 5.25 N-, O- and S-heteroatom ^{11}C-methylation reactions based on [^{11}C]CH$_3$I and/or [^{11}C]CH$_3$OTf

[207] or in a circulation process where the [^{11}C]CH$_4$ is circularly pumped through the iodination system until complete iodination [208].

Alternatively, the [^{11}C]CH$_4$ can be produced in situ in the target and used directly for the iodination process. This variant saves one reaction step and thus time. Furthermore, the in situ production of [^{11}C]CH$_4$ in the target generally provides higher specific radioactivity. To date, the highest reported specific radioactivity of [^{11}C]CH$_3$I was 4,700 GBq/μmol and was obtained from iodination of in situ produced [^{11}C]CH$_4$ in a single pass reaction [209, 210]. Due to that fact, an easier automation of the process and more convenient ongoing maintenance of the synthesis system, the 'dry' method almost superseded the 'wet' alternative for [^{11}C]CH$_3$I productions. Particularly, when high specific radioactivity is required as for PET studies of receptor systems in the CNS, the 'dry' process is the method of choice for the [^{11}C]CH$_3$I production.

In some cases, [^{11}C]CH$_3$I is not reactive enough for sufficient ^{11}C-methylation and a more reactive ^{11}C-methylation agent is needed [211]. Hence, [^{11}C]CH$_3$I can be converted to the more reactive [^{11}C]CH$_3$OTf by means of silver triflate at elevated temperatures. The ^{11}C-methylation with [^{11}C]CH$_3$OTf generally offers higher RCY in reduced reaction times and at lower temperatures in comparison to the [^{11}C]CH$_3$I methylation as it has already been demonstrated for several important ^{11}C-labelled PET radiopharmaceuticals [212–215].

Generally, ^{11}C-labelling via methylation is performed as N-, O- or S-heteroatom ^{11}C-methylation using the desmethyl precursors. Accordingly, the routinely used ^{11}C-labelled PET radiopharmaceuticals [N-methyl-^{11}C]flumazenil [210, 216, 217], [O-methyl-^{11}C]raclopride [218, 219] or L-[S-methyl-^{11}C] methionine [203, 220] are prepared via N-, O- or S-^{11}C-methylation, respectively (see Fig. 5.25).

Heteroatom ^{11}C-methylation reactions are usually carried out in solvents such as dimethylformamide, dimethylsulfoxide or acetonitrile. The ^{11}C-methylation agents is directly transferred into the solution which contains the desmethyl precursor and mostly a base such as sodium hydroxide, sodium hydride, potassium carbonate or tetrabutylammonium hydroxide. ^{11}C-

Methylations are normally completed within 10 min under elevated temperatures.

Solid phase: Over the years, the basic reaction conditions have not been changed so much, but several interesting and innovative technical improvements have been developed. As a consequence, most of the radiosyntheses of the routinely employed ^{11}C-labelled PET radiopharmaceuticals can be performed on solid-phase. As resin or solid phase material, commercially available C-18 solid-phase-extraction (SPE) cartridges can be applied. The cartridges are loaded with precursor, base and small amounts of solvent and the ^{11}C-methylation agent is passed through the cartridge by a gentle stream of nitrogen or helium. The reactions are normally efficient at ambient temperature and completed after short reaction times. The ^{11}C-labelled product is eluted from the cartridge with an appropriate solvent and often it is directly eluted into a loop of the HPLC system for the subsequent purification. For example, the 5-HT$_{1A}$ antagonist ^{11}C]WAY 100635 have been prepared and isolated within 25 min synthesis time in good yields of ~40% (related to ^{11}C]CH$_3$I, not decay corrected) [221]. Several important ^{11}C-labelled PET radiopharmaceuticals have also shown applicability for solid-phase-supported radiosynthesis [222–224].

Loop method: A further development of the solid-phase supported radiosyntheses is the so-called loop method. A conventional HPLC loop is coated with a film of the precursor solution and the ^{11}C-methylation agent is passed through by a gentle stream of nitrogen or helium. Subsequently, the loop content is washed out and simultaneously injected into the HPLC system. The method saves reaction time and reduces the technical assembly to a bare minimum. A variety of ^{11}C-labelled radiopharmaceuticals can be prepared by this convenient and fast method [225–229].

Another technical advancement which has recently entered the PET radiochemistry field is the microfluidic radiosyntheses systems. The systems are based on continuous-flow microreactors and use only micro- or nanolitre volumes. Some systems have been developed so far (see Sect. 5.2) and have already been successfully applied for ^{11}C-labelling of several carboxylic acid esters [230].

[11]C–C bond reactions: [11]C]CH$_3$I can also be applied in ^{11}C–C bond formation reactions. Due to the short half-life, the most limiting factor is the reaction/synthesis time of such ^{11}C–C bond formations. Nonetheless, there are several examples of C–C bond formations applied in ^{11}C-labelling using ^{11}C]CH$_3$I. Some examples can be found for the use of ^{11}C]CH$_3$I in Wittig reactions as its corresponding triphenylphosphorane ^{11}C]CH$_2$PPh$_3$ [231] or triphenylarsonium ^{11}C]CH$_2$ArPh$_3$ [232]. Most examples of various ^{11}C–C bond formation reactions can be found for ^{11}C-labelled amino acids using methods like enzymatic ^{11}C–C bond formations [233, 234] or enantioselective ^{11}C–C bond formations based on Schiff-base Ni-complexes as chiral auxiliaries [235, 236]. Furthermore, such multi-step radiosyntheses of ^{11}C–C bond formations towards ^{11}C-labelled amino acids have been shown to be transferable into automated synthesis systems [237]. However, besides amino acids, also several other pharmacologically relevant substances have been ^{11}C-labelled by C–C bond formations [238–243].

Other approaches for ^{11}C–C bond formations are palladium-supported cross-coupling reactions which have been developed for various ^{11}C-labelled radiopharmaceuticals. The most prominent representatives of these reaction type are the Stille reaction [244–247], the Suzuki cross coupling reaction [245, 247, 248] and the Sonogashira reaction [248, 249]. The Stille reaction is the most intensively employed variant of palladium-catalysed ^{11}C–C bond formations (see Fig. 5.26)

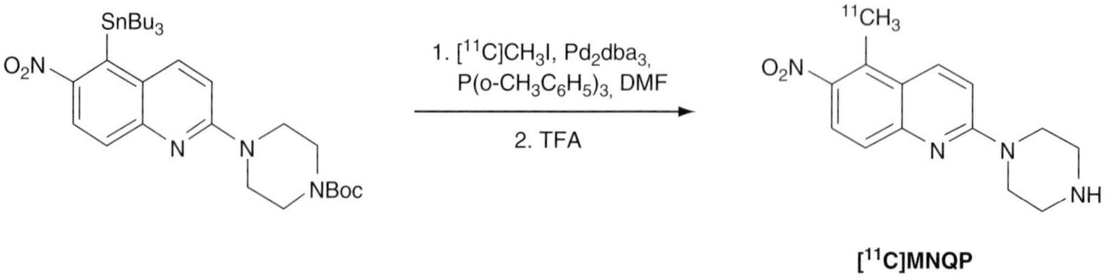

Fig. 5.26 Radiosynthesis of the serotonin transporter ligand 5-^{11}C]methyl-6-nitroquipazine (^{11}C]MNQP) using ^{11}C]CH$_3$I in a palladium-catalysed Stille reaction

and has proven its applicability for many ^{11}C-labelled PET radiopharmaceuticals [245–248, 250–254].

Most ^{11}C-labelling procedures are clearly based on [^{11}C]CH$_3$I as the most versatile ^{11}C-labelling synthon or precursor. The most convenient methods are the very fast N-, O- and S-heteroatom ^{11}C-methylation reactions which can be accomplished even with simple technical equipment such as a conventional HPLC loop in case of a [^{11}C]CH$_3$I loop reaction. Furthermore, also multi-step radiosyntheses like ^{11}C–C bond formations have been proven as useful ^{11}C-labelling strategy. Particularly, the palladium-promoted ^{11}C–C bond formations have broadened the applicability of ^{11}C-labelling towards PET radiopharmaceuticals.

5.2.4 Fast Reactions for Oxygen-15 and Nitrogen-13

The half-lives of 2 and 10 min of the extremely short-lived positron emitter oxygen-15 and nitrogen-13, respectively, allow only very fast conversions without time-consuming labelling procedures. Moreover, in PET imaging using ^{15}O- or ^{13}N-labelled radiopharmaceuticals, only simple physiological processes with very fast kinetics such as perfusion or blood flow can be studied.

The extremely short half-life of oxygen-15 allows only very fast online reactions in terms of radiochemistry. A number of nuclear reactions exist for the production of oxygen-15, but the most commonly used method is the ^{14}N(d,n)^{15}O nuclear reaction [255]. The target material is aluminium and the target content is a mixture of nitrogen and 0.2–1.0% of oxygen. An example for such an online reaction is the preparation of the perfusion tracer [^{15}O]water. The target release is mixed with hydrogen and passed over a palladium/activated charcoal catalyst at 200°C to give [^{15}O]water [256, 257]. Another ^{15}O-labelled perfusion and blood flow tracer is n-[^{15}O]butanol [258]. In this case, a solid phase-supported (cartridge extraction) reaction of tri-n-butylborane and the target released c.a. [^{15}O]O$_2$ furnishes the n-[^{15}O]butanol. The radiosyntheses of ^{15}O-labelled PET radiopharmaceuticals are restricted to such fast online processes and the application of ^{15}O-tracers in PET imaging is limited to perfusion or blood flow studies.

The general production route to nitrogen-13 is the ^{16}O(p,α)^{13}N nuclear reaction [259]. The nitrogen-13 is

obtained in the form of ^{13}N-labelled nitrites and nitrates, which are subsequently reduced to [^{13}N] ammonia by titanium(III)chloride or Devarda's alloy in alkaline medium [260]. Another method uses additional ethanol in the target gas as radical scavenger to avoid nitrite and nitrate formation [261]. This method leads directly to [^{13}N]ammonia.

[^{13}N]NH$_3$ is a perfusion tracer and the most commonly used ^{13}N-labelled PET radiopharmaceutical in PET imaging. In addition to the direct clinical applications of [^{13}N]NH$_3$, there are a few examples of ^{13}N-labelled compounds which derive from [^{13}N]NH$_3$, but generally without clinical relevance. The L-[^{13}N] amino acids L-[^{13}N]LEU, L-[^{13}N]VAL and L-[^{13}N] GLU were ^{13}N-labelled via an enzyme-supported amino acid synthesis and used for investigations of their pharmacokinetics in the myocardium [262]. The half-life of 10 min of nitrogen-13 offers a little bit more flexibility than does oxygen-15, but its half-life is still unsuitable for extensive radiosyntheses.

5.2.5 Non-standard Positron Emitters

5.2.5.1 Labelling Using Radioiodine

From more than 30 radioactive isotopes of iodine, only iodine-120 and iodine-124 have suitable properties for use as PET radionuclides. However, the low abundance of positron emission (56% for ^{120}I and 22% for ^{124}I), their high positron energies (4.1 MeV for ^{120}I and 2.1 MeV for ^{124}I) and an extensive production route make them less attractive for routine PET imaging. Significantly more importance in nuclear medicine and general life science have iodine-123 (100% EC, 159 keV γ-line [main]) as SPECT nuclide, iodine-125 (100% EC, 35 keV γ-line [main]) for long-term in vitro studies and radioimmunoassays and the β^--emitter iodine-131 as nuclide in radiotherapy of thyroid gland and tumours. Because of the convenient longer half-life ($T_{1/2} = 8.02$ days), the well-detectable γ-line of 364 keV (85.5%) and the good availability, ^{131}I lends itself as model isotope for radiotracer development.

The main pathways for radioiodine labelling can be classified into four general procedures [10, 263–264]:

- Direct electrophilic radioiodination
- Electrophilic demetallation

- Non-isotopic exchange (nucleophilic labelling)
- Prosthetic group labelling (indirect method)

5.2.5.2 Direct Electrophilic Radioiodination

The direct electrophilic substitution is the most commonly used radioiodination method. A lot of various techniques are available, which lead to high RCY in uncomplicated labelling reactions and which can be often carried out at room temperature. Due to its high volatility, low reactivity and the need for carrier addition, molecular iodine (I_2) is excluded for the n.c.a. scale. These problems to achieve reactive electrophilic species are easily circumvented by an in situ oxidation of iodide, which is obtained straight from the target. The generally used oxidants are Chloramine-T (CAT; *para*-tosylchloramide sodium), Iodogen[TM] (1,3,4,6-tetrachloro-3α,6α-diphenylglycouril) and *N*-halogen-succinimides.

The exact chemical nature and oxidation state of the iodinating species are not fully clarified so far. In case of aqueous solutions with strong acidic conditions, a hypoiodite, and for neutral and alkaline conditions, an iodine-analogue of, for example, CAT are postulated [265]. Due to the insignificant differences in their redox potentials, the choice of the proper oxidant is depended on the reaction conditions and the character of the iodine substrate. CAT allows oxidations in homogeneous aqueous solutions, whereas Iodogen[TM] is insoluble in water and thus it is the proper substance for a heterogenic reaction route, which is advantageous for oxidation-sensitive precursors. In the group of *N*-halogensuccinimides *N*-chlorotetrafluoro-succinimide (NCTFS), *N*-chlorosuccinimide (NCS) and rarely *N*-bromosuccinimide (NBS) are applied for in situ oxidation [266, 267]. When using NCS in trifluoromethane sulphonic acid, even deactivated aromatic compounds can be labelled with radioiodine in acceptable RCY [268]. Besides these oxidants, conventional oxidising reagents are in use, such as hydrogen peroxide, respectively, peracids [269] and metal cations (Ag^+, Tl^{3+}, Pb^{4+} and Ce^{4+}) [270]. Rather unconventional, but also useful are enzymatic [271] or electrochemical [272] methods for oxidation. As a disadvantage, the electrophilic radioiodination may raise the problem of a regio-unselective attack, as a result of which isomeric derivatives may occur.

5.2.5.3 Electrophilic Demetallation

Contrary to the direct electrophilic procedure, the electrophilic demetallation provides an almost regiospecific radioiodination. Especially for automated syntheses, it offers simple purification and isolation of the radiotracer and is therefore the first choice. Nonetheless, the syntheses of the organometallic precursors may become complex and extensive [273]. Suitable precursors for demetallation radioiodine-labelling are organometallic compounds of thallium [274], boron [275], mercury [276] and particularly, the organometallics of the elements of the group IVb. Of these, an exceptional position is taken by the organotins, which show, many times, excellent RCY in very short reaction time (few minutes); generally the RCY increases with Si < Ge < Sn [277]. Currently, the radioiodo-destannylation is the most suitable radioiodination procedure and thus is the most commonly employed method.

5.2.5.4 Non-isotopic Exchange (Nucleophilic Labelling)

Another labelling procedure for regiospecific radioiodine introduction is the non-isotopic exchange. Non-isotopic exchange is generally Cu(I)-catalysed and is suitable for electron-rich as well as for electron-deficient aromatic molecules [278]. In case of iodine-for-bromine exchange, high specific activities are available. In Cu(I)-promoted reactions, the readiness of the displacement follows the nucleofugality of the halogens ($I^- > Br^- > Cl^-$). In the Cu(I)-mediated substitution mechanism, a quadratic-planar complex was suggested, including Cu(I) as coordinated central atom, whereby the activation energy for the substitution process is reduced and the iodine can be introduced [279]. In variations, the Cu(I)-salts are in situ synthesised by a mild reduction of Cu(II)-salts (reducing agent: ascorbic acid, bisulphite or Sn(II)-compounds). Hereby, Cu_2SO_4 is more applicable than the use of copper halides, because the formation of halogenated side products is excluded. One of the important advantages is the much easier precursor preparation and their high stability. Moreover, it is again a highly regiospecific labelling route for radioiodine. In comparison to the electrophilic radioiodination, disadvantages are relatively high reaction temperatures of up to 180°C and vastly longer reaction times up to hours. In given cases, the separation and isolation of the radiotracer provokes difficulties due to its chemical and physical similarities to the bromine precursor.

5.2.5.5 Prosthetic Group Labelling

If molecules are sensitive to oxidative reagents or functional groups for iodination are lacking, the above-mentioned direct radioiodination methods fail. As an alternative, small molecules can be radioiodinated as labelling synthons and subsequently coupled with the desired compound. This is principally the same procedure as for the ^{18}F-labelling via prosthetic groups (cf. Sect. 5.4.3.1).

The first approach on prosthetic groups for radioiodination was the so-called Bolton–Hunter reagent, N-succinimidyl-3-(4-hydroxyphenyl)propionate (SHPP), an activated ester as labelling synthon for proteins via coupling with a free amino function, normally of the amino acid lysine [280, 281]. It is still widely used for radioiodination of proteins and macromolecules; thus a ^{124}I-labelled VEGF antibody (VEGF = vascular endothelial growth factor) for measuring angiogenesis was recently radioiodinated via a derivative of the Bolton–Hunter reagent [282]. The Bolton–Hunter principle for radioiodination of proteins led to further developments of prosthetic groups such as methyl-p-hydroxybenzimidate (Wood reagent) which is an activated imidate ester and also a versatile and convenient radioiodination synthon [283]. In addition, aldehydes, isothiocyanates [284] and activated α-carbonyl halides [285] are further prosthetic groups for labelling via free amino functions.

In case of aldehydes, the radioiodo-tyramine-cellobiose is an important compound which, for example, was used for labelling monoclonal antibodies [286]. Several other coupling methods of prosthetic groups with functional groups of proteins or complex molecules are known. Another common example for suitable functions is the thiol group of cysteine, where appropriate prosthetic groups are malimide derivatives [287].

5.2.5.6 Labelling Using Radiobromine

In case of positron emitting radioisotopes of bromine, three nuclides are suitable for PET imaging, ^{75}Br

($T_{1/2}$ = 98 min, 75% β$^+$), ^{76}Br ($T_{1/2}$ = 16.2 h, 57% β$^+$) and ^{77}Br ($T_{1/2}$ = 57 h, 0.7% β$^+$). Among these nuclides, the most preferred one is bromine-76. It has a longer and more convenient half-life than bromine-75 and a much higher β$^+$-abundance than bromine-77. Bromine-77 is more attractive for radiotherapy than for PET imaging as it decays also by Auger electron-emission [288–291]. It has been demonstrated that bromine-77 is highly lethal when it is incorporated into DNA of mammalian cells [289].

In small medical cyclotrons, bromine-76 can be produced via the ^{76}Se(p,n)^{76}Br nuclear reaction using a Cu$_2$Se target. The bromine-76 is isolated from the target by a dry distillation process and usually trapped in alkaline solution [292]. In the same way as radioiodine, for electrophilic demetallation reactions (mostly destannylations), radiobromine can be easily oxidised in situ using oxidants such as CAT, NCS or simply hydrogen peroxide in combination with acetic acid. As an example, the proliferation marker [^{76}Br]bromofluorodeoxyuridine has been radiobrominated via in situ oxidation by CAT and electrophilic destannylation of the corresponding trimethyltin precursor [293–295]. An alternative radiobromination method is the nucleophilic non-isotopic exchange. Again the conditions of nucleophilic radioiodination reactions are transferable, thus Cu(II)-mediated exchange reactions are particularly suitable. According to this, a ^{76}Br-labelled derivative of epibatidine was synthesised for PET imaging studies of the nicotinic acetylcholine receptor system [296].

In general, radiobromine is less available than radioiodine, due to more complicated target work-up and isolation procedures. In the radiochemistry of radiobromine, methods from radioiodine labelling can often be directly adopted and the radiochemistry is more convenient to accomplish than fluorine-18 labelling. Predominantly, the electrophilic destannylation reactions are employed for radiobromination chemistry. However, a few ^{76}Br-labelled radiopharmaceuticals have been developed to date [294–301], but they have only little relevance in clinical PET imaging.

5.2.5.7 Complexes for Labelling with Metallic PET Radionuclides

Among the metallic positron emitters which are suitable for PET imaging, the production routes can be

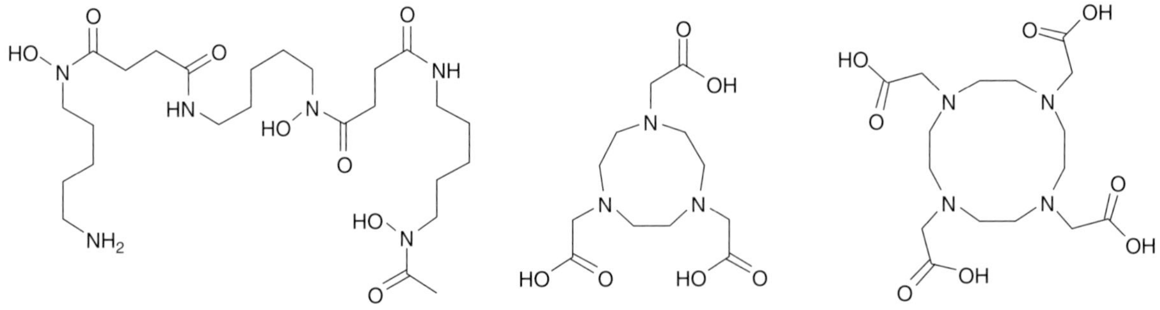

Desferrioxamine-B   **NOTA**   **DOTA**

Fig. 5.27 Chelator systems for labelling with metallic nuclides such as gallium-68

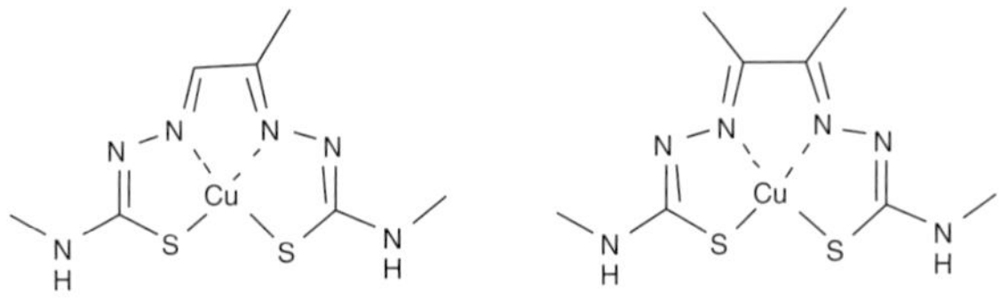

Cu-PTSM   **Cu-ATSM**

Fig. 5.28 Chelator systems for (radio)copper

divided into cyclotron-produced nuclides such as copper-64, titanium-45, yttrium-86 or zirconium-89 and generator-produced nuclides such as gallium-68, rubidium-82, or copper-62. The main advantage of the latter is clearly their availability which is not limited to facilities with an on-site cyclotron. Gallium-68 ($T_{1/2}$ = 68 min) is available from the ^{68}Ge-^{68}Ga generator. In a similar manner, rubidium-82 ($T_{1/2}$ = 1.3 min) can be obtained from the ^{82}Sr-^{82}Rb generator and copper-62 ($T_{1/2}$ = 10 min) from the ^{62}Zn-^{62}Cu generator. Especially, gallium-68 has more and more drawn the attention of radiopharmaceutical research, due to its favourable nuclear characteristics.

In terms of radiochemistry, labelling with metallic nuclides is based on chelatoring systems which are coupled to biomolecules or which have interesting biological properties themselves. Prominent examples of chelating systems for gallium-68 are DOTA (1,4,7,10-tetraazacyclododecane-N,N',N'',N'''-tetraacetic acid), NOTA (1,4,7-triazacyclononane-N,N',N''-triacetic acid) and DFO (desferrioxamine-B) (see Fig. 5.27). The latter was used as an octreotide conjugate forming a ^{68}Ga-labelled octreotide derivative for tumour imaging of somatostatin receptor-positive tumours [302]. Octreotide was also ^{68}Ga-labelled

using the DOTA and the NOTA system; however, of these, the most promising candidate is the DOTA conjugate [^{68}Ga-DOTA, Tyr^3]octreotide ([^{68}Ga]DOTA-TOC) [26, 303–305].

In a similar manner, radiocopper forms complexes such as Cu-PTSM (pyruvaldehyde-bis(N^4-methythiosemicarbazone)) or Cu-ATSM (diacetyl-bis(N^4-methylthiosemicarbazone)) (see Fig. 5.28) [306–309]. These Cu-complexes are both employed in the clinics. ^{62}Cu-labelled PTSM is used as perfusion and blood flow agent for heart and brain, whereas ^{62}Cu-labelled ATSM has been shown to accumulate in hypoxic tumour cells.

5.3 Conclusions

A variety of labelling methods has already been developed, but some methods are only suitable for certain radionuclides and they are often limited in their applicability. On the other hand, more and more molecules of biological or pharmacological interest are discovered and pose new challenges to radiolabelling and radiochemistry. Consequently, the development and improvement of new labelling strategies and methods for PET radiopharmaceuticals are of paramount interest. In particular, the expansion of the labelling methods for fluorine-18 as the most commonly used and preferred radionuclide in PET imaging are of great importance.

However, many PET radiopharmaceuticals have been developed and a few of them found the way into clinical routine. PET chemistry forms the basis of PET radiopharmaceuticals and PET imaging and will always be a major contributor to the success of the growing field of this molecular imaging modality.

References

1. Lawrence EO, Livingston MS (1932) The production of high speed light ions without the use of high voltages. Phys Rev 40:19–35
2. Herzog H (2001) In vivo functional imaging with SPECT and PET. Radiochim Acta 89:203–214
3. Ido T, Wan C-N, Casella V, Fowler JS, Wolf AP, Reivich M, Kuhl DE (1978) Labeled 2-deoxy-D-glucose analogs. ^{18}F-labeled 2-deoxy-2-fluoro-D-glucose, 2-deoxy-2-fluoro-D-mannose and ^{14}C-2-deoxy-2-fluoro-D-glucose. J Labeled Compd Radiopharm 14:175–182
4. Coleman RE (2000) FDG imaging. Nucl Med Biol 27:689–690
5. Reske SN, Kotzerke J (2001) FDG-PET for clinical use. Eur J Nucl Med 28:1707–1723
6. Gambhir SS, Czerni J, Schwimmer J, Silverman DHS, Coleman RE, Phelps ME (2001) A tabulated summary of FDG PET literature. J Nucl Med 42:1S–93S
7. Adam MJ (2002) Radiohalogenated carbohydrates for use in PET and SPECT. J Labelled Compd Radiopharm 45:167–180
8. Shiue C-Y, Welch MJ (2004) Update on PET radiopharmaceuticals: life beyond fluorodeoxyglucose. Radiol Clin N Am 42:1033–1053
9. Couturier O, Luxen A, Chatal J-F, Vuillez J-P, Rigo P, Hustinx R (2004) Fluorinated tracers for imaging cancer with positron emission tomography. Eur J Nucl Med Mol Imaging 31:1182–1206
10. Adam MJ, Wilbur DS (2005) Radiohalogens for imaging and therapy. Chem Soc Rev 34:153–163
11. Schubiger PA, Lehmann L, Friebe M (eds) (2007) PET chemistry – the driving force in molecular imaging. Springer, Berlin
12. Van Dongen GAMS, Visser GWM, Lub-De Hooge MN, Vries D, Perk LR (2007) Immuno-PET: a navigator in monoclonal antibody development and applications. Oncologist 12:1279–1390
13. Dehdashti F, Mintun MA, Lewis JS, Bradley J, Govindan R, Laforest R, Welch MJ, Siegel BA (2003) In vivo assessment of tumor hypoxia in lung cancer with ^{60}Cu-ATSM. Eur J Nucl Med Mol Imaging 30:844–850
14. Herzog H, Qaim SM, Tellmann L, Spellerberg S, Kruecker D, Coenen HH (2006) Assessment of the short-lived non-pure positron-emitting nuclide ^{120}I for PET imaging. Eur J Nucl Med Mol Imaging 33:1249–1257
15. Laforest R, Rowland DJ, Welch MJ (2002) MicroPET imaging with nonconventional isotopes. IEEE Trans Nucl Sci 49:2119–2126
16. Qaim SM (2001) Nuclear data relevant to the production and application of diagnostic radionuclides. Radiochim Acta 89:223–232
17. Magill J, Pfennig G, Galy J (2006) The Karlsruhe chart of the nuclides, 7th edn. ISBN 92-79-02175-3
18. Plenevaux A, Guillaume M, Brihaye C, Lemaire C, Cantineau R (1990) Chemical processing for production of no-carrier-added Selenium-73 from germanium and arsenic targets and synthesis of L-2-amino-4-([^{73}Se]methylseleno) butyric acid (L-[^{73}Se] selenomethionine). Appl Radiat Isot 41:829–835
19. Emert J, Blum T, Hamacher K, Coenen HH (2001) Alternative syntheses of [73, 75Se]selenoethers exemplified for homocysteine[73, 75Se]selenolactone. Radiochim Acta 89:863–866
20. Müller K, Faeh C, Diederich F (2007) Fluorine in pharmaceuticals: looking beyond intuition. Science 317:1881–1886
21. Hagmann WK (2008) The many roles for fluorine in medicinal chemistry. J Med Chem 51:4359–4369
22. Love WD, Romney RB, Burgh GE (1954) A comparison of the distribution of potassium and exchangeable rubidium in the organs of dog using rubidium 86. Cir Res 2:112–122
23. Selwyn AP, Allan RM, L'Abbate A, Horlock P, Camici P, Clark J, óBrien HA, Grant PM (1982) Relation between regional myocardial uptake of rubidium-82 and perfusion: absolute reduction of cation uptake in ischemia. Am J Cardiol 50:112–121
24. Gould KL (1991) PET perfusion imaging and nuclear cardiology. J Nucl Med 32:579–606
25. Machac J, Bacharach SL, Bateman TM, Bax JJ, Beanlands R, Bengel F, Bergmann SR, Brunken RC, Case J, Delbeke D, DiCarli MF, Garcia EV, Goldstein RA, Gropler RJ, Travin M, Patterson R, Schelbert HR (2006) Positron emission tomography myocardial perfusion and glucose metabolism imaging. J Nucl Cardiol 13:e121–e151
26. Hofmann M, Oei M, Boerner AR, Maecke H, Geworski L, Knapp WH, Krause T (2005) Comparison of Ga-68-DOTATOC and Ga-68-DOTANOC for radiopeptide PET. Nuklearmedizin 44:A58
27. Lasne MC, Perrio C, Rouden J, Barré L, Roeda D, Dollé F, Crouzel C (2002) Chemistry of β$^+$-emitting compounds based on Fluorine-18. Topics Curr Chem 222:201–258
28. Wester HJ (2003) ^{18}F-labeling chemistry and labeled compounds. In: Rösch F (ed) Handbook of nuclear chemistry. Kluwer, Dordrecht, pp 167–209
29. Coenen HH (2007) Fluorine-18 labelling methods: features and possibilities of basic reactions. In: Schubiger PA, Lehmann L, Friebe M (eds) PET chemistry – the driving force in molecular imaging. Springer, Berlin, pp 15–50
30. Ametamey SM, Honer M, Schubiber PA (2008) Molecular imaging with PET. Chem Rev 108:1501–1516

31. Miller PW, Long NJ, Vilar R, Gee AD (2008) Synthesis of 11C, 18F, 15O, and 13N radiolabels for positron emission tomography. Angew Chem Int Ed 47:8998–9033

32. Qaim SM, Clark JC, Crouzel C, Guillaume M, Helmeke HJ, Nebeling B, Pike VW, Stöcklin G (1993) PET radionuclide production. In: Stöcklin G, Pike VW (eds) Radiopharmaceuticals for positron emission tomography – methodological aspects. Kluwer, Dordrecht, pp 1–43

33. Guillaume M, Luxen A, Nebeling B, Argentini M, Clark JC, Pike VW (1991) Recommendations for Fluorine-18 production. Appl Radiat Isot 42:749–762

34. Namavari M, Bishop A, Satyamurthy N, Bida G, Barrio JR (1992) Regioselective radiofluorodestannylation with [^{18}F]F$_2$, and [^{18}F]CH$_3$COOF: a high yield synthesis of 6-[^{18}F]fluoro-L-dopa. Appl Radiat Isot 43:989–996

35. De Vries EFJ, Luurtsema G, Brüssermann M, Elsinga PH, Vaalburg W (1999) Fully automated synthesis module for the high yield one-pot preparation of 6-[^{18}F]fluoro-L-DOPA. Appl Radiat Isot 51:389–394

36. Wallach O (1886) Über das Verhalten einiger Diazo- und Diazoamidoverbindungen. Justus Liebig Ann Chem 235:242–255

37. Balz G, Schiemann G (1927) Über aromatische Fluorverbindungen, I.: Ein neues Verfahren zu ihrer Darstellung. Chem Ber 60:1186–1190

38. Atkins HL, Christmann DR, Fowler JS, Hauser W, Hoyte RM, Kloper JF, Lin SS, Wolfe AP (1972) Organic radiopharmaceuticals labelled with isotopes of short half-life. V. ^{18}F-labeled 5- and 6-fluorotryptophan. J Nucl Med 13:713–719

39. Tewson TJ, Welch MJ (1979) Preparation of fluorine-18 aryl fluorides: piperidyl triazenes as a source of diazonium salts. J Chem Soc Chem Commun 1149–1150

40. Hess E, Blessing G, Coenen HH, Qaim SM (2000) Improved target system for production of high purity [18F]fluorine via the 18O(p, n)18F reaction. Appl Radiat Isot 52:1431–1440

41. Bauer A, Zilles K, Matusch A, Holzmann C, Riess O, von Hörsten S (2005) Regional and subtype selective changes of neurotransmitter receptor density in a rat transgenic for the Huntington's disease mutation. J Neurochem 94:639–650

42. Ametamey SM, Honer M, Schubiger PA (2008) Molecular imaging with PET. Chem Rev 108:1501–1516

43. Fowler JS, Shiue CY, Wolf AP, Salvador AP, MacGregor RR (1982) Synthesis of ^{18}F-labeled acetyl hypofluoride for radiotracer synthesis. J Labelled Compd Radiopharm 19:1634–1635

44. Chirakal R, Firnau G, Schrobigen GJ, MacKay J, Garnett ES (1984) The synthesis of [^{18}F]xenon difluoride from [^{18}F] fluorine gas. Appl Radiat Isot 35:401–404

45. Constantinou M, Aigbirhio FI, Smith RG, Ramsden CA, Pike VW (2001) Xenon difluoride exchanges fluoride under mild conditions: a simple preparation of [^{18}F] xenon difluoride for PET and mechanistic studies. J Am Chem Soc 123:1780–1781

46. Satyamurthy N, Bida GT, Phelps ME, Barrio J (1990) N-[^{18}F]Fluoro-N-alkylsulfonamides: novel reagents for mild and regioselective radiofluorination. Appl Radiat Isot 41:733–738

47. Shiue CY, Salvadori AP, Wolf AP, Fowler JS, MacGregor RR (1982) A new improved synthesis of 2-deoxy-2-[^{18}F] fluoro-D-glucose from ^{18}F-labeled acetyl hypofluorite. J Nucl Med 23:899–903

48. Ehrenkaufer RE, Potocki JF, Jewett DM (1984) Simple synthesis of F-18-labeled 2-fluoro-2-deoxy-D-glucose. J Nucl Med 25:333–337

49. Levy S, David RE, Livni E (1982) A new method using anhydrous [^{18}F]fluoride to radiolabel 2- [^{18}F]fluoro-2-deoxy-D-glucose. J Nucl Med 23:918–922

50. Bida TG, Satyamurthy N, Barrio JR (1984) The synthesis of 2-[F-I8]fluoro-2-deoxy-D-glucose using glycals: a reexamination. J Nucl Med 25:1327–1334

51. Korytnyk W, Valentekovic-Horvat S (1980) Reactions of glycals with xenon fluoride: an improved synthesis of 2-deoxy- 2- fluoro-saccharides. Tetrahedron Lett 21: 1493–1496

52. Shiue C-Y, To K-C, Wolf AP (1983) A rapid synthesis of 2-deoxy-2-fluoro-D-glucose from xenon difluoride suitable for labelling with ^{18}F. J Label Comp Radiopharm 20:157–162

53. Sood S, Firnau G, Garnett ES (1983) Radiofluorination with xenon difluoride: a new high yield synthesis of [^{18}F] 2-fluoro-2-deoxy-D-glucose. J Nucl Med 24:718–721

54. Strauss LG, Conti PS (1991) The application of PET in clinical oncology. J Nucl Med 32:623–648

55. Dimitrakopoulou-Strauss A, Strauss LG, Schlag P, Hohenberger P, Mühler M, Oberdorfer F, van Kaick G (1998) Fluorine-18-fluorouracil to predict therapy response in liver metastases from colorectal carcinoma. J Nucl Med 39:1197–1202

56. Oberdorfer F, Hofmann E, Maier-Borst W (1989) Preparation of ^{18}F-labelled 5-fluorouracil of very high purity. J Labelled Compd Radiopharm 27:137–145

57. Firnau G, Chirakal R, Garnett ES (1984) Aromatic radiofluorination with [^{18}F]fluorine gas: 6-[^{18}F]fluoro-L-Dopa. J Nucl Med 25:1228–1233

58. Coenen HH, Franken F, Kling P, Stöcklin G (1988) Direct electrophilic radiofluorination of phenylalanine, tyrosine and dopa. Appl Radiat Isot 39:1243–1250

59. Chirakal R, Vasdev N, Schrobilgen GJ, Nahmias C (1999) Radiochemical and NMR spectroscopic investigation of the solvent effect on the electrophilic elemental fluorination of L-DOPA: synthesis of [^{18}F]5-Fluoro-L-DOPA. J Fluorine Chem 99:87

60. Adam MJ, Jivan S (1988) Synthesis and purification of L-6-[^{18}F]Fluorodopa. Appl Radiat Isot 39:1203–1206

61. Luxen A, Perlmutter M, Bida GT, Van Moffaert G, Cook JS, Satyamurthy N, Phelps ME, Barrio JR (1990) Remote, semiautomated production of 6-[^{18}F]fluoro-L-dopa for human studies with PET. Appl Radiat Isot 41:275–281

62. Szajek LP, Channing MA, Eckelman WC (1998) Automated synthesis 6-[^{18}F]fluoro-L-DOPA using polystyrene supports with 6-mercuric of modified bound DOPA precursors. Appl Radiat Isot 49:795–804

63. Dollé F, Demphel S, Hinnen F, Fournier D, Vaufrey F, Crouzel C (1998) 6-[^{18}F]Fluoro-L-DOPA by radiofluorodestannylation: a short and simple synthesis of a new labelling precursor. J Labelled Compd Radiopharm 41:105–114

64. Füchtner F, Angelberger P, Kvaternik H, Hammerschmidt F, Simovc P, Steinbach J (2002) Aspects of 6-[^{18}F]fluoro-L-DOPA preparation: precursor synthesis, preparative HPLC purification and determination of radiochemical purity. Nucl Med Biol 29:477–481

65. Bergman J, Solin O (1997) Fluorine-18-labeled fluorine gas for synthesis of tracer molecules. Nucl Med Biol 24:677–683

66. Coenen HH, Klatte B, Knöchel A, Schüller M, Stöcklin G (1986) Preparation of n.c.a. 17-[^{18}F]fluoroheptadecanoic acid in high yields via aminopolyether supported, nucleophilic fluorination. J Labelled Compd Radiopharm 23:455–467

67. Hamacher K, Coenen HH, Stöcklin G (1986) Efficient stereospecific synthesis of no-carrier-added 2-[^{18}F]-fluoro-2-deoxy-D-glucose using aminopolyether supported nucleophilic substitution. J Nucl Med 27:235–238

68. Alexoff D, Schlyer DJ, Wolf AP (1989) Recovery of [^{18}F] Fluoride from [^{18}O]water in an electrochemical cell. Appl Radiat Isot 40:1–6

69. Hamacher K, Hirschfelder T, Coenen HH (2002) Electrochemical cell for separation of [^{18}F]Fluoride from irradiated O-18-water and subsequent no-carrier-added nucleophilic Fluorination. Appl Radiat Isot 56:519–523

70. Kim DW, Choe YS, Chi DY (2003) A new nucleophilic fluorine-18 labeling method for aliphatic mesylates: reaction in ionic liquids shows tolerance for water. Nucl Med Biol 30:345–350

71. Kim HW, Jeong JM, Lee YS, Chi DY, Chung KH, Lee DS, Chung JK, Lee MC (2004) Rapid synthesis of [^{18}F]FDG without an evaporation step using an ionic liquid. Appl Radiat Isot 61:1241–1246

72. Kim DW, Ahn D-S, Oh Y-H, Lee S, Kil HS, Oh SJ, Lee SJ, Kim JS, Ryu JS, Moon DH, Chi SY (2006) A new class of S$_N$2 reactions catalyzed by protic solvents: facile fluorination for isotopic labeling of diagnostic molecules. J Am Chem Soc 128:16394–16397

73. Martin SJ, Eisenbarth JA, Wagner-Utermann U, Mier W, Henze M, Pritzkow H, Haberkorn U, Eisenhut M (2002) A new precursor for the radiosynthesis of [^{18}F]FLT. Nucl Med Biol 29:263–273

74. Kämäräinen E-L, Kyllönen T, Nihtilä O, Björk H, Solin O (2004) Preparation of fluorine-18-labelled fluoromisonidazole using two different synthesis methods. J Labelled Compd Radiopharm 47:37–45

75. Hamacher K, Coenen HH (2002) Effcient routine production of the ^{18}F-labelled amino acid O-(2-[^{18}F]fluoroethyl)-L-tyrosine. Appl Radiat Isot 57:205–212

76. Krasikova RN, Kuznetsova OF, Fedorova OS, Maleev VI, Saveleva VM, Belokon YN (2008) No carrier added synthesis of O-(2′-[^{18}F]fluoroethyl)-l-tyrosine via a novel type of chiral enantiomerically pure precursor, Ni^{II} complex of a (S)-tyrosine Schiff base. Bioorg Med Chem 16:4994–5003

77. DeGrado TR, Baldwin SW, Wang S, Orr MD, Liao RP, Friedman HS, Reiman R, Price DT, Coleman RE (2001) Synthesis and evaluation of ^{18}F-labeled choline analogs as oncologic PET tracers. J Nucl Med 42:1805–1814

78. Angeli G, Speranza M, Wolf AP, Shiue CY, Fowler JS, Watanabe M (1984) New developments in the synthesis of no-carrier-added (nca) ^{18}F-labeled aryl fluorides using the nucleophilic aromatic substitution reaction. J Labelled Compd Radiopharm 21:1223–1225

79. Hamacher K, Hamkens W (1995) Remote controlled one-step production of ^{18}F-labeled butyrophenone neuroleptics exemplified by the synthesis of n.c.a. [^{18}F]N-methylspiperone. Appl Radiat Isot 46:911–916

80. Katsifis A, Hamacher K, Schnittler J, Stöcklin G (1993) Optimization studies concerning the direct nucleophilic fluorination of butyrophenone neuroleptics. Appl Radiat Isot 44:1015–1020

81. Lemaire C, Cantineau R, Guillaume M, Plenevaux A, Christiaens L (1991) Fluorine-18-altanserin: a radioligand for the study of serotonin receptors with PET: radiolabeling and in vivo biologic behavior in rats. J Nucl Med 32:2266–2272

82. Shiue C-Y, Shiue GG, Mozley D, Kung M-P, Zhuang Z-P, Kim H-J, Kung HF (1997) p-[^{18}F]-MPPF: a potential radioligand for PET studies of 5-HT$_{1A}$ receptors in humans. Synapse 25:147–154

83. Le Bars D, Lemaire C, Ginovart N, Plenevaux A, Aerts J, Brihaye C, Hassoun W, Leviel V, Mekhsian P, Weissmann D, Pujol JF, Luxen A, Comar D (1998) High yield radiosynthesis and preliminary in vivo evaluation of p-[^{18}F] MPPF, a fluoro analog of WAY-100635. Nucl Med Biol 25:343–350

84. Irie T, Fukushi K, Ido T (1982) Synthesis of ^{18}F-6-flouropurine and ^{18}F-6-flouro-9-β-D-ribofuranosylpurine. Int J Appl Radiat Isot 33:445–448

85. Knust EJ, Müller-Platz C, Schüller M (1982) Synthesis, quality control and tissue distribution of 2-[^{18}F]-nicotinic acid diethylamide, a potential agent for regional cerebral function studies. J Radioanal Chem 74:283–291

86. Dollé F (2005) Fluorine-18-labelled fluoropyridines: advances in radiopharmaceutical design. Curr Pharm Des 11:3221–3235

87. Horti A, Ravert HT, London ED, Dannals RF (1996) Synthesis of a radiotracer for studying nicotinic acetylcholine receptors: (+/−)-exo-2-(2-[^{18}F]fluoro-5-pyridyl)-7-azabicyclo[2.2.1]heptane. J Labelled Compd Radiopharm 38:355–365

88. Ding Y-S, Liang F, Fowler JS, Kuhar MJ, Carroll FI (1997) Synthesis of [^{18}F]norchlorofluoroepibatidine and its N-methyl derivative: new PET ligands for mapping nicotinic acetylcholine receptors. J Labelled Compd Radiopharm 39:827–832

89. Dolci L, Dollé F, Valette H, Vaufrey F, Fuseau C, Bottlaender M, Crouzel C (1999) Synthesis of a fluorine-18 labeled derivative of epibatidine for in vivo nicotinic acetylcholine receptor PET imaging. Bioorg Med Chem 7:467–479

90. Horti A, Scheffel U, Stathis M, Finley P, Ravert HT, London ED, Dannals RF (1997) Fluorine-18-FPH for PET imaging of nicotinic acetylcholine receptors. J Nucl Med 38:1260–1265

91. Dolle F, Valette H, Bottlaender M, Hinnen F, Vaufrey F, Guenther I, Crouzel C (1998) Synthesis of 2-[^{18}F]fluoro-3-[2(S)-2-azetidinylmethoxy]pyridine, a highly potent radioligand for in vivo imaging central nicotinic acetylcholine receptors. J Labelled Compd Radiopharm 41:451–463

92. Ding Y-S, Liu N, Wang T, Marecek J, Garza V, Ojima I, Fowler JS (2000) Synthesis and evaluation of 6-[^{18}F]

fluoro-3-(2(S)-azetidinylmethoxy)pyridine as a PET tracer for nicotinic acetylcholine receptors. Nucl Med Biol 27:381–389

93. Beer H-F, Haeberli M, Ametamey S, Schubiger PA (1995) Comparison of two synthetic methods to obtain N-(2-aminoethyl)-5-[^{18}F]fluoropyridine-2-carboxamide, a potential MAO-B imaging tracer for PET. J Labelled Compd Radiopharm 36:933–945

94. Moerlein SM, Perlmutter JS, Markham J, Welch MJ (1997) In vivo kinetics of [^{18}F](N-Methyl)benperidol: a novel PET tracer for assessment of dopaminergic D2-like receptor binding. J Cereb Blood Flow Metab 17:833–845

95. Ryzhikov NN, Seneca N, Krasikova RN, Gomzina NA, Shchukin E, Fedorova OS, Vassiliev DA, Gulyás B, Hall H, Savic I, Halldin C (2005) Preparation of highly specific radioactivity [^{18}F]flumazenil and its evaluation in cynomolgus monkey by positron emission tomography. Nucl Med Biol 32:109–116

96. Stone-Elander S, Elander N (2002) Microwave applications in radiolabelling with short-lived positron-emitting radionuclides. J Labelled Compd Radiopharm 45:715–746

97. Hwang D-R, Moerlein SM, Lang L, Welch MJ (1987) Application of microwave technology to the synthesis of short-lived radiopharmaceuticals. J Chem Soc Chem Commun 1799–1801

98. Stone-Elander S, Elander N (1993) Fast chemistry in microwave fields: nucleophilic ^{18}F-radiofluorinations of aromatic molecules. Appl Radiat Isot 44:889–893

99. Ding Y-S, Shiue C-Y, Fowler JS, Wolf AP, Plenevaux A (1990) No-carrier-added (NCA) aryl [^{18}F]fluorides via the nucleophilic aromatic substitution of electron-rich aromatic rings. J Fluorine Chem 48:189–206

100. Chakraborty PK, Kilbourn MR (1991) [^{18}F]Fluorination/decarbonylation: new route to aryl [^{18}F]fluorides. Appl Radiat Isot 42:1209–1213

101. Plenevaux A, Lemaire L, Palmer AJ, Damhaut P, Comar D (1992) Synthesis of non-activated ^{18}F-fluorinated aromatic compounds through nucleophilic substitution and decarboxylation reactions. Appl Radiat Isot 42:1035–1040

102. Reddy GN, Haeberli M, Beer H-F, Schubiger PA (1993) An improved synthesis of no-carrier-added (NCA) 6-[^{18}F]Fluoro-l-DOPA and its remote routine production for PET investigations of dopaminergic systems. Appl Radiat Isot 44:645–649

103. Hostetler ED, Jonson SD, Welch MJ, Katzenellenbogen JA (1999) Synthesis of 2-[^{18}F]fluoroestradiol, a potential diagnostic imaging agent for breast cancer: strategies to achieve nucleophilic substitution of an electron-rich aromatic ring with [^{18}F]F$^-$. J Org Chem 64:178–185

104. Pike VW, Aigbirhio FI (1995) Reactions of cyclotron-produced [^{18}F]fluoride with diaryliodonium salts – a novel single-step route to no-carrier-added [^{18}F]fluoroarenes. J Chem Soc Chem Commun 2215–2216

105. Ross TL, Ermert J, Hocke C, Coenen HH (2007) Nucleophilic ^{18}F-fluorination of heteroaromatic iodonium salts with no-carrier-added [^{18}F]fluoride. J Am Chem Soc 129:8018–8025

106. Wüst FR, Carlson KE, Katzenellenbogen JA (2003) Synthesis of novel arylpyrazolo corticosteroids as potential ligands for imaging brain glucocorticoid receptors. Steroids 68:177–191

107. Zhang MR, Kumata K, Suzuki K (2007) A practical route for synthesizing a PET ligand containing [^{18}F]fluorobenzene using reaction of diphenyliodonium salt with [^{18}F]F$^-$. Tetrahedron Lett 48:8632–8635

108. Okarvi SM (2001) Recent progress in fluorine-18 labelled peptide radiopharmaceuticals. Eur J Nuc Med 28:929–938

109. Wester H-J, Schottelius M (2007) Fluorine-18 labeling of peptides and proteins. In: Schubiger PA, Lehmann L, Friebe M (eds) PET chemistry – the driving force in molecular imaging. Springer, Berlin, pp 79–111

110. Dollé F (2007) [^{18}F]Fluoropyridines: from conventional radiotracers to labeling of macromolecules such as proteins and oligonuclides. In: Schubiger PA, Lehmann L, Friebe M (eds) PET chemistry – the driving force in molecular imaging. Springer, Berlin, pp 113–157

111. Müller-Platz CM, Kloster G, Legler G, Stöcklin G (1982) [^{18}F]fluoroacetate: an agent for introduction no-carrier-added Fluorine-18 into Urokinase without loss of biological activity. J Labelled Compd Radiopharm 19:1645–1646

112. Block D, Coenen HH, Stöcklin G (1988) N.c.a. ^{18}F-fluoroacylation via fluorocarboxylic acid esters. J Labelled Compd Radiopharm 25:185–200

113. Jacobson KA, Furlano DC, Kirk KL (1988) A prosthetic group for the rapid introduction of fluorine into peptides and functionalized drugs. J Fluor Chem 39:339–347

114. Guhlke S, Coenen HH, Stöcklin G (1994) Fluoroacylation agents based on small n.c.a. [^{18}F]fluorocarboxylic acids. Appl Radiat Isot 45:715–727

115. Guhlke S, Wester H-J, Burns C, Stöcklin G (1994) (2-[^{18}F]fluoropropionyl-(D)phe^1)-octreotide, a potential radiopharmaceutical for quantitative somatostatin receptor imaging with PET: synthesis, radiolabeling, in vitro validation and biodistribution in mice. Nucl Med Biol 21:819–825

116. Garg PK, Garg S, Zalutsky MR (1991) Fluorine-18 labeling of monoclonal antibodies and fragments with preservation of immunoreactivity. Bioconjugate Chem 2:44–49

117. Vaidyanathan G, Bigner DD, Zalutsky MR (1992) Fluorine-18 labeled monoclonal antibody fragments: a potential approach for combining radioimmunoscintigraphy and positron emission tomography. J Nucl Med 33:1535–1541

118. Vaidyanathan G, Zalutsky MR (1992) Labeling proteins with fluorine-18 using N-succinimidyl 4-[^{18}F]fluorobenzoate. Nucl Med Biol 19:275–281

119. Vaidyanathan G, Zalutsky MR (1994) Improved synthesis of N-succinimidyl-4-[^{18}F]fluorobenzoate and its application to the labeling of a monoclonal antibody fragment. Bioconjugate Chem 5:352–356

120. Lang L, Eckelman WC (1994) One-step synthesis of ^{18}F-labeled [^{18}F]-N-succinimidyl-4-(fluoromethyl)benzoate for protein labelling. Appl Radiat Isot 45:1155–1163

121. Wester H-J, Hamacher K, Stöcklin G (1996) A comparative study of n.c.a. Fluorine-18 labeling of proteins via acylation and photochemical conjugation. Nucl Med Biol 23:365–372

122. Lang L, Eckelman WC (1997) Labeling proteins at high specific activity using N-succinidyl 4-[^{18}F](fluoromethyl)benzoate. Appl Radiat Isot 48:169–173

123. Kilbourn MR, Dence CS, Welch MJ, Mathias CJ (1987) Fluorine-18 labeling of proteins. J Nucl Med 28:462–470

124. Block D, Coenen HH, Stöcklin G (1988) N.c.a. ^{18}F-fluor-oalkylation of H-Acidic compounds. J Labelled Compd Radiopharm 25:201–216

125. Glaser M, Karlsen H, Solbakken M, Arukwe J, Brady F, Luthra SK, Cuthbertson A (2004) ^{18}F-fluorothiols: a new approach to label peptides chemoselectively as potential tracers for positron emission tomography. Bioconjugate Chem 15:1447–1453

126. Shai Y, Kirk KL, Channing MA, Dunn BB, Lesniak MA, Eastman RC, Finn RD, Roth J, Jacobson KA (1989) Fluorine-18 labeled insulin: a prosthetic group methodology for incorporation of a positron emitter into peptides and proteins. Biochem 28:4801–4806

127. Dollé F, Hinnen F, Vaufrey F, Tavitian B, Crouzel C (1997) A general method for labeling oligodeoxynucleo-tides with ^{18}F for in vivo PET imaging. J Labelled Compd Radiopharm 39:319–330

128. Haradahira T, Hasegawa Y, Furuta K, Suzuki M, Wata-nabe Y, Suzuki K (1998) Synthesis of a F-18 labeled analog of antitumor prostaglandin delta 7-PGA1 methyl ester using p-^{18}F]fluorobenzylamine. Appl Radiat Isot 49:1551–1556

129. Jelinski M, Hamacher K, Coenen HH (2002) C-Terminal ^{18}F-fluoroethylamidation exemplified on [Gly-OH[9]] oxy-tocin. J Labelled Compd Radiopharm 45:217–229

130. Bettio A, Honer M, Müller C, Brühlmeier M, Müller U, Schibli R, Groehn V, Schubiger PA, Ametamey SM (2006) Synthesis and Preclinical evaluation of a folic acid derivative labeled with ^{18}F for PET Imaging of folate receptor-positive tumors. J Nucl Med 47:1153–1160

131. Shiue CY, Watanabe M, Wolf AP, Fowler JS, Salvadori P (1984) Application of the nucleophilic substitution reac-tion to the synthesis of No-carrier-added ^{18}F]fluoroben-zene and other ^{18}F-labeled aryl fluorides. J Labelled Compd Radiopharm 21:533–547

132. Downer JB, McCarthy TJ, Edwards WB, Anderson CJ, Welch MJ (1997) Reactivity of p-^{18}F]fluorophenacyl bro-mide for radiolabeling of proteins and peptides. Appl Radiat Isot 48:907–916

133. Poethko T, Schottelius M, Thumshirn G, Hersel U, Herz M, Henriksen G, Kessler H, Schwaiger M, Wester H-J (2004) Two-step methodology for high-yield routine radiohalogenation of peptides: ^{18}F-labeled RGD and octreotide analogs. J Nucl Med 45:892–902

134. Poethko T, Schottelius M, Thumshirn G, Herz M, Haubner R, Henriksen G, Kessler H, Schwaiger M, Wester H-J (2004) Chemoselective pre-conjugate radiohalogenation of unprotected mono- and multimeric peptides via oxime formation. Radiochim Acta 92:317–327

135. Lange CW, VanBrocklin HF, Taylor SE (2002) Photocon-jugation of 3-azido-5-nitrobenzyl-^{18}F]fluoride to an oli-gonucleotide aptamer. J Labelled Compd Radiopharm 45:257–268

136. Kolb HC, Finn MG, Sharpless KB (2001) Click chemistry: diverse chemical function from a few good reactions. Angew Chem Int Ed 40:2004–2021

137. Marik J, Sutcliffe JL (2006) Click for PET: rapid prepara-tion of [18F]fluoropeptides using CuI catalyzed 1, 3-dipo-lar cycloaddition. Tetrahedron Lett 47:6681–6684

138. Glaser M, Robins EG (2009) 'Click labelling' in PET radio-chemistry. J Labelled Compd Radiopharm 52:407–414

139. Ross TL (2010) Recent advances in Fluorine-18 radio-pharmaceuticals: the click chemistry approach applied to Fluorine-18. Curr Radiopharm 3:200–221

140. Ramenda T, Bergmann R, Wüst FR (2007) Synthesis of 18F-labelled neurotensin(8–13) via copper-mediated 1, 3-dipolar [3+2]cycloaddition reaction. Lett Drug Des Disc 4:279–285

141. Becaud J, Karramkam M, Mu L, Schubiger PA, Ametamey SM, Smits R, Koksch B, Graham K, Cyr JE, Dinkelborg L, Suelzle D, Stellfeld T, Brumby T, Lehmann L, Srinivasan A (2008) Development of new direct meth-ods for ^{18}F-labeling of peptides. J Labelled Compd Radio-pharm 50:S215

142. Ting R, Adam MJ, Ruth TJ, Perrin DM (2005) Arylfluor-oborates and alkylfluorosilicates as potential PET imaging agents: high-yielding aqueous biomolecular ^{18}F-labeling. J Am Chem Soc 127:13094–13095

143. Schirrmacher R, Bradtmöller G, Schirrmacher E, Thews O, Tillmanns J, Siessmeier T, Buchholz HG, Bartenstein P, Wängler B, Niemeyer CM, Jurkschat K (2006) ^{18}F-labeling of peptides by means of an organosi-licon-based fluoride acceptor. Angew Chem Int Ed 45:6047–6050

144. Schirrmacher E, Wängler B, Cypryk M, Bradtmöller G, Schäfer M, Eisenhut M, Jurkschat K, Schirrmacher R (2007) Synthesis of p-(Di-tert-butyl[18]F]fluorosilyl)benz-aldehyde (^{18}F]SiFA-A) with high specific activity by isotopic exchange: a convenient labeling synthon for the ^{18}F-labeling of N-amino-oxy derivatized peptides. Bio-conjugate Chem 18:2085–2089

145. Mu L, Höhne A, Schubiger PA, Ametamey SM, Graham K, Cyr JE, Dinkelborg L, Stellfeld T, Srinivasan A, Voigtmann U, Klar U (2008) Silicon-based building blocks for one-step ^{18}F-radiolabeling of peptides for PET imaging. Angew Chem Int Ed 47:4922–4925

146. Wüst FR (2007) Fluorine-18 labelling of small molecules: the use of ^{18}F-labeled aryl fluorides derived from no-carrier-added ^{18}F]fluoride as labeling precursors. In: Schubiger PA, Lehmann L, Friebe M (eds) PET chemistry – the driving force in molecular imaging. Springer, Berlin, pp 51–78

147. Wilson AA, Dannals RF, Ravert HT, Wagner HN (1990) Reductive amination of ^{18}F]fluorobenzaldehydes: radio-synthesis of 2-^{18}F]- and 4-^{18}F]fluorodexetimides. J Labelled Compd Radiopharm 28:1189–1199

148. Negash K, Morton TE, VanBrocklin HF (1997) ^{18}F] Fluorobenzyltrozamicol: an efficient synthetic approach. J Labe Compd Radiopharm 40:40–42

149. Mishani E, McCarthy TJ, Brodbeck R, Dence DS, Krause JE, Welch MJ (1997) Synthesis and evaluation of a fluo-rine-18 labeled NK-1 antagonist. J Labelled Compd Radiopharm 40:653–655

150. Lee SY, Choe YS, Kim YR, Paik JY, Choi BW, Kim SE (2004) Synthesis and evaluation of 5, 7-dihydro-3[2-[1-(4-[18F]fluorobenzyl]-4-piperidinyl]ethyl]-6H-pyrrolo[3, 2-f] -1, 2-benzisoxazol-6-ome for in vivo mapping of acetyl-cholinesterase. Nucl Med Commun 25:591–596

151. Mäding P, Füchtner F, Hilger CS, Halks-Miller M, Horuk R (2004) ^{18}F-labelling of a potent nonpeptide CCR1 antag-onist for the diagnosis of the Alzheimer's disease. J Labelled Compd Radiopharm 47:1053–1054

152. Ryu EK, Choe YS, Park EY, Pail EY, Kim YR, Lee KH, Choi Y, Kim SE, Kim BT (2005) Synthesis and evaluation of 2-[18F]fluoro-CP-118, 954 for the in vivo mapping of acetylcholinesterase. Nucl Med Biol 32:185–191

153. Hatano K, Ido T, Iwata R (1991) The Synthesis of *o*- and *p*-[^{18}F]fluorobenzyl bromides asn their application to the preparation of labelled neuroleptics. J Labelled Compd Radiopharm 29:373–380

154. Dence CS, John CS, Bowen WD, Welch MJ (1997) Synthesis and evaluation of [^{18}F] labelled benzamide: high affinity sigma receptor ligands for PET imaging. Nucl Med Biol 24:333–340

155. Mach RH, Elder ST, Morton TE, Nowak PA, Evora PH, Scripko JG, Luedtke RR, Unsworth CD, Filtz T, Rao AV, Molinoff PB, Ehrenkaufer RLE (1993) The use of 4[^{18}F]fluorobenzyl iodide (FBI) in PET radiotracer synthesis: model alkylation studies and its application in the design of dopamine D_1 and D_2 receptor-based imaging agents. Nucl Med Biol 20:777–794

156. Iwata R, Pascali C, Bogni A, Horvath G, Kovacs Z, Yanai K, Ido T (2000) A new, convenient method for the preparation of 4-[^{18}F]fluorobenzyl halides. Appl Radiat Isot 52:87–92

157. Lemaire C, Damhaut P, Plenevaux A, Comar D (1994) Enantioselective synthesis of 6-[Fluorine-18]-fluoro-L-Dopa from no-carrier-added Fluorine-18-fluoride. J Nucl Med 35:1996–2002

158. Lemaire C, Gillet S, Guillouet S, Plenevaux A, Aerts J, Luxen A (2004) Highly enantioselective synthesis of no-carrier-added 6-[^{18}F]fluoro-L-dopa by chiral phase-transfer alkylation. Eur J Org Chem 2899–2904

159. Piarraud A, Lasne MC, Barrè L, Vaugois JM, Lancelot JC (1993) Synthesis of no-carrier-added [^{18}F]GBR 12936 via Wittig reaction for use in adopamine reuptake site study. J Labelled Compd Radiopharm 32:253–254

160. Gerster S, Wüst FR, Pawelke B, Bergmann R, Pietzsch J (2005) Synthesis and biodistribution of a ^{18}F-labelled resveratrol derivative for small animal positron emission tomography (PET). Amino Acids 29:415–428

161. Lemaire C, Guillaume M, Christiaens L, Palmer AJ, Cantineau R (1987) A new route for the synthesis of [^{18}F]fluoroaromatic substituted amino acids: no-carrier-added *L-p*-[^{18}F]fluorophenylalanine. Appl Radiat Isot 38:1033–1038

162. Ding YS, Fowler JS, Gatley SJ, Dewey SL, Wolf AP (1991) Synthesis of high specific activity (+)- and (-)-6-[^{18}F]fluoronorepinephrine via the nucleophilic aromatic substitution reaction. J Med Chem 34:767–771

163. Langer O, Dolle F, Valette H, Halldin C, Vaufrey F, Fuseau C, Coulon C, Ottaviani M, Någren K, Bottlaender M, Maziere B, Crouzel C (2001) Synthesis of high-specific-radioactivity 4- and 6-[^{18}F]fluorometaraminol-PET tracers for the adrenergic nervous system of the heart. Bioorg Med Chem 9:677–694

164. Banks WR, Hwang DR, Borcher RD, Mantil JC (1993) Production optimization of a bifunctional fluorine-18-labelled radiopharmaceutical intermediate: fluorine-18-fluoroacetophenone. J Labelled Compd Radiopharm 32:101–103

165. Kochanny MJ, VanBrocklin HF, Kym PR, Carlson KE, O'Neil JP, Bonasera TA, Welch MJ, Katzenellenbogen JA (1993) Fluorine-18-labeled progestin ketals: synthesis and target tissue uptake selectivity of potential imaging agents for receptor-positive breast tumors. J Med Chem 36:1120–1127

166. Allain-Barbier L, Lasne MC, Perrio-Huard C, Moreau B, Barrè L (1998) Synthesis of 4-[^{18}F]Fluorophenyl-alkenes and -arenes via palladium-catalyzed coupling of 4-[^{18}F]Fluoroiodobenzene with vinyl and aryl tin reagents. Acta Chem Scand 52:480–489

167. Forngren T, Andersson Y, Lamm B, Långström B (1998) Synthesis of [4-^{18}F]-1-bromo-4-fluorobenzene and its use in palladium-promoted cross-coupling reactions with organostannanes. Acta Chem Scand 52:475–479

168. Marrière E, Rouden J, Tadino V, Lasne MC (2000) Synthesis of analogues of (-)-cytisine for in vivo studies of nicotinic receptors using positron emission tomography. Org Lett 2:1121–1124

169. Wüst FR, Kniess T (2004) Synthesis of ^{18}F-labelled nucleosides using Stille cross-coupling reactions with [4-^{18}F]fluoroiodobenzene. J Labelled Compd Radiopharm 47:457–468

170. Wüst FR, Höhne A, Metz P (2005) Synthesis of ^{18}F-labelled COX-2 inhibitors via Stille reaction with 4-[^{18}F]fluoroiodobenzene. Org Biomol Chem 3:503–507

171. Wüst FR, Kniess T (2003) Synthesis of 4-[^{18}F]fluoroiodobenzene and its applicationin the Sonogashira cross-coupling reaction with terminal alkynes. J Labelled Compd Radiopharm 46:699–713

172. Steiniger B, Wüst FR (2006) Synthesis of ^{18}F-labelled biphenyls via Suzuki cross-coupling with 4-[^{18}F]fluoroiodobenzene. J Labelled Compd Radiopharm 49:817–827

173. Marrière E, Chazalviel L, Dhilly M, Toutain J, Perrio C, Dauphin F, Lasne MC (1999) Synthesis of [^{18}F]RP 62203, a potent and selective serotonine 5-HT$_{2A}$ receptor antagonist and biological evaluation with ex-vivo autoradiography. J Labelled Compd Radiopharm 42:S69–S71

174. Wüst FR, Kniess T (2005) Synthesis of ^{18}F-labelled sigma-2 receptor ligands for positron emission tomograpy (PET) via *latN*-arylation with 4-[^{18}F]fluoroiodobenzene. J Labelled Compd Radiopharm 48:31–43

175. Ludwig T, Gail R, Coenen HH (2001) New ways to n.c.a. radiofluorinated aromatic compounds. Isotop Lab Compds 7:358–361

176. Gail R, Coenen HH (1994) A one step preparation of the n. c.a. fluorine-18-labelled synthons: 4-fluorobromo-benzene and 4-fluoroiodobenzene. Appl Radiat Isot 45:105–111

177. Gail R, Hocke C, Coenen HH (1997) Direct n.c.a. ^{18}F-fluorination of halo- and alkylarenes via corresponding diphenyliodonium salts. J Labelled Compd Radiopharm 40:50–52

178. Shah A, Pike VW, Widdowson DA (1998) The synthesis of [^{18}F]Fluoroarenes from the reaction of cyclotron-produced [^{18}F]fluoride ion with diaryliodonium salts. J Chem Soc Perkin Trans 1:2043–2046

179. Ermert J, Hocke C, Ludwig T, Gail R, Coenen HH (2004) Comparison of pathways to the versatile synthon of no-carrier-added 1-bromo-4-[^{18}F]fluorobenzene. J Labelled Compd Radiopharm 47:429–441

180. Shiue C-Y, Fowler JS, Wolf AP, Watanabe M, Arnett CD (1985) syntheses and specific activity determinations of

no-carrier-added fluorine-18-labeled neuroleptic drugs. J Nucl Med 26:181–186

181. Collins M, Lasne MC, Barre L (1992) Rapid synthesis of N, N′-disubstituted piperazines. Application to the preparation of no carrier added 1-(4-[18F]fluorophenyl)piperazine and of an [18F]-selective ligand of serotoninergic receptors (5HT2 antagonist). J Chem Soc Perkin Trans 1:3185–3188

182. VanBrocklin HF, O'Neil JP, Hom DL, Gibbs AR (2001) Synthesis of [18F]fluoroanilines: precursors to [18F]fluoroanilinoquilazolines. J Labelled Compd Radiopharm 44: S880–S882

183. Olma S, Ermert J, Coenen HH (2005) Preparation of n.c.a. [18F]fluorophenylureas. J Labelled Compd Radiopharm 48:S175

184. Vasdev N, Dorff PN, Gibbs AR, Nandanan E, Reid LM, O'Neil JP, VanBrocklin HF (2005) Synthesis of 6-acrylamido-4-(2-[18F]fluoroanilino)quinazoline: a prospective irreversible EGFR binding probe. J Labelled Compd Radiopharm 48:109–115

185. Seimbille Y, Phelps ME, Czernin J, Silverman DHS (2005) Fluorine-18 labeling of 6, 7-disubstituted anilinoquinazoline derivatives for positron emission tomography (PET) imaging of tyrosine kinase receptors: synthesis of 18F-Iressa and related molecular probes. J Labelled Compd Radiopharm 48:829–843

186. Kirk KL, Creveling CR (1984) The chemistry and biology of ring-fluorinated biogenic amines. Med Res Rev 4: 189–220

187. Barrè L, Barbier L, Lasne MC (1993) Investigation of possible routes to no-carrier-added 4-[18F]fluorophenol. Labelled Compd Radiopharm 35:167–168

188. Ludwig T, Ermert J, Coenen HH (2002) 4-[18F]fluoroarylalkylethers via an improved synthesis of n.c.a. 4-[18F] fluorophenol. Nucl Med Biol 29:255–262

189. Stoll T, Ermert J, Oya S, Kung HF, Coenen HH (2004) Application of n.c.a. 4-[18F]fluorophenol in diaryl ether syntheses of 2-(4-[18F]fluorophenoxy)-benzylamines. J Labelled Compd Radiopharm 47:443–455

190. Ludwig T, Ermert J, Coenen HH (2001) Synthesis of the dopamine-D4 receptor ligand 3-(4-[18F]fluorophenoxy) propyl-(2-(4-tolyloxy)ethyl)amine via optimised n.c.a. 4-[18F]fluorophenol. J Labelled Compd Radiopharm 44: S1–S3

191. Casella V, Christman DR, Ido T, Wolf AP (1978) Excitation-function for N-14 (p, alpha) C-11 reaction up to 15-MeV. Radiochim Acta 25:17–20

192. Buckley KR, Huser J, Jivan S, Chun KS, Ruth TJ (2000) 11C-methane production in small volume, high pressure gas targets. Radiochim Acta 88:201–205

193. Buckley KR, Jivan S, Ruth TJ (2004) Improved yields for the in situ production of [11C]CH4 using a niobium target chamber. Nucl Med Biol 31:825–827

194. Ferrieri RA, Wolf AP (1983) The chemistry of positron emitting nucleogenic (hot) atoms with regard to preparation of labelled compounds of practical utility. Radiochim Acta 34:69–83

195. Wolf AP, Redvanly CS (1977) Carbon-11 and radiopharmaceuticals. Appl Radiat Isot 28:29–48

196. Schirbel A, Holschbach MH, Coenen HH (1999) N.c.a. [11C]CO2 as a safe substitute for phosgene in the carbonylation of primary amines. J Labelled Compd Radiopharm 42:537–551

197. Pike VW, Horlock PL, Brown C, Clarck JC (1984) The remotely controlled preparation of a 11C-labelled radiopharmaceutical – [1-11C]acetate. Appl Radiat Isot 35:623–627

198. Kruijer PS, Ter Linden T, Mooij R, Visser FC, Herscheid JDM (1995) A practical method for the preparation of [11C]acetate. Appl Radiat Isot 46:317–321

199. Långström B, Kihlberg T, Bergstrom M, Antoni G, Bjorkman M, Forngren BH, Forngren T, Hartvig P, Markides K, Yngve U, Ogren M (1999) Compounds labelled with short-lived beta +-emitting radionuclides and some applications in life sciences. The importance of time as a parameter. Acta Chem Scand 53:651–669

200. Antoni G, Kihlberg T, Långström B (2003) 11C: labelling chemistry and labelled compounds. In: Vertes A, Nagy S, Klencsar Z (eds) Handbook of nuclear chemistry, vol 4, Radiochemistry and Radiopharmaceutical chemistry in life science. Kluwer, Dordrecht, pp 119–165

201. Comar D, Maziere M, Crouzel M (1973) Synthesis and metabolism of 11C-chlorpromazine methiodide. Radiopharm Labeled Compd 7:461–469

202. Långström B, Lunqvist H (1976) The preparation of [11C]methyl iodide and its use in the synthesis of [11C] methyl-L-methionine. Appl Radiat Isot 27:357–363

203. Oberdorfer F, Hanisch M, Helus F, Maier-Borst W (1985) A new procedure for the preparation of 11C-labelled methyl iodide. Appl Radiat Isot 36:435–438

204. Holschbach MH, Schüller M (1993) A new simple on-line method for the preparation of n.c.a. [11C]methyl iodide. Appl Radiat Isot 44:779–780

205. Larsen P, Ulin J, Dahlstrom K (1995) A new method for production of 11C-labelled methyl iodide from [11C]methane. J Labelled Compd Radiopharm 37:73–75

206. Link JM, Clark JC, Larsen P, Krohn KA (1995) Production of [11C]methyl iodide by reaction of [11C]CH4 with I2. J Labelled Compd Radiopharm 37:76–78

207. Link JM, Krohn KA, Clark JC (1997) Production of [11C] CH3I by single pass reaction of [11C]CH4 with I2. Nucl Med Biol 24:93–97

208. Larsen P, Ulin J, Dahlstrom K, Jensen M (1997) Synthesis of [11C]Iodomethane by iodination of [11C]methane. Appl Radiat Isot 48:153–157

209. Noguchi J, Suzuki K (2003) Automated synthesis of the ultra high specific activity of [11C]Ro15-4513 and its application in an extremely low concentration region to an ARG study. Nucl Med Biol 30:335–343

210. Zhang MR, Suzuki K (2005) Sources of carbon which decrease the specific activity of [11C]CH3I synthesized by the single pass I2 method. Appl Radiat Isot 62:447–450

211. Jewett DM (1992) A simple synthesis of [11C]methyl triflate. Appl Radiat Isot 43:1383–1385

212. Någren K, Müller L, Halldin C, Swahn CG, Lehikoinen P (1995) Improved synthesis of some commonly used PET radioligands by the use of [11C]methyl triflate. Nucl Med Biol 22:235–239

213. Någren K, Halldin C, Müller L, Swahn CG, Lehikoinen P (1995) Comparison of [11C]methyl triflate and [11C] methyl iodide in the synthesis of PET radioligands such as [11C]beta-CIT and [11C]beta-CFT. Nucl Med Biol 22:965–979

214. Lundkvist C, Sandell J, Någren K, Pike VW, Halldin C (1998) Improved synthesis of the PET radioligands [11C] FLB 457, [11C]MDL 100907 and [11C]β-CIT-FE, by the use of [11C]methyl triflate. J Labelled Compd Radiopharm 41:545–556

215. Någren K, Halldin C (1998) Methylation of amide and thiol functions with [11C]methyl triflate, as exemplied by [11C]NMSP, [11C]Flumazenil and [11C]Methionine. J Labelled Compd Radiopharm 41:831–841

216. Maziere M, Hantraye P, Prenant C, Sastre J, Comar D (1984) Synthesis of ethyl 8-fluoro-5, 6-dihydro5- [11C] methyl-6-oxo-4H-imidazo[1, 5-a] [1, 4]benzodiazepine-3-carboxylate (RO 15.1788–11C): a specific radioligand for the in vivo study of central benzodiazepine receptors by positron emission tomography. Appl Radiat Isot 35:973–976

217. Suzuki K, Inoue O, Hashimoto K, Yamasaki T, Kuchiki M, Tamate K (1985) Computer-controlled large scale production of high specific activity [11C]RO 15-1788 for PET studies of benzodiazepine receptors. Appl Radiat Isot 36:971–976

218. Farde L, Ehrin E, Eriksson L, Greitz T, Hall H, Hedstrom C-G, Litton J-E, Sedvall G (1985) Substituted benzamides as ligands for visualization of dopamine receptor binding in the human brain by positron emission tomography. Proc Natl Acad Sci USA 82:3863–3867

219. Farde L, Hall H, Ehrin E, Sedvall G (1986) Quantitative analysis of D_2 dopamine receptor binding in the living human brain by PET. Science 231:258–261

220. Långström B, Antoni G, Gullberg P, Halldin C, Malmborg P, Någren K, Rimland A, Svärd H (1987) Synthesis of L- and D-[methyl-11C]methionine. J Nucl Med 28:1037–1040

221. Wilson AA, DaSilva JN, Houle S (1996) Solid-phase synthesis of [11C]WAY 100635. J Labelled Compd Radiopharm 38:149–154

222. Iwata R, Pascali C, Yuasa M, Yanai K, Takahashi T, Ido T (1992) On-line [11C]methylation using [11C]methyl iodide for the automated preparation of 11C-radiopharmaceuticals. Appl Radiat Isot 43:1083–1088

223. Pascali C, Bogni A, Iwata R, Decise D, Crippa F, Bombardieri E (1999) High effciency preparation of L-[S-methyl-11C]methionine by on-column [11C]methylation on C18 Sep-Pak. J Labelled Compd Radiopharm 42:715–724

224. Pascali C, Bogni A, Iwata R, Cambie M, Bombardieri E (2000) [11C]Methylation on a C18 Sep-Pak cartridge: a convenient way to produce [N-methyl-11C]choline. J Labelled Compd Radiopharm 43:195–203

225. Watkins GL, Jewett DM, Mulholland GK, Kilbourn MR, Toorongian SA (1988) A captive solvent method for rapid N-[11C]methylation of secondary amides: application to the benzodiazepine, 4′-chlorodiazepam (RO5-4864). Appl Radiat Isot 39:441–444

226. Wilson AA, Garcia A, Jin L, Houle S (2000) Radiotracer synthesis from [11C]-iodomethane: a remarkable simple captive solvent method. Nucl Med Biol 27:529–532

227. Iwata R, Pascali C, Bogni A, Miyake Y, Yanai K, Ido T (2001) A simple loop method for the automated preparation of [11C]raclopride from [11C]methyl triflate. Appl Radiat Isot 55:17–22

228. Iwata R, Pascali C, Bogni A, Yanai K, Kato M, Ido T, Ishiwata K (2002) A combined loop-SPE method for the automated preparation of [11C]doxepin. J Labelled Compd Radiopharm 45:271–280

229. Studenov AR, Jivan S, Adam MJ, Ruth TJ, Buckley KR (2004) Studies of the mechanism of the in-loop synthesis of radiopharmaceuticals. Appl Radiat Isot 61:1195–1201

230. Lu S-Y, Watts P, Chin FT, Hong J, Musachio JL, Briard E, Pike VW (2004) Syntheses of 11C- and 18F-labeled carboxylic esters within a hydrodynamically-driven micro-reactor. Lab Chip 4:523–525

231. Kihlberg T, Gullberg P, Langström B (1990) [11C]Methylenetriphenylphosphorane, a new 11C precursor, used in a one-pot Wittig synthesis of [beta-11C]styrene. J Labelled Compd Radiopharm 28:1115–1120

232. Zessin J, Steinbach J, Johannsen B (1999) Synthesis of triphenylarsonium [11C]methylide, a new 11C-precursor. Application in the preparation of [2-11C]indole. J Labeled Compd Radiopharm 42:725–736

233. Bjurling P, Watanabe Y, Tokushige M, Oda T, Langström B (1989) Syntheses of beta-11C-labeled L-tryptophan and 5-hydroxy-L-tryptophan using a multi-enzymatic reaction route. J Chem Soc Perkin Trans 1:1331–1334

234. Ikemoto M, Sasaki M, Haradahira T, Yada T, Omura H, Furuya Y, Watanabe Y, Suzuki K (1999) Synthesis of L-[beta-11C]amino acids using immobilized enzymes. Appl Radiat Isot 50:715–721

235. Fasth KJ, Langström B (1990) Asymmetric synthesis of L-[beta-11C]amino acids using a chiral nickel-complex of the Schiff-base of (S)-O-[(N-benzylprolyl)-amino]benzophenone and glycine. Acta Chem Scand 44:720–725

236. Mosevich IK, Kuznetsova OF, Vasil'ev DA, Anichkov AA, Korsakov MV (1999) Automated synthesis of [3-11C]-L-alanine involving asymmetric alkylation with (CH3I)-11C of the nickel complex of the Schiff base derived from glycine and (S)-2-N-(N-benzylprolyl)amino-benzophenone. Radiochemistry 41:273–280

237. Harada N, Nishiyama S, Sato K, Tsukada H (2000) Development of an automated synthesis apparatus for L-[3-11C] labeled aromatic amino acids. Appl Radiat Isot 52: 845–850

238. Kihlberg T, Langström B (1994) Cuprate-mediated 11C-C coupling reactions using Grignard-reagents and 11C alkyl iodides. Acta Chem Scand 48:570–577

239. Hostetler ED, Fallis S, McCarthy TJ, Welch MJ, Katzenellenbogen JA (1998) Improved methods for the synthesis of [omega-11C]palmitic acid. J Org Chem 63: 1348–1351

240. Wuest F, Dence CS, McCarthy TJ, Welch MJ (2000) A new approach for the synthesis of [11C]-labeled fatty acids. J Labelled Compd Radiopharm 43:1289–1300

241. Conti PS, Alauddin MM, Fissekis JR, Schmall B, Watanabe KA (1995) Synthesis of 2′-fluoro-5-[11C]-methyl-1-beta-D-arabinofuranosyluracil ([11C]-FMAU) – a potential nucleoside analog for in-vivo study of cellular proliferation with PET. Nucl Med Biol 22:783–789

242. De Vries EFJ, van Waarde A, Harmsen MC, Mulder NH, Vaalburg W, Hospers GAP (2000) [11C]FMAU and [18F] FHPG as PET tracers for herpes simplex virus thymidine kinase enzyme activity and human cytomegalovirus infections. Nucl Med Biol 27:113–119

243. Karramkam M, Demphel S, Hinnen F, Trognon C, Dolle F (2003) Methylation of the thiophene ring using carbon-11-labelled methyl iodide: formation of 3-[^{11}C]methylthiophene. J Labelled Compd Radiopharm 46:255–261

244. Andersson Y, Cheng AP, Langström B (1995) Palladium-promoted coupling reactions of [^{11}C]methyl-iodide with organotin and organoboron compounds. Acta Chem Scand 49:683–688

245. Samuelsson L, Langström B (2003) Synthesis of 1-(2'-deoxy-2'-fluoro-beta-D-arabinofuranosyl)-[methyl-^{11}C]thymine ([^{11}C]FMAU) via a Stille cross-coupling reaction with [^{11}C]methyl iodide. J Labelled Compd Radiopharm 46:263–272

246. Madsen J, Merachtsaki P, Davoodpour P, Bergström M, Langström B, Andersen K, Thomsen C, Martiny L, Knudsen GM (2003) Synthesis and biological evaluation of novel carbon-11-labelled analogues of citalopram as potential radioligands for the serotonin transporter. Bioorg Med Chem 11:3447–3456

247. Huang YY, Narendran R, Bischoff F, Guo NN, Zhu ZH, Bae SA, Lesage AS, Laruelle M (2005) A positron emission tomography radioligand for the in vivo labeling of metabotropic glutamate 1 receptor: (3-ethyl-2-[^{11}C] methyl-6-quinolinyl) (cis-4-methoxycyclohexyl)methanone. J Med Chem 48:5096–5099

248. Wüst F, Zessin J, Johannsen B (2003) A new approach for 11C-C bond formation: synthesis of 17 alpha-(3'-[11C] prop-1-yn-1-yl)-3-methoxy-3, 17 beta-estradiol. J Labelled Compd Radiopharm 46:333–342

249. Wuest FR, Berndt M (2006) ^{11}C-C bond formation by palladium-mediated cross-coupling of alkenylzirconocenes with [^{11}C]methyl iodide. J Labelled Compd Radiopharm 49:91–100

250. Bjorkman M, Doi H, Resul B, Suzuki M, Noyori R, Watanabe Y, Langström B (2000) Synthesis of a ^{11}C-labelled prostaglandin F-2 alpha analogue using an improved method for Stille reactions with [^{11}C]methyl iodide. J Labelled Compd Radiopharm 43:1327–1334

251. Sandell J, Halldin C, Sovago J, Chou YH, Gulyas B, Yu MX, Emond P, Nagren K, Guilloteau D, Farde L (2002) PET examination of [^{11}C]5-methyl-6-nitroquipazine, a radioligand for visualization of the serotonin transporter. Nucl Med Biol 29:651–656

252. Langer O, Forngren T, Sandell J, Dolle F, Langström B, Nagren K, Halldin C (2003) Preparation of 4-[^{11}C]methyl-metaraminol, a potential PET tracer for assessment of myocardial sympathetic innervation. J Labelled Compd Radiopharm 46:55–65

253. Hamill TG, Krause S, Ryan C, Bonnefous C, Govek S, Seiders TJ, Cosford NDP, Roppe J, Kamenecka T, Patel S, Gibson RE, Sanabria S, Riffel K, Eng WS, King C, Yang XQ, Green MD, óMalley SS, Hargreaves R, Burns HD (2005) Synthesis, characterization, and first successful monkey imaging studies of metabotropic glutamate receptor subtype 5 (mGluR5) PET radiotracers. Synapse 56:205–216

254. Hosoya T, Sumi K, Doi H, Wakao M, Suzuki M (2006) Rapid methylation on carbon frameworks useful for the synthesis of ^{11}CH$_3$-incorporated PET tracers: Pd(0)-mediated rapid coupling of methyl iodide with an alkenyl-tributylstannane leading to a 1-methylalkene. Org Biomol Chem 4:410–415

255. Clark JC, Crouzel C, Meyer GJ, Strijckmans K (1987) Current methodology for oxygen-15 production for clinical use. Appl Radiat Isot 38:597–600

256. Welch MJ, Kilbourn MR (1985) A remote system for routine production of oxygen-15 radiopharmaceuticals. J Labelled Compd Radiopharm 22:1193–1200

257. Meyer GJ, Osterholz A, Hundeshagen H (1986) O-15-water constant infusion system for clinical routine application. J Labelled Compd Radiopharm 23:1209–1210

258. Kabalka GW, Lambrecht RM, Sajjad M, Fowler JS, Kunda SA, McCollum GW, MacGregor R (1985) Synthesis of ^{15}O-labeled butanol via organoborane chemistry. Appl Radiat Isot 36:853–855

259. Sajjad M, Lambrecht RM, Wolf AP (1986) Cyclotron isotopes and radiopharmaceuticals 37. exitation-functions for the O-16(p, alpha)N-13 and N-14(p, pn)N-13 reactions. Radiochim Acta 39:165–168

260. Vaalburg W, Kamphuis JA, Beerling-van der Molen HD, Reiffers S, Rijskamp A, Woldring MG (1975) An improved method for the cyclotron production of ^{13}N-ammonia. Appl Radiat Isot 26:316–318

261. Wieland B, Bida G, Padgett H, Hendry G, Zippi E, Kabalka G, Morelle J-L, Verbruggen R, Ghyoot M (1991) In target production of ^{13}N-ammonia via proton irradiation of aqueous ethanol and acetic acid mixtures. Appl Radiat Isot 42:1095–1098

262. Barrio JR, Baumgartner FJ, Henze E, Stauber MS, Egbert JE, MacDonald NS, Schelbert HR, Phelps ME, Liu F-T (1983) Synthesis and myocardial kinetics of N-13 and C-11 labeled branched-chain L-amino acids. J Nucl Med 24:937–944

263. Seevers RH, Counsell RE (1982) Radioiodination techniques for small organic molecules. Chem Rev 82:575–590

264. Coenen HH, Mertens J, Mazière B (2006) Radioiodination reactions for radiopharmaceuticals – compemdium for effective synthesis strategies. Springer, Dordrecht

265. Jirousek L (1981) On the chemical nature of iodinating species. J Radioanal Chem 65:139–154

266. Coenen HH, El-Wetery AS, Stöcklin G (1981) Further studies on practically carrier-free 123I-iodination and 75, 77Br-bromination of aromatic substrates. J Labelled Compd Radiopharm 18:114–115

267. Youfeng H, Coenen HH, Petzold G, Stöcklin G (1982) A comparative study of radioiodination of simple aromatic compounds via N-halosuccinimides and chloramine-t in TFAA. J Labelled Compd Radiopharm 19:807–819

268. Mennicke E, Holschbach M, Coenen HH (2000) Direct N.C.A. electrophilic radioiodination of deactivated arenes with N-chlorosuccinimide. J Labelled Compd Radiopharm 43:721–737

269. Moerlein SM, Mathis CA, Yano Y (1987) Comparative evaluation of electrophilic aromatic iododemetallation techniques for labeling radiopharmaceuticals with iodine-122. Appl Radiat Isot 38:85–90

270. Mennicke E, Hennecken H, Holschbach M, Coenen HH (1998) Thallium-tris(trifluoroacetate): a powerful reagent for the N.C.A: radioiodination of weakly activated arenes. Eur J Nucl Med 25:843–845

271. Morrison M, Bayse GS (1970) Catalysis of iodination by lactoperoxidase. Biochem 9:2995–3000

272. Moore DH, Wolf W (1978) Electrochemical radioiodination of estradiol. J Labelled Compd Radiopharm 15:443–450

273. Moerlein SM, Beyer W, Stöcklin G (1988) No-carrier-added radiobromination and radioiodination of aromatic rings using in situ generated peracetic acid. J Chem Soc Perkin Trans 1:779–786

274. McKillop A, Taylor EC, Fowler JS, Zelesko MJ, Hunt JD, McGillivray G (1969) Thallium in organic synthesis. X. A one-step synthesis of aryl iodides. Tetrahedron Lett 10:2427–2430

275. Kabalka GW, Varma RS (1989) The synthesis of radiolabeled compounds via organometallic intermediates. Tetrahedron 45:6601–6621

276. Flanagan RJ (1991) The *synthesis of halogenated radiopharmaceuticals using organomercurials.* In: Emran AM (ed) New trends in radiopharmaceutical synthesis quality assurance and regulatory control. Plenum, New York, pp 279–288

277. Moerlein SM, Coenen HH (1985) Regiospecific no-carrier-added radiobromination and radioiodination of aryltrimethyl Group IVb organometallics. J Chem Soc Perkin Trans 1:1941–1947

278. Lindley J (1984) Tetrahedron report number 163: copper assisted nucleophilic substitution of aryl halogen. Tetrahedron 40:1433–1456

279. Clark JH, Jones CW (1987) Reverse halogenation using supported copper(I) iodide. J Chem Soc Chem Commun 1409–1411

280. Bolton AE, Hunter WM (1973) The labelling of proteins to high specific radioactivities by conjugation to a ^{125}I-containing acylating agent. Application to the radioimmunoassay. Biochem J 133:529–533

281. Rudinger J, Ruegg U (1973) Appendix: preparation of N-succinimidyl 3-(4-hydroxyphenyl)propionate. Biochem J 133:538–539

282. Glaser M, Carroll VA, Collinbridge DR, Aboagye EO, Price P, Bicknell R, Harris AL, Luthra SK, Brady F (2002) Preparation of the iodine-124 derivative of the Bolton-Hunter reagent ([124I]I-SHPP) and its use for labelling a VEGF antibody as a PET tracer. J Labelled Compd Radiopharm 45:1077–1090

283. Wood FT, Wu MM, Gerhart JJ (1975) The radioactive labeling of proteins with an iodinated amidination reagent. Anal Biochem 69:339–349

284. Ram S, Fleming E, Buchsbaum DJ (1992) Development of radioiodinated 3 iodophenylisothiocyanate for coupling to monoclonal antibodies. J Nucl Med 33:1029

285. Khawli LA, Chen FM, Alaudin MM, Stein AL (1991) Radioiodinated monoclonal-antibody conjugates – synthesis and comparable-evaluation. Antibody Immunoconj Radiopharm 4:163–182

286. Ali SA, Eary JF, Warren SD, Krohn KA (1988) Synthesis and radioiodinationof tyramine cellobiose for labeling monoclonal antibodies. Nucl Med Biol 15:557–561

287. Khawli LA, van de Abeele AD, Kassis AI (1992) N-(m-[125I]iodophenyl)maleimide: an agent for high yield radiolabeling of antibodies. Nucl Med Biol 19:289–295

288. Kassis AI, Adelstein SJ, Haydock S, Sastry KSR, McElvany KD, Welch MJ (1982) Lethality of Auger electrons from the decay of bromine-77 in the DNA of mammalian cells. Radiat Res 90:362–373

289. DeSombre ER, Hughes A, Mease RC, Harpet PV (1990) Comparison of the distribution of bromine-77-bromovinyl steroidal and triphenylethylene estrogens in the immature rat. J Nucl Med 31:1534–1542

290. DeSombre ER, Hughes A, Gatley SJ, Schwartz JL, Harper PV (1990) Receptordirected radiotherapy: a new approach to therapy of steroid receptor positive cancers. Prog Clin Biol Res 322:295–309

291. Downer JB, Jones LA, Engelbach JA, Lich LL, Mao W, Carlson KE, Katzenellenbogen JA, Welch MJ (2001) Comparison of animal models for the evaluation of radiolabeled androgens. Nucl Med Biol 28:613–626

292. Tolmachev V, Lövqvist A, Einarsson L, Schultz J, Lundqvist H (1998) Production of [76]Br by a low-energy cyclotron. Appl Radiat Isot 49:1537–1540

293. Bergström M, Lu L, Fasth KJ, Wu F, Bergström-Pettermann E, Tolmachev V, Hedberg E, Cheng A, Langstrom B (1998) In vitro and animal validation of bromine-76-bromodeoxyuridine as a proliferation marker. J Nucl Med 39:1273–1279

294. Ryser JE, Blauenstein P, Remy N, Weinreich R, Hasler PH, Novak-Hofer I, Schubiger PA (1999) [76Br]Bromodeoxyuridine, a potential tracer for the measurement of cell proliferation by positron emission tomography, in vitro and in vivo studies in mice. Nucl Med Biol 26:673–679

295. Lu L, Bergström M, Fasth K-J, Långström B (2000) Synthesis of [76Br]bromofluorodeoxyuridine and its validation with regard to uptake, DNA Incorporation, and excretion modulation in rats. J Nucl Med 41:1746–1752

296. Kassiou M, Loc'h C, Dolle F, Musachio JL, Dolci L, Crouzel C, Dannals RF, Mazière B (2002) Preparation of a bromine-76 labelled analogue of epibatidine: a potent ligand for nicotinic acetylcholine receptor studies. Appl Radiat Isot 57:713–717

297. Foged C, Halldin C, Loc'h C, Maziere B, Pauli S, Maziere M, Hansen HC, Suhara T, Swahn CG, Karlsson P, Farde L (1997) Bromine-76 and carbon-11 labeled NNC 13–8199, metabolically stable benzodiazepine receptor agonists as radioligands for positron emission tomography. Eur J Nucl Med 24:1261–1267

298. Lovqvist A, Sundin A, Ahlstrom H, Carlsson J, Lundqvist H (1997) Pharmacokinetics and experimental PET imagingn of a bromine-76-labeled monoclonal anti-CEA antibody. J Nucl Med 38:395–401

299. Loc'h C, Halldin C, Bottlaender M, Swahn CG, Moresco RM, Maziere M, Farde L, Maziere B (1996) Preparation of [76Br]FLB 457 and [76Br]FLB 463 for examination of striatel and extrastriatal dopamine D-2 receptors with PET. Nucl Med Biol 23:813–819

300. Wu F, Yngvu U, Hedberg E, Honda M, Lu L, Eriksson B, Watanabe Y, Bergstrom M, Langstrom B (2000) Distribution of 76Br-labeled antisense oligonucleotides of different length determined ex vivo in rats. Eur J Pharm Sci 10:179–186

301. Winberg KJ, Persson M, Malmstrom PU, Sjoberg S, Tolmachev V (2004) Radiobromination of anti-HER2/neu/ErB-2 monoclonal antibody using the p-isothiocyanatobenzene derivative of the [76Br]undecahydro-bromo-7, 8-dicarbanido-undecaborate(1-) ion. Nucl Med Biol 31:425–433

302. Smith-Jones PM, Stolz B, Bruns C, Albert R, ReistHW FR, Maecke HR (1994) Gallium-67/gallium-68-[DFO]-octreotide – a potential radiopharmaceutical for PET imaging of somatostatin receptor-positive tumors: synthesis and radiolabeling in vitro and preliminary in vivo studies. J Nucl Med 35:317–325

303. Hofmann M, Maecke H, Börner A, Weckesser E, Schöffski P, Oei M, Schumacher J, Henze M, Heppeler A, Meyer G, Knapp W (2001) Biokinetics and imaging with the somatostatin receptor PET radioligand ^{68}Ga-DOTA-TOC: preliminary data. Eur J Nucl Med 28:1751–1757

304. Kowalski J, Henze M, Schuhmacher J, Maecke HR, Hofmann M, Haberkorn U (2003) Evaluation of positron emission tomography imaging using [^{68}Ga]-DOTA-D-Phe[1]-Tyr[3]-octreotide in comparison to [^{111}In]-DTPAOC SPECT. First results in patients with neuroendocrine tumors. Mol Imaging Biol 5:42–48

305. Henze M, Dimitrakopoulou-Strauss A, Milker-Zabel S, Schuhmacher J, Strauss LG, Doll J, Maecke HR, Eisenhut M, Debus J, Haberkorn U (2005) Characterization of ^{68}Ga-DOTA-D-Phe[1]-Tyr[3]-octreotide kinetics in patients with meningiomas. J Nucl Med 46:763–769

306. Green MA, Klippenstein DL, Tennison JR (1988) Copper (II)bis(thiosemicarbazone) complexes as potential tracers for evaluation of cerebral and myocardial blood flow with PET. J Nucl Med 29:1549–1557

307. Takahashi N, Fujibayashi Y, Yonekura Y, Welch MJ, Waki A, Tsuchida T, Sadato N, Sugimoto K, Itoh H (2000) Evaluation of [62]Cu labeled diacetyl-bis(N[4]-methylthiosemicarbazone) in hypoxic tissue in patients with lung cancer. Ann Nucl Med 14:323–328

308. Dehdashti F, Mintun MA, Lewis JS (2003) In vivo assessment of tumour hypoxiy in lung cancer with [60]Cu-ATSM. Eur J Nucl Med Mol Imaging 30:844–850

309. Haynes NG, Lacy JL, Nayak N, Martin CS, Dai D, Mathias CJ, Green MA (2000) Performance of a [62]Zn/[62]Cu generator in clinical trials of PET perfusion agent [62]Cu-PTSM. J Nucl Med 41:309–314

PET Chemistry: Radiopharmaceuticals

6

Tobias L. Roß and Simon M. Ametamey

Contents

6.1 PET Radiopharmaceuticals in the Clinics – Precursors

Although many radiolabelled compounds for PET imaging have been developed so far, only a few have reached the status of a clinically established and routinely used PET radiopharmaceutical. At the early stage of development, a reasonable medical indication is obviously fundamental for a PET radiopharmaceuti-

cal to be further considered as clinically relevant. However, besides a favourable in vivo behaviour and appropriate imaging characteristics, certain criteria have to be fulfilled, such as a fast, straightforward and reliable radiosynthesis; an assured stability of the label as well as of the compound itself and a good availability of a suitable precursor. In particular, the ease and reliability of the radiochemistry is critical as the radiopharmaceutical needs to be available on demand in sufficient amounts. The precursors play the decisive role in the radiochemical approach as they specify the radiosynthetic route. Furthermore, the accessibility of the appropriate precursors is important for the applicability of radiosynthesis. Today, most precursors of the commonly used PET radiopharmaceuticals are commercially available and provided as approved medical products by suppliers such as ABX – advanced biochemical products GmbH Germany [1].

6.1.1 ^{18}F-Labelled PET Radiopharmaceuticals and Their Precursors

Fluorine-18 is clearly the most important radionuclide employed in clinical PET imaging. While it is available in large quantities, it also has further optimal physical and chemical properties for PET imaging. In its [^{18}F]FDG form it probably contributed most to the success of PET imaging in clinical diagnostics. Since the development of [^{18}F]FDG in the 1970s, it has become the most important and most commonly used PET radiopharmaceutical in nuclear medicine. However, during the past 30 years, several other useful ^{18}F-labelled PET radiopharmaceuticals have been

T.L. Roß (✉)
Radiopharmaceutical Chemistry, Institute of Nuclear Chemistry, Johannes Gutenberg-University Mainz, Fritz-Strassmann-Weg 2, D-55128, Mainz, Germany
e-mail: ross@uni-mainz.de
S.M. Ametamey
Animal Imaging Center-PET, Center for Radiopharmaceutical Sciences of ETH, PSI and USZ, ETH-Hönggerberg, D-CHAB IPW HCI H427, Wolfgang-Pauli-Str. 10, CH-8093, Zurich, Switzerland
e-mail: amsimon@ethz.ch

M.M. Khalil (ed.), *Basic Sciences of Nuclear Medicine*, DOI: 10.1007/978-3-540-85962-8_6,
© Springer-Verlag Berlin Heidelberg 2011

designed and some have been further developed to routine PET radiopharmaceuticals in nuclear medicine clinics. In the following paragraphs, some representative examples of clinically employed ^{18}F-labelled PET radiopharmaceuticals are outlined. Furthermore, their general production routes and most commonly used precursors are described.

6.1.1.1 ^{18}F]NaF

As mentioned earlier, ^{18}F-labelled sodium fluoride is the simplest form of a ^{18}F-labelled radiopharmaceutical and it was shown already in 1940 in in vitro tests that ^{18}F]NaF is uptaken by bone and dentine structures [2]. Since the 1960s, ^{18}F]NaF has been used in the nuclear medicine clinics for skeletal scintigraphy to identify malignant and benign mass in bones [3, 4]. N.c.a. [18]F]NaF can be produced directly by elution of the trapped ^{18}F]fluoride from the anionic exchange resin (solid phase extraction cartridge systems) using potassium carbonate solution. The obtained ^{18}F]fluoride solution can be used directly for administration.

6.1.1.2 2-^{18}F]Fluorodeoxyglucose (^{18}F]FDG)

[18]FDG is the most important ^{18}F-labelled PET radiopharmaceutical, and its availability, broad applicability, and increasing use have made it a diagnostic method accepted worldwide. [18]FDG is most widely used as a diagnostic compound in oncology [5], but there are many more indications and applications for this versatile radiopharmaceutical [6–9]. The first approach towards 2-^{18}F]FDG was based on an electrophilic ^{18}F-labelling with only low yields and in a mixture with the stereoisomer 2-^{18}F]fluorodeoxymannose (see Chap. 5, Fig. 5.1) [10]. In the 1980s, a new precursor, mannose triflate (1,3,4,6-tetra-O-acetyl-2-O-trifluoro-methanesulfonyl-beta-D-mannopyranose, TATM) (see Fig. 6.1) [11], for an efficient nucleophilic n.c.a. ^{18}F-labelling of 2-^{18}F]FDG became available and is still the precursor of choice

for routine productions of n.c.a. [18]F]FDG with yields of up to 40–50 GBq per batch. Generally, TATM is n.c.a. ^{18}F-fluorinated in the Kryptofix2.2.2©/K2CO3 system in acetonitrile. The subsequent hydrolysis using hydrochloric acid provides ^{18}F]FDG in high radiochemical yields of ~50–70%. Recently, the deprotection procedure has been optimised by changing to an alkaline system [12–14]. The alkaline system sufficiently removes all acetyl protection groups already at 40°C in 0.3 N NaOH in less than 5 min. The reaction conditions must be strictly kept to reduce an alkaline epimerisation on the C-2 position towards 2-^{18}F]fluorodeoxymannose to a minimum [13].

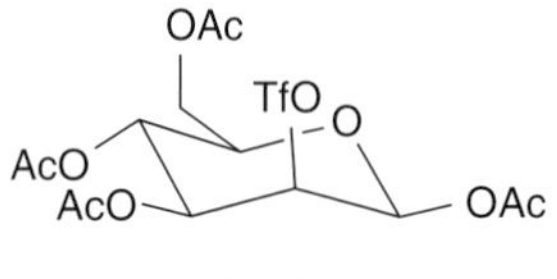

6.1.1.3 6-^{18}F]Fluoro-L-DOPA (^{18}F]F-DOPA)

Similar to [18]FDG, the first ^{18}F-labelling approaches to ^{18}F]F-DOPA were based on direct electrophilic ^{18}F-labelling using ^{18}F]F2 and L-DOPA as precursor (see Chap. 5, Fig. 5.2). This method led to a mixture of the three possible regioisomers 2-, 5- and 6-^{18}F]F-DOPA and gave only 21% RCY of the desired 6-^{18}F]F-DOPA. The introduction of the 6-trimethyltin precursor for electrophilic ^{18}F-fluorodemetallations offered enhanced ^{18}F-labelling with regioselective ^{18}F-introduction and higher RCY (see Chap. 5, Fig. 5.3) [15]. The electrophilic ^{18}F-fluorodemetallation reaction for 6-^{18}F]F-DOPA was further developed and optimised, and is now applicable as a fully automated version [16–19]. Attempts for a nucleophilic approach of n.c.a. ^{18}F-labelling of 6-^{18}F]F-DOPA have been made, but even the most promising ones are multi-step radiosyntheses using chiral auxiliaries and thus make automation difficult (Chap. 5, Fig. 5.17) [20, 21]. Consequently, the commonly used production route is still the electrophilic ^{18}F-fluorodemetallation using the trimethyltin precursor which is available in a few different versions with varying protection groups (see Fig. 6.2).

6-^{18}F]fluoro-L-DOPA is the second ranked ^{18}F-labelled PET radiopharmaceutical after [18]FDG. It is the PET tracer of choice for studies of the dopaminergic system [22], particularly for studies of changes in the presynaptic dopaminergic nerve terminals in Parkinson's disease [23, 24]. Furthermore, 6-^{18}F]F-DOPA has also shown applicability in oncology for detecting neuroendocrine tumours where a visualisation using ^{18}F]FDG PET imaging is not feasible [25].

Fig 6.1 Mannose triflate precursor for radiosynthesis of n.c.a. [18]F]FDG

TATM

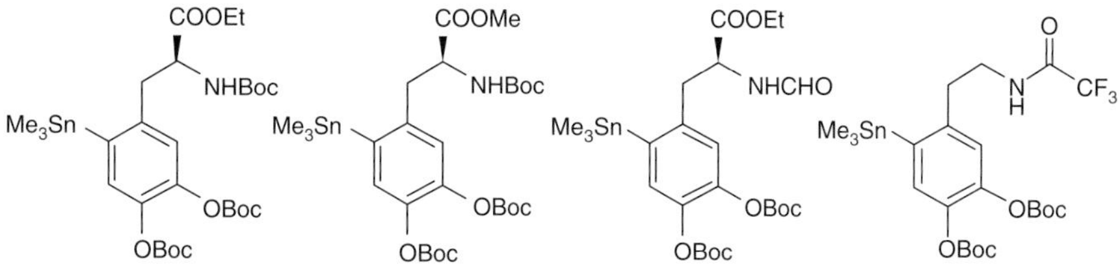

Fig. 6.2 Most important precursors for electrophilic radiofluorination of 6-[^{18}F]F-DOPA by regioselective ^{18}F-fluorodestannylation

6.1.1.4 O-(2-[^{18}F]Fluoroethyl)-L-Tyrosine ([^{18}F]FET)

[^{18}F]FET is a ^{18}F-labelled amino acid derivative and is routinely used for PET imaging of brain tumours as it has only minor uptake in normal brain and provides excellent tumour-to-background contrast [26]. Furthermore, it is not uptaken by inflammatory tissue like ^{18}FDG and allows a more exact detection of tumour mass and size in general tumour imaging [27]. In combination with magnetic resonance imaging (MRI), PET imaging of cerebral gliomas using [^{18}F]FET significantly enhanced the diagnostic assessment [28]. The first radiosynthesis was based on a two-step ^{18}F-labelling using the primary precursor ethyleneglycol-1,2-ditosylate [29]. After ^{18}F-labelling and a semi-preparative HPLC purification, the 2-[^{18}F]fluoroethyltosylate was coupled to the unprotected (S)-tyrosine to give [^{18}F]FET. The two-step method could be circumvented by the advancement of a new precursor, (2 S)-O-(2′-tosyloxyethyl)-N-trityl-tyrosine-tert-butyl ester (TET) for a direct ^{18}F-labelling (see Fig. 6.3) [30]. Although the precursor for direct ^{18}F-labelling offers a shorter, more convenient and more efficient preparation of [^{18}F]FET, both methods are routinely used. A very recently developed precursor is based on a chiral Ni(II) complex of a (S)-tyrosine Schiff base and led to an enantiomerically pure (S)-2-[^{18}F]FET and furthermore, this approach could avoid toxic TFA in the hydrolysis step [31].

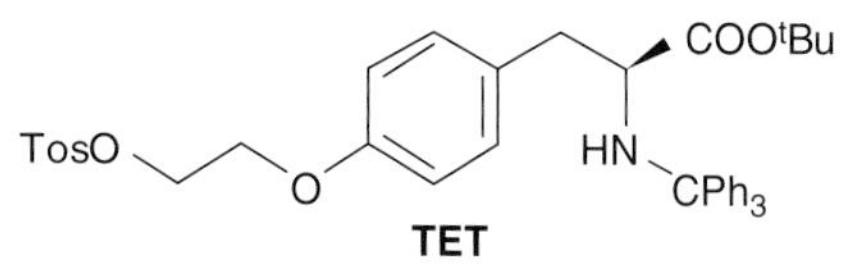

6.1.1.5 3-Deoxy-3′-[^{18}F]fluorothymidine ([^{18}F]FLT)

This ^{18}F-labelled thymidine derivative is a substrate of the thymidine kinase-1 (TK1) and thus phosphorylated and trapped in the cell [32]. The TK1 is correlated with cell proliferation as its designated substrate thymidine is essential for DNA and RNA synthesis. Hence, [^{18}F]FLT can be used for PET imaging of cell prolif-

Fig 6.3 Precursor TET for the direct ^{18}F-labelling of [^{18}F]FET

eration and of tumours with increased TK1 levels [33]. [^{18}F]FLT has proven clinical importance, even in comparison with [^{18}F]FDG in several tumour imaging studies [34–40]. The first radiosynthesis of 3-Deoxy-3′-[^{18}F]fluorothymidine gave only low RCY of 7% [41]. Several improvements of the radiosynthesis, precursors and the HPLC systems for purifications have increased the availability of [^{18}F]FLT [42–47], but still, the radiosynthesis remains tedious and causes difficulties in routine productions [47]. The most commonly used precursors for ^{18}F-labeling of [^{18}F]FLT are depicted in Fig. 6.4.

6.1.1.6 16α-[^{18}F]Fluoro-17β-Estradiol ([^{18}F]FES)

^{18}F-labelled estrogens have been developed as PET radiopharmaceuticals for imaging the estrogen hormone receptor [48]. The estrogen receptor expression is a crucial factor in breast cancer development and critical for the response of endocrine therapies [49, 50]. The first ^{18}F-labelled derivatives of estrogen were the 4-[^{18}F]fluoroestranone and the 4-[^{18}F]Fluoro-estradiol which were achieved only in low radiochemical yields of ~3% [51, 52]. Several other ^{18}F-labelled estrogen derivatives have been developed and evaluated preclinically [53–57]. However, the most promising candidate and, today, routinely used ^{18}F-labelled estrogen derivative is the 16α-[^{18}F]Fluoro-17β-estradiol ([^{18}F]FES) [54, 55]. The synthesis and preparation methods for [^{18}F]FES have been improved and automated and [^{18}F]FES can be achieved in radiochemical yields of 70% within 60 min synthesis time [58–60]. As precursor, the cyclic sulphate

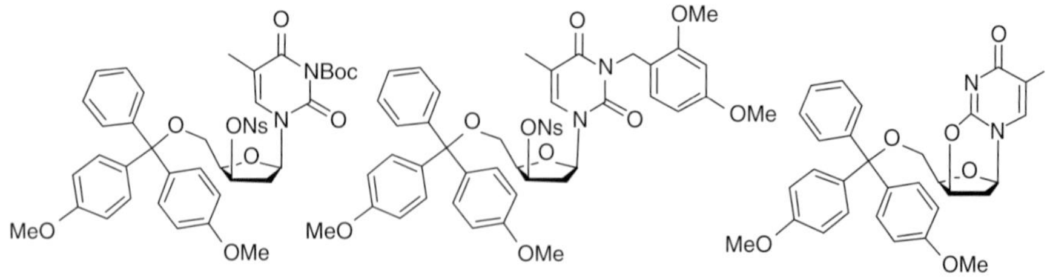

Fig 6.4 Various precursors
for the ^{18}F-labelling of
[^{18}F]FLT

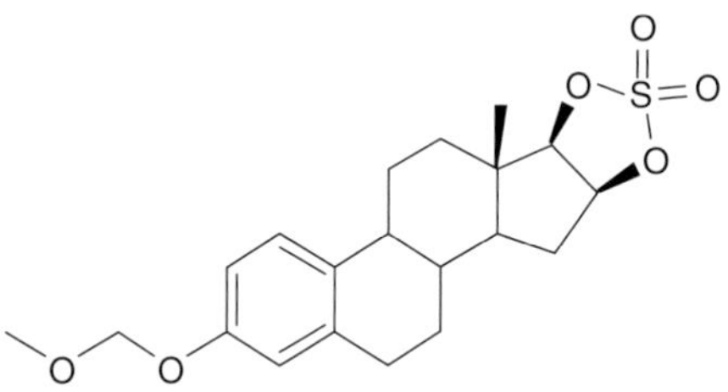

Fig. 6.5 Cyclic sulphate precursor for the ^{18}F-labelling of [^{18}F]FES

3-O-methoxymethyl-16β,17β-O-sulfuryl-estra-1,3,5(10)-triene-3,16β,17β-triol (see Fig. 6.5) has prevailed and is commonly employed. After radio-fluorination, a hydrolysis step using 1 N HCl yields the 16α-[^{18}F]Fluoro-17β-estradiol. The product is then purified by semi-preparative HPLC and formulated.

6.1.1.7 [^{18}F]Fluorocholine ([^{18}F]FCH)

The ^{11}C-labelled derivative of choline, [^{11}C]choline, was found to be a suitable radiopharmaceutical for tumour imaging, especially for prostate cancer [61, 62]. As a consequence, also the ^{18}F-labelled derivative [^{18}F]fluorocholine was developed and showed similarly good imaging characteristics in PET tumour imaging [61, 63, 64]. Furthermore, [^{18}F]FCH was also found to clearly visualise brain tumours [65] and in comparison with [^{18}F]FDG, it gave better PET images for brain tumours, prostate cancer, lung cancer, head and neck cancer [64]. Generally, [^{18}F]fluorocholine can be obtained in RCY of 20–40% from a coupling reaction of N,N-dimethyl-ethanolamine with the ^{18}F-labelling synthon [^{18}F]fluorobromomethane ([^{18}F]FBM) (see Fig. 6.6) [63]. The ^{18}F-labelling of [^{18}F]FBM is based on the precursor dibromomethane, and [^{18}F]FBM is isolated by a subsequent gas chromatography purification [66, 67].

6.1.1.8 [^{18}F]Fluoromisonidazole ([^{18}F]F-MISO)

[^{18}F]F-MISO (1H-1-(3-[^{18}F]Fluoro-2-hydroxypropyl)-2-nitroimidazole) is used as an indicator for the oxygenation status of cells as is accumulated in hypoxic tissue. Particularly in oncologic radiotherapy and chemotherapy, hypoxia is of major interest for the therapy prognosis [68–70]. Although [^{18}F]F-MISO shows some unfavourable pharmacological characteristics such as slow clearance from norm-oxygenated cells (background) and a relatively moderate uptake in hypoxic cells in general, it is the most widely used PET radiopharmaceutical for imaging hypoxic tumours. Recently, other hypoxia PET tracers have been developed and showed very promising results, but they have not reached the clinics yet [71–73]. Generally, two variants of the radiosynthesis towards [^{18}F]F-MISO are available [74–79]. The first successful attempts of an efficient radiolabelling of [^{18}F]F-MISO were based on a two-pot reaction. The primary precursor (2R)-(-)glycidyl tosylate (GOTS) was labelled with [^{18}F]fluoride to yield [^{18}F]epifluorohydrin ([^{18}F]EPI-F) which subsequently reacted with 2-nitroimidazole (2-NIM) in a nucleophilic ring opening to give [^{18}F]F-MISO in RCY of 20–40% (see Fig. 6.7) [75, 76]. The development of a direct ^{18}F-labelling of [^{18}F]F-MISO in one-pot has made radiosynthesis of this PET radiopharmaceutical more convenient and reliable [77, 78]. Starting from the precursor 1-(2′-nitro-1′-imidazolyl)-2-O-tetrahydropyranyl-3-O-toluenesulphonyl-propanediol (NITTP) (see Fig. 6.7), [^{18}F]F-MISO can be obtained in an one-pot procedure within 70–90 min [77–79]. Both approaches are capable for [^{18}F]F-MISO preparation, while the one-pot method usually gives RCY of 35–40% and it is much more suitable for automated routine productions [74]. Furthermore, the radiosynthesis based on the NITTP precursor is normally more reliable and more robust.

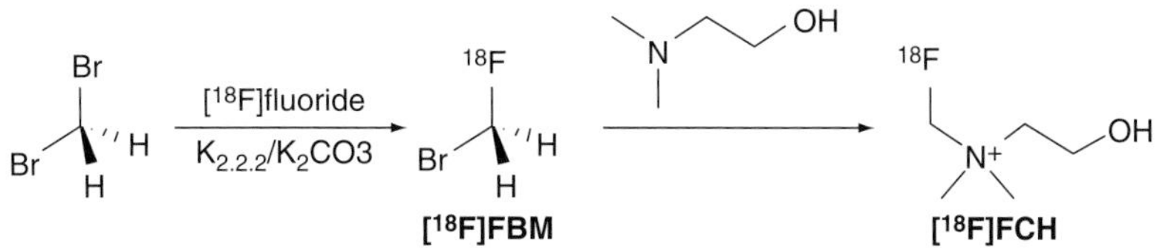

Fig. 6.6 Preparation of [^{18}F]choline via the ^{18}F-labelling synthon [^{18}F]FBM

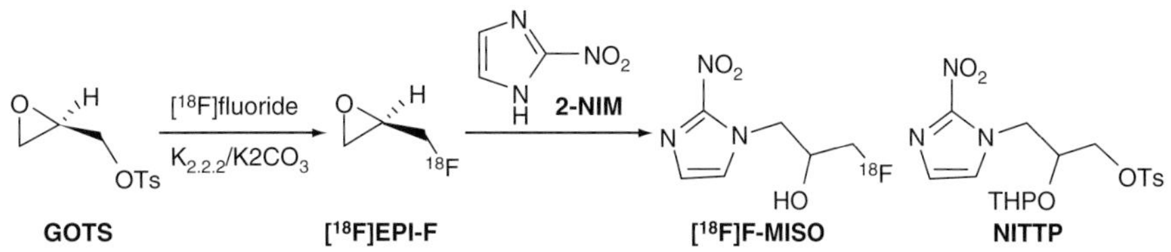

Fig. 6.7 Preparation of [^{18}F]F-MISO using a two-pot radiosynthesis (left hand side) and the precursor NITTP for the one-step ^{18}F-labelling procedure (right hand side)

6.1.1.9 [^{18}F]Altanserin

This ^{18}F-labelled PET radiopharmaceutical is the most widely used PET tracer for studies of the 5-HT$_{2A}$ receptor system as it is, so far, the most suitable ^{18}F-labelled 5-HT$_{2A}$ receptor ligand. Among other ^{18}F-labelled ligands for this receptor system, [^{18}F] altanserin shows the highest affinity to 5-HT$_{2A}$ receptors and a good selectivity over the other receptor systems, dopamine D$_2$, histamine H$_1$, adrenergic α_1 and α_2 and opiate receptor sites (μ-opiate) [80, 81]. [^{18}F]Altanserin can be obtained from direct ^{18}F-labelling of the appropriate nitro precursor (nitro-altanserin) (see Fig. 6.8) with good RCY in a one-step procedure. As no functional groups are present which need to be protected, the radiopharmaceutical is readily available after HPLC purification [82, 83].

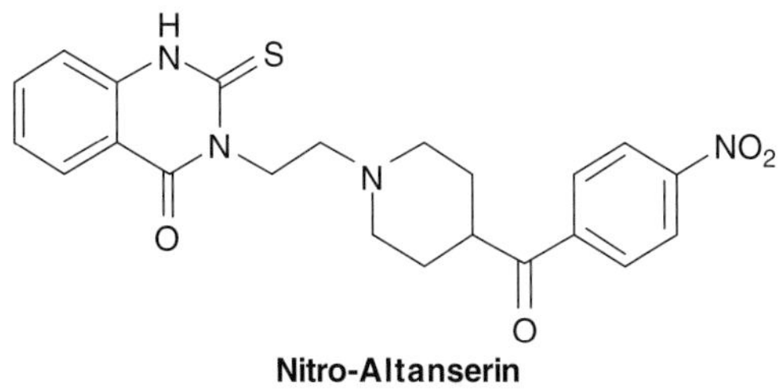

Fig. 6.8 Nitro-precursor for the direct ^{18}F-labelling of [^{18}F]altanserin

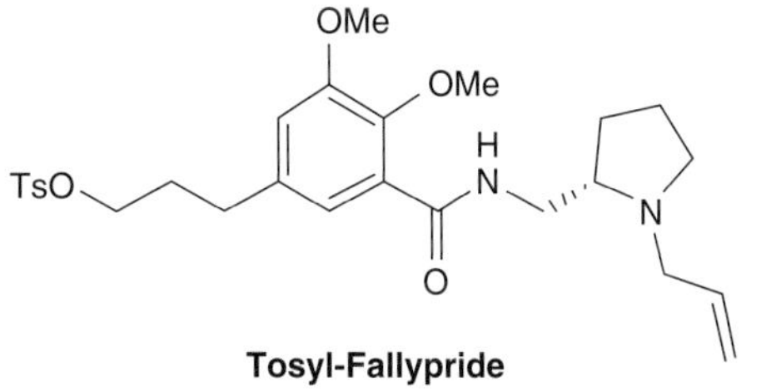

Fig. 6.9 'Tosyl-Fallypride' as precursor for one-step ^{18}F-labelling of [^{18}F]fallypride

6.1.1.10 [^{18}F]Fallypride

This ^{18}F-labelled derivative of benzamide neuroleptics has a high affinity (reversible binding) to dopamine D$_2$ receptors. [^{18}F]Fallypride is widely used as PET radiopharmaceutical for investigations of the dopamine D$_2$ receptor system and allows PET imaging of both striatal and extrastriatal dopamine D$_2$ receptors [84–88]. The ^{18}F-radiolabelling using the 'Tosyl-Fallypride' precursor (see Fig. 6.9) is a one-step ^{18}F-labelling procedure and provides [^{18}F]fallypride in good RCY of 20–40% [89].

6.1.2 ^{11}C-Labelled PET Radiopharmaceuticals and Their Precursors

Carbon-11 is particularly suited for labelling compounds with short biological half-lives. Compared to fluorine-18, the short physical half-life of ^{11}C permits repeated investigations in the same subject and within short intervals. Labelling is mainly by isotopic

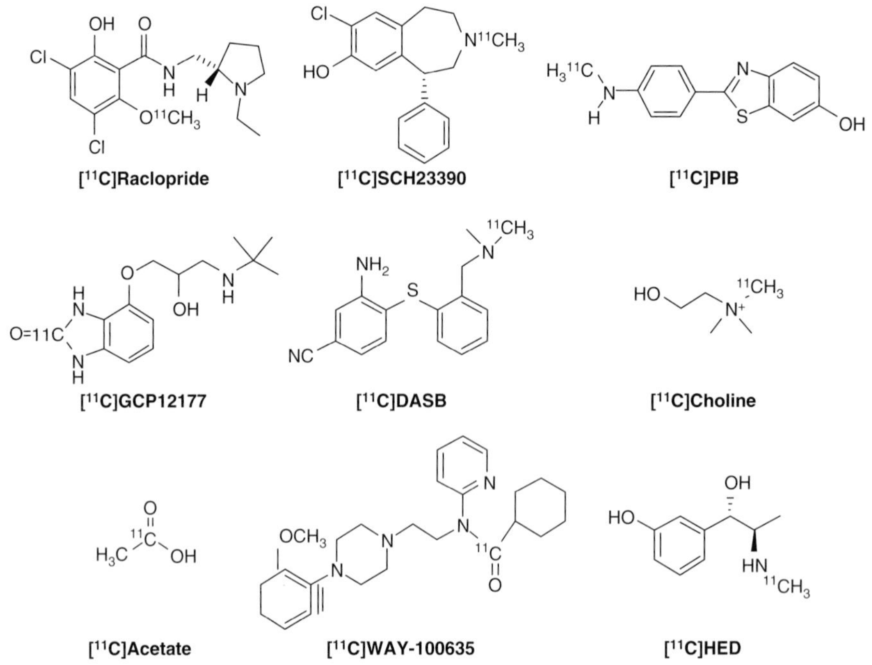

Fig. 6.10 Examples of commonly used and clinically established ^{11}C-labelled PET radiopharmaceuticals

[^{11}C]Raclopride   [^{11}C]SCH23390   [^{11}C]PIB

[^{11}C]GCP12177   [^{11}C]DASB   [^{11}C]Choline

[^{11}C]Acetate   [^{11}C]WAY-100635   [^{11}C]HED

substitution, but unlike ^{18}F labelled radiopharmaceuticals, carbon-11 labelled compounds can be prepared and used only in PET centres with a cyclotron and radiochemistry facility. As such carbon-11 labelled compounds are not commercially available. In Fig. 6.10, the structures of some established and commonly used carbon-11 labelled radiopharmaceuticals are shown, which have found routine application in clinical PET studies. All the compounds are prepared starting from the commercially available desmethyl or normethyl precursors. A large number of carbon-11 labelled radiopharmaceuticals have been reported in the literature, but only a handful of these have been shown to have clinical utility (see Chap. 5, Table 5.1). Procedures for the preparation of some representative examples of these radiopharmaceuticals are described.

6.1.2.1 [^{11}C]Raclopride

Of all benzamide derivatives reported to date, ^{11}C-raclopride is the most widely used PET ligand for the investigation of postsynaptic striatal D2/D3 receptors in humans. It has been used to image D2/D3 receptors in patients with Parkinson's disease, Huntington's disease, and schizophrenia, for determining receptor occupancy of antipsychotic drugs as well as for the

indirect measurement of dopamine concentrations in the synaptic cleft. Raclopride can be labelled by O-methylation with ^{11}C-methyl iodide or ^{11}C-methyltriflate (see Chap. 5, Fig. 5.24). Another approach involves N-ethylation with ^{11}C-ethyl iodide; however, due to the longer reaction time and a lower specific radioactivity, O-methylation is the preferred method for routine synthesis [90]. O-methylation was performed by using 5 M NaOH as the base in dimethylsulfoxide at 80°C for 5 min. ^{11}C-raclopride is purified by reversed phase HPLC using a μ-Bondapak C-18 column (Waters, 300 × 7.8 mm, 10 μm) with acetonitrile/0.01 M phosphoric acid (30/70) as the mobile phase. After formulation, the product is filtered through 0.22 μm Millipore membrane filter to give a sterile and pyrogen-free product. The total synthesis time is around 40–45 min and specific activities are in the range of 20–100 GBq/μmol depending on the synthesis method and the production route of ^{11}C-methyl iodide (i.e. 'wet' or 'dry' method).

6.1.2.2 [^{11}C]Flumazenil

^{11}C-labelled flumazenil is routinely used in clinical PET studies for the visualisation of central benzodiazepine receptors. It has high affinity for the

GABA$_A$ receptors and has been employed in PET studies mainly for the localisation of epileptic foci. ^{11}C-flumazenil has been labelled with carbon-11 by N-methylation with ^{11}C-methyl iodide or esterification with ^{11}C-ethyl iodide. For routine synthesis, N-methylation with ^{11}C-methyl iodide is the method of choice (Chap. 5, Fig. 5.24). [^{11}C]flumazenil is purified by reversed phase HPLC using a μ-Bondapak C-18 column (Waters, 300 × 7.8 mm, 10 μm) with acetonitrile/0.01 M phosphoric acid (25/75) as the mobile phase [91]. After formulation, the product is filtered through 0.22 μm Millipore membrane filter to give a sterile and pyrogen-free product. The total synthesis time is around 40–45 min and specific activities are in the range of 20–100 GBq/μmol.

6.1.2.3 L-[S-Methyl-^{11}C]Methionine

Methionine, labelled in its methyl position and named L-[S-methyl-^{11}C]-methionine, is a widely used amino acid for the detection of tumours using PET imaging. The uptake of L-[S-methyl-^{11}C]-methionine reflects several processes including transport, protein synthesis and transmethylation.

A number of synthetic pathways leading to L-[S-methyl-^{11}C]-methionine have been reported [92, 93]. The most simple and commonly used synthetic approach utilises the L-homocysteine thiolactone method. This method involves the in situ ring opening of L-homocysteine thiolactone by sodium hydroxide and the subsequent alkylation of the sulphide anion of L-homocysteine with ^{11}C-methyl iodide or ^{11}C-methyltriflate (Chap 5, Fig. 5.24). The final product is purified by HPLC, formulated and filtered through a 0.22 μm Millipore membrane filter to give a sterile and pyrogen-free product. The total synthesis time is around 40–45 min and although, unlike brain receptors, high specific radioactivities are not required, practical values obtained after the radiosynthesis are in the range of other ^{11}C-labelled compounds (Table 6.1).

6.1.3 ^{15}O- and ^{13}N-Labelled PET Radiopharmaceuticals

Oxygen-15 ($T_{1/2}$ = 2 min) has been used mainly for the labelling of oxygen, water and butanol. Of all these

Table 6.1 Established ^{11}C-labelled PET radiopharmaceuticals and their clinical applications

^{11}C-radiopharmaceutical	Target	Reference
[^{11}C]Flumazenil	Central benzodiazepine receptors	[94]
[^{11}C]WAY-100635	5-HT$_{1A}$ receptors	[95]
[^{11}C]PIB	Amyloid deposits	[96]
[^{11}C]raclopride	D2-receptor occupancy	[97]
[^{11}C]SCH23390	D1-receptor occupancy	[98]
[^{11}C]DASB	SERT	[99]
[^{11}C]methionine	Amino acid uptake	[100–102]
[^{11}C]choline	Cell membrane synthesis	[97]
[^{11}C]acetate	Oxygen metabolism	[103]
[^{11}C]HED	Presynaptic uptake-1 and storage	[104, 105]
[^{11}C]GP 12177	β-Adrenoceptors	[104, 105]

three compounds, ^{15}O-labelled water and butanol have found widespread application as myocardial and brain perfusion imaging agents.

6.1.3.1 [^{15}O]Water

A number of nuclear reactions exist for the production of oxygen-15, but the most commonly used method is the ^{14}N(d,n)^{15}O nuclear reaction [106]. The target material is aluminium and the target content is a mixture of nitrogen and 0.2–1.0% of oxygen. [^{15}O]water is then produced by reacting hydrogen with [^{15}O]O$_2$ (formed from the exchange reaction with carrier oxygen) over palladium-alumina catalyst at 200°C. The [^{15}O]water vapour formed is trapped in sterile isotonic saline and filtered through a 0.22 μm Millipore membrane filter.

6.1.3.2 [^{15}O]Butanol

n-[^{15}O]Butanol is prepared by the reaction of tri-n-butyl borane with [^{15}O]O$_2$ produced via the ^{14}N (d,n)^{15}O nuclear reaction. Alumina is used as a solid support for the tri-n-butyl borane. After the reaction, the labelled product is washed from the cartridge with water. Further purification is achieved by passing the product through a C-18 cartridge and eluting over a sterile filter with 10% ethanol/saline [107].

6.1.3.3 [^{13}N]Ammonia

Nitrogen-13 ($T_{1/2} = 10$ min) is prepared via the $^{16}O(p,\alpha)^{13}N$ nuclear reaction [108]. The material is usually aluminium, but targets made of nickel or titanium are in use. Of all compounds labelled with nitrogen-13, [^{13}N]ammonia is most commonly used for PET studies. Two methods exist for its production. The first method involves the reduction of ^{13}N-labelled nitrites/nitrates, formed during the proton irradiation, with either titanium(III) chloride or hydroxide or Devarda's alloy in alkaline medium [109]. After distillation, trapping in acidic saline solution and sterile filtration, [^{13}N]ammonia is ready for human application. The second method prevents the in situ oxidation of ^{13}N to ^{13}N-labelled nitrites/nitrates through the addition of ethanol as a radical scavenger to the target content [109]. Thereafter, the target content is passed through a small cation exchanger. [^{13}N] ammonium ions trapped on the cartridge are eluted with saline and the solution containing the product is then passed through a sterile filter. [^{13}N]Ammonia is used mainly for myocardial perfusion studies.

6.1.4 Other PET Radiopharmaceuticals

As an alternative to carbon-11 and fluorine-18, the most commonly used PET radionuclides, metallic positron emitters have gained acceptance also as radionuclides for the labelling of biomolecules. Apart from ^{64}Cu, most of the metallic positron emitters including ^{82}Rb, ^{68}Ga and ^{62}Cu are generator-produced isotopes. An advantage of generators is the fact that PET studies can be performed without an on-site cyclotron.

Rubidium-82 ($T_{1/2} = 1.3$ min) is produced from the strontium-82 (^{82}Sr)-^{82}Rb generator system. The ^{82}Sr-^{82}Rb generator system (Cardiogen-82®) is commercially available from Bracco Diagnostics, Princeton, NJ. [^{82}Rb]RbCl is used in clinical routine for cardiac perfusion measurements.

Gallium-68 ($T_{1/2} = 68$ min) is produced from the ^{68}Ge-^{68}Ga generator system. The generator is made up of a matrix of Sn(IV), Ti(IV) and Zr(IV) oxides in a glass column. The ^{68}Ga is eluted from the column with 0.005 M EDTA or 1 M HCl (mostly). When, however, the ^{68}Ga is eluted with EDTA, prior dissociation of the [^{68}Ga]EDTA complex is necessary, provided [^{68}Ga]EDTA is not the desired radiopharmaceutical. [^{68}Ga]EDTA is used mainly for brain tumour imaging as perfusion agent. For other ^{68}Ga-based radiopharmaceuticals, the ^{68}Ga needs to be available for chelating and thus the acidic elution with HCl is more favourable [110]. The most prominent examples of clinically used ^{68}Ga-radiopharmaceuticals are [^{68}Ga]DOTA-TOC and [^{68}Ga]DOTA-NOC, which have found application as imaging agents for somatostatin receptor-positive tumours [111, 112].

Copper-62 ($T_{1/2} = 10$ min) is produced from the ^{62}Zn-^{62}Cu generator system. In this generator system, ^{62}Zn is loaded on a Dowex 1 × 10 anion exchange column and the ^{62}Cu is eluted with 2 M HCl. Two well-known copper-62 radiopharmaceuticals are [^{62}Cu]ATSM (Diacetyl-bis(N^4-methylthiosemicarbazone)) and [^{62}Cu]PTSM (Pyruvaldehyde-bis(N^4-methylthiosemicarbazone)). [^{62}Cu]ATSM is being used in the clinic as a hypoxia imaging agent [113–115]. [^{62}Cu]PTSM has found application as a myocardial and brain perfusion PET imaging agent [116].

6.2 Automated Radiosyntheses – Modules

Semi-automated and automated processes have always been part of radiochemical methods or syntheses. This is due to the fact that one major concern in radio- and nuclearchemistry is to keep the radiation dose to personnel at a minimum. Accordingly, automation is favourable and generally preferable as many of these automated operations process large amounts of radioactivity which are excluded for a direct manual handling. Particularly,, for short-lived radionuclides such as carbon-11, nitrogen-13, oxygen-15 and fluorine-18, the required amounts of radioactivity in routine productions are very high and call for fully remote-controlled operations. Furthermore, automated reaction steps or procedures are generally more reliable and thus more reproducible than manual radiosyntheses. In addition, automated processes save time and therefore enhance product yields and efficiency. Today, the radiosyntheses of almost all routine PET radiopharmaceuticals are fully automated and are performed in so-called modules.

The first radiosynthesis modules were self-constructed and made of several remote-controlled valves, solvent reservoirs, radiation detectors and reactors or heating systems. The components were connected by tubes and lines from conventional HPLC systems. The radiosyntheses were carried out by manual switching of the valves. Today, the modules are computer-controlled, and the reaction steps of a radiosynthesis are programmed, while the basic concept of the hardware has not changed much [117].

After a module is equipped with precursor, solvents and reagents, the radionuclide is transferred directly from the target into the module and the radiosynthesis is started. During the procedure, (radio)detectors and other probes in the module monitor the course of radioactivity, temperature, pressure and further reaction parameters which are all usually recorded by the computer.

Depending on the system, different radiosyntheses can be programmed. If they are all based on the same radiochemical principle (e.g. a two-step radiosynthesis consisting of a radiolabelling step and a subsequent deprotection step), only basic parameters such as temperature and time need to be re-programmed. For more complex radiosyntheses, more changes are required and the radiosynthesis module has to be technically adapted to meet the demands of the new procedure. Consequently, in routine productions for clinical use on daily basis, each PET radiopharmaceutical is produced in a specifically designed module.

Several commercial module-based synthesis systems have been marketed so far. The first systems were available for [18F]FDG and have clearly contributed to the success and commercialisation of [18F]FDG [117–119]. Some examples of manufacturers and vendors of radiosynthesis modules and their corresponding synthesis modules for [18F]FDG productions are outlined in Table 6.2.

Automated radiosynthesis devices are commercially available for almost every clinically relevant PET radiopharmaceutical such as [18F]FDG, [18F]FLT, [18F]F-DOPA, [11C]CH$_3$I or [13N]NH$_3$. Furthermore, systems which are more flexible and adaptable for different radiosyntheses have been developed. The so-called modular systems offer a

Table 6.2 Examples of vendors of automated radiosynthesis apparatuses and their systems for [18F]FDG

Company	Radiosynthesis module for [18F]FDG
CTI Molecular Imaging/ Siemens Healthcare	CPCU (chemistry process control unit)
GE Medical Systems (Nuclear Interface Module)	TRACERlab Fx$_{FDG}$
Raytest Isotopenmessgeräte GmbH	SynChrom F18 FDG
Eckert & Ziegler Strahlen- und Medizintechnik AG	Modular-Lab for FDG
EBCO Industries Ltd./ Advanced Cyclotrons	Radiochemistry modules (FDG synthesis)
Bioscan	FDG-plus synthesiser

broad adaptability and high flexibility towards more complex radiosyntheses and individual method development. Various small components, generally designed for certain processes or reaction steps, are combined and assembled according to the desired radiosynthetic route. In contrast, the so-called 'black boxes', which generally allow only one type of radiosynthesis, need more service and maintenance, for example, cleaning procedures and the radiosyntheses have to be programmed and developed by the customers.

Recently, new approaches using micro-reactors and microfluidic systems have emerged in the field [120, 121]. Such microscale reactions benefit from very small amounts of precursors while they still give high yields after very short reaction times. The first systems have proven applicability and have shown satisfying results for the production of some ^{11}C-labelled [122–124] and ^{18}F-labelled [122] PET radiopharmaceuticals. As [18F]FDG is the most widely employed PET radiopharmaceutical in nuclear medicine, the radiosynthesis of [18F]FDG is commonly used as a benchmark test for those microfluidic systems. The development of these systems is still in its infancy, but the proof-of-principle has been made.

6.3 Quality Control of PET Radiopharmaceuticals

As PET radiopharmaceuticals are administered to humans, they need to fulfil certain test criteria before

Table 6.3 Quality control tests for PET radiopharmaceuticals

Quality control test	Criteria or subject of test	Test method
Biological tests		
Sterility	Injected volume needs to be sterile	Incubation over 2 weeks (bacteria growth)
Pyrogenicity	Batch needs to be apyrogenic	Limulus amebocyte lysate (LAL) test[a]
Physicochemical tests		
Appearance	Colour/clarity–turbidity	Visual inspection
Isotonicity	Injected volume needs to be isotonic	Osmometry (cryoscopy)
pH	7.4 (ideal) and slightly lower or higher	pH meter
Radionuclidic purity	Radionuclides must be pure prior to use	γ-spectroscopy and further radioanalytics
Chemical purity	Impurities or solvent traces need to be removed or proved to be harmless	Chemical analytics, frequently HPLC or GC
Radiochemical purity	Individual limits[b]	Radiochromatography (HPLC and TLC)

[a]Quick test for pyrogens based on coagulation of the lysate of amebocytes from the blood of the horseshoe crab (Limulus Polyphemus).
[b]Generally, for PET radiopharmaceuticals, there are individual limits/specifications set by the national pharmacopeia or the authorities of the corresponding country.

they are authorised for administration. In comparison to normal drugs, some test results cannot be obtained before administration due to the short half-lives of the radionuclides used for PET radiopharmaceuticals. In such cases, so-called dry runs for validation are performed. The full batch of a PET radiopharmaceutical production is used for tests and thereby, the method and procedure of production can be validated. In general, all productions, methods and test procedures have to be validated in accordance with GMP guidelines.

Quality control tests for PET radiopharmaceuticals can be divided into two subtypes: biological tests and physicochemical tests [125]. A list of required tests for PET radiopharmaceuticals is outlined in Table 6.3 (see Chap. 4).

In general, the biological tests need prolonged time and cannot be analysed before the administration of the PET radiopharmaceutical. These tests are performed 'after the fact' or for validation of the production process in dry runs.

The quality control tests for PET radiopharmaceuticals in clinical routine are regulated by the national law of the corresponding country. Responsible authorities usually provide guidelines such as pharmacopeia with clear specifications for routine productions of PET radiopharmaceuticals in clinical use.

6.4 PET Radiopharmaceuticals in Drug Development

During the development of new drugs, many questions and decisions have to be answered and made, respectively. Some of them are crucial and serve as knock-out criteria for the drug candidates. In pharmaceutical industry and the drug development field, three main concepts are classified: 'Proof of Target (POT),' 'Proof of Mechanism (POM)' and 'Proof of Concept (POC)' [126]. The available methods to give such proofs are limited and the field of PET imaging offers great opportunities for that. However, only a few examples can be found where PET radiopharmaceuticals have been employed as biomarkers in drug development.

Examples for the use of a PET tracer for the POT can be found in the development of therapeutics for neurodegenerative diseases. In the development of a new dopamine D2 receptor antagonist (ziprasidone, CP-88,059-01), the receptor occupancy of a dopamine D2 receptor antagonist, ziprasidone (CP-88,059-01) was determined using [^{11}C]raclopride [127]. In the same manner, the dopamine D_2 and D_3 receptor occupancy were studied by PET imaging using [^{11}C]raclopride during the development of a potential antipsychotic drug (aripiprazole, OPC 14597) [128]. In both studies, the displacement of the radiolabelled receptor ligand by the drug candidates gave the proof of target interaction. If, in a later stage, PET imaging results correlate with the clinical outcome, it could be further used as proof of concept.

In oncology, PET imaging is commonly used for the diagnosis and staging of cancers and has also shown potential in therapy monitoring. PET imaging using [^{18}F]FDG can visualise changes in tumour metabolism and thus can show therapy effects at a very early stage. Consequently, [^{18}F]FDG PET imaging can give the proof of mechanism as it can provide information of the tumour response to a new drug. This has been demonstrated in patients with gastrointestinal tumours treated with new kinase inhibitors as the [^{18}F]FDG uptake into the tumours was significantly reduced already after one cycle of treatment [129, 130].

Most information can be obtained if the drug candidate itself is radiolabelled. This strategy is not always adaptable and limited to structures which allow the authentic introduction of a radionuclide. However, a radiolabelled drug candidate gives information about the full pharmacokinetics and can answer many crucial questions at once.

PET imaging is particularly suitable for several questions in drug development. However, PET imaging has been used in drug development only to a small extent until now, but it is gaining more and more acceptance. Besides neurosciences and oncology, the use of PET imaging in drug development can be expected to grow further and also to emerge in other fields of drug development.

6.5 Conclusions

[^{18}F]FDG is the best clinically known and the most successful PET radiopharmaceutical. Due to the clinical utility of [^{18}F]FDG, PET imaging has grown rapidly and PET has become a powerful imaging technique. It is one of the leading technologies in molecular imaging. Besides [^{18}F]FDG, a number of PET radiopharmaceuticals have also found application as routine imaging agents in the clinic. Most of these radiopharmaceuticals can be produced in automated synthesis modules and quite a number of

^{18}F-labelled radiopharmaceuticals are commercially available for those clinics lacking an on-site cyclotron or radiochemistry facility. Nonetheless, for a vast majority of new targets there are currently no PET imaging probes. Radiochemists are therefore challenged to develop appropriate imaging probes for these new targets. The hope is also that those PET radiopharmaceuticals currently under development and in preclinical evaluation will find their way very rapidly into the clinics.

References

1. ABX – advanced biochemical products GmbH Germany, http://www.abx.de, Radeberg, Germany
2. Volker JF, Hodge HC, Wilson HJ, Van Voorhis SN (1940) The adsorption of fluorides by enamel, dentin, bone and hydroxyapatite as shown by the radioactive isotope. J Biol Chem 134:543–548
3. Blau M, Nagler W, Bender MA (1962) Fluorine-18: a new isotope for bone scanning. J Nucl Med 3:332–334
4. Grant FD, Fahey FH, Packard AB, Davis RT, Alavi A, Treves ST (2008) Skeletal PET with ^{18}F-Fluoride: applying new technology to an old tracer. J Nucl Med 49:68–78
5. Kumar R, Alavi A (2005) Clinical applications of fluorodeoxyglucose–positron emisson tomography in the management of malignant melanoma. Curr Opin Oncol 17:154–159
6. Coleman RE (2000) FDG imaging. Nucl Med Biol 27:689–690
7. Reske SN, Kotzerke J (2001) FDG-PET for clinical use. Eur J Nucl Med 28:1707–1723
8. Gambhir SS, Czerni J, Schwimmer J, Silverman DHS, Coleman RE, Phelps ME (2001) A tabulated summary of FDG PET literature. J Nucl Med 42:1S–93S
9. Adam MJ (2002) Radiohalogenated carbohydrates for use in PET and SPECT. J Labelled Compd Radiopharm 45:167–180
10. Ido T, Wan C-N, Casella V, Fowler JS, Wolf AP, Reivich M, Kuhl DE (1978) Labeled 2-deoxy-D-glucose analogs. ^{18}F-labeled 2-deoxy-2-fluoro-D-glucose, 2-deoxy-2-fluoro-D-mannose and ^{14}C-2-deoxy-2-fluoro-D-glucose. J Labeled Compd Radiopharm 14:175–182
11. Hamacher K, Coenen HH, Stöcklin G (1986) Efficient stereospecific synthesis of no-carrier-added 2-[^{18}F]-fluoro-2-deoxy-D-glucose using aminopolyether supported nucleophilic substitution. J Nucl Med 27:235–238
12. Füchtner FF, Steinbach J, Mäding P, Johannsen B (1996) Basic hydrolysis of 2-[18F]fluoro-1, 3, 4, 6-tetra-O-acetyl-D-glucose in the preparation of 2-[18F]fluoro-2-deoxy-D-glucose. Appl Radiat Isot 47:61–66
13. Meyer G-J, Matzke KH, Hamacher K, Füchtner FF, Steinbach P, Notohamiprodjo G, Zijlstra S (1999) Stability

of 2-[18f9fluoro-deoxy-D-glucose towards epimerisation under alkaline conditions. Appl Radiat Isot 51:37–41

14. Beuthien-Baumann B, Hamacher K, Oberdorfer F, Steinbach J (2000) Preparation of fluorine-18 labelled sugars and derivatives and their application as tracer for positron-emission-tomography. Carbohydr Res 327:107–118

15. Namavari M, Bishop A, Satyamurthy N, Bida G, Barrio JR (1992) Regioselective radiofluorodestannylation with [18F]F2, and [18F]CH3COOF: a high yield synthesis of 6-[18F]Fluoro-L-dopa. Appl Radiat Isot 43:989–996

16. De Vries EFJ, Luurtsema G, Brüssermann M, Elsinga PH, Vaalburg W (1999) Fully automated synthesis module for the high yield one-pot preparation of 6-[18F]fluoro-L-DOPA. Appl Radiat Isot 51:389–394

17. Adam MJ, Jivan S (1988) Synthesis and purification of L-6-[18F]fluorodopa. Appl Radiat Isot 39:1203–1206

18. Luxen A, Perlmutter M, Bida GT, Van Moffaert G, Cook JS, Satyamurthy N, Phelps ME, Barrio JR (1990) Remote, semiautomated production of 6-[18F]Fluoro-L-dopa for human studies with PET. Appl Radiat Isot 41:275–281

19. Szajek LP, Channing MA, Eckelman WC (1998) Automated synthesis 6-[18F]fluoro-L-DOPA using polystyrene supports with 6-mercuric of modified bound DOPA precursors. Appl Radiat Isot 49:795–804

20. Lemaire C, Damhaut P, Plenevaux A, Comar D (1994) Enantioselective synthesis of 6-[Fluorine-18]-Fluoro-L-Dopa from no-carrier-added fluorine-18-fluoride. J Nucl Med 35:1996–2002

21. Lemaire C, Gillet S, Guillouet S, Plenevaux A, Aerts J, Luxen A (2004) Highly enantioselective synthesis of no-carrier-added 6-[18F]Fluoro-L-dopa by chiral phase-transfer alkylation. Eur J Org Chem 2899–2904

22. Garnett ES, Firnau G, Nahmias C (1983) Dopamine visualized in the basal ganglia of living man. Nature 305: 137–138

23. Volkow ND, Fowler JS, Gatley SJ, Logan J, Wang G-J, Ding Y-S, Dewey S (1996) PET evaluation of the dopamine system of the human brain. J Nucl Med 37:1242–1256

24. Lee CS, Samii A, Sossi V, Ruth TJ, Schulzer M, Holden JE, Wudel J, Pal PK, De La Fuente-Fernandez R, Calne DB, Stoessl AJ (2000) In vivo positron emission tomographic evidence for compensatory changes in presynaptic dopaminergic nerve terminals in Parkinson's disease. Ann Neurol 47:493–503

25. Becherer A, Szabó M, Karanikas G, Wunderbaldinger P, Angelberger P, Raderer M, Kurtaran A, Dudczak R, Kletter K (2004) Imaging of advanced neuroendocrine tumors with 18F-FDOPA PET. J Nucl Med 45:1161–1167

26. Langen K-J, Hamacher K, Weckesser M, Floeth F, Stoffels G, Bauer D, Coenen HH, Pauleit D (2006) O-(2-[18F]fluoroethyl)-L-tyrosine: uptake mechanisms and clinical applications. Nucl Med Biol 33:287–294

27. Kaim AH, Weber B, Kurrer MO, Westera G, Schweitzer A, Gottschalk J, von Schulthess GK, Buck A (2002) 18F-FDG and 18F-FET uptake in experimental soft tissue infection. Eur J Nucl Med Mol Imaging 29:648–654

28. Pauleit D, Floeth F, Hamacher K, Riemenschneider MJ, Reifenberger G, Müller H-W, Zilles K, Coenen HH, Langen K-J (2005) O-(2-[18F]fluoroethyl)-L-tyrosine PET combined with MRI improves the diagnostic assessment of cerebral gliomas. Brain 128:678–687

29. Wester H-J, Herz M, Weber W, Heiss P, Senekowitsch-Schmidtke R, Schwaiger M, Stöcklin G (1999) Synthesis and radiopharmacology of O-(2-[18F]fluoroethyl)-L-tyrosine for tumor imaging. J Nucl Med 40:205–212

30. Hamacher K, Coenen HH (2002) Effcient routine production of the 18F-labelled amino acid O-(2-[18F]fluoroethyl)-L-tyrosine. Appl Radiat Isot 57:205–212

31. Krasikova RN, Kuznetsova OF, Fedorova OS, Maleev VI, Saveleva TF, Belokon YN (2008) No carrier added synthesis of O-(2'-[18F]fluoroethyl)-l-tyrosine via a novel type of chiral enantiomerically pure precursor, Ni^{II} complex of a (S)-tyrosine schiff base. Bioorg Med Chem 16:4994–5003

32. Kong XB, Zhu QY, Vidal PM, Watanabe KA, Polsky B, Armstrong D, Ostrander M, Lang SA Jr, Muchmore E, Chou TC (1992) Comparisons of anti-human immunodeficiency virus activities, cellular transport, and plasma and intracellular pharmacokinetics of 3'-fluoro-3'-deoxythymidine and 3'-azido-3'-deoxythymidine. Antimicrob Agents Chemother 36:808–818

33. Shields AF, Grierson JR, Dohmen BM, Machulla H-J, Stayanoff JC, Lawhorn-Crews JM, Obradovich JE, Muzik O, Mangner TJ (1998) Imaging proliferation in vivo with [F-18]FLT and positron emission tomography. Nat Med 4:1334–1336

34. Mier W, Haberkorn U, Eisenhut M (2002) [F-18]FLT; portrait of a proliferation marker. Eur J Nucl Med Mol Imaging 29:165–169

35. Buck AK, Halter G, Schirrmeister H, Kotzerke J, Wurziger I, Glatting G, Mattfeldt T, Neumaier B, Reske SN, Hetzel M (2003) Imaging proliferation in lung tumors with PET: 18F-FLT versus 18F-FDG. J Nucl Med 44:1426–1431

36. Francis DL, Visvikis D, Costa DC, Arulampalam THA, Townsend C, Luthra SK, Taylor I, Ell PJ (2003) Potential impact of [18F]3'-deoxy-3'-fluorothymidine versus [18F]fluoro-2-deoxy-d-glucose in positron emission tomography for colorectal cancer. Eur J Nucl Med Mol Imaging 30:988–994

37. Van Waarde A, Cobben DCP, Suurmeijer AJH, Maas B, Vaalburg W, de Vries EFJ, Jager PL, Hoekstra HJ, Elsinga PH (2004) Selectivity of 18F-FLT and 18F-FDG for differentiating tumor from inflammation in a rodent model. J Nucl Med 45:695–700

38. Chen W, Cloughesy T, Kamdar N, Satyamurthy N, Bergsneider M, Liau L, Mischel P, Czernin J, Phelps ME, Silverman DHS (2005) Imaging proliferation in brain tumors with 18F-FLT PET: comparison with 18F-FDG. J Nucl Med 46:945–952

39. Shields AF (2006) Positron emission tomography measurement of tumor metabolism and growth: its expanding role in oncology. Mol Imag Biol 8:141–150

40. Yamamoto Y, Nishiyama Y, Kimura N, Ishikawa S, Okuda M, Bandoh S, Kanaji N, Asakura M, Ohkawa M (2008) Comparison of 18F-FLT PET and 18F-FDG PET for preoperative staging in non-small cell lung cancer. Eur J Nucl Med Mol Imaging 35:236–245

41. Wilson IK, Chatterjee S, Wolf W (1991) Synthesis of 3'-fluoro-3'-deoxythymidine and studies of its 18F-radiolabeling, as a tracer for the noninvasive monitoring of the biodistribution of drugs against AIDS. J Fluorine Chem 55:283–289

42. Kim DW, Ahn D-S, Oh Y-H, Lee S, Kil HS, Oh SJ, Lee SJ, Kim JS, Ryu JS, Moon DH, Chi SY (2006) A new class of S_N2 reactions catalyzed by protic solvents: facile fluorination for isotopic labeling of diagnostic molecules. J Am Chem Soc 128:16394–16397

43. Martin SJ, Eisenbarth JA, Wagner-Utermann U, Mier W, Henze M, Pritzkow H, Haberkorn U, Eisenhut M (2002) A new precursor for the radiosynthesis of [18F]FLT. Nucl Med Biol 29:263–273

44. Grierson JR, Shields AF (2000) Radiosynthesis of 3'-deoxy-3'-[18F]fluorothymidine: [18F]FLT for imaging of cellular proliferation in vivo. Nucl Med Biol 27: 143–156

45. Machulla H-J, Blocher A, Kuntzsch M, Piert M, Wei R, Grierson JR (2000) Simplified labeling approach for synthesizing 3'-deoxy-3'-[18F]fluorothymidine ([18F]flt). J Radioanal Nucl Chem 243:843–846

46. Yun M, Oh SJ, Ha H-J, Ryu JS, Moon DH (2003) High radiochemical yield synthesis of 3'-deoxy-3'-[18F] fluorothymidine using (5'-O-dimethoxytrityl-2'-deoxy-3'-O-nosyl-β-D-threo pentofuranosyl)thymine and its 3-N-BOC-protected analogue as a labeling precursor. Nucl Med Biol 30:151–157

47. Windhorst AD, Klein PJ, Eisenbarth J, Oeser T, Kruijer PS, Eisenhut M (2008) 3'-Sulfonylesters of 2, 5'-anhydro-1-(2-deoxy-β-D-threo-pentofuranosyl)thymine as precursors for the synthesis of [18F]FLT: syntheses and radiofluorination trials. Nucl Med Biol 35:413–423

48. Mintun MA, Welch MJ, Siegel BA, Mathias CJ, Brodack JW, McGuire AH, Katzenellenbogen JA (1988) Breast cancer: PET imaging of estrogen receptors. Radiology 169:45–48

49. Dehdashti F, Mortimer JE, Siegel BA, Griffeth LK, Bonasera TJ, Fusselman MJ, Detert DD, Cutler PD, Katzenellenbogen JA, Welch MJ (1995) Positron tomographic assessment of estrogen receptors in breast cancer: comparison with FDG-PET and in vitro receptor assays. J Nucl Med 36:1766–1774

50. Sundararajan L, Linden HM, Link JM, Krohn KA, Mankoff DA (2007) 18F-fluoroestradiol. Sem Nucl Med 37:470–476

51. Palmer AJ, Widdowson DA (1979) The preparation of 18F-labelled 4-fluoroestrone and 4-fluoroestradiol. J Labeled Compd Radiopharm 16:14–16

52. Eakins MN, Palmer AJ, Waters SL (1979) Studies in the rat with 18f-4-fluoro-oestradiol and 18f-4-fluoro-oestrone as potential prostate scanning agents: comparison with 125i–2-iodo-oestradiol and 125i–2, 4-di-iodo-oestradiol. Int J Appl Radiat Isot 30:695–700

53. Heiman DF, Senderoff SG, Katzenellenbogen JA, Neeley RJ (1980) Estrogen-receptor based imaging agents. 1. synthesis and receptor-binding affinity of some aromatic and d-ring halogenated estrogens. J Nucl Med 23:994–1002

54. Kiesewetter DO, Katzenellenbogen JA, Kilbourn MR, Welch MJ (1984) Synthesis of 16-fluoroestrogens by unusually facile fluoride ion displacement reactions: prospects for the preparation of fluorine-18 labeled estrogens. J Org Chem 49:4900–4905

55. Kiesewetter DO, Kilbourn MR, Landvatter SW, Heiman DF, Katzenellenbogen JA, Welch MJ (1984) Preparation of four fluorine-18-labeled estrogens and their selective uptakes in target tissues of immature rats. J Nucl Med 25:1212–1221

56. Van Brocklin HF, Carlson KE, Katzenellenbogen JA, Welch MJ (1993) 16β-([18F]Fluoro)estrogens: systematic investigation of a new series of fluorine-18-labeled estrogens as potential imaging agents for estrogen-receptor-positive breast tumors. J Med Chem 36: 1619–1629

57. Benard F, Ahmed N, Beauregard JM, Rousseau J, Aliaga A, Dubuc C, Croteau E, van Lier JE (2008) [F-18]fluorinated estradiol derivatives for oestrogen receptor imaging: impact of substituents, formulation and specific activity on the biodistribution in breast tumour-bearing mice. Eur J Nucl Med Mol Imaging 35:1473–1479

58. Römer J, Steinbach J, Kasch H (1996) Studies on the synthesis of 16 alpha-[F-18]fluoroestradiol. Appl Radiat Isot 47:395–399

59. Römer J, Füchtner F, Steinbach J, Johanssen B (1999) Automated production of 16α-[F-18]fluoroestradiol for breast cancer imaging. Nucl Med Biol 26:473–479

60. Mori T, Kasamatsu S, Mosdzianowski C, Welch MJ, Yonekura Y, Fujibayashi Y (2006) Automatic synthesis of 16α-[F-18]fluoro-17β-estradiol using a cassette-type [F-18]fluorodeoxyglucose synthesizer. Nucl Med Biol 33:281–286

61. DeGrado TR, Baldwin SW, Wang S, Orr MD, Liao RP, Friedman HS, Reiman R, Price DT, Coleman RE (2001) Synthesis and evaluation of 18F-labeled choline analogs as oncologic pet tracers. J Nucl Med 42:1805–1814

62. Hara T, Kosaka N, Shinoura N, Kondo T (1997) PET imaging of brain tumor with [methyl-11C]choline. J Nucl Med 38:842–824

63. DeGrado TR, Coleman RE, Wang S, Baldwin SW, Orr MD, Robertson CN, Polascik TJ, Price DT (2000) Synthesis and evaluation of 18F-labeled choline as an oncologic tracer for positron emission tomography: initial findings in prostate cancer. Cancer Res 61:110–117

64. Hara T (2001) 18F-Fluorocholine: a new oncologic PET tracer. J Nucl Med 12:1815–1817

65. Kwee SA, Coel MN, Lim J, Ko JP (2004) Combined use of F-18 fluorocholine positron emission tomography and magnetic resonance spectroscopy for brain tumour evaluation. J Neuroimaging 14:285–289

66. Coenen HH, Colosimo M, Schüller M, Stöcklin G (1985) Preparation of N. C. A. [18F]-CH2BrF via aminopolyether supported nucleophilic substitution. J Labelled Compd Radiopharm 23:587–595

67. Eskola O, Bergman J, Lehikoinen P, Ögren M, Långström B, Solin O (1999) Synthesis of 18F-bromofluoromethane [18F]FCH2Br; fluoromethylation reagent with high specific radioactivity. J Labelled Compd Radiopharm 42:S543–S545

68. Rasey JS, Koh W-J, Evans ML, Peterson LM, Lewellen TK, Graham MM, Krohn KA (1996) Quantifying regional hypoxia in human tumors with positron emission tomography of [18F]fluoromisonidazole: a pretherapy study of 37 patients. Int J Radiat Oncol Biol Phys 36:417–428

69. Lui R-S, Chu L-S, Yen S-H, Chang C-P, Chou K-L, Wu L-C, Chang C-W, Lui M-T, Chen KY, Yeh S-H (1996) Detection of anaerobic odontogenic infections by fluorine-18 fluoromisonidazole. Eur J Nucl Med Mol Imaging 23:1384–1387

70. Rajendran JG, Wilson DC, Conrad EU, Peterson LM, Bruckner JD, Rasey JS, Chin LK, Hofstrand PD, Grierson JR, Eary JF, Krohn KA (2003) [^{18}F]FMISO and [^{18}F]FDG PET imaging in soft tissue sarcomas: correlation of hypoxia, metabolism and VEGF expression. Eur J Nucl Med Mol Imaging 30:695–704

71. Lewis JS, Welch MJ (2001) PET imaging of hypoxia. Q J Nucl Med 45:183–188

72. Lehtiö K, Oikonen V, Nyman S, Grönroos T, Roivainen A, Eskola O, Minn H (2003) Quantifying tumour hypoxia with fluorine-18 fluoroerythronitroimidazole ([^{18}F]FET-NIM) and PET using the tumour to plasma ratio. Eur J Nucl Med Mol Imaging 30:101–108

73. Barthel H, Wilson H, Collingridge DR, Brown G, Osman S, Luthra SK, Brady F, Workman P, Price PM, Aboagye EO (2004) In vivo evaluation of [18F]fluoroetanidazole as a new marker for imaging tumour hypoxia with positron emission tomography. Brit J Cancer 90:2232–2242

74. Kämäräinen E-L, Kyllönen T, Nihtilä O, Björk H, Solin O (2004) Preparation of fluorine-18-labelled fluoromisonidazole using two different synthesis methods. J Labelled Compd Radiopharm 47:37–45

75. Grierson JR, Link JM, Mathis CA, Rasey JS, Krohn KA (1989) A radiosynthesis of fluorine-18 fluoromisonidazole. J Nucl Med 30:343–350

76. McCarthy TJ, Dence CS, Welch MJ (1993) Application of microwave heating to the synthesis of [^{18}F]fluoromisonidazole. Appl Radiat Isot 44:1129–1132

77. Lim J-L, Berridge MS (1993) An efficient radiosynthesis of [^{18}F]fluoromisonidazole. Appl Radiat Isot 44:1085–1091

78. Patt M, Kuntzsch M, Machulla HJ (1999) Preparation of [18F]fluoromisonidazole by nucleophilic substitution on THP-protected precursor: yield dependence on reaction parameters. J Radioanal Nucl Chem 240:925–927

79. Oh SJ, Chi DY, Mosdzianowski C, Kim JY, Gil HS, Kang SH, Ryu JS, Moon DH (2005) Fully automated synthesis of [^{18}F]fluoromisonidazole using a conventional [^{18}F]FDG module. Nucl Med Biol 32:899–905

80. Crouzel C, Guillaume M, Barré L, Lemaire C, Pike VW (1992) Ligands and tracers for PET studies of the 5-HT system – current status. Nucl Med Biol 19:857–870

81. Pike VW (1995) Radioligands for PET studies of central 5-HT receptors and re-uptake sites – current status. Nucl Med Biol 22:1011–1018

82. Lemaire C, Cantineau R, Guillaume M, Plenevaux A, Christiaens L (1991) Fluorine-18-altanserin: a radioligand for the study of serotonin receptors with PET: radiolabeling and in vivo biologic behavior in rats. J Nucl Med 32:2266–2272

83. Lemaire C, Cantineau R, Christiaens L, Guillaume M (1989) N.c.a. radiofluorination of altanserin: apotential serotonin receptor-binding radiopharamceutical for positron emission tomography. J Labelled Compd Radiopharm 26:336–337

84. Mukherjee J, Yang Z-Y, Lew R, Brown T, Kronmal S, Cooper MD, Seiden LS (1997) Evaluation of d-amphetamine effects on the binding of dopamine D-2 receptor radioligand, F-18-fallypride in nonhuman primates using positron emission tomography. Synapse 27:1–13

85. Mukherjee J, Yang Z-Y, Brown T, Lew R, Wernick M, Ouyang X, Yasillo N, Chen C-T, Mintzer R, Cooper M (1999) Preliminary assessment of extrastriatal dopamine d-2 receptor binding in the rodent and nonhuman primate brains using the high affinity radioligand, ^{18}F-fallypride. Nucl Med Biol 26:519–527

86. Christian BT, Narayanan TK, Shi BZ, Mukherjee J (2000) Quantitation of striatal and extrastriatal D-2 dopamine receptors using PET imaging of [F-18]fallypride in nonhuman primates. Synapse 38:71–79

87. Slifstein M, Narendran R, Hwang DR, Sudo Y, Talbot PS, Huang YY, Laruelle M (2004) Effect of amphetamine on [F-18]fallypride in vivo binding to D-2 receptors in striatal and extrastriatal regions of the primate brain: single bolus and bolus plus constant infusion studies. Synapse 54:46–63

88. Riccardi P, Baldwin R, Salomon R, Anderson S, Ansari MS, Li R, Dawant B, Bauernfeind A, Schmidt D, Kessler R (2008) Estimation of baseline dopamine D-2 receptor occupancy in striatum and extrastriatal regions in humans with positron emission tomography with [F-18] fallypride. Biol Psychiatry 63:241–244

89. Mukherjee J, Yang Z-Y, Das MK, Brown T (1995) Fluorinated benzamide neuroleptics – III. Development of (S)-N-[(1-allyl-2-pyrrolidinyl)methyl]-5-(3-[18F]fluoropropyl)-2, 3-dimethoxybenzamide as an improved dopamine D-2 receptor tracer. Nucl Med Biol 22:283–296

90. Farde L, Pauli S, Hall A, Eriksson L, Halldin C, Hörgberg T, Nilsson L, Sjögren I, Stone-Elander S (1988) Stereoselective binding of ^{11}C-raclopride in living human brain – a search for extrastriatal D2 receptors by PET. Psychopharmacology 94:471–478

91. Halldin C, Stone-Elander S, Thorell J-O, Pearson A, Sedvall G (1988) ^{11}C-labelling of Ro 15-1788 in two different positions, and also ^{11}C-labelling of its main metabolite Ro 153890 for PET studies of benzodiazepine receptors. Appl Radiat Isot 39:993–997

92. Långström B, Lunqvist H (1976) The preparation of [^{11}C]methyl iodide and its use in the synthesis of [^{11}C] methyl-L-methionine. Appl Radiat Isot 27:357–363

93. Långström B, Antoni G, Gullberg P, Halldin C, Malmborg P, Någren K, Rimland A, Svärd H (1987) Synthesis of L- and D-[methyl-^{11}c]methionine. J Nucl Med 28: 1037–1040

94. Guadagno JV, Donnan GA, Markus R, Gillard JH, Baron JC (2004) Imaging the ischaemic penumbra. Curr Opin Neurol 17:61–67

95. Savic I, Lindström P, Gulyas B, Halldin C, Andree B, Farde L (2004) Limbic reduction of 5-HT$_{1A}$ receptor binding in human temporal lobe epilepsy. Neurology 62:1343–1351

96. Klunk WE, Engler H, Nordberg A, Wang YM, Blomqvist G, Holt DP, Bergstrom M, Savitcheva I, Huang GF, Estrada S, Ausen B, Debnath ML, Barletta J, Price JC, Sandell J, Lopresti BJ, Wall A, Koivisto P, Antoni G, Mathis CA, Langstrom B (2004) Imaging brain amyloid in Alzheimer's disease with Pittsburgh compound-B. Ann Neurol 55:306–319

97. Tian M, Zhang H, Oriuchi N, Higuchi T, Endo K (2004) Brain tumour imaging with comparison of ^{11}C-choline PET and FDG PET for the differential diagnosis of malignant tumors. Eur J Nucl Med 31:1064–1072

98. Farde L, Halldin C, Stone-Elander S, Sedvall G (1987) PET analysis of human dopamine receptor subtypes using

c-11 sch 23390 and c-11 raclopride. Psychopharmacology 92:278–284

99. Houle S, Ginovart N, Hussey D, Meyer JH, Wilson AA (2000) Imaging the serotonin transporter with positron emission tomography: initial human studies with [^{11}C] DAPP and [^{11}C]DASB. Eur J Nucl Med Mol Imaging 27:1719–1722

100. Strauss LG, Conti PS (1991) The application of PET in clinical oncology. J Nucl Med 32:623–648

101. Derlon JM (1998) The in vivo metabolic investigation of brain gliomas with positron emission tomography. Adv Tech Stand Neursurg 24:41–76

102. Bombardieri E, Carriago I, Conzales P, Serafini A, Turner JH, Virgolini I, Maffioli L (1999) Main diagnostic applications in oncology. Eur J Nucl Med 26:BP21–BP27

103. Oyama N, Miller TR, Dehdashti F, Siegel BA, Fischer KC, Michalski JM, Kibel AS, Andriole GL, Picus J, Welch MJ (2003) ^{11}C-acetate PET imaging of prostate cancer: detection of recurrent disease at PSA relapse. J Nucl Med 44:549–555

104. Schäfers M, Dutka D, Rhodes CG, Lammertsma AA, Hermansen F, Schober O, Camici PG (1998) Myocardial presynaptic and postsynaptic autonomic dysfunction in hypertropic cardiomyopathy. Circ Res 82:57–62

105. Wichter T, Schäfers M, Rhodes CG, Borggrefe M, Lerch H, Lammertsma AA, Hermansen F, Schober O, Breithardt G, Camici PG (2000) Abnormalities of cardiac sympathetic innervation in arrhythmogenic right ventricular cardiomyopathy: quantitative assessment of presynaptic norepinephrine reuptake and postsynaptic ß-adrenergic receptor density with positron emission tomography. Circulation 101:1552–1558

106. Clark JC, Crouzel C, Meyer GJ, Strijckmans K (1987) Current methodology for oxygen-15 production for clinical use. Appl Radiat Isot 38:597–600

107. Berridge MS, Cassidy EH, Terris AH (1990) A routine, automated synthesis of oxygen-15 labelled butanol for positron emission tomography. J Nucl Med 31:1727–1731

108. Sajjad M, Lambrecht RM, Wolf AP (1986) Cyclotron isotopes and radiopharmaceuticals 37. Exitation-functions for the O-16(p, alpha)N-13 and N-14(p, pn)N-13 reactions. Radiochim Acta 39:165–168

109. Wieland B, Bida G, Padgett H, Hendry G, Zippi E, Kabalka G, Morelle J-L, Verbruggen R, Ghyoot M (1991) In target production of ^{13}N-ammonia via proton irradiation of aqueous ethanol and acetic acid mixtures. Appl Radiat Isot 42:1095–1098

110. Rösch F, Riss PJ (2010) The renaissance of ^{68}Ge/^{68}Ga radionuclide generators initiates new developments in ^{68}Ga radiopharmaceutical chemistry. Curr Topics Med Chem 10: (in press)

111. Hofmann M, Oei M, Boerner AR, Maecke H, Geworski L, Knapp WH, Krause T (2005) Comparison of Ga-68-DOTATOC and Ga-68-DOTANOC for radiopeptide PET. Nuklearmedizin 44:A58

112. Henze M, Dimitrakopoulou-Strauss A, Milker-Zabel S, Schuhmacher J, Strauss LG, Doll J, Maecke HR, Eisenhut M, Debus J, Haberkorn U (2005) Characterization of ^{68}Ga-DOTA-D-Phe^1-Tyr^3-octreotide kinetics in patients with meningiomas. J Nucl Med 46:763–769

113. Green MA, Klippenstein DL, Tennison JR (1988) Copper (II)bis(thiosemicarbazone) complexes as potential tracers for evaluation of cerebral and myocardial blood flow with PET. J Nucl Med 29:1549–1557

114. Takahashi N, Fujibayashi Y, Yonekura Y, Welch MJ, Waki A, Tsuchida T, Sadato N, Sugimoto K, Itoh H (2000) Evaluation of ^{62}Cu labeled diacetyl-bis(N^4-methylthiosemicarbazone) in hypoxic tissue in patients with lung cancer. Ann Nucl Med 14:323–328

115. Dehdashti F, Mintun MA, Lewis JS (2003) In vivo assessment of tumour hypoxiy in lung cancer with ^{60}Cu-ATSM. Eur J Nucl Med Mol Imaging 30:844–850

116. Haynes NG, Lacy JL, Nayak N, Martin CS, Dai D, Mathias CJ, Green MA (2000) Performance of a ^{62}Zn/^{62}Cu generator in clinical trials of PET perfusion agent ^{62}Cu-PTSM. J Nucl Med 41:309–314

117. Satyamurthy N, Phelps ME, Barrio JR (1999) Electronic generators for the production of positron-emitter labelled radiopharmaceuticals: Where would PET be without them? Clin Posit Imag 2:233–253

118. Alexoff DL (2003) Automation for the synthesis and application of PET radiopharmaceuticals. In: Welch MJ, Redvanly CS (eds) Handbook of radiopharmaceuticals. Radiochemistry and application. Wiley, Chichester, pp 283–305

119. Krasikova R (2007) Synthesis modules and automation in F-18 labeling. In: Schubiger PA, Lehmann L, Friebe M (eds) PET chemistry – the driving force in molecular imaging. Springer, Berlin, pp 289–316

120. Lucignani G (2006) Pivotal role of nanotechnologies and biotechnologies for molecular imaging and therapy. Eur J Nucl Med Mol Imaging 33:849–851

121. Pike VW, Lu SY (2007) Micro-reactors for pet tracer labeling. In: Schubiger PA, Lehmann L, Friebe M (eds) PET chemistry – the driving force in molecular imaging. Springer, Berlin, pp 271–287

122. Brady F, Luthra SK, Gillies JM, Geffery NT (2003) Use of microfabricated devices. PCT WO 03/078358 A2

123. Lu SY, Watts P, Chin FT, Hong J, Musachio JL, Briard E, Pike VW (2004) Syntheses of ^{11}C- and ^{18}F-labeled carboxylic esters within a hydrodynamically driven microreactor. Lab Chip 4:523–525

124. Gillies JM, Prenant C, Chimon GN, Smethurst GJ, Perrie W, Hamblett I, Dekker B, Zweit J (2006) Microfluidic reactor for the radiosynthesis of PET radiotracers. Appl Radiat Isot 64:325–332

125. Saha GB (2004) Fundamentals of nuclear pharmacy, 5th edn. Springer, New York

126. Littman BH, Williams SA (2005) The ultimate model organism: progress in experimental medicine. Nat Rev Drug Discov 4:631–638

127. Bench CJ, Lammertsma AA, Dolan RJ, Grasby PM, Warrington SJ, Gunn K, Cuddigan M, Turton DJ, Osman S, Frackowiak RSJ (1993) Dose dependent occupancy of central dopamine D2 receptors by the novel neuroleptic CP-88, 059–01: a study using positron emission tomography and 11C-raclopride. Psychopharmacology 112:308–314

128. Yokoi F, Gründer G, Biziere K, Stephane M, Dogan AS, Dannals RF, Ravert H, Suri A, Bramer S, Wong DF (2002)

Dopamine D-2 and D-3 receptor occupancy in normal humans treated with the antipsychotic drug aripiprazole (OPC 14597): a study using positron emission tomography and [C-11]raclopride. Neuropsychopharmacology 27:248–259

129. Joensuu H, Roberts PJ, Sarlomo-Rikala M, Andersson LC, Tervahartiala P, Tuveson D, Silberman SL, Capdeville R, Dimitrijevic S, Druker B, Demetri GD (2001) Effect of the tyrosine kinase inhibitor STI571 in a patient with ameta-static gastrointestinal stromal tumor. New Engl J Med 344:1052–1056

130. Demetri GD, George S, Heinrich MC, Fletcher JA, Fletcher CDM, Desai J, Cohen DP, Scigalla P, Cherrington JM, Van Den Abbeele AD (2003) Clinical activity and tolerability of the multi-targeted tyrosine kinase inhibitor SU11248 in patients with metastatic gastrointestinal stromal tumor (GIST) refractory to imatinib mesylate. Proc Am Soc Clin Oncol 22:3273

Radiation Dosimetry: Definitions and Basic Quantities

Michael G. Stabin

Contents

7.1 Introduction

The discovery of X-rays by Roentgen in 1895 began a new era in medicine. The first uses of ionizing radiation permitted the noninvasive visualization of internal structures of the body, which was quite revolutionary. Later in 1924, de Hevesy and colleagues performed studies of the kinetics of lead-210 (^{210}Pb) and bismuth-210 (^{210}Bi) in animals, introducing the idea of the use of radioactive substances to investigate dynamic processes in the body and study physiological, as opposed to only anatomical, information [1].

This science grew steadily for many years, and the Society of Nuclear Medicine was organized 30 years later, to facilitate the exchange of information by professionals in this field. Most applications of the science of nuclear medicine are *diagnostic*, i.e., evaluating body structures and internal processes to diagnose diseases and guide medical response to potential human health issues. Radiopharmaceuticals used in nuclear medicine have also been applied for many decades in *therapeutics*, i.e., exploiting the ability of ionizing radiation to destroy potentially harmful tissues in the body (e.g., cancer or inflamed joints). A radiation dose analysis is a necessary element of the safety analysis to permit the use of either diagnostic or therapeutic radiopharmaceuticals. For diagnostic compounds, the US Food and Drug Administration (FDA) evaluates a number of safety parameters during the approval process for new pharmaceuticals; internal dose assessment (or "dosimetry") is one of the key areas of evaluation. During the various phases of the drug approval process, radiation dose estimates are generated, and average values will be included with the product information package that accompanies radioactive drugs that are brought successfully to market. These dose estimates are not often used directly in day-to-day practice in the clinic, but are often referred to when comparing advantages and disadvantages of possible competing drug products, by radioactive drug research committees (RDRCs) in evaluating safety concerns in research protocols, and other situations.

7.1.1 Practice of Internal Dosimetry

In therapeutic applications, physicians *should* perform a patient-specific evaluation of radiation doses to tumors and normal tissues in order to design a

M.G. Stabin
Department of Radiology and Radiological Sciences Vanderbilt University, 1161 21st Avenue South, Nashville, TN 37232-2675,
e-mail: michael.g.stabin@vanderbilt.edu

M.M. Khalil (ed.), *Basic Sciences of Nuclear Medicine*, DOI: 10.1007/978-3-540-85962-8_7,
© Springer-Verlag Berlin Heidelberg 2011

treatment protocol that maximizes the dose to malignant tissues while maintaining doses to healthy tissues at acceptable levels (i.e., below thresholds for direct deleterious effects). This is done routinely in external radiation therapy treatment planning, but unfortunately, dose assessment is not routinely practiced in most clinics at present in the administration of radiopharmaceuticals for therapy. All patients are generally treated with the same or similar amounts of activity, without regard to their specific biokinetic characteristics. Many investigators have called for dose assessment to become a routine part of the practice of radiopharmaceutical therapy [2–6]' in the interests of improving patient care.

7.1.2 Responsibilities

The patient/physician relationship involves trust, the weighing and balancing of a number of risks and benefits of possible procedures, discussion of personal information, and other delicate issues such as personal, ethical, and religious standards. Physicists provide information that the physician must understand and convey to his/her patients, and thus play a peripheral, but still important, part of the process of the delivery of medical care involving radioactive substances. In diagnostic applications, the physicist is rather removed from the process, having previously provided dose calculations to regulatory and other bodies for their evaluations of the use of radiopharmaceuticals in clinical practice and research. In radiopharmaceutical therapy, however, the physicist should be more involved in the future, as is true for external beam therapy, and much useful experience can be gained that will ultimately result in better and more durable patient outcomes [6].

7.2 Basic Quantities and Units

Accurate quantification of the various terms involved in our theoretical calculations is important to obtaining an acceptable outcome. Many of the conversions that occur in the use of quantities in the atomic world have very large or very small exponents (e.g., there are 1.6×10^{-13} J in 1 MeV). Thus, when unit conversions are performed, involving multiplication and/or division,

small errors in values of a conversion constant may result in *enormous* errors in our final calculation. Common sense must be applied in the choice of the number of significant figures shown in presented dose estimates; the final value should also be rounded to a *sensible* number of significant figures. Roger Cloutier once quipped that "I only use one significant digit in reporting internal dose values because you can't use any fewer!" [7] In internal dose assessments, a number of modeling assumptions and simplifications are usually applied to solve a problem. Numerous uncertainties exist in the input values as well as the applicability of the values and the models used. Providing organ dose or effective dose values to ten significant figures is simply unreasonable. Final answers for any radiopharmaceutical dose estimate should be given to two or three significant figures, no more.

7.2.1 Administered Activity

The quantity "Activity" is defined as the number of nuclear transformations per unit time occurring in a given sample of radioactive material. The units are nuclear transformations/unit time. Special units include:

Curie (Ci) = 3.7×10^{10} transformations/s

Becquerel (Bq) = 1 transformation/s

Two other quantities are also defined: The radioactive decay constant (λ) is the rate constant for radioactive atoms undergoing spontaneous nuclear transformation. Its units are inverse time, (s^{-1}, for example). The radioactive half-life is the time needed for one half of the atoms in a sample of radioactive material to undergo transformation. Mathematically, the half-life is $\ln(2)/\lambda = 0.693/\lambda$. Its units are time (seconds, for example).

7.2.2 Absorbed Dose

Absorbed Dose is the energy absorbed per unit mass of any material (i.e., not only human tissue). Absorbed dose (D) is defined as:

$$D = \frac{d\varepsilon}{dm}$$

where $d\varepsilon$ is the mean energy imparted by ionizing radiation to matter in a volume element of mass dm. The units of absorbed dose are energy per unit mass, e.g., erg/g, J/kg, or others. Special units include the rad (equal to 100 erg/g), the gray (Gy) (1 J/kg). 1 Gy = 100 rad. The word "rad" was originally an acronym meaning "radiation absorbed dose." The rad is being replaced by the SI unit value, the gray (Gy), which is equal to 100 rad. Note that "rad" and "gray" are collective quantities; one does not need to place an "s" after them to indicate more than one.

Closely related to absorbed dose is the quantity kerma, which is actually an acronym meaning "kinetic energy released in matter." Kerma is given as

$$K = \frac{dE_{Tr}}{dm}$$

dE_{Tr} is the sum of the initial kinetic energies of all the charged ionizing particles liberated by uncharged ionizing particles in a material of mass dm. Kerma has the same units and special units as absorbed dose, but is a measure of energy *liberated*, rather than energy *absorbed*. The two will be equal under conditions of charged particle equilibrium, and assuming negligible losses by bremsstrahlung radiation.

7.2.3 Linear Energy Transfer

The quantity Linear Energy Transfer (LET) is given as:

$$LET = \frac{dE_L}{dl}$$

where dE_L is the average energy locally imparted to a given medium by a charged particle passing through a length of medium dl. The units of LET are often given as keV/μm, although any units may be used. LET is an important parameter used in characterizing energy deposition in radiation detectors and in biological media in which we wish to study the effects of different types of radiation.

7.2.4 Relative Biological Effectiveness (RBE)

When the effects of other radiations on the same cell population to produce the same endpoint are studied, it is often observed that all radiation does not produce the same effects at the same dose levels as this "reference" radiation. If a dose D' of a given radiation type produces the same biological endpoint in a given experiment as a dose D of our reference radiation, we can define a quantity called the Relative Biological Effectiveness (RBE) [8] as:

$$RBE = \frac{D}{D'}$$

So, for example, if a dose of 1 Gy of the reference radiation produces a particular cell survival level, but only 0.05 Gy of alpha radiation produces the same level of cell killing, the RBE for alpha particles in this experiment is given as 20.

RBE is closely related to radiation LET. High LET radiations generally have high RBEs (250 kVp X-rays are generally considered to be low LET radiation). The relationship of the two variables is not directly linear, but there is clearly a positively correlated relationship of RBE with LET, until very high LET values are reached, where "overkill" of cells causes the RBE not to increase so quickly.

The reader may have noted that in the numerical example chosen above, the RBE for alpha particles is exactly equal to the currently recommended value of w_R, the radiation weighting factor used in radiation protection. This was done intentionally. Values of w_R are very closely tied to RBE values; however, they are NOT exactly equal. Generally, conservative values of RBE were used to set the values assigned for w_R values (also formerly called "quality factors"). RBE values are highly dependent on the experimental conditions (cell type, radiation type, radiation dose rate) and the biological endpoint defined for study in which they were defined. Radiation weighting factors, on the other hand, are chosen operational quantities to be applied to a type of radiation in all situations.

7.2.5 Radiation Weighting Factor and Equivalent Dose

The quantity equivalent dose ($H_{T,R}$) has been defined to account for differences in the effectiveness of different types of radiation in producing biological damage:

$$H_{T,R} = w_R D_{T,R}$$

where $D_{T,R}$ is the dose delivered by radiation type R averaged over a tissue or organ T and w_R is the radiation weighting factor for radiation type R.

The weighting factor w_R is really dimensionless, so fundamentally, the units are the same as absorbed dose (energy/mass). Operationally, however, we distinguish using the special units of the rem (which is the D(rad) $\times w_R$) and sievert (Sv) (equal to the D(Gy) $\times w_R$). As 1 Gy = 100 rad, 1 Sv = 100 rem.

Note that like rad and gray, the rem and sievert are collective terms; one need not speak of "rems" and "sieverts", although this may be heard in common speech and even observed in publications. Also note that units that incorporate a person's name (Roentgen, Gray, Sievert) are given in lower case when spelled out completely, but with the first letter capitalized when given as the unit abbreviation (e.g., "sievert" and "Sv").

Equivalent dose is defined for ANY kind of radiation, but ONLY in human tissue. The recommended values of the radiation weighting factor have varied somewhat over the years, as evidence from biological experiments has been given and interpreted. The current values recommended by the International Commission on Radiological Protection [9] are shown in Table 7.1 (note that values for neutrons are not given, as they are not often of interest in internal dosimetry).

The weighting factor of 20 for alpha particles is reasonable for radiation protection purposes, but some radiobiological evidence indicates that this value may be too conservative for use in radiopharmaceutical

Table 7.1 Radiation weighting factors recommended by the ICRP [9]

Type of radiation	w_R
Photons, all energies	1
Electrons and muons	1
Protons and charged pions	2
Alpha particles, fission fragments, heavy ions	20

therapy, and may be as low as five [10] or even one [11] The contrary argument applies to the use of Auger emitters, for which literature values indicate a range of potential RBEs greater than 1, particularly if the emitters are closely associated with cellular DNA [12] Clearly, more investigation and guidance from regulatory and international advisory bodies are needed for the application of these values to internal dosimetry therapy.

7.2.6 Tissue Weighting Factor and Effective Dose

The International Commission on Radiological Protection (ICRP), in its 1979 description of radiation protection quantities and limits for radiation workers [13] defined a new dosimetry quantity, the *effective dose equivalent* (H_e or EDE). The ICRP subsequently renamed this quantity *effective dose* (E) in 1991 [14] and the weighting factors were again updated in ICRP Publication 103 [9]. Certain organs or organ

Table 7.2 Weighting factors recommended by the ICRP for calculation of the effective dose

Organ	ICRP 30 (1979)	ICRP 60 (1991)	ICRP 103 (2007)
Gonads	0.25	0.20	0.08
Red marrow	0.12	0.12	0.12
Colon		0.12	0.12
Lungs	0.12	0.12	0.12
Stomach		0.12	0.12
Bladder		0.05	0.04
Breasts	0.15	0.05	0.12
Liver		0.05	0.04
Esophagus		0.05	0.04
Thyroid	0.03	0.05	0.04
Skin		0.01	0.01
Bone surfaces	0.03	0.01	0.01
Brain			0.01
Salivary glands			0.01
Remainder	0.30	0.05	0.12

systems were assigned dimensionless weighting factors (Table 7.2) which are a function of their assumed relative radiosensitivity for expressing fatal cancers or genetic defects.

Here is an example calculation using the tissue weighting factors from ICRP 60 and some assumed individual organ equivalent doses:

Organ	Weighting Factor	Equivalent Dose (mSv)	Weighted dose Equivalent (mSv)
Liver	0.05	0.53	0.0265
Kidneys	0.005	0.37	0.00185
Ovaries	0.20	0.19	0.038
Red marrow	0.12	0.42	0.0504
Bone surfaces	0.01	0.55	0.0055
Thyroid	0.05	0.05	0.0025
Total (effective dose)			0.125

The assumed radiosensitivities were derived from the observed rates of expression of these effects in various populations exposed to radiation. Multiplying an organ's dose equivalent by its assigned weighting factor gives a "weighted dose equivalent." The *sum of weighted dose equivalents* for a given exposure to radiation is the effective dose:

$$E = \sum_T H_T \times w_T$$

The effective dose is meant to represent the equivalent dose which, if received uniformly by the whole body, would result in the same total risk as that actually incurred by a given actual nonuniform irradiation. It is *entirely different* from the dose equivalent to the "whole body" that is calculated using dose conversion factors for the total body. "Whole body" doses are basically meaningless in nuclear medicine applications, as nonuniform and localized energy deposition is simply averaged over the mass of the whole body (70 kg). Thus, if a radiopharmaceutical concentrates heavily in a few organs, all of the energy absorbed by these (and other) organs is divided by the mass of the whole body to obtain the "whole body" dose. This quantity is not meaningful in internal dose assessment, unless the radionuclide distribution is nearly uniform, as, for example, for intakes of ^3H_2O, or ^{137}Cs. The goal of nuclear medicine is to administer compounds that selectively concentrate in particular organs or regions of the body for diagnostic or therapeutic purposes, so "whole body" dose is not a descriptive or useful quantity to calculate. Table 7.3 summarizes some of the dose quantities of interest in nuclear medicine dosimetry.

Some have objected to the use of the effective dose quantity in nuclear medicine, due to the uncertainties involved and the fact that the quantity was derived for use with a radiation worker population [15] The ICRP itself, however, as well as many other international organizations, has affirmed that the quantity is useful for nuclear medicine applications, the associated uncertainties notwithstanding. It is clearly more useful in evaluating and comparing doses between radiopharmaceuticals with different distribution and retention patterns in the body. It is very important, however, to recognize the *limitations* on its use:

Table 7.3 Summary of nuclear medicine dose quantities

Quantity	Units	Comments
Individual organ dose (absorbed dose or equivalent dose)	Gy or Sv	Doses to all available organs and tissues in the standardized phantoms should be routinely reported.
Maximum dose organ (absorbed dose or equivalent dose)	Gy or Sv	The individual organ that receives the highest dose per unit activity administered or per study should be considered in study design and execution.
Whole body dose (absorbed dose or equivalent dose)	Gy or Sv	Useful *only* if all organs and tissues in the body receive an approximately uniform dose. Rarely of value for radiopharmaceuticals. Most useful in external dose assessment.
Effective dose	Sv	Risk weighted effective whole body dose. Gives the equivalent dose uniform to the whole body that theoretically has the same risk as the actual, nonuniform dose pattern received.

- The quantity should *never be used in situations involving radiation therapy*, as it is related to the evaluation of stochastic risks from exposures involving low doses and dose rates.
- It should *not be used to evaluate the risk to a given individual*; its application is to populations which receive doses at these levels.

If one accepts the quantity, with all of its inherent assumptions and uncertainties, however, it provides some useful features:

- As just noted, it allows direct comparison of different radiopharmaceuticals which may have completely different radiation dose patterns. For example, compare the use of ^{201}Tl chloride with ^{99m}Tc Sestamibi for use in myocardial imaging studies. There are many variables that enter into a discussion of which agent is preferable for these studies, and we will not review all of them here. But just from a radiation dose standpoint, if one uses, for example, 74 MBq (2 mCi) of ^{201}Tl chloride, the two highest dose organs are the thyroid, which may receive about 40 mGy (4 rad) and the kidneys, which may receive about 30 mSv (3 rem) [16] One might instead use 740 MBq (20 mCi) of ^{99m}Tc Sestamibi, in which case, the two highest dose organs are the gallbladder, which may receive about 29 mSv (2.9 rem) and the kidneys, which may receive about 27 mSv (2.7 rem) (rest patients) [17] The kidney doses are similar, but is 40 mGy to the thyroid more acceptable than 29 mGy to the gallbladder? The effective dose for ^{201}Tl chloride is 11.5 mSv (1.15 rem) and for ^{99m}Tc Sestamibi is 6.7 mSv (0.67 rem). So, strictly from a dose standpoint, the use of ^{99m}Tc Sestamibi appears more desirable, although this was not immediately obvious by looking at the highest dose organs.
- Effective doses from radiopharmaceuticals may be added to those received from other procedures outside of nuclear medicine. For example, if a typical value of an effective dose for a lumbar spine x-ray is 2.1 mSv (0.21 rem), and a subject has had two such exams recently and then receives a ^{99m}Tc Sestamibi heart scan, the total effective dose is estimated as $6.7 + (2 \times 2.1) = 11$ mSv (1.1 rem).
- A popular way to explain radiation risks in a simple way that many members of the public can understand is to express the dose in terms of equivalent years of exposure to background radiation [18] Estimates of background radiation dose rates vary, but if one chooses 3 mSv/year (300 mrem/

year) as an example, then the ^{99m}Tc Sestamibi study discussed above may be thought of as equivalent in total risk to slightly more than 2 years of exposure to natural background radiation.

7.2.7 Specific Energy

It is a generally accepted axiom that the cell nucleus is the critical target for either cell death or transformation (some arguments about dose to other cell structures, such as the mitochondria, being important have been raised, but are controversial). As the target size that we estimate the dose to becomes small, and as the dose becomes low, variations in dose may become very large, and average values become less meaningful. Thus, in many cases, it becomes more meaningful to express the absorbed dose as a *stochastic* quantity instead of as a single average value. The *stochastic quantity* that is the corollary to the average absorbed dose in macrodosimetry (the subject addressed previously in this chapter) is called the *specific energy* (z). It is defined as the quotient of e over m, where e is the energy imparted by ionizing radiation to matter of mass m:

$$z = \frac{e}{m}$$

The mean absorbed dose in a specified volume, D, is the mean value of z over all possible values:

$$D = \bar{z}$$

7.2.8 Cumulated Activity

Total dose over some period of integration (usually from the time of administration to infinity) requires calculation of the time integral of the time–activity curve for all important organs. Time–activity curves may have many forms; a very general function is shown here:

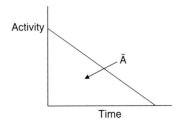

Regardless of the shape of the time–activity curve, its integral, however obtained, *will have units of the number of total nuclear transitions* (activity, which is transitions per unit time, multiplied by time). Common units for activity are Bq or MBq, and time may be given in seconds or hours. A Bq-s is numerically equal to one disintegration.

7.2.9 Radiation Dosimeters

Some interest has been shown using thermoluminescent dosimeters (TLD) to measure internal doses. These devices generally have a wide relatively flat response independent of energy, and a wide linear sensitivity to dose. These have been used mostly in inanimate phantoms, but have been used in animal studies, and have been proposed for some human applications. These are integrating devices and read out the dose absorbed between the time implanted and the time when retrieved from the subject. Small thermoluminescent dosimeters (TLDs) have been very useful in anthropomorphic phantoms in calibration of diagnostic and therapeutic external radiation sources, and attempts were made to place them into small animals, principally in tumors to measure accumulated radiation doses over time [19–21] Glass-encapsulated MOSFET detectors have been successfully used for radiation dosimetry with IMRT, and RIT [22, 23] and are under continued development. This kind of device may be of value in the validation of absorbed dose estimates from external beam and from internal emitter therapy, such as with ^{90}Y spheres currently being used in nuclear medicine therapy.

References

1. Early PJ (1995) Use of diagnostic radionuclides in medicine. Health Phys 69:649–661
2. Siegel JA, Stabin MG, Brill AB (2002) The importance of patient-specific radiation dose calculations for the administration of radionuclides in therapy. Cell Mol Biol (Noisy-le- grand) 48(5):451–459
3. Thierens HM, Monsieurs MA, Bacher K (2005) Patient dosimetry in radionuclide therapy: the whys and the wherefores. Nucl Med Commun 26(7):593–599
4. Brans B, Bodei L, Giammarile F, Linden O, Luster M, Oyen WJG, Tennvall J (2007) Clinical radionuclide therapy dosimetry: the quest for the "Holy Gray". Eur J Nucl Med Mol Imaging 34:772–786
5. Jonsson H, Mattsson S (2004) Excess radiation absorbed doses from non-optimised radioiodine treatment of hyperthyroidism. Radiat Prot Dosim 108(2):107–114
6. Stabin MG (2008) The case for patient-specific dosimetry in radionuclide therapy. Cancer Biotherapy Radiopharmaceut 23(3):273–284
7. Stabin M (2006) Nuclear medicine dosimetry, Review article. Phys Med Biol 51:R187–R202
8. NCRP (1990) The relative biological effectiveness of radiations of different quality. NCRP Report No. 104, National Council on Radiation Protection and Measurements, Bethesda
9. International Commission on Radiological Protection (2007) Recommendations of the ICRP. ICRP Publication 103. Ann ICRP 37(2–3):64
10. U.S. Department of Energy (1996) Proceedings, workshop – alpha emitters for medical therapy – Denver, Colorado, 30–31 May 1996. http://www.ornl.gov/RDF/BSMTH/denver/minutes_2.html. Accessed Feb 2002
11. Fisher DR, Frazier ME, Andrews TK Jr (1985) Energy distribution and the relative biological effects of internal alpha emitters. Radiat Prot Dosim 13(1–4):223–227
12. Humm JL, Howell RW, Rao DV (1994) AAPM Report No. 49, Dosimetry of Auger-electron-emitting radionuclides. Med Phys 21(12), December 1994
13. International Commission on Radiological Protection (1979) Limits for intakes of radionuclides by workers. ICRP Publication 30, Pergamon, New York
14. International Commission on Radiological Protection (1991) 1990 Recommendations of the International Commission on Radiological Protection. ICRP Publication 60, Pergamon, New York
15. Poston JW (1993) Application of the effective dose equivalent to nuclear medicine patients. The MIRD Committee. J Nucl Med 34(4):714–716
16. Thomas SR, Stabin MG, Castronovo FP (2005) Radiation-absorbed dose from 201Tl-thallous chloride. J Nucl Med 46 (3):502–508
17. International Commission on Radiological Protection (1988) Radiation dose to patients from radiopharmaceuticals. ICRP Publication 53, Pergamon, New York
18. Cameron JR (1991) A radiation unit for the public. Phys Soc News 20:2
19. Demidecki AJ, Williams LE, Wong JY et al (1993) Considerations on the calibration of small thermoluminescent dosimeters used for measurement of beta particle absorbed doses in liquid environments. Med Phys 20:1079–1087
20. Yorke ED, Williams LE, Demidecki AJ et al (1993) Multicellular dosimetry for beta-emitting radionuclides: autoradiography, thermoluminescent dosimetry and three-dimensional dose calculations. Med Phys 20:543–550
21. Jarnet D, Denizot B, Hindre F, Venier-Julienne MC, Lisbona A, Bardies M, Jallet P (2004) New thermoluminescent dosimeters (TLD): optimization and characterization of TLD threads sterilizable by autoclave. Phys Med Biol 49:1803
22. Gladstone DJ, Lu XQ, Humm JL et al (1994) A miniature MOSFET radiation dosimeter probe. Med Phys 21:1721–1728
23. Gladstone DJ, Chin LM (1995) Real-time, in vivo measurement of radiation dose during radioimmunotherapy in mice using a miniature MOSFET dosimeter probe. Radiat Res 141:330–335

Radiation Dosimetry: Formulations, Models, and Measurements

8

Michael G. Stabin

Contents

8.1 Introduction

As measurements of doses received by internal tissues of the body cannot be made, internal dose estimates must be performed via calculations and the use of theoretical models. Standardized models of the human body, and often standardized models of radiopharmaceutical behavior in the body, are employed to describe and predict the radiation doses received by various tissues in the body. The use of agreed-upon standardized models will result in calculations that are traceable and reproducible, but one must bear in mind that calculated dose estimates are only as good as the input assumptions and models employed as input to the calculations. One must also remember that these calculated doses are doses to a *model*, not a patient. In diagnostic applications, this is generally acceptable. All input data has some associated uncertainty, and the calculated results reflect the inherent uncertainty in the data as well as those related to the application of standardized models of the body to a variety of patients who vary substantially in size, age, and other physical characteristics (this subject is discussed in detail later in this chapter). When the radiation doses are relatively low, this kind of uncertainty is tolerable, because if calculated answers are not entirely accurate, the consequences for the patient will be small or even nonexistent (depending on what one believes about radiation risk at low doses and dose rates). In therapeutic applications, however, more attention to accuracy and precision is needed, as with these higher doses, the chances of reaching or exceeding an organ's threshold for expressing radiation damage are more significant.

The use of model-based dosimetry for therapy with radiopharmaceuticals should soon be abandoned and replaced with patient-specific modeling efforts that consider both patient-individualized anatomic and physiologic characteristics of the patient, as has been done in external beam radiotherapy for decades (this subject is also treated in more detail below). Such attention to detail requires significantly more effort in data gathering and dosimetric modeling, but the effort is worthwhile in providing the patient with a better quality of care and possibilities for a positive outcome from the therapy. Radiopharmaceutical therapy *must*

M.G. Stabin
Department of Radiology and Radiological Sciences, Vanderbilt University, 1161 21st Avenue South, Nashville TN 37232-2675, USA
e-mail: michael.g.stabin@vanderbilt.edu

M.M. Khalil (ed.), *Basic Sciences of Nuclear Medicine*, DOI: 10.1007/978-3-540-85962-8_8,
© Springer-Verlag Berlin Heidelberg 2011

move beyond its current practice of administering the same or similar quantities of drug to all subjects, without consideration of dosimetry, and become more like external beam radiotherapy, employing patient-specific evaluations of the radiation dose to all tissues of interest.

Gathering data for dose calculations requires that subjects spend perhaps 10–40 min lying still in the nuclear medicine camera bed, which of course involves some discomfort and difficulty; then data analyses require some time to complete. A balance is always needed between high-quality scientific analyses and logistical concerns. An absolute minimum of data is required (as shown below) to establish the radiopharmaceutical biokinetics. Additional data may be taken as is possible, given the consent of the physician and patient and availability of the counting systems. During the approval phases of both diagnostic and therapeutic radiopharmaceuticals, this balance is usually achievable, and reasonably good dosimetry is usually performed. The present practice of gathering no data at all for therapy patients needs to be upgraded to a system in which at least the minimum amount of data for a dose analysis is taken.

8.2 Basic Principles of Radiation Safety

Philosophical principles: The practice of radiation protection involves three fundamental principles:

1. *Justification* – no practice should be undertaken unless sufficient benefit to the exposed individuals will offset the radiation detriment.
2. *Optimization* – the magnitude of individual doses, the number of people exposed, and the likelihood of incurring exposures should be kept as low as reasonably achievable (ALARA), economic and social factors being taken into account.
3. *Limitation* – the exposure of individuals should be subject to dose limits. These limits are designed to prevent deterministic effects and to reduce stochastic effects to an "acceptable" level.

Internal dose calculations are part of an overall system of radiation protection. For radiation workers, radiation dose limits are prescribed and enforced by regulatory agencies, as discussed in Chapter 7. For nuclear

medicine patients, no numerical dose limits apply. In the United States, the US Food and Drug Administration (FDA) approves radioactive drugs for use in the general population. Certainly, radiation dose is a consideration in the approval of a radiopharmaceutical, but no strict numerical limits are applied in the approval process. For human volunteers participating in studies of radiopharmaceutical biokinetics and dosimetry (again, in the US), numerical dose limits are applied to the doses received by individual organs and the whole body, and are specified in 21CFR361. In the daily practice of nuclear medicine, physicians should balance potential risks of the use of radioactive drugs against their potential benefits, for both diagnostic and therapeutic procedures, with more importance being placed on the latter, as discussed above.

8.3 Internal Radiation Dose Calculation Systems

A generic equation for cumulative internal dose can be shown as:

$$D_T = \frac{k \sum_S \widetilde{A}_S \sum_i n_i E_i \phi_i (T \leftarrow S)}{m_T}$$

where D_T is the absorbed dose to a target region T (rad or Gy). $\widetilde{A}_S$ is the number of nuclear transitions in source region S, or "cumulated activity" (perhaps given as µCi-h or MBq-s). This is the area under the time-activity curve for any region (see Chap. 7) in the body that accumulates a significant amount of activity and is designated as a "source" region. n_i = number of radiations with energy E_i emitted per nuclear transition. E_i = energy per radiation (MeV). $\phi(T \leftarrow S)$ = fraction of energy emitted in source region S that is absorbed in the target region T. m_T = mass of target region T (g or kg). k = some proportionality constant (rad-g/µCi-h-MeV or Gy-kg/MBq-s-MeV).

The numerical value of k reflects the units chosen for the other terms in the equation. Various groups have developed versions of this equation for use in their dosimetry systems.

8.3.1 System of the US Society of Nuclear Medicine's Medical Internal Radiation Dose (MIRD) Committee

The equation for absorbed dose given in the MIRD system [1] is:

$$D_{r_k} = \sum_h \tilde{A}_h \, S(r_k \leftarrow r_h)$$

In this equation, r_k represents a target region and r_h represents a source region. The use of the subscripts "h" and "k" for "source" and "target" is unusual. The cumulated activity, $\tilde{A}$, is as defined above; all other terms were combined in the factor "S":

$$S(r_k \leftarrow r_h) = \frac{k \sum_i n_i \, E_i \, \phi_i (r_k \leftarrow r_h)}{m_{r_k}}$$

In the MIRD equations, the factor k is 2.13, which gives doses in rad, from activity in microcuries, mass in grams, and energy in MeV. The MIRD system, which to date, still depends on non-SI units, was developed primarily for use in estimating radiation doses received by patients from administered radiopharmaceuticals; it was not intended to be applied to a system of dose limitation for workers.

8.3.2 The International Commission on Radiological Protection (ICRP)

The ICRP has developed two comprehensive internal dosimetry systems intended for use in protecting radiation workers. ICRP publication II [2] was the basis for the first set of complete radiation protection regulations in the USA (Code of Federal Regulations (CFR), Title 10, Chap. 20, or 10CFR20). These regulations were replaced (completely) only in 1994 when a revision of 10CFR20 incorporated many of the new procedures and results of the ICRP 30 series [3]. Both of these systems, dealing with occupational exposures, used equivalent dose as their main dose parameter.

In the ICRP II system, the dose equivalent rate was given by the expression:

$$H = \frac{51.2 \, A \, \xi}{m}$$

The term ξ contains several of the terms in our generic equation above.

$$\xi = \sum_i n_i \, E_i \, \phi_i \, Q_i$$

The ICRP developed a system of limitation of concentrations in air and water for employees from this equation and assumptions about the kinetic behavior of radionuclides in the body. These were the well-known maximum permissible concentrations (MPCs). Employees could be exposed to these concentrations on a continuous basis and not receive an annual dose rate to the so-called critical organ that exceeded established annual dose limits.

In the ICRP 30 system, the cumulative dose equivalent was given as:

$$H_{50,T} = 1.6 \times 10^{-10} \sum_S U_S \, SEE(T \leftarrow S)$$

In this equation, T represents a target region and S represents a source region. The factor SEE is:

$$SEE = \frac{\sum_i n_i \, E_i \, \phi_i (T \leftarrow S) \, Q_i}{m_T}$$

The factor U_s is another symbol for cumulated activity, and the factor 1.6×10^{-10} is k. Note that the symbol Q (quality factor), used in some of the early ICRP manuals, is shown here instead of the current notation w_R (radiation weighting factor). As in ICRP II, this equation was used to develop a system of dose limitation for workers, but unlike the ICRP II system, limits are placed on *activity intake during a year, which would prevent cumulative doses* (not continuous dose rates) from exceeding established limits. These quantities of activity were called annual limits on intake (ALIs); derived air concentrations (DACs), which are directly analogous to MPCs for air, were calculated from ALIs. More recent ICRP documents (e.g., ICRP 71 [4]) changed the formulation somewhat. For example, the equivalent dose at age t in target organ or tissue T due to an intake of a radionuclide at age t_0 may be given as:

$$\dot{H}(t, t_0) = \sum_S q_s(t, t_0) \, SEE(T \leftarrow S; t)$$

$q_s(t,t_0)$ = the activity of the radionuclide in source organ S at age t after intake at age t_0 (Bq), SEE

$(T \leftarrow S, t_0)$ = the Specific Effective Energy, as defined in Chap. 7, except that the energy is given in J and mass is given in kg, so the units of dose are Gy without the need for a unit conversion factor.

The ICRP uses multicompartment models to describe the kinetics of the movement of radioactive material through the respiratory and gastrointestinal tracts, which then permit entry of material into the systemic circulation, where its movements are treated with individual biokinetic models for each element, and sometimes for more than one form of each element. Much detail about these model systems are not given here, but are detailed elsewhere [5]. Once the biokinetic model for an element (including the kinetics of the intake component (lung or GI)) is characterized, U_S values may be calculated for all of the important source regions, and dose estimates are obtained by multiplying them by the appropriate dose conversion factors (SEEs), as shown above. To calculate an SEE, one needs decay data, data on standard organ masses, and the "absorbed fractions" for photons. In the ICRP system, doses are calculated, as are amounts of activity that would give permissible annual doses to workers. The dose conversion factors are usually calculated as 50-year committed dose (Sv) per Bq of intake (by inhalation or ingestion). Knowing our annual dose limits in Sv, we can thus calculate the number of Bq that are permissible to take in during 1 year of work. There are two dose limits that must be satisfied at the same time – the stochastic limit (50 mSv effective whole body) and the nonstochastic limit (500 mSv to any organ). The permissible amount of activity for any element that may be taken in during one working year (the Annual Limit on Intake, ALI) is that amount that will satisfy both limits and choose the smaller of the two values as our controlling limit.

Example

Calculate the ALI and the DAC for inhalation of class D ^{32}P. Solution of the biokinetic model gives the following values for the number of disintegrations in various source organs for a 1 Bq intake:

Lungs	1.8×10^4
ULI contents	1.4×10^3
LLI contents	2.5×10^3
Cortical bone	1.5×10^5
Trabecular bone	1.5×10^5
Other tissues	2.8×10^5

Dose conversion factors (SEEs) may be taken from ICRP 30 (or later documents, but this example is continued as it is still the basis for regulations in the USA), and solve for the H_{50} values as follows:

$$H_{50,\text{gonads}} = 1.6 \times 10^{-10} \frac{\text{Sv g}}{\text{MeV}} \times 2.8 \times 10^5 \frac{\text{transf}}{\text{Bq intake}}$$
$$\times 9.9 \times 10^{-6} \frac{\text{MeV}}{\text{g transf}} = 4.4 \times 10^{-10} \frac{\text{Sv}}{\text{Bq}}$$

$$H_{50,\text{breasts}} = 1.6 \times 10^{-10} \frac{\text{Sv g}}{\text{MeV}} \times 2.8 \times 10^5 \frac{\text{transf}}{\text{Bq intake}}$$
$$\times 9.9 \times 10^{-6} \frac{\text{MeV}}{\text{g transf}} = 4.4 \times 10^{-10} \frac{\text{Sv}}{\text{Bq}}$$

$$H_{50,\text{marrow}} = 1.6 \times 10^{-10} \frac{\text{Sv g}}{\text{MeV}} \times 2.8 \times 10^5 \frac{\text{transf}}{\text{Bq intake}}$$
$$\times 9.9 \times 10^{-6} \frac{\text{MeV}}{\text{g transf}} + 1.6 \times 10^{-10} \frac{\text{Sv g}}{\text{MeV}}$$
$$\times 1.5 \times 10^5 \frac{\text{transf}}{\text{Bq intake}}$$
$$\times 2.3 \times 10^{-4} \frac{\text{MeV}}{\text{g transf}} = 6.0 \times 10^{-9} \frac{\text{Sv}}{\text{Bq}}$$

$$H_{50,\text{lungs}} = 1.6 \times 10^{-10} \frac{\text{Sv g}}{\text{MeV}} \times 2.8 \times 10^5 \frac{\text{transf}}{\text{Bq intake}}$$
$$\times 9.9 \times 10^{-6} \frac{\text{MeV}}{\text{g transf}} + 1.6 \times 10^{-10} \frac{\text{Sv g}}{\text{MeV}}$$
$$\times 1.8 \times 10^4 \frac{\text{transf}}{\text{Bq intake}}$$
$$\times 6.9 \times 10^{-4} \frac{\text{MeV}}{\text{g transf}} = 2.4 \times 10^{-9} \frac{\text{Sv}}{\text{Bq}}$$

$$H_{50,ULI} = 1.6 \times 10^{-10} \frac{\text{Sv g}}{\text{MeV}} \times 2.8 \times 10^5 \frac{\text{transf}}{\text{Bq intake}}$$
$$\times 9.9 \times 10^{-6} \frac{\text{MeV}}{\text{g transf}} + 1.6 \times 10^{-10} \frac{\text{Sv g}}{\text{MeV}}$$
$$\times 1.4x10^3 \frac{\text{transf}}{\text{Bq intake}}$$
$$\times 1.6 \times 10^{-3} \frac{\text{MeV}}{\text{g transf}} = 8.0 \times 10^{-10} \frac{\text{Sv}}{\text{Bq}}$$

$$H_{50,LLI} = 1.6 \times 10^{-10} \frac{\text{Sv g}}{\text{MeV}} \times 2.8 \times 10^5 \frac{\text{transf}}{\text{Bq intake}}$$
$$\times 9.9 \times 10^{-6} \frac{\text{MeV}}{\text{g transf}} + 1.6 \times 10^{-10} \frac{\text{Sv g}}{\text{MeV}}$$
$$\times 2.5 \times 10^3 \frac{\text{transf}}{\text{Bq intake}}$$
$$\times 2.6 \times 10^{-3} \frac{\text{MeV}}{\text{g transf}} = 1.5 \times 10^{-9} \frac{\text{Sv}}{\text{Bq}}$$

$$H_{50,\text{bone surfaces}} = 1.6 \times 10^{-10} \frac{\text{Sv g}}{\text{MeV}}$$

$$\times 2.8 \times 10^5 \frac{\text{transf}}{\text{Bq intake}} \times 9.9$$

$$\times 10^{-6} \frac{\text{MeV}}{\text{g transf}} + 1.6 \times 10^{-10} \frac{\text{Sv g}}{\text{MeV}}$$

$$\times 1.5 \times 10^5 \frac{\text{transf}}{\text{Bq intake}} \times 8.7$$

$$\times 10^{-5} \frac{\text{MeV}}{\text{g transf}} + 1.6 \times 10^{-10} \frac{\text{Sv g}}{\text{MeV}}$$

$$\times 1.5 \times 10^5 \frac{\text{transf}}{\text{Bq intake}} \times 1.4$$

$$\times 10^{-4} \frac{\text{MeV}}{\text{g transf}} = 5.9 \times 10^{-9} \frac{\text{Sv}}{\text{Bq}}$$

Having the individual $\times H_{50}$ values, we can choose the appropriate tissue weighting factors for each organ and also calculate the effective dose equivalent, using the ICRP 30 tissue weighting factors:

Organ	H_{50}	w_T	$w_T \times H_{50,T}$
Gonads	4.4×10^{-10}	0.25	1.1×10^{-10} Sv/Bq
Breast	4.4×10^{-10}	0.15	6.6×10^{-11} Sv/Bq
Red marrow	6.0×10^{-9}	0.12	7.2×10^{-10} Sv/Bq
Lungs	2.4×10^{-9}	0.12	2.9×10^{-10} Sv/Bq
Bone surface cells	5.9×10^{-9}	0.03	1.8×10^{-10} Sv/Bq
ULI	8.0×10^{-10}	0.06	4.8×10^{-11} Sv/Bq
LLI	1.5×10^{-9}	0.06	9.0×10^{-11} Sv/Bq
			$\Sigma = 1.5 \times 10^{-9}$ Sv/Bq

Now we need to calculate our two possible intake values (called Annual Limits on Intake, or ALIs). For the stochastic ALI, we divide the stochastic dose limit into the effective dose (the sum of the right hand column). For the nonstochastic ALI, we divide the nonstochastic limit into the highest of the dose/intake values for the individual organs:

$$\text{ALI}_{\text{stochastic}} = \frac{0.05 \frac{\text{Sv}}{\text{year}}}{1.5 \times 10^{-9} \frac{\text{Sv}}{\text{Bq}}} = 3.3 \times 10^7 \frac{\text{Bq}}{\text{year}}$$

$$\text{ALI}_{\text{non-stochastic}} = \frac{0.5 \frac{\text{Sv}}{y}}{6.0 \times 10^{-9} \frac{\text{Sv}}{\text{Bq}}} = 8.3 \times 10^7 \frac{\text{Bq}}{y}$$

As the stochastic limit is less than the nonstochastic limit, this becomes the limiting value, and is our actual ALI (3.3×10^7 Bq). Calculation of an air concentration that a worker may breathe continuously for a working year without exceeding the dose limit is obtained by dividing the ALI by the amount of air breathed in a year (2,400 m^3, based on a breathing rate of 0.02 m^3/min):

$$\text{DAC} = \frac{3.3 \times 10^7 \text{ Bq}}{2,400 \text{ m}^3} = 1.4 \times 10^4 \frac{\text{Bq}}{\text{m}^3}$$

Important Notes.

- If one takes in exactly one ALI of any nuclide, one is exposed exactly at the dose limit, and may have no other sources of exposure during that year. Thus, the true compliance equation is:

$$\sum \frac{\text{Intake}}{\text{ALI}_i} + \frac{H_{\text{ext}}}{50 \text{ mSv}} \leq 1.0$$

- The DAC gives the concentration that may be present continuously throughout a (2,000 h) working year. Thus, the true limit on air concentrations is based on the idea of DAC-hours – if one is exposed to 2,000 DAC-hours in a year, one takes in exactly 1 ALI by inhalation, and is thus exposed exactly at the dose limit. Another form of the compliance equation may thus be:

$$\sum \frac{\text{Intake}}{\text{ALI}_i} + \sum \frac{\text{DAC} - \text{hours}}{2,000} + \frac{H_{\text{ext}}}{50 \text{ mSv}} \leq 1.0$$

One may thus be exposed to a level of 2,000 DACs for 1 h and still be within permissible dose limits! This again assumes that the individual had no external radiation exposures during the year, and had no other intakes, either by inhalation or ingestion, during that year.

8.3.3 Practical Considerations

Radiation workers have defined dose limits, for deep and shallow doses, for the whole body, individual organs, and extremities (hands and feet) [6]. Declared pregnant workers adhere to lower dose limits, to protect the unborn child. When working with sources of radiation, simple procedures such as awareness of time, distance, and shielding (TDS) principles can greatly reduce radiation dose. Other references treat these subjects in more depth than is possible here [7]. Safe administration of radiopharmaceuticals to nuclear medicine patients is also a subject of considerable depth, including subjects such as use in children and pregnant women, release of radioactive subjects, communication of risks and benefits, and doses and risks from extravasations; many of these topics have been addressed in other works [7, 35].

8.3.4 RADAR

In the early twenty-first century, an electronic resource was established on the internet to provide rapid, worldwide dissemination of important dose quantities and data. The RAdiation Dose Assessment Resource (RADAR) established a web site (www.doseinfo-radar.com), and provided a number of publications on the data and methods used in the system. The RADAR system [8] has perhaps the simplest representation of the cumulative dose equation:

$$D_T = \sum_S N_S \times DF(\mathrm{T} \leftarrow \mathrm{S})$$

where N_S is the number of disintegrations that occur in a source organ, and DF(T←S) is:

$$DF(\mathrm{T} \leftarrow \mathrm{S}) = \frac{k \sum_i n_i E_i \phi_i (\mathrm{T} \leftarrow \mathrm{S})}{m_T}$$

The DF is conceptually similar to the "S value" defined in the MIRD system or the "SEE" factor of the ICRP system. The number of disintegrations is the integral of a time-activity curve for a source region ($\tilde{A}_S$ in the generic equation).

RADAR members have produced compendia of decay data, dose conversion factors, and catalogued standardized dose models for radiation workers and nuclear medicine patients, among other resources. They also produced the OLINDA/EXM [9] personal computer software code, which used the equations shown here and the input data from the RADAR site. This code was basically a revised version of the MIR-DOSE [10] software, which implemented the MIRD method for internal dose calculations (but was not in any way associated with the MIRD Committee itself). The RADAR site and OLINDA/EXM software implement all of the most current and widely accepted models and methods for internal dose calculations, and are constantly updated to reflect changes that occur in the science of internal dose assessment. The structure of the RADAR schema is summarized in Fig. 8.1.

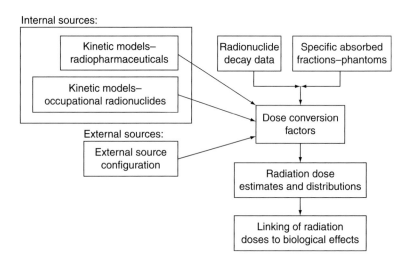

Fig. 8.1 An overview of the structure of the RADAR schema

8.3.5 Anthropomorphic Models for Standardized Dose Calculations

The current state of the art in full body anthropomorphic phantoms is based on the original Fisher-Snyder whole body and organ phantom [11]. This phantom used a combination of geometric shapes – spheres, cylinders, cones, etc. – to create a simple representation of the body and its internal structures. Monte Carlo computer programs were used to simulate the transport of photons through these various structures in the body, whose atomic composition and density were based on data provided in the original ICRP report on Reference Man [12]. This report provided various anatomical data assumed to represent the average working adult male in the Western hemisphere, and has been recently updated [13]. Using this phantom, absorbed fractions for adults based on activity residing in any organ and irradiating any other organ were calculated and published [11], and dose conversion factors were published [14] in the 1970s for this single model. Later, Cristy and Eckerman [15] modified the adult male model somewhat and developed models for a series of individuals of different size and age. Six phantoms were developed, which were assumed to represent children of ages 0 (newborn), 1-year, 5-year, 10-year, and 15-year-olds, and adults of both sexes.

8.3.6 Absorbed Fractions and Dose Conversion Factors

Absorbed fractions for photons at discrete energies were published for these phantoms, which contained approximately 25 source and target regions. Tables of S values were never published, but ultimately were made available in the MIRDOSE computer software [16]. Stabin et al. developed a series of phantoms for the adult female, both nonpregnant and at three stages of pregnancy [17]. These phantoms modeled the changes to the uterus, intestines, bladder, and other organs that occur during pregnancy, and included specific models for the fetus, fetal soft tissue, fetal skeleton, and placenta. S values for these phantoms were also made available through the MIRDOSE software [16]. A number of authors have developed

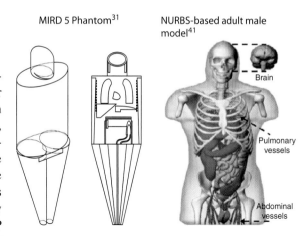

MIRD 5 Phantom[31]   NURBS-based adult male model[41]

Brain

Pulmonary vessels

Abdominal vessels

Fig. 8.2 Comparison of the realism of the traditional body models with those being used to support current dose modeling efforts

more realistic phantoms using image-based methods to replace the stylized models of the 1970s with voxel-based [18–20] or the use of mathematical methods like nonuniform rational B-splines (NURBS) [21]. An example of modeling efforts involved with more realistic whole body and organ models is shown in Fig. 8.2.

Spiers et al. at the University of Leeds [22] first established electron absorbed fractions (AFs) for bone and marrow in a healthy adult male, which were used in the dose factors (DFs), or S values, in MIRD Pamphlet No. 11 [14]. Eckerman re-evaluated this work and extended the results to derive DFs for fifteen skeletal regions in six models representing individuals of various ages [23]. The results were used in the MIRDOSE 3 software [14] to provide mean marrow dose, regional marrow dose, and dose-volume histograms for different individuals. This model was updated and improved employing more realistic assumptions of energy absorption at low electron energies [24].

For many years, the only source of dose factors for use in practical calculations were found in MIRD Pamphlet 11 [14], in which factors were given for about 25 organs, but only in the adult male phantom, for 117 radionuclides. The MIRDOSE code provided dose factors for over 240 radionuclides, for about 25 organs as well, but in the entire Cristy–Eckerman and Stabin et al. pediatric, adult, and pregnant female phantoms series (10 phantoms). Siegel and Stabin [8] then calculated dose factors for over 800 radionuclides for:

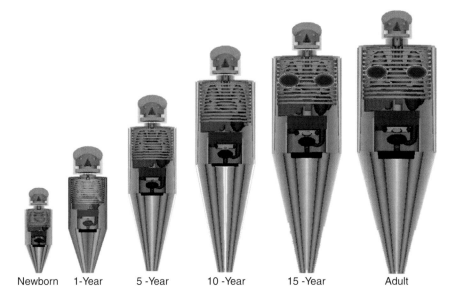

Fig. 8.3 Frontal views of the revised ORNL phantoms: newborn, 1-year, 5-year, 10-year, 15-year, and adult. Skin and muscle are made semitransparent for clear viewing of internal organs and the skeleton. (From Ref. [51]) Reprinted with permission from IOP publishing and the corresponding author

Newborn   1-Year   5 -Year   10 -Year   15 -Year   Adult

1. All source and target regions in the six models in the Cristy/Eckerman phantom series [15] (see Fig. 8.3)
2. All source and target regions in the four models in the Stabin et al. pregnant female phantoms series [17]
3. All target regions in the Watson and Stabin peritoneal cavity model [25]
4. All target regions in the Stabin prostate gland model [26]
5. All source and target regions in the six models of the MIRD head and brain model [27]
6. All source and target regions in the MIRD regional kidney model [28]
7. The unit density sphere models of Stabin and Konijnenberg [29]

These dose factors were based on decay data from the Brookhaven National Laboratory resource (http://www.nndc.bnl.gov/) [30], and are useful for implementation in the dose equations described above. These dose conversion factors use the child, adult, and pregnant woman phantoms and bone and marrow models described above, and included standard modeling assumptions, as were described in that paper. Examples of absorbed fractions and dose factors are given in the Stabin and Siegel document [8], and on the RADAR internet web site (www.doseinfo-radar.com).

8.4 Doses for Nuclear Medicine Patients

Dose calculations for nuclear medicine patients depend on development of a kinetic model, based on measurements made in animal or human studies, and employment of appropriate dose conversion factors. Radionuclides in nuclear medicine are bound to a very wide variety of compounds, and a separate kinetic model must be developed for each compound; this involves the proper design and execution of experiments in either animals or humans to obtain the necessary data to build a kinetic model. To design and execute a good kinetic study, one needs to collect the correct data, enough data, and express the data in the proper units. The basic data needed are the fraction (or percent) of administered activity in important source organs and excreta samples. We shall discuss later how these data are gathered from an animal or human study.

8.4.1 Data Sampling

It is very important, in either type of study, to take enough samples to characterize both the distribution and retention of the radiopharmaceutical over the course of the study. One must gather enough data to study early and late intake and washout phases, collect data over at least three effective half times of the radiopharmaceutical, collect at least two time points per phase of uptake or clearance, account for 100% of the activity at all times, and account for all major paths of excretion (urine, feces, exhalation, etc.). Some knowledge of the expected kinetics of the pharmaceutical are needed for a good study design before data collection begins. For example, the spacing of the measurements and the time of the initial measurement will be greatly different if we are studying a ^{99m}Tc-labeled renal agent 95% of which is cleared from the body in 180 min or an ^{131}I labeled antibody 80% of which clears in the first day and the remaining 20% over the next 2 weeks. The characterization of excretion is essential to a complete dosimetric evaluation, as the excretory organs (intestines, urinary bladder) are in many cases, the organs which receive the highest absorbed doses, as 100% of the activity (minus decay) will eventually pass through one or both of these pathways at different rates. If excretion is not quantified, the modeler must make the assumption that the compound is retained in the body and removed only by radioactive decay. For very short-lived radionuclides, this may not be a problem and in fact may be quite accurate. For moderately long-lived nuclides, this can cause an overestimate of the dose to most body organs and an underestimate of the dose to the excretory organs, perhaps significantly.

8.4.2 Extrapolation of Animal Data

Data for kinetic studies are generally derived from animal studies, usually performed for submission of an application for approval to the Food and Drug Administration in the United States for use of a so-called Investigational New Drug (IND), and human studies, usually performed in Phase I, II, or III of approval of a New Drug Application (NDA). In an animal study, the radiopharmaceutical is administered to a number of animals for which organ, whole body, and excretion data may be collected. Animal data must be somehow extrapolated to obtain dose estimates for humans. The extrapolation of animal data to humans is not an exact science. Crawford and Richmond [31] and Wegst [32] studied some of the strengths and weaknesses of various extrapolation methods

proposed in the literature. One method of extrapolating animal data is the % kg/g method [33]. In this method, the animal organ data need to be reported as percentage of injected activity per gram of tissue, and the animal whole body weight must be known. The extrapolation to humans then uses the human organ and whole body weight, as follows:

$$
\left[\left(\frac{\%}{g_{organ}} \right)_{animal} \times \left(kg_{TBweight} \right)_{animal} \right]
$$
$$
\times \left(\frac{g_{organ}}{kg_{TBweight}} \right)_{human}
$$
$$
= \left(\frac{\%}{organ} \right)_{human}
$$

8.4.3 Activity Quantitation

In human studies, data are collected with a nuclear medicine gamma camera. Quantification of data gathered with these cameras is rather involved. Projection images (anterior and posterior, typically) of the patient are developed and processed. As this is a projection image, the actual depth of the object within the patient is not known. One may draw regions of interest (ROIs) around images of objects that will be recognizable as internal organs or structures; the number of counts in a ROI, however, cannot be used directly to calculate how much activity is in the organ. A number of corrections is needed to the observed number of counts to obtain a reliable estimate of activity in this object [34]. To remove uncertainties about the depth of the object, usually images are taken in front of and behind the patient, and a geometric mean of the two values is taken. This geometric mean has been shown to be relatively independent of depth for most radionuclides of interest, and thus this quantity is thought to be the most reliable for use in quantitation. Other degrading factors such as attenuation and scatter can be tackled by using a transmission source and an appropriate scatter correction technique.

After scatter correction has been applied, the activity of the source within the ROI is thus given by:

$$
A_{ROI} = \sqrt{\frac{I_A I_P}{e^{-\mu_e t}} \frac{f_j}{C}}
$$

where I_A and I_P are the Anterior and Posterior counts in the region, μ_e is the effective attenuation coefficient, t is the average patient thickness over the ROI, f_j is the source self-attenuation coefficient (given as $[(\mu_e\,t/2)/\sinh(\mu_e\,t/2)]$, but which is rarely of much impact in the calculation and so is usually neglected), and C is a source calibration factor (cts/s/Bq), obtained by counting a source of known activity in air. Thus, activity in identifiable regions of the body, like liver, spleen, kidneys, etc. may be determined at individual times. ROIs may also be drawn over the entire body, to track the retention and excretion of the compound in the body. Excreta samples may also be taken to study excretion pathways. If only a single excretion pathway is important, knowledge of whole body clearance may be used to explain excretion. Single Photon Emission Computed Tomography (SPECT) or Positron Emission Tomography (PET) methods may also be used to obtain quantitative data for dosimetry studies. This takes considerably more effort, both in data gathering and analysis, and is employed by fewer investigators.

8.4.4 Data Analysis

Once kinetic data are obtained, analysis of the data involves estimation of the area under the time-activity curve to obtain the number of disintegrations (N or $\tilde{A}$) in all important source regions. In general, there are three levels of complexity that our analysis can take:

8.4.4.1 Direct Integration

One can directly integrate under the actual measured values by a number of methods. This does not give much information about your system, but it does allow you to calculate the area under the time-activity curve rather easily. The most common method used is the Trapezoidal Method, simply approximating the area by a series of trapezoids.

8.4.4.2 Least Squares Analysis

In this application, one attempts to fit curves of a given shape to the data. The curves are represented by mathematical expressions which can be directly integrated. The most common approach is to attempt to charac-

terize a set of data by a series of exponential terms, as many systems are well represented by this form, and exponential terms are easy to integrate. In general, the approach is to minimize the sum of the squared distance of the data points from the fitted curve. The curve will have the form:

$$A(t) = a_1 e^{-b_1 t} + a_2 e^{-b_2 t} + \cdots$$

The method evaluates the squared difference between each point and the solution of the fitted curve at that point, and minimizes this quantity by taking the partial derivative of this expression with respect to each of the unknowns a_i and b_i and setting it equal to zero. Once the ideal estimates of a_i and b_i are obtained, the integral of $A(t)$ from zero to infinity is simply:

$$\int_0^\infty A(t)dt = \frac{a_1}{b_1} + \frac{a_2}{b_2} + \ldots$$

If the coefficients a_i are in units of activity, this integral represents cumulated activity (the units of the b_i are time^{-1}).

8.4.4.3 Compartmental Models

The situation frequently arises that you either know quite a bit about the biological system under investigation or you would like to know in greater detail how this system is working. In this case, you can describe the system as a group of compartments linked through transfer rate coefficients. Solving for $\tilde{A}$ of the various compartments involves solving a system of coupled differential equations describing transfer of the tracer between compartments and elimination from the system. The solution to the time activity curve for each compartment will usually be a sum of exponentials, but not obtained by least squares fitting each compartment separately, but by varying the transfer rate coefficients between compartments until the data are well fit by the model.

8.4.4.4 Dose Calculation Steps

As outlined with examples by Stabin [35], dose calculations proceed with the selection of an appropriate standardized anthropomorphic model, extrapolation of animal data (in preclinical studies), or quantification of human imaging data, a thorough kinetic analysis, and finally, dose calculations using established, standardized methods, as described above. The reader is referred to the longer discussion of these topics in this publication, with several worked out numerical examples.

8.4.4.5 Uncertainties in Internal Dose Calculations

All dose calculation must begin with an estimation of the amount of activity as a function of time in a source region. As noted above, activity in source regions for radiopharmaceuticals is generally determined in one of two ways (a) experiments in animal models with extrapolation of the observed results to humans and (b) measurements in human subjects (volunteers or patients) with calculation of dose estimates, either general dose estimates for reference individuals or specific dose estimates for the individual patient. In all cases, one begins with a measurement of counts of a radioactive source which contains an inherent and well-known statistical uncertainty.

Converting counts to disintegrations requires application of a calibration factor (e.g., Bq-s/count), which is based on measured counts of a radioactive source in some experimental situation in which other uncertainties may be introduced but are not often reported (e.g., measurement errors in adding volume of a standard to a calibration device, errors in making estimates of distances or time differences, or performance of dose calibrators).

Sparks and Aydogan [36] discussed the quality of extrapolation of animal data to humans, for 11

radionuclides in 33 radiopharmaceuticals, for which data for 115 organs were available both for extrapolated animal data and subsequent measurements in human subjects. Table 8.1 shows their observations; they found that animal data generally *under*predicted the actual number of disintegrations (and thus organ self dose) seen in human subjects, and that the accuracy of the extrapolation was not particularly strong. No strong preference was seen for any particular extrapolation method, but what was most striking was the general lack of accuracy of the extrapolated data. Not until a factor of 10 tolerance was given were the estimates predictive in close to 90% of the cases.

In human studies, after administration of the radiopharmaceutical, a series of images are made with nuclear medicine imaging systems (gamma cameras) and counts are extracted from the images and related to absolute activity values via calibration factors. Siegel et al. [37] discuss many of the strengths and weaknesses of the various data gathering methods used in nuclear medicine. Influences on the quality of the data include inherent system energy resolution, degradation of this spatial resolution due to collimator septal penetration by high-energy photons (if present in the decay scheme), data loss due to scatter and attenuation, and the inherent statistical variability in any measurement of any radioactive source (see Chap. 14).

Stabin [38] performed an analysis of uncertainty in the various terms of the dose equation shown above, including in activity measurements and integrations. The conclusions regarding these other quantities are summarized in Table 8.2 and discussed here:

- The factor k has zero uncertainty. It is simply an analytical quantity based on known conversion constants. It includes the various factors that are

Table 8.1 Percent of time that different scaling methods were successful in predicting human biokinetics from animal data within specified uncertainty levels [36]. "Mass" scaling means extrapolation of animal data based on organ concentrations and body mass, as shown in the Kirschner et al. [33] equation above, "time" scaling means extrapolation of the time scale based on differences in body mass and assumed metabolic rates

Extrapolation type	Uncertainty level					
	±25%	±50%	±2X	±4X	±10X	±20X
None	18%	30%	39%	62%	84%	92%
Mass	8%	18%	40%	66%	85%	93%
Time	21%	32%	50%	74%	88%	91%
Mass and time	8%	21%	46%	79%	94%	97%

Table 8.2 Summary of sources of uncertainty in dose estimate

Variable	Uncertainty	Remarks	Publications
k	Zero uncertainty	An analytical quantity used mainly to match among units	Stabin [38]
n_i and E_i	Negligible when compared with other variables		Stabin [38]
AF or (SAF) and mass terms	(~5% or less) uncertainty is reduced by applying large number of photon histories in the simulation process (i.e., reduction of statistical error)	The uncertainty is particularly large when a patient geometry is significantly different from the assumed reference man/women model.	Stabin [38]
Biokinetic parameters Inherent in $\tilde{A}_S$ (Fractional uptake and T_b)	10–20% when adjustments are done to account for individual kinetics.		Stabin [38]
Biokinetics + organ mass	Could result in doubling in 95% confidence intervals around median value of dose estimates of most organ		Stabin[38]
Effective whole body dose	20–40%	Differences in tissue sensitivities (w_T) at different ages	Stabin [38]
Data extrapolation to human	Uncertainty in extrapolation methods cannot be quantitatively assessed	Observations suggest considerable underestimation of human organ uptake and dose	Aydogan et al. [41]

needed to obtain the dose in the desired units, from the units employed for the other variables.

- The uncertainty in the terms n_i and E_i is very low and mostly negligible, in comparison with uncertainties in the other terms in the equation.

- The other three terms in the equation, namely ϕ (or AF), $\tilde{A}_S$ and m, contribute the vast majority of the uncertainty to internal dose calculations for radiopharmaceuticals.

- The absorbed fraction and mass terms used in most internal dose calculations are based on standardized individuals, i.e., reference man, reference woman, reference pediatric individuals, and so on. When standardized phantoms are used with Monte Carlo radiation transport simulation codes to obtain absorbed fraction (AF) values (or "specific absorbed fractions," SAFs, which are equal to the absorbed fraction divided by the mass of the target region), the absolute uncertainty in the calculated AFs or SAFs can be limited (to ~5% or less) simply by performing a large number of particle histories. Thus, the inherent uncertainty is small, and somewhat comparable to that for the decay data. However, the application of these SAFs and

organ mass values to individuals who are not well represented by the population median value will thus be in error by as much as the individual's body geometry varies from the median, at least tens of percent.

- The biokinetic parameters inherent in calculation of $\tilde{A}_S$, namely fractional uptake and effective half-time in organs and the body, vary substantially between individuals. Variability of a factor of 2 or more is reasonable to assume for the kinetics of any given radiopharmaceutical, if applying a general biokinetic model to any individual in the nuclear medicine patient population. If a specific study of an individual is performed to determine the particular kinetics for that individual, and care is taken to adjust doses for cases in which organ volumes are known to vary from those of the reference individuals, final doses may have uncertainties as low as 10–20%. But in the general case, uptake and clearance of radiopharmaceuticals varies substantially between individuals, and although the mean or median values may be quite reliable, the uncertainty for any given subject is substantial. Two examples from the literature are shown in

Fig. 8.4 Uptake and retention of 99mTc-RP527, a gastrin-releasing peptide (GRP) agonist for the visualization of GRP receptor–expressing malignancies in various subjects, as reported by Van de Wiele et al. [39]. Reprinted with permission of the Society of Nuclear Medicine

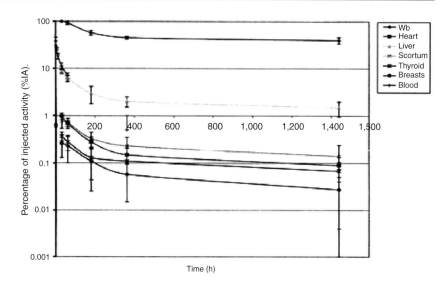

Fig. 8.5 Cumulative excretion of Ho-166 DOTMP in twelve subjects (six males and six females) with multiple myeloma. (From Ref. [40]) Reprinted with permission of the Society of Nuclear Medicine

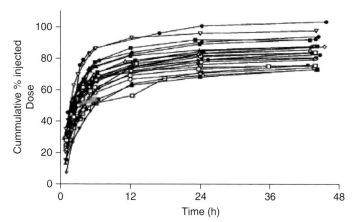

Figs. 8.4 and 8.5 from Van de Wiele [39] and Breitz et al. [40].

- Another source of uncertainty in reported estimates of effective whole body dose involves changes in the recommended tissue weighting factors at different times by the ICRP. This may introduce an additional uncertainty of up to 20–40% in reported values of effective dose for diagnostic radiopharmaceuticals.

Aydogan et al. [41] evaluated the uncertainty in dose estimates for an ^{123}I labeled brain imaging agent (IPT) in seven healthy adult subjects (five males, two females). They reported uncertainties in the fitted biokinetic coefficients and specific absorbed fractions, as obtained by first order error propagation (FOEP) and Latin Hypercube Sampling (LHS) methods. They concluded that variability in individual biokinetics and

in mass could account for a doubling in the 95% confidence intervals around the point (median) dose estimates for most organs. They stated that absorbed doses that any given patient in the broad nuclear medicine population receives may be up to twice as large as reported mean. Figure 8.6 shows their predicted 95% confidence interval for dose to the liver using their LHS modeling and taking into account all sources of uncertainty.

8.5 Image-Based, 3D Patient-Specific, Dosimetry

Several of the efforts to use image data to perform dose calculations, as described above, include the 3D-ID code from the Memorial Sloan-Kettering Cancer

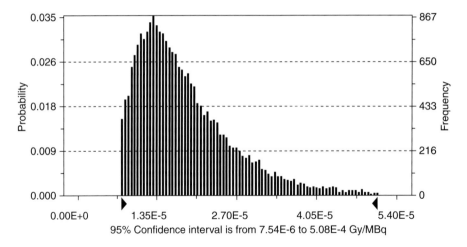

Fig. 8.6 An example of absorbed dose distribution (with 95% confidence). It shows the uncertainty in dose estimates for an ^{123}I-labeled brain imaging agent (IPT) in seven healthy adult subjects (five males, two females) (Taken from Ref. [41])

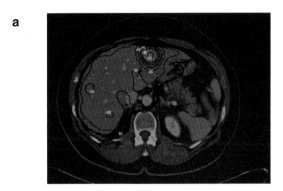

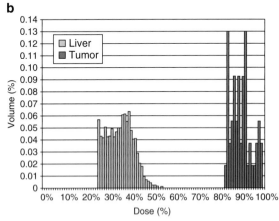

Center [42], the SIMDOS code from the University of Lund [43], the RTDS code at the City of Hope Medical Center [44], the RMDP code from the Royal Marsden Hospital [45] and the DOSE3D code [46]. Neither has a particularly robust and well-supported electron transport code, as is available in EGS [47], MCNP [48], or GEANT [49]. The PEREGRINE code [50] has also been proposed for three-dimensional, computational dosimetry and treatment planning in radioimmunotherapy. The promise of this type of code is great, in providing three dimensional, image-based dose calculations to the nuclear medicine physician which may be used in patient-specific treatment planning in radiopharmaceutical therapy (see Fig. 8.7). The challenge, as noted above, is finding broad clinical acceptance for these approaches and a move away from the approach to therapy involving a uniform administration of activity to all patients, with no consideration of radiation dose. Further discussion about patient-specific dosimetry can be found in Chap. 14.

Fig. 8.7 Example of 3D dose distributions. (**a**) Calculated dose distribution after administration of ^{131}I-MIBG superimposed on axial CT scan. (**b**) Differential dose volume histogram for normal liver and metastasis. (From Strigari et al. [51]). Reprinted with kind permission from Medical Physics

References

1. Loevinger R, Budinger T, Watson E (1988) MIRD primer for absorbed dose calculations. Society of Nuclear Medicine, New York
2. International Commission on Radiological Protection (1960) Report of committee II on permissible dose for internal radiation. *Health Phys.* 3

3. International Commission on Radiological Protection (1979) Limits for Intakes of Radionuclides by Workers. ICRP Publication 30, Pergamon, New York

4. International Commission on Radiological Protection (1996) Age-dependent doses to members of the public from intake of radionuclides: Part 4, inhalation dose coefficients. ICRP Publication 71, Pergamon, New York

5. Stabin MG (2008) Radiation protection and dosimetry, an introduction to health physics. Springer, New York

6. United States Nuclear Regulatory Commission, Part 20, Title 10, Code of Federal Regulations

7. Cormack J, Towson JET, Flower MA (2004) Radiation protection and dosimetry in clinical practice. In: Ell PJ, Gambhir SS (eds) Nuclear medicine in clinical diagnosis and treatment, 3rd edn. Churchill Livingston, Philadelphia, PA, pp 1871–1902

8. Stabin MG, Siegel JA (2003) Physical models and dose factors for use in internal dose assessment. Health Phys 85 (3):294–310

9. Stabin MG, Sparks RB, Crowe E (2005) OLINDA/EXM: the second-generation personal computer software for internal dose assessment in nuclear medicine. J Nucl Med 46:1023–1027

10. Stabin MG (1996) MIRDOSE: personal computer software for internal dose assessment in nuclear medicine. J Nucl Med 37(3):538–546

11. Snyder W, Ford M, Warner G (1978) Estimates of specific absorbed fractions for photon sources uniformly distributed in various organs of a heterogeneous phantom. MIRD Pamphlet No. 5, revised, Society of Nuclear Medicine, New York

12. International Commission on Radiological Protection (1975) *Report of the Task Group on Reference Man.* ICRP Publication 23, Pergamon, New York, NY

13. International Commission on Radiological Protection (2003) Basic anatomical and physiological data for use in radiological protection: reference values. ICRP Publication 89, Pergamon, New York, NY

14. Snyder W, Ford M, Warner G, Watson S (1975) "S," absorbed dose per unit cumulated activity for selected radionuclides and organs, MIRD Pamphlet No. 11, Society of Nuclear Medicine, New York, NY

15. Cristy M, Eckerman K (1987) Specific absorbed fractions of energy at various ages from internal photons sources. ORNL/TM-8381 V1-V7. Oak Ridge National Laboratory, Oak Ridge, TN

16. Stabin M (1996) MIRDOSE – the personal computer software for use in internal dose assessment in nuclear medicine. J Nucl Med 37:538–546

17. Stabin M, Watson E, Cristy M, Ryman J, Eckerman K, Davis J, Marshall D, Gehlen K (1995) Mathematical models and specific absorbed fractions of photon energy in the nonpregnant adult female and at the end of each trimester of pregnancy. ORNL Report ORNL/TM-12907

18. Yoriyaz H, Stabin MG, dos Santos A (2001) Monte Carlo MCNP-4B-based absorbed dose distribution estimates for patient-specific dosimetry. J Nucl Med 42(4): 662–669

19. Petoussi-Henss N, Zankl M, Fill U, Regulla D (2002) The GSF family of voxel phantoms. Phys Med Biol 47(1): 89–106

20. Lee C, Williams JL, Lee C, Bolch WE (2005) The UF series of tomographic computational phantoms of pediatric patients. Med Phys 32(12):3537–3548

21. Segars JP (2001) Development and Application of the New Dynamic NURBS-based Cardiac-Torso (NCAT) Phantom, PhD dissertation. The University of North Carolina

22. Spiers FW, Whitwell JR, Beddoe AH (1978) Calculated dose factors for radiosensitive tissues in bone irradiated by surface-deposited radionuclides. Phys Med Biol 23:481–494

23. Eckerman K, Stabin M (2000) Electron absorbed fractions and dose conversion factors for marrow and bone by skeletal regions. Health Phys 78(2):199–214

24. Stabin MG, Eckerman KF, Bolch WE, Bouchet LG, Patton PW (2002) Evolution and status of bone and marrow dose models cancer biotherapy and radiopharmaceuticals 17 (4):427–434

25. Watson EE, Stabin MG, Davis JL, Eckerman KF (1989) A model of the peritoneal cavity for use in internal dosimetry. J Nucl Med 30:2002–2011

26. Stabin MG (1994) A model of the prostate gland for use in internal dosimetry. J Nucl Med 35(3):516–520

27. Bouchet L, Bolch W, Weber D, Atkins H, Poston J Sr (1999) MIRD pamphlet no 15: radionuclide S values in a revised dosimetric model of the adult head and brain. J Nucl Med 40:62S–101S

28. Bouchet LG, Bolch WE, Blanco HP, Wessels BW, Siegel JA, Rajon DA, Clairand I, Sgouros G (2003) MIRD pamphlet no. 19: absorbed fractions and radionuclide S values for six age-dependent multiregion models of the kidney. J Nucl Med 44:1113–1147

29. Stabin MG, Konijnenberg M (2000) Re-evaluation of absorbed fractions for photons and electrons in small spheres. J Nucl Med 41:149–160

30. Stabin MG, da Luz CQPL (2002) New decay data for internal and external dose assessment. Health Phys 83 (4):471–475

31. Crawford DJ, Richmond CR (1981) Epistemological considerations in the extrapolation of metabolic data from non-humans to humans. In: Watson E, Schlafke-Stelson A, Coffey J, Cloutier R (eds) Third International Radiopharmaceutical Dosimetry Symposium. US Department of Health, Education, and Welfare, pp 191–197

32. Wegst A (1981) Collection and presentation of animal data relating to internally distributed radionuclides. In: Watson E, Schlafke-Stelson A, Coffey J, Cloutier R (eds) Third International Radiopharmaceutical Dosimetry Symposium. US Dept of Health, Education, and Welfare, pp 198–203

33. Kirschner A, Ice R, Beierwaltes W (1975) Radiation dosimetry of [131]I-19-iodocholesterol: the pitfalls of using tissue concentration data, the author's reply. J Nucl Med 16(3): 248–249

34. Siegel J, Thomas S, Stubbs J et al (1999) MIRD pamphlet no 16 – techniques for quantitative radiopharmaceutical biodistribution data acquisition and analysis for use in human radiation dose estimates. J Nucl Med 40:37S–61S

35. Stabin MG (2008) Fundamentals of nuclear medicine dosimetry. Springer, New York

36. Sparks RB, Aydogan B (1999) Comparison of the effectiveness of some common animal data scaling techniques in estimating human radiation dose. In: Oak Ridge TN, Stelson

A, Stabin M, Sparks R (eds) Sixth International Radiopharmaceutical Dosimetry Symposium. pp 705–716

37. Siegel JA, Thomas SR, Stubbs JB, Stabin MG, Hays MT, Koral KF, Robertson JS, Howell RW, Wessels BW, Fisher DR, Weber DA, Brill AB (1999) MIRD pamphlet no. 16: techniques for quantitative radiopharmaceutical biodistribution data acquisition and analysis for use in human radiation dose estimates. J Nucl Med 4037S–4061S

38. Stabin M (2008) Uncertainties in internal dose calculations for radiopharmaceuticals. J Nucl Med 49:853–860

39. Van de Wiele C, Dumont F, Dierckx RA, Peers SH, Thornback JR, Slegers G, Thierens H (2001) Biodistribution and dosimetry of 99mTc-RP527, a gastrin-releasing peptide (GRP) agonist for the visualization of GRP receptor–expressing malignancies. J Nucl Med 42:1722–1727

40. Breitz HB, Wendt WE III, Stabin MG, Shen S, Erwin WD, Rajendran JG, Eary JF, Durack L, Delpassand E, Martin W, Meredith RF (2006) 166Ho-DOTMP radiation-absorbed dose estimation for skeletal targeted radiotherapy. J Nucl Med 47:534–542

41. Aydogan B, Sparks RB, Stubbs JB, Miller LF (1999) Uncertainty analysis for absorbed dose from a brain receptor agent. In: Oak Ridge TN, Stelson A, Stabin M, Sparks R (eds) Sixth International Radiopharmaceutical Dosimetry Symposium. pp 732–740

42. Kolbert KS, Sgouros G, Scott AM, Bronstein JE, Malane RA, Zhang J, Kalaigian H, McNamara S, Schwartz L, Larson SM (1997) Implementation and evaluation of patient-specific three-dimensional internal dosimetry. J Nucl Med 38:301–308

43. Yuni KD, Scott JW, Michael Ljungberg, Kenneth FK, Kenneth Zasadny, Mark SK (2005) Accurate dosimetry in 131I radionuclide therapy using patient-specific, 3-dimensional methods for SPECT reconstruction and absorbed dose calculation. J Nucl Med 46:840–849

44. Liu A, Williams L, Lopatin G, Yamauchi D, Wong J, Raubitschek A (1999) A radionuclide therapy treatment planning and dose estimation system. J Nucl Med 40:1151–1153

45. Guy MJ, Flux GD, Papavasileiou P, Flower MA, Ott RJ (2003) RMDP: a dedicated package for I-131 SPECT quantification, registration and patient-specific dosimetry. Cancer Biother Radiopharm 18(1):61–69

46. Clairand I, Ricard M, Gouriou J, Di Paola M, Aubert B (1999) DOSE3D: EGS4 Monte Carlo code-based software for internal radionuclide dosimetry. J Nucl Med 40:1517–1523

47. Bielajew A, Rogers D (1987) PRESTA: the parameter reduced electron-step transport algorithm for electron monte carlo transport. Nucl Instrum Methods B18:165–181

48. Briesmeister JF (ed) (2000) MCNP – A General Monte Carlo N-Particle Transport Code, Version 4C. LA-13709-M, Los Alamos National Laboratory

49. Allison J, Amako K, Apostolakis J, Araujo H, Arce Dubois P, Asai M, Barrand G, Capra R, Chauvie S, Chytracek R, Cirrone GAP, Cooperman G, Cosmo G, Cuttone G, Daquino GG, Donszelmann M, Dressel M, Folger G, Foppiano F, Generowicz J, Grichine V, Guatelli S, Gumplinger P, Heikkinen A, Hrivnacova I, Howard A, Incerti S, Ivanchenko V, Johnson T, Jones F, Koi T, Kokoulin R, Kossov M, Kurashige H, Lara V, Larsson S, Lei F, Link O, Longo F, Maire M, Mantero A, Mascialino B, McLaren I, Mendez Lorenzo P, Minamimoto K, Murakami K, Nieminen P, Pandola L, Parlati S, Peralta L, Perl J, Pfeiffer A, Pia MG, Ribon A, Rodrigues P, Russo G, Sadilov S, Santin G, Sasaki T, Smith D, Starkov N, Tanaka S, Tcherniaev E, Tome B, Trindade A, Truscott P, Urban L, Verderi M, Walkden A, Wellisch JP, Williams DC, Wright D, Yoshida H (2006) Geant4 developments and applications. IEEE Trans Nucl Sci 53(1):270–278

50. Lehmann J, Hartmann Siantar C, Wessol DE, Wemple CA, Nigg D, Cogliati J, Daly T, Descalle MA, Flickinger T, Pletcher D, Denardo G (2005) Monte Carlo treatment planning for molecular targeted radiotherapy within the MINERVA system. Phys Med Biol 50(5):947–958

51. Lidia Strigari, Marco D'Andrea, Carlo Ludovico Maini, Rosa Sciuto, Marcello Benassi (2006) Biological optimization of heterogeneous dose distributions in systemic radiotherapy. Medical Physics 33(6):1857–1866

Radiobiology: Concepts and Basic Principles

9

Michael G. Stabin

Contents

9.1 Introduction

Very soon after the discovery of radiation and radioactivity short- and long-term negative effects of radiation on human tissue were observed. Adverse effects of X-rays were observed by Thomas Edison, William J. Morton, and Nikola Tesla; they independently reported eye irritations from experimentation with X-rays and fluorescent substances. These effects were thought to be eye strain, or possibly due to exposure to ultraviolet radiation. Elihu Thomson (an American physicist) deliberately exposed the little finger of his left hand to X-rays for several days, for a short time each day, and observed pain, swelling, stiffness, erythema, and blistering in the finger, which was clearly and immediately related to the radiation exposure. William Herbert Rollins (a Boston dentist) demonstrated that X-rays could kill guinea pigs and result in the death of offspring when guinea pigs were irradiated while pregnant. Henri Becquerel received a skin burn from a radium source given to him by the Curies that he carried in a vest pocket at times. He once was reported to have said: "I love this radium but I have a grudge against it!" The first death in an X-ray pioneer attributed to cumulative overexposure was to C.M. Dally in 1904. Radiologists and other physicians who used X-rays in their practices before health physics practices were common had a significantly higher rate of leukemia than their colleagues. A particularly tragic episode in the history of the use of radiation and in the history of industrialism was the acute and chronic biological damage suffered by the Radium Dial Painters [1]. Radium was used in luminous paints in the early 1900s. In factories where luminous dial watches were made, workers (mainly women) would sharpen the tips of their paint brushes with their lips, and thus ingested large amounts of radium. They had increased amounts of bone cancer (carcinomas in the paranasal sinuses or the mastoid structures, which are very rare, and were thus clearly associated with their exposures, as well as cancers in other sites) and even spontaneous fractures in their jaws and spines from cumulative radiation injury. Others died of anemia and other causes.

9.2 Stochastic Versus Nonstochastic Effects

There are two broad categories of radiation-related effects in humans, *stochastic* and *nonstochastic*.

M.G. Stabin
Department of Radiology and Radiological Sciences, Vanderbilt University, 1161 21st Avenue South, Nashville, TN 37232–2675, USA
e-mail: michael.g.stabin@vanderbilt.edu

M.M. Khalil (ed.), *Basic Sciences of Nuclear Medicine*, DOI: 10.1007/978-3-540-85962-8_9,
© Springer-Verlag Berlin Heidelberg 2011

There are three important characteristics that distinguish them.

9.2.1 Nonstochastic Effects

Nonstochastic effects (now officially called "deterministic effects," previously also called "acute effects") are effects that are generally observed soon after exposure to radiation. As they are "nonstochastic" in nature, they will always be observed (if the dose threshold is exceeded), and there is generally no doubt that they were caused by the radiation exposure. The major identifying characteristics of nonstochastic effects are:

1. There is a *threshold* of dose below which the effects will not be observed.
2. Above this threshold, the *magnitude* of the effect increases with dose.
3. The effect is *clearly associated* with the radiation exposure.

Examples include:

- Erythema (reddening of the skin)
- Epilation (loss of hair)
- Depression of bone marrow cell division (observed in counts of formed elements in peripheral blood)
- Nausea, vomiting, diarrhea (NVD) – often observed in victims after an acute exposure to radiation
- Central nervous system (CNS) damage
- Damage to the unborn child (physical deformities), microcephaly (small head size at birth), mental retardation

When discussing nonstochastic effects, it is important to note that some organs are more radiosensitive than others. The so-called law of Bergonie and Tribondeau [2] states that cells tend to be radiosensitive if they have three properties:

- Cells have a high division rate.
- Cells have a long dividing future.
- Cells are of an unspecialized type.

A concise way of stating the law might be to say that "the radiosensitivity of a cell type is proportional to its rate of division and inversely proportional to its degree of specialization." So, rapidly dividing and unspecialized cells, as a rule, are the most radiosensitive. Two important examples are cells in the red marrow and in the developing embryo/fetus. In the case of marrow, a number of *progenitor* cells which, through many generations of cell division, produce a variety of different functional cells that are very specialized (e.g., red blood cells, lymphocytes, leukocytes, platelets). Some of these functional cells do not divide at all, and are thus themselves quite radioresistant. However, if the marrow receives a high dose of radiation, damage to these progenitor cells is very important to the health of the organism. As we will see shortly, if these cells are affected, in a short period this will be manifested in a measurable decrease in the number of formed elements in the peripheral blood. If the damage is severe enough, the person may not survive. If not, the progenitor cells will eventually repopulate and begin to replenish the numbers of the formed elements, and subsequent blood samples will show this recovery process.

In the fetus, organs and systems develop at different rates. At the moment of conception, of course, we have one completely undifferentiated cell that becomes two cells after one division, then four then eight, and so on. As the rapid cell division proceeds, groups of cells "receive their assignments" and differentiate to form organs and organ systems, still with a very rapid rate of cell division. At some point, individual organs become well defined and formed, and cell division slows as the fetus simply adds mass. But while differentiation and early rapid cell division is occurring, these cells are quite radiosensitive, and a high dose to the fetus may cause fetal death, or damage to individual fetal structures. This is discussed further below. On the other hand, in an adult, cells of the CNS (brain tissue, spinal cord, etc.) are very highly specialized and have very low, or no, rate of division. The CNS is thus particularly radioresistant. One important nonstochastic effect is death. This results from damage to the bone marrow (first), then to the gastrointestinal tract, then to the nervous system.

9.2.2 Stochastic Effects

Stochastic effects are effects that are, as the name implies, probabilistic. They may or may not occur in any given exposed individual. These effects generally manifest many years, even decades, after the radiation exposure (and were once called "late effects"). Their major characteristics, in direct contrast with those for nonstochastic effects, are:

1. A *threshold* may not be observed.
2. The *probability* of the effect increases with dose.
3. You *cannot definitively associate* the effect with the radiation exposure.

Examples include:

- Cancer induction
- Genetic effects (offspring of irradiated individuals)

9.3 Cellular Response and Survival

Much information on the biological effects of radiation has been obtained for many years through the use of direct experiments on cell cultures. It is of course far easier to control the experiment and the variables involved when the radiation source can be carefully modulated, the system under study can be simple and uniform, and the results can be evaluated over almost any period of time desired (days to weeks, or even over microseconds, such as in the study of free radical formation and reaction [3]). After exposure of a group of cells to radiation, the most common concept to study is that of cell survival. Typically, the natural logarithm of the surviving fraction of irradiated cells is plotted against the dose received.

As shown in Fig. 9.1, the simplest survival curve is a single exponential, and can be formulated as:

$$S = S_0 \, e^{-D/D_0}$$

Here S is the surviving fraction, S_0 is the original number of cells irradiated, D is the dose received, and D_0 is the negative reciprocal of the slope of the curve, and is called the mean lethal dose. When cells receive dose D_0, the surviving fraction is 0.37, which is $1/e$. This dose may also be referred to as the D_{37} dose, just as we define the LD_{50}, the lethal dose of radiation that will kill half of a population. Generally speaking, particles with a high linear energy transfer (LET) will show this form of a survival curve, while those

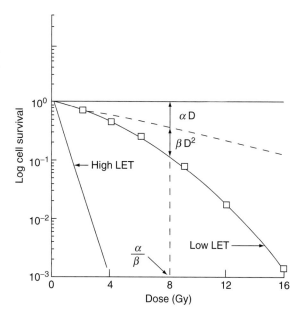

Fig. 9.1 Typical cell survival curve after exposure to low and high LET radiation. From Annals of the ICRP, Volume 37, Issues 2-4, Pages 1-332 , 2007 with permission

of low LET will have a more complicated curve, of the form:

$$S = S_0 \left[1 - \left(1 - e^{-D/D_0} \right)^n \right]$$

Here n is the assumed number of targets that need to be hit in order to inactivate a cell. If $n = 1$, the equation reduces to the simpler form shown above. The usual curve, however, has a "shoulder," indicating that a certain amount of dose must be received before any significant effect on cell survival is seen. At higher doses, the curve attains the usual linear shape with slope $-1/D_0$. If the linear portion is extrapolated back to zero dose, it will intercept the y-axis at the "extrapolation number" n, which is numerically equal to the number of targets assumed to be relevant to the cells' survival.

Several factors affect the shape of the dose–response function other than the LET of the radiation, including:

- *Dose rate* – the LD_{50} of a population of cells will clearly increase as the dose rate at which a fixed dose D is delivered is decreased. Cells have a considerable capacity to repair radiation damage, and if time is allowed for repair, more radiation can be tolerated.

- *Dose fractionation* – if cells are given a cumulative dose D, but instead of being delivered all at once, it is delivered in *N* fractions of *D/N* each, the cell survival curve will show a *series of shoulders* linked together, because cellular repair is again ongoing between fractions. This is a strategy used in radiation therapy procedures to allow healthy tissues time for repair while still delivering an ultimately lethal dose to the tumor tissues.
- *Presence of oxygen* – dissolved oxygen in tissue causes the tissue to be sensitive to radiation. Hypoxic cells have been shown to be considerably more radioresistant. The effect of oxygen is sometimes expressed as the "oxygen enhancement ratio" (OER), which is the ratio of the slope of the straight portion of the cell survival curve with and without oxygen present.

Another expression of the standard model of cell survival gives the fraction of cells surviving the irradiation (SF) as a function of the dose delivered (D):

$$\ln(\text{SF}) = -\alpha D - \beta D^2$$

where α and β are disease- or even patient-specific parameters related to radiosensitivity, and the ratio of these parameters determines the shape of the cell survival curve. A dose protraction factor, G, has been added to this model [4, 5] to accommodate the effect on cell kill by the change in absorbed dose rate:

$$G = \frac{2}{D^2} \int_0^\infty \dot{D}(t) \int_0^t \dot{D}(t') e^{-\mu(t-t')} \mathrm{d}t' \mathrm{d}t$$

where μ is the constant of sublethal damage repair and t' is a time point during the treatment prior to time t. The biologically effective dose (BED) [6, 7] has been defined as:

$$\text{BED} = -\frac{\ln(\text{SF})}{\alpha}$$

This quantity is defined for external beam radiotherapy and therapy with radiopharmaceuticals using the following equations:

For external beam radiotherapy:

$$\text{BED}_{\text{EBT}} = D_{\text{EBT}} \left(1 + \frac{D_{\text{EBT}}/n}{\alpha/\beta} \right)$$

and for radiopharmaceuticals (including the decay constant, λ, for the radionuclide and a term μ related to cellular response rate to radiation damage:

$$\text{BED}_{\text{TRT}} = D_{\text{TRT}} \left(1 + \frac{D_{\text{TRT}}\lambda}{(\mu + \lambda)(\alpha/\beta)} \right)$$

It has been shown that that these radiobiological arguments may be employed to combine radionuclide and external beam radiotherapy [8].

9.3.1 Mechanisms of Radiation Damage to Biological Systems

Radiation interactions with aqueous systems can be described as occurring in four principal stages:

1. Physical
2. Prechemical
3. Early chemical
4. Late chemical

In the *physical* stage of water radiolysis, a primary charged particle interacts through elastic and inelastic collisions. Inelastic collisions result in the ionization and excitation of water molecules, leaving behind ionized (H_2O^+) and excited (H_2O^*) molecules, and unbound subexcitation electrons ($e_{-\text{sub}}$). A subexcitation electron is one whose energy is not high enough to produce further electronic transitions. By contrast, some electrons produced in the interaction of the primary charged particle with the water molecules may have sufficient energy themselves to produce additional electronic transitions. These electrons may produce secondary track structures (delta rays), beyond that produced by the primary particle. All charged particles can interact with electrons in the water both individually and collectively in the condensed, liquid phase. The initial passage of the particle, with the production of ionized and excited water molecules and subexcited electrons in the local track region (within a few hundred angstroms), occurs within about 10^{-15} s. From this time until about 10^{-12} s, in the *prechemical* phase, some initial reactions and rearrangements of these species occur. If a water molecule is ionized, this results in the creation of an ionized water molecule and a free electron. The free electron rapidly attracts other water molecules, as the slightly polar molecule has a positive and negative pole, and the positive pole is attracted to the electron. A group of water molecules thus clusters around the electron, and it is known as a "hydrated electron" and is designated as e_{aq}^-. The water molecule dissociates immediately:

$$H_2O \rightarrow H_2O^+ + e_{aq}^- \rightarrow H^+ + OH \cdot + e_{aq}^-$$

In an excitation event, an electron in the molecule is raised to a higher energy level. This electron may simply return to its original state, or the molecule may break up into an H and an OH radical (a radical is a species that has an unpaired electron in one of its orbitals – the species is not necessarily charged, but is highly reactive).

$$H_2O \rightarrow H \cdot + OH \cdot$$

The free radical species and the hydrated electron undergo dozens of other reactions with each other and other molecules in the system. Reactions with other commonly encountered molecules in aqueous systems are shown in Table 9.1. Reactions with other molecules have been studied and modeled by various investigators as well [9–12].

The *early chemical* phase, extending from ~10^{-12} to ~10^{-6} s, is the time period within which the species can diffuse and react with each other and with other molecules in solution. By about 10^{-6} s most of the

Table 9.1 Comparison of reaction rate coefficients and reaction radii for several reactions of importance to radiation biology[a]

Reaction	k (10^{10} M^{-1} s^{-1})	R (nm)
$H \cdot + OH \cdot \rightarrow H_2O$	2.0	0.43
$e_{aq}^- + OH \rightarrow OH^-$	3.0	0.72
$e_{aq}^- + H + H_2O \rightarrow H_2 + OH^-$	2.5	0.45
$e_{aq}^- + H_3O^+ \rightarrow H \cdot + H_2O$	2.2	0.39
$H \cdot + H \cdot \rightarrow H_2$	1.0	0.23
$OH \cdot + OH \cdot \rightarrow H_2O_2$	0.55	0.55
$2e_{aq}^- + 2H_2O \rightarrow H_2 + 2OH^-$	0.5	0.18
$H_3O^+ + OH^- \rightarrow 2H_2O$	14.3	1.58
$e_{aq}^- + H_2O_2 \rightarrow OH^- + OH \cdot$	1.2	0.57
$OH + OH^- \rightarrow H_2O + O^-$	1.2	0.36

[a]k is the reaction rate constant and R is the "reaction radius" for the specified reaction. The use of these concepts is explained in the physical chemistry literature

original track structure is lost, and any remaining reactive species are so widely separated that further reactions between individual species are unlikely [5]. From 10^{-6} s onward, referred to as the *late chemical* stage, calculation of further product yields can be made by using differential rate-equation systems which assume uniform distribution of the solutes and reactions governed by reaction-rate coefficients. Cells clearly have mechanisms for repairing DNA damage. If damage occurs to a single strand of DNA, it is particularly easy for the cells to repair this damage, as information from the complementary chain may be used to identify the base pairs needed to complete the damaged area. "Double strand breaks" are more difficult to repair, but cellular mechanisms do exist that can affect repair here also.

9.3.2 Bystander Effect

Other recent interesting experimental evidence has shown that energy deposition alone cannot always predict the occurrence of cellular changes, but that in some conditions, cells that have received no direct energy deposition from radiation may demonstrate a biological response, the so-called bystander effect. Brooks notes that "[t]he potential for bystander effects may impact risk from nonuniform distribution of dose or energy in tissues and raises some very interesting questions as to the validity of such calculations." Hall [13] notes that "[t]he plethora of data now available concerning the bystander effect fall into two quite separate categories, and it is not certain that the two groups of experiments are addressing the same phenomenon." Those two categories are:

1. *Medium transfer experiments* – a number of independent studies [13] have shown that irradiated cells may have secreted some molecule into the culture medium that was capable of killing cells when that medium was placed in contact with unirradiated cells. This bystander effect can be seen at radiation doses as low as 0.25 mGy, and does not appear to be significantly increased up to doses of 10 Gy. Medium transfer experiments have shown an increase in neoplastic transformation as well as genomic instability in cells that have not themselves been irradiated.

2. *Microbeam irradiation experiments* – accurately directed beams of radiation have facilitated the exposure of only specified cells in a culture medium to radiation, but effects in other, unirradiated, cells have been observed. Hall discusses a striking experiment, in which human fibroblasts were irradiated with microbeams of alpha particles, with cells of one population lightly stained with cyto-orange, a cytoplasmic vital dye, while cells of another population were lightly stained blue with a nuclear vital dye. The two cell populations were mixed and allowed to attach to the culture dish, and the computer controlling the accelerator was programmed to irradiate only blue-stained cells with ten alpha particles directed at the centroid of the nucleus. The cells were fixed and stained 48 h later, at which time micronuclei and chromosome bridges were visible in a proportion of the nonhit (i.e., orange-stained) cells.

Other studies have shown interesting effects, such as one involving irradiation of the lung base in rats, but in which an increase in the frequency of micronuclei was found in the shielded lung apex [10]. On the other hand, radiation of the lung apex did not result in an increase in the chromosome damage in the shielded lung base. This suggests that a factor was transferred from the exposed portion of the lung to the shielded part and that this transfer has direction from the base to the apex of the lung. In another experiment, exposure of the left lung resulted in a marked increase in micronuclei in the unexposed right lung. Experiments suggest that bystander effects are limited to the organ irradiated, and have been demonstrated primarily in experiments with alpha particles. These results challenge the traditional notion of the relationship of dose and effects.

9.4 Relevance of Radiation Biology to Radionuclide Therapy

9.4.1 Thyroid Disease

Clinical applications of dosimetry in radionuclide therapy vary in their application. Standardized methodologies have not been agreed upon, and results of different investigators may be difficult to compare.

The advent of multimodality imaging (single photon emission computed tomography (SPECT)/CT or positron emission tomography (PET)/CT) and the incorporation of patient-specific 3D image in the dosimetric calculations along with radiobiolgical modeling will lead to a better characterization of radiation dosimetry during therapy applications. There is clear evidence that dosimetry can prove to be of practical benefit in clinical practice, but many physicians remain skeptical of the need for dosimetry in routine practice, although it is required in the clinical trial phase of new drug approval.

Maxon et al. [14, 15] used a dosimetric approach in the treatment of thyroid disease and concluded that a reliable response of the diseased tissue is not likely unless the radiation reaches or exceeds 85 Gy. Kobe et al. [16] evaluated the success of the treatment of Graves' disease in 571 subjects, with the goal of delivering 250 Gy to the thyroid, with the end-point measure being the elimination of hyperthyroidism, evaluated 12 months after the treatment. Relief from hyperthyroidism was achieved in 96% of patients who received more than 200 Gy, even for those with thyroid volumes > 40 ml. Individually tailored patient thyroid dosimetry was made to the targeted total dose, with ultrasound measurement of subject thyroid mass and adjustment of the procedure to account for differences between observed effective retention half-times between studies involving the tracer activity and the therapy administration. Two groups asserted that an absorbed therapeutic dose can be predicted by a prior tracer administration with a reasonable degree of accuracy that would enable patient-specific treatment planning [17, 18], and it has further been shown that the rate of hypothyroidism resulting from the treatment of Graves' disease with radioiodine is correlated with the absorbed dose [19]. Dorn et al. [20] found that with lesion doses above 100 Gy were needed to ensure a complete response (CR) in their population of over 120 subjects treated for differentiated thyroid cancer. Jonsson and Mattsson [21] compared theoretical levels of activity that could be given to patients using patient-specific dose calculations and actual practice in nearly 200 cases of the use of radioiodine to treat Graves' disease at one institution. They showed that "most of the patients were treated with an unnecessarily high activity, as a mean factor of 2.5 times too high and in individual patients up to eight times too high, leading to an unnecessary radiation exposure both for the patient, the family and the public." Pauwels et al. found a convincing relationship in their study of 22 patients with ^{90}Y Octreother [22] (an anti-somato-statin peptide) employing PET imaging with ^{86}Y to characterize the in vivo kinetics of the agent. In the treatment of thyroid cancer, treatments are mostly based on fixed activities rather than absorbed doses, although some have employed a dose-based approach [23, 24].

9.4.2 Other Diseases

I-131 meta-iodobenzylguanidine (mIBG) has been used for many years for the treatment of adult and pediatric neuroendocrine tumors, including pheochro-mocytoma, paraganglioma, and neuroblastoma. In studies in which dosimetry has been performed it has been shown that significant variations occur in absorbed doses to the whole body, normal organs, and tumors if a fixed administered activity approach is used [24, 25].

The use of monoclonal antibodies for the treatment of cancer, particularly the use of monoclonal anti-bodies (mAbs) against non-Hodgkin's lymphoma, has been widely studied [26–28]. Two products, Bexxar and Zevalin, employing an anti-CD20 anti-body, have been approved by the United States Food and Drug Administration (US FDA) for the treatment of relapsed or refractory B-cell non-Hodgkin's lym-phoma. Bexxar uses ^{131}I as the radionuclide, and Zevalin employs the longer-range beta emitter ^{90}Y. In the treatment with Bexxar, at least whole-body dose is evaluated with a target dose of 0.75 Gy [29] (which is really to limit marrow toxicity); with Zeva-lin, unfortunately, no dosimetry is performed [30]. Peptide therapy for neuroendocrine tumors has been investigated, primarily in Europe, including somatostatin analogues such as the compound DOTA-DPhe(1)-Tyr(3)-octreotide (DOTATOC). A few dosi-metric studies have been performed [31–32]. Barone et al. [33] evaluated kidney dose from administrations of 8.1 GBq – 22.9 GBq of ^{90}Y DOTATOC and, cal-culating the BED instead of just absorbed dose, found a strong correlation between BED and creatinine clearance.

9.5 Conclusion

Our understanding of radiation biology from internal emitters requires considerable attention in the years to come. Improving this understanding can only come if careful dosimetry is performed with many therapy patients, as dose/effect relationships cannot be studied at all if there is no calculation of dose. Providing better and more durable outcomes for cancer patients requires more aggressive and optimized therapy, which again is not possible without careful and accurate dosimetry. A recent analysis [34] showed that:

- Widely accepted and automated methods, with rel-atively easy adjustment for patient-specific organ masses and use of individual patient kinetic data, are of similar cost and difficulty to those used in other therapeutic modalities.
- The use of a dosimetry-based approach will result in better patient outcomes, improving the quality of medical care for patients and reducing costs for the institutions involved.
- Careful use of patient-individualized dose calcula-tions will produce calculated radiation dose esti-mates that correlate well with observed effects. Such data, as they accumulate with the increased application of patient-specific techniques, will con-tinually improve our understanding of the link between radiation dose and effect, and the success rates of these techniques.

A paradigm shift is needed in the nuclear medicine clinic to accommodate these changes and improve patient therapy. The question is not *whether* we should perform individualized dosimetry for radionuclide therapy patients, but *how* we will perform it.

References

1. Mullner R (1989) Deadly glow. The radium dial worker trag-edy. American Public Health Association, Washington DC
2. Bergonie J, Tribondeau L (1906) De quelques resultats de la Radiotherapie, et esaie de fixation d'une technique ratio-nelle. Comptes Rendu des Seances de l'Academie des Sciences 143:983–985
3. Jonah CD, Miller JR (1977) Yield and decay of the OH radical from 100 ps to 3 ns. J Phys Chem 81:1974–1976
4. Sachs RK, Hahnfeld P, Brenner DJ (1997) The link between low-LET dose-response relations and the underlying

kinetics of damage production/repair/misrepair. Int J Radiat Biol 72:351–374

5. Lea DE, Catcheside DG (1942) The mechanism of the induction by radiation of chromosome abberations in tradescantia. J Genet 44:216–245

6. Barendson GW (1982) Dose fractionation, dose-rate and iso-effect relationships for normal tissue responses. Int J Radiat Oncol Biol Phys 8:1981–1987

7. Fowler JF (1989) The linear-quadratic formula and progress in fractionated radiotherapy. Br J Radiol 62:679–694

8. Bodey RK, Evans PM, Flux GD (2004) Application of the linear-quadratic model to combined modality radiotherapy. Int J Radiat Oncol Biol Phys 59(1):228–241

9. Pimblott SM, LaVerne JA (1997) Stochastic simulation of the electron radiolysis of water and aqueous solutions. J Phys Chem A 101:5828–5838

10. Becker D, Sevilla MD, Wang W, LaVere T (1997) The role of waters of hydration in direct-effect radiation damage to DNA. Radiat Res 148:508–510

11. Wright HA, Magee JL, Hamm RN, Chatterjee A, Turner JE, Klots CE (1985) Calculations of physical and chemical reactions produced in irradiated water containing DNA. Radiat Prot Dosimetry 13:133–136

12. Turner JE, Hamm RN, Ritchie RH, Bolch WE (1994) Monte Carlo track-structure calculations for aqueous solutions containing biomolecules. Basic Life Sci 63:155–166

13. Hall Eric J (2003) The Bystander effect. Health Phys 85(1):31–35

14. Maxon HR, Englaro EE, Thomas SR, Hertzberg VS, Hinnefeld JD, Chen LS et al (1992) Radioiodine-131 therapy for well-differentiated thyroid-cancer – a quantitative radiation dosimetric approach – outcome and validation in 85 patients. J Nucl Med 33(6):1132–1136

15. Maxon HR (1999) Quantitative radioiodine therapy in the treatment of differentiated thyroid cancer. Q J Nucl Med 43(4):313–323

16. Kobe C, Eschner W, Sudbrock F, Weber I, Marx K, Dietlein M, Schicha H (2008) Graves' disease and radioiodine therapy: is success of ablation dependent on the achieved dose above 200 Gy? Nuklearmedizin 47(1): 13–17

17. Canzi C, Zito F, Voltini F, Reschini E, Gerundini P (2006) Verification of the agreement of two dosimetric methods with radioiodine therapy in hyperthyroid patients. Med Phys 33(8):2860–2867

18. Carlier T, Salaun PY, Cavarec MB, Valette F, Turzo A, Bardies M, Bizais Y, Couturier O (2006) Optimized radioiodine therapy for Graves' disease: two MIRD-based models for the computation of patient-specific therapeutic I-131 activity. Nucl Med Commun 27(7):559–566

19. Grosso M, Traino A, Boni G, Banti E, Della Porta M, Manca G, Volterrani D, Chiacchio S, AlSharif A, Borso E, Raschilla R, Di Martino F, Mariani G (2005) Comparison of different thyroid committed doses in radioiodine therapy for Graves' hyperthyroidism. Cancer Biother Radiopharm 20(2):218–223

20. Dorn R, Kopp J, Vogt H, Heidenreich P, Carroll RG, Gulec SA (2003) Dosimetry-guided radioactive iodine treatment in patients with metastatic differentiated thyroid cancer: largest safe dose sing a risk-adapted approach. J Nucl Med 44:451–456

21. Jonsson H, Mattsson S (2004) Excess radiation absorbed doses from non-optimised radioiodine treatment of hyperthyroidism. Radiat Prot Dosim 108(2):107–114

22. Pauwels S, Barone R, Walrand S, Borson-Chazot F, Valkema R, Kvols LK, Krenning EP, Jamar F (2005) Practical dosimetry of peptide receptor radionuclide therapy with ^{90}Y-labeled somatostatin analogs. J Nucl Med 46(1 (Suppl)):92S–98S

23. Furhang EE, Larson SM, Buranapong P, Humm JL (1999) Thyroid cancer dosimetry using clearance fitting. J Nucl Med 40(1):131–136

24. Maxon HR, Thomas SR, Samaratunga RC (1997) Dosimetric considerations in the radioiodine treatment of macrometastases and micrometastases from differentiated thyroid cancer. Thyroid 7(2):183–187

25. Monsieurs M, Brans B, Bacher K, Dierckx R, Thierens H (2002) Patient dosimetry for I-131-MIBG therapy for neuroendocrine tumours based on I-123-MIBG scans. Eur J Nucl Med Mol Imaging 29(12):1581–1587

26. Flux GD, Guy MJ, Papavasileiou P, South C, Chittenden SJ, Flower MA, Meller ST (2003) Absorbed dose ratios for repeated therapy of neuroblastoma with I-131 mIBG. Cancer Biother Radiopharm 18(1):81–87

27. DeNardo GL, DeNardo SJ, Shen S, DeNardo DA, Mirick GR, Macey DJ, Lamborn KR (1999) Factors affecting I-131-Lym-1 pharmacokinetics and radiation dosimetry in patients with non-Hodgkin's lymphoma and chronic lymphocytic leukemia. J Nucl Med 40(8): 1317–1326

28. Linden O, Tennvall J, Cavallin-Stahl E, Darte L, Garkavij M, Lindner KJ, Ljungberg M, Ohlsson T, Sjogreen K, Wingardh K, Strand SE (1999) Radioimmunotherapy using I-131-labeled anti-CD22 monoclonal antibody (LL2) in patients with previously treated B-cell lymphomas. Clin Cancer Res 5(10):3287S–3291S

29. Chatal JF, FaivreChauvet A, Bardies M, Peltier P, Gautherot E, Barbet J (1995) Bifunctional antibodies for radioimmunotherapy. Hybridoma 14(2):125–128

30. Wahl RL, Kroll S, Zasadny KR (1998) Patient-specific whole-body dosimetry: principles and a simplified method for clinical implementation. J Nucl Med 39(8):14S–20S

31. Wiseman GA, White CA, Sparks RB, Erwin WD, Podoloff DA, Lamonica D, Bartlett NL, Parker JA, Dunn WL, Spies SM, Belanger R, Witzig TE, Leigh BR (2001) Biodistribution and dosimetry results from a phase III prospectively randomized controlled trial of Zevalin (TM) radioimmunotherapy for low-grade, follicular, or transformed B-cell non-Hodgkin's lymphoma. Crit Rev Oncol Hematol 39(1–2):181–194

32. Cremonesi M, Ferrari M, Chinol M, Bartolomei M, Stabin MG, Sacco E, Fiorenza M, Tosi G, Paganelli G (2000) Dosimetry in radionuclide therapies with Y-90-conjugates: the IEO experience. Q J Nucl Med 44(4):325–332

33. Barone R, Walrand S, Valkema R, Kvols L, Smith C, Krenning EP, Jamar F, Pauwels S (2002) Correlation between acute red marrow (RM) toxicity and RM exposure during Y-90-SMT487 therapy. J Nucl Med 43:1267

34. Stabin MG (2008) The case for patient-specific dosimetry in radionuclide therapy. Cancer Biother Radiopharm 23(3): 273–284

Part III

SPECT and PET Imaging Instrumentation

Elements of Gamma Camera and SPECT Systems

10

Magdy M. Khalil

Contents

10.1 Introduction

Nuclear medicine provides noninvasive imaging tools to detect a variety of human diseases. The two major components of these imaging procedures are radio-pharmaceuticals and an imaging system. The latter is a position-sensitive detector that relies on detecting gamma photons emitted from the administered

M.M. Khalil
Biological Imaging Centre, MRC/CSC, Imperial College London, Hammersmith Campus, Du Cane Road, W12 0NN London, UK
e-mail: magdy.khalil@imperial.ac.uk

radionuclide. Many single-photon and positron emitters are used in the nuclear medicine clinic. The radiopharmaceuticals are designed for tracing many pathophysiologic as well as molecular disorders and utilize the penetrating capability of gamma rays to functionally map the distribution of the administered compound within different biological tissues. The imaging systems used for detection of radionuclide-labeled compounds are special devices called scintillation cameras or positron emission tomographic (PET) scanners. These devices have passed through a number of developments since their introduction in the late 1960s and have had a significant impact on the practice and diagnostic quality of nuclear medicine.

The birth of nuclear medicine instrumentation dates to 1925; Blumgert and his coworker Otto C. Yens had modified the cloud chamber to measure the circulation time using an arm-to-arm method [1]. They used a mixture of radium decay products that emit beta and gamma rays. Blumgert postulated some assumptions for designing a detector or measurement technique that still hold true when compared with requirements of today: The technique must be objective and noninvasive and have the capability to measure the arrival of the substance automatically [1]. In 1951, Benedict Cassen introduced the rectilinear scanner to register a distribution of radioactivity accumulated in a human body. To scan a given area of interest, the scanner moves along a straight line collecting activity point by point. The scanner then moves over a predetermined distance and moves back in the opposite direction to span an equivalent length. This process is continued until the device scans the desired area of interest. Images are formed by a mechanical relay printer that prints the acquired events in a dot style. Initially, the scanner was used to scan iodine-131 in thyroid patients [2]. A major drawback of the

M.M. Khalil (ed.), *Basic Sciences of Nuclear Medicine*, DOI: 10.1007/978-3-540-85962-8_10,
© Springer-Verlag Berlin Heidelberg 2011

rectilinear scanner was the long acquisition time since radiation events are registered point by point in a sequential manner, taking 60–90 min to determine the outline of the thyroid gland [2]. Low contrast and spatial resolution of the formed images were also disadvantages of the rectilinear scanner.

In 1953, Hal Anger (at the Donner Laboratory of the Lawrence Berkeley Laboratory, USA) developed the first camera in which a photographic x-ray film was in contact with an NaI(Tl) intensifying screen. He used a pinhole collimation and small detector size to project the distribution of gamma rays onto the scintillation screen [3]. Initially, the camera was used to scan patients administered therapeutic doses of [131]I. A disadvantage of this prototype was the small field of view of the imaging system (4-in. diameter). Moreover, good image quality was difficult to obtain unless high doses were administered along with long exposure times. In 1958, Anger succeeded in developing the first efficient scintillation camera, which was then called by his name, the Anger camera. Marked progress in detection efficiency was realized as he used an NaI(Tl) crystal, photomultiplier tubes (PMTs), and a larger field of view.

Recent years have witnessed remarkable advances in the design of the gamma camera and single-photon emission computed tomographic (SPECT) systems. These were not only concerned with clinical scanners but also small-animal SPECT systems, providing a new era of molecular and imaging innovations using compounds labeled with single-photon emitters. Unlike PET, SPECT compounds in theory can provide images with high spatial resolution and the ability to follow the tracer uptake over more time intervals, including hours and days. PET imaging lacks such a property due to the short half-lives of most tracers. In contrast to PET scanners, dual tracer imaging capability can be easily achieved using SPECT compounds and a gamma camera system equipped with a multichannel analyzer.

While most of the present and commercially available gamma cameras are based largely on the original design made by Anger using sodium iodide crystal, successful trials of new imaging systems that suit either specific imaging requirements or improved image quality and enhanced diagnostic accuracy are emerging. One of these changes is the trend toward manufacturing a semiconductor gamma camera with performance characteristics superior to those achieved by the conventional design. Organ-specific or dedicated designs are now well recognized in cardiac as well as scintimammography. Both imaging procedures were shown to be superior, with such systems realizing better imaging quality and enhancement of lesion detectability. When these approaches were implemented and introduced into the clinic, significant changes in data interpretation and diagnostic outcome were achieved.

For breast imaging, a miniaturized version of the gamma camera based either on semiconductor technology or scintillation detectors has been commercially available. Another example is the cardiac-specific gamma camera, and a growing number of dedicated cardiac systems have been under development (some of them are combined with computed tomography [CT]) to improve the detection task. The developments in this area are concerned not only with hardware components but also some successful approaches to improve diagnostic images using resolution recovery and subsequent reduction of imaging time or administered dose. It has become possible that some imaging systems can perform cardiac scanning in a significantly shorter scanning time than conventionally used. The utility of SPECT systems is increasing with the addition of anatomical imaging devices such as CT and magnetic resonance imaging (MRI), and this is covered in some detail in the last few sections of the chapter.

Now, there is also interest in using semiconductor photodetectors to replace the historical PMTs to provide compactness, portability, and reduction of space requirements along with features that allow incorporation in multimodality imaging devices. The next generation of SPECT and PET devices will exploit these characteristics to overcome the current performance limitations of both imaging modalities.

10.2 The Gamma Camera

10.2.1 Theory

The gamma camera is a medical radiation detection device of various hardware components such that each component has a specific role in the photon detection process. It is outside the scope of the chapter to describe all these elements and their detailed functions. However, the principal components of the imaging system are described in addition to their relative contribution to image formation. Generally, these components are the collimator, crystal, PMT, preamplifier, amplifier, pulse height analyzer (PHA), position circuitry, computer system for data correction and image analysis, and ultimately a monitor for image display.

Briefly, once the patient has been injected and prepared for imaging, the first hardware component that is met by the incident photons is the collimator. The collimator determines the directionality of the incident photons and accordingly forms the hardware role in outlining the activity distribution within different organs. The accepted photons then interact with the detector crystal to produce scintillation light photons. The photomultiplier converts the light pulse into an electronic signal. Through a number of steps that involve an identification of the photon energy and event positioning, the scintillation site is determined, which in turn reflects the spatial position of the emitted photons.

The heart of the scintillation camera is a position-sensitive detector that can localize the interaction sites where incident photons imparted their energy. The conventional design of the gamma camera consists of a continuous structure of a scintillation crystal mapped by an array of PMTs. The last component is not a point or pencil-like photodetector, and size, shape, and the number of PMTs vary among manufacturers. Another point that should be mentioned is that the scintillation light emits a narrow beam of light photons; however, it diverges and spreads over the crystal and appears at the PMT end as a cone shape, illuminating more than one PMT. Most often, one PMT receives the maximum amount of light produced by the scintillation event; therefore, the site of interaction could be determined based on a single PMT signal [4]. The original design proposed by Anger is shown in Fig. 10.1.

To spatially determine a distribution of radioactivity inside a human organ, an electronic circuit that is able to localize the position of the emitted gamma radiations must exist in the detection system. The inclusion of all PMT signals should theoretically yield better precision in positioning measurements. However, as the distant PMTs receive little light, they contribute with less certainty to the identification process, leading to increased noise. This can be treated by a thresholding process, by which the tube signals below a set value are either ignored or the tubes are adjusted by a threshold value [5, 6].

The output of the PMTs is mapped by a network of electric resistors. The resistors are weighted according to the spatial position of the PMTs in the x- and y-axes of the coordinate system of the array. This helps to identify the spatial position of an event based on the relative amount of current received by each resistor. The classical method of event positioning determination is the Anger logic centroid approach, by which each event results in four signals $X-$, $X+$, $Y-$, and $Y+$, and then applying a simple formula per coordinate to obtain the spatial position within the 2D (two-dimensional) matrix [1].

In the analog design of the gamma camera, three signals are detected. Two signals indicate the spatial position (X, Y), and one signal indicates the energy of the incident photon, Z-signal, or pulse height. The three signals are a mathematical analysis of the PMT output identified according to the positive and negative direction of the x ($x+$ and $x-$) and y ($y+$ and $y-$) coordinates. The energy is proportional to the amount of light produced in the crystal and with the energy deposited by the gamma radiation and computed by summing all the output signals of the involved PMTs. The position signal is divided by the energy signal so that the spatial coordinate signals become more independent of the energy signal. However, this simple process for event localization suffers from nonuniform spatial behavior, differences in PMT gain, and edge packing problems, which occurs when the scintillation event becomes close to the crystal edge. In the last situation, the positioning algorithm fails to accurately position the scintillation event as the light distribution from the scintillation site is asymmetric or truncated, leading to improper PMT position weighting and loss of spatial resolution. Furthermore, these problems associated with the detector peripheral regions cause loss of detection efficiency and a reduction of the imaging field of view. In gamma camera-based coincidence systems, this phenomenon could result in malfunctioning detector areas corrupting the reconstruction process.

In the digital gamma camera, the signal of the PMT is digitized by what is called an analog-to-digital converter (ADC). Further detector development has resulted in a process of digitizing the signal directly at the preamplifier output to couple each PMT to a

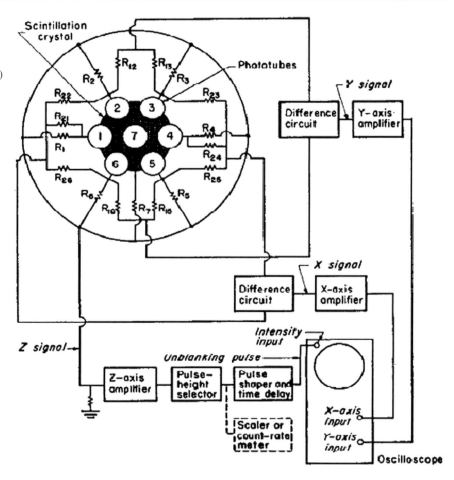

single ADC. In this situation, position information is no longer established using resistors and a summation circuit, but the localization circuitry has been totally replaced by a dedicated onboard computer [7].

After signal digitization, the determination of pulse position on the crystal is achieved using the "normalized position-weighted sum" circuit, in a fashion similar to the analog camera "Anger logic circuit," or by picking up a correction factor from lookup tables constructed previously in a calibration test. This process is implemented through a software program using mathematical algorithms. Other event-positioning methods were developed, such as detailed crystal mapping, Gaussian fitting, neural networks, maximum likelihood estimation, and distance-weighted algorithms applied in an iterative manner [5, 8]. The lookup correction tables contain information regarding the spatial distortion or camera nonlinearity for accurate determination of event position during routine patient acquisition. In the calibration process, the PMT response is calibrated to a spatial activity distributing with a well-defined pattern on the crystal surface [9].

10.2.2 Collimators

Gamma radiation emitted from a radioactive source are uniformly distributed over a spherical geometry. They are not like light waves, which can be focused into a certain point using optical lenses. Gamma radiation emitted from an administered radionuclide into a patient is detected by allowing those photons that pass through a certain direction to interact with the crystal. By this concept, we can collect and outline the radioactivity distributed within different tissues by a multi-hole aperture or what is called a collimator.

The collimator is an array of holes and septa designed with a specific geometric pattern on a slab of lead. The geometric design of the holes and septa determines the collimator type and function. Unfortunately, most gamma radiation emitted from an injected radionuclide cannot be detected by the gamma camera since many gamma rays do not travel in the directions provided by collimator holes. This is in great part due to the small solid angle provided by the collimator area in addition to the area occupied by the septal thickness. In the detection process for gamma rays, approximately 1 of every 100,000 photons is detected by the detector system, which is relatively inefficient process for gamma ray detection, leading to poor count statistics [10]. The collimator material is often made of lead due to its attenuation and absorption properties. Lead has a high atomic number ($Z = 82$) and high density (11.3 g/cm^3), providing a mass absorption coefficient of 2.2 cm^2/g at 140 keV associated with Tc-99m emission.

To obtain a better count rate performance, a reduction of collimator resolution cannot be avoided. On the other hand, collimators with better spatial resolution tend to reduce sensitivity at the cost of improving image details. Therefore, there is often a trade-off that should be made to the geometric dimensions of the holes and septa. The collimation system has an important role in spatial resolution, sensitivity, and count rate of acquired data; it affects the spatial properties and signal-to-noise ratio of the acquired scintigraphic images.

Different types and designs were proposed and operating in nuclear medicine laboratories. However, the general types of collimators used in nuclear medicine imaging are parallel hole, converging, diverging, and a special type known as a pinhole collimator, which has proved valuable in small animal imaging with superb intrinsic spatial resolution. The main differences among these types, as mentioned, are their geometric dimensions, including shape, size, and width of the collimator holes. Figures 10.2–10.4 show different types of collimators used in nuclear medicine clinics.

Parallel-hole collimators: The holes and septa of parallel-hole collimators are parallel to each other, providing a chance for those photons that fall perpendicular to the crystal surface to be accepted (Fig.10.2a). The image size projected by the parallel-hole collimator onto the crystal is 1:1 since it does not offer any geometric magnification to the acquired images. The most common types of parallel-hole collimator are

- Low-energy all-purpose (LEAP) (or low-energy general- purpose, LEGP) collimator
- Low-energy high-resolution (LEHR) collimator
- Low-energy high-sensitivity (LEHS) collimator
- Medium- and high-energy (ME and HE, respectively) collimators

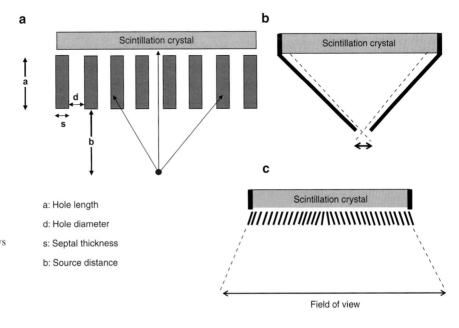

a: Hole length

d: Hole diameter

s: Septal thickness

b: Source distance

Fig. 10.2 Three different types of collimator. (**a**) Shows the parallel geometry along with definition of collimator holes and septa. (**b**) Pinhole geometry. (**c**) Divergent collimator

Fig. 10.3 Three different types of parallel-hole collimators: low-energy high-resolution, low-energy general-purpose, and low-energy high-sensitivity collimators. *FWHM* full width at half maximum

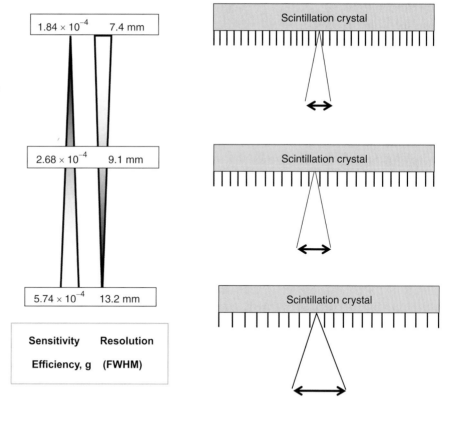

Fig. 10.4 Cone beam and fan beam collimators. For the former, all holes focus at a single point, while in the latter all holes at the same transaxial slice look at the same focal point

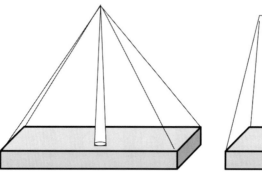
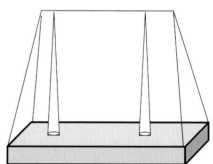

Focal point   Focal line

LEHR collimators provide a small acceptance angle by the aid of their narrow and longer holes. This helps to resolve fine details and improves the spatial resolution of the acquired images. Moreover, it tends to keep resolution at a distance and hence is recommended in cardiac SPECT imaging due to the varying distance of the heart from the surface of the detector.

For *LEGP collimators*, **the** hole diameter is relatively larger, and the acceptance angle is wider than for the high-resolution (HR) collimator. It provides greater sensitivity and lower spatial resolution characteristics as opposed to the LEHR collimator. LEGP collimators are useful in examinations that require a high count rate (e.g., dynamic studies) to improve sensitivity while spatial resolution is not so influential to the interpretation of the images. Table 10.1 compares the general purpose (GP) and HR collimators for a commercially available gamma camera system [11].

The difference in geometric dimensions of the hole diameter and length in addition to the septal thickness of both collimators results in a significant improvement of the sensitivity of the GP collimator over the HR collimator with minimal loss in resolution measurements. In Table 10.1, notice that the GP collimator provides a count rate efficiency about 50% greater than that of the HR collimator. It should be pointed out that manufacturers have their own special designs and label them differently. Collimator specifications given, for example, to a GP collimator might be completely different from those given by another manufacturer to the same type of collimator [12].

LEHS collimators: This type of collimators provides good count rate capabilities and produces images with low statistical noise if compared with other collimators given the same acquisition time. However, this is achieved by trading off the resolution properties of the acquired images. In other words, the improvement in sensitivity is obtained at the cost of compromising the detectability of fine structures. Figure 10.3 shows the trade-off between spatial resolution and sensitivity in collimator design.

HE and ME collimators: Medium-energy radionuclides in nuclear medicine such as gallium-67 and In-111 and high-energy radionuclides such as I-131 and Fluorodeoxyglucose-F18 (FDG) have high penetrating power and thus could penetrate collimator septa, causing higher background images and could adversely affect spatial contrast. ME and HE collimators have increased septal thickness and provide a lower transparency to high-energy gamma photons than lower-energy collimators. However, radionuclide studies that use ME and HE collimators manifest lower spatial resolution by degrading small-size lesions. As a result, lower quantitative accuracy is achieved by partial volume averaging [13]. Nevertheless, ME collimators were recommended over LE collimators in studies that required low-energy photons (e.g., iodine-123) if there

were other emissions of higher-energy gamma rays to lessen septal penetration artifacts and improve quantitative accuracy. Some manufacturers overcame the problem by introducing new collimators with a special design that are able to maintain resolution and sensitivity of the examination while providing lower septal penetration [13].

Converging and diverging collimators have a field of view different from parallel-hole collimators with the same exit plane size. The converging collimators have a smaller field of view, whereas the diverging ones offer a larger field of view than that provided by parallel-hole collimators. In diverging collimators, the direction of the holes diverges from the point of view of the back surface of the collimator (the face opposing the crystal). They are used in cameras with a small field of view so that they can lessen large organs to be projected onto the camera crystal (Fig. 10.2c).

In *converging collimators*, the holes are converging from the perspective of the back surface of the collimator. Cone beam and fan beam are special types of gamma camera collimators; the former has one focal point for all collimator holes that lies at a certain distance away from the collimator surface and is called the focal point. The focal length is minimal at the center of the collimator and increases gradually as it goes to the periphery. In the fan beam collimator, each row of collimator holes has its own focal point, and all the focal points form a focal line for the entire collimator. As such, it has parallel collimation along the axial direction of the subject and converging collimation within each slice, providing independent and nonoverlapping projection profiles. This geometry allows for a simplified slice-by-slice image reconstruction to be applied. Cone beam geometry, however, complicates image reconstruction by involving the holes axially and transaxially. Both collimators are shown in Fig. 10.4.

A converging collimator provides a magnified view of small objects found at locations between the collimator surface and the focal point/line with relative improvement in count sensitivity, which is maximum at the focal site. They are of particular interest in brain

Table 10.1 Characteristics of two different collimators: low-energy general-purpose (GP) and high-resolution (HR) collimators[a]

Collimator	Hole diameter (mm)	Septal thickness (mm)	Hole length (mm)	Resolution at 15 cm (mm)	Relative efficiency
GP	1.40	0.18	25.4	11.5	1.0
HR	2.03	0.13	54.0	9.5	0.52

[a]Taken from Ref. [11].

tomographic imaging and in some other applications. Resolution of the converging collimator is maximum at the surface and decreases with an increase in source distance, while the sensitivity increases gradually from the collimator surface until the source reaches the focal point. This is because the fraction of holes that can see the object at a near distance increases with an increase in object distance; therefore, the object at larger distances is seen by more holes, resulting in improved sensitivity. Magnification takes place only in one direction, typically the transverse direction, and the cone beam collimator magnifies along the axial direction as well [14]. The drawbacks of converging collimators are reduced field of view and data insufficiency for 3D (three-dimensional) reconstruction.

Pinhole collimator: The pinhole collimator is an important type that is used frequently in nuclear medicine laboratories, especially in small-organ imaging, such as thyroid and parathyroid scanning (Fig. 10.2b). Also, it has useful applications in skeletal extremities, bone joints, and the pediatric population. It is a cone-shaped structure made of lead, tungsten, and platinum and has an aperture of a few millimeters in diameter (2–6 mm). In the small-animal pinhole collimator, the aperture size can go decrease to 1–2 mm or even less to meet the resolution requirements imposed by small structures and minute tracer uptake [15]. The collimator length that extends from the back surface to the point of the aperture is 20–25 cm. Image formation can be described using lens equations in the sense that the acquired data reveal an inverted and magnified image. The pinhole collimator provides a magnified image of small objects, yielding an appearance that reflects an improvement in spatial resolution.

10.2.3 Crystal

Scintillation crystal is the second component that encounters the incident photons after passing the collimator holes. There are some favorable properties based on which the crystal needs to be selected before implementation in gamma camera design. Scintillators of high density, high atomic number, short decay time, high light output, and low cost are desired and allow better imaging performance. However, there is no ideal detector material in the field of diagnostic radiology; most often, the selected material has some

Table 10.2 Properties of scintillation crystals used in gamma camera

	Na(Tl)	CsI(Tl)	CsI(Na)
Z_{eff}	3.67	54	54
Density (g/cm^3)	50	4.51	4.51
Decay time (ns)	230	1,000	630
Photon yield (keV)	38	45–52[a]	39
Refraction index	1.85	1.8	1.84
Hygroscopic	Yes	Slightly	yes
Peak emission (nm)	415	540	420

[a]CsI(Tl) is poorly matched to the response of photomultiplier tube (PMT). However, the scintillation yield is much higher when measured by photodiodes with extended response into the red region of the spectrum [20].

desired features that make it preferred over alternatives. Table 10.2 lists the most common crystals used in gamma camera design.

The most commonly used detector material for the gamma camera is the thallium-activated sodium iodide [NaI(Tl)] crystal. It utilizes the scintillation phenomenon to convert gamma rays into light quanta that can be amplified by a PMT to produce a detectable electronic signal. Scintillation occurs when the incident photon interacts with the crystal material to produce photoelectrons or Compton scattering. The resulting electrons from photoelectric or Compton interactions travel short distances within the crystal to produce more interactions in a form of excitations or ionizations of the crystal atoms and molecules. These excited products are deexcited by converting to the ground state by releasing scintillation light.

A continuous large slab of sodium iodide crystal is the conventional structure that is used in most gamma camera designs. The crystal thickness can be 3/8 in., 5/8 in., or even larger for high detection efficiency [16]. A pixilated or segmented version of scintillation crystals has also been utilized in small SPECT systems using photosensitive PMTs as photodetectors and parallel or pinhole imaging geometry, yielding high-resolution tomographic images. Segmentation of the scintillation crystal allows the spatial resolution of the imaging system to be improved to an extent determined mainly by the segmentation size. Nevertheless, this comes with a reduction of count sensitivity, increased costs, and degraded energy resolution [17]. It is often used in small field-of-view, organ specific-systems or in small-animal scanners. Another option that can be considered as an intermediate solution between continuous and segmented or pixilated crystals is partially slotted crystals, which have been investigated to produce better energy resolution than fully pixilated crystals and improved detection sensitivity while maintaining the spatial resolution at better levels with an appropriate data analysis [18, 19]. Additional features provided by such systems are their relative ease and cheap manufacturing costs.

The NaI(Tl) crystal is formed by adding a controlled amount of thallium to a pure sodium iodide crystal during growth. The addition of thallium makes the NaI crystal scintillate at room temperature since pure a NaI crystal works at a low temperature under nitrogen cooling [9, 20]. Some precautions are taken into account during the design of the NaI(Tl) crystal. It must be sealed in an airtight enclosure, usually aluminum, to avoid exposure to air owing to its hygroscopic properties. Exposing the crystal to air can cause yellow spots, which can develop heterogeneous light transmission.

Thallium-activated cesium iodide, CsI(Tl), is slightly denser than sodium iodide crystal and better suited if coupled to photodiodes as the emission wavelength is shifted to higher values, at which the response of PMTs is relatively weaker. It therefore does not properly fit the requirements imposed by PMTs, which need light quanta of shorter wavelengths. A pixilated CsI(Tl) crystal has been tested in a miniaturized gamma camera with the collimator matching the detector array and size suitable for breast imaging. The system showed good performance characteristics, such as an improved spatial resolution, high detection efficiency, and better scatter rejection (~8% full width at half maximum [FWHM] at 140 keV) [21]. The CsI(Tl) crystal has also been utilized in a pixilated fashion and coupled with silicon photodiode in a commercial design developed as a dedicated cardiac tomograph. Cardius 3 XPO is manufactured by Digirad and consists of 768 pixilated Cs(Tl) crystals coupled to individual silicon photodiodes and digital Anger electronics for signal readout [22].

Sodium-activated cesium iodide, CsI(Na), has an emission spectrum similar to NaI(Tl) that suits PMT response, with comparable light yield and relatively slow decay time. It has been utilized in small-animal SPECT scanners in pixilated 5-mm thickness (21×52 pixels of 2.5×2.5 mm) coupled to photosensitive PMTs [23]. The system provided an intrinsic spatial resolution of 2.5 mm, intrinsic energy resolution of 35% (at 140 keV), and intrinsic sensitivity of 42% using an energy width of 35% at 140 keV. Comparison of partially slotted CsI(Na) and CsI(Tl) crystals revealed the superior performance of the latter in terms of detection efficiency and spatial and energy resolution [19].

Yttrium aluminum perovskite (YALO3:Ce) is a nonhygroscopic scintillation crystal with the structure of the perovskite and is called YAP. It has a density of 5.37 g/cm^3, an effective atomic number of 34–39, and light output of 40% relative to NaI(Tl) and is used for gamma as well as annihilation coincidence detection [24]. Lanthanum bromide (LaBr:Ce) is a fast scintillator (short decay time, 16 ns) with high light output. These characteristics are suitable for time-of-flight applications in PET scanners (see Chap. 11). High light yield is an important parameter that improves the certainty of photon statistics and serves to improve system spatial and energy resolution. The crystal has been evaluated using a flat-panel, photosensitive PMT; it showed good imaging performance for single-photon applications with superior energy resolution (6–7.5%) and spatial resolution of 0.9 mm. The detection efficiency was also high, yielding 95% at 140-keV photon energy [25–27].

While SPECT and PET can be combined into one imaging device known as hybrid SPECT/PET camera, there are some modifications that have to be implemented in electronic circuitry and crystal thickness. The latter should be adapted to improve photon detection efficiency. The NaI(Tl) crystal is an efficient scintillator for low-energy photons; it is greater than 95% for 140 keV. However, its response against 511 keV is significantly poorer as it shows a coincidence detection efficiency of about 10%.

Some manufacturers have used the traditional scintillation crystal by increasing the thickness up to 25 mm, while others have modified the crystal so that the back surface of the crystal is grooved, allowing detection of single-photon emitters to be maintained. Meanwhile, the system is efficiently able to image patients injected with medium- and high-energy radiotracers. However, all the major suppliers are currently providing PET scanners with a more efficient performance, which have a cylindrical-type design.

StarBrite crystal, developed by Bicron Corporation (Newbury, OH), is a dual-function 1-in. thick crystal that serves to improve the detection efficiency of medium- and high-energy photons and has been incorporated in some commercial designs [16, 28] (see Fig. 10.5). The slots at the back surface of the NaI(Tl) crystal are machined to prevent light diffusion, reducing the impact of wide-angle reflected light. This also maintains a uniform light collection as a function of position, achieving better intrinsic spatial resolution (4 mm) [29, 30]. In performance evaluation with other systems, this design provided a good compromise in terms of spatial resolution and sensitivity for ^{111}In ProstaScint® SPECT imaging. However, the

collimator-crystal pair combined with system electronics work together to determine the overall system spatial resolution and sensitivity given a particular detection task.

In humans, visual perception is the ability to interpret information and surroundings from visible light reaching the eye. In a similar way, the light released from the scintillator after the interaction of the incident radiation with the detector system needs an interpretation process. This process in the gamma camera is implemented by the readout component or photodetectors that lie in close proximity to the back surface of the scintillation crystal. A remarkable feature of the design made by Anger is the photomultiplier mapping of the detector crystal together with the mathematical logic he used in event identification.

10.2.4 Photomultiplier Tube

The PMT is an important hardware component in the detection system of the gamma camera. Its main function is to convert the scintillation photons to a detectable electronic signal. The PMT as shown in Fig. 10.6 is a vacuum tube consisting of an entrance window, a photocathode, focusing electrodes, electron multiplier (dynodes), and anode. The PMT has a long history in many applications, including medical as well as other fields such as high-energy physics, spectrophotometry,

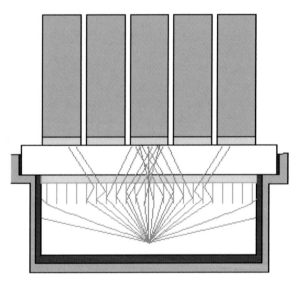

Fig. 10.5 StarBrite. (Courtesy of Saint-Gobain Crystals)

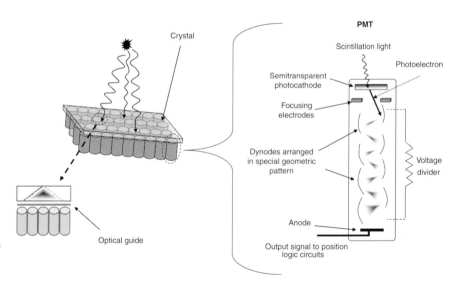

Fig. 10.6 Photon interaction and conversion to electronic signal

and is widely used in many SPECT and PET imaging systems.

10.2.4.1 Photocathode

The photocathode is a photo-emissive surface usually consisting of bialkali metals with low work functions and weakly bound valence electrons. The photocathode receives the scintillation light from the crystal, such as an NaI(Tl), by a wavelength of 415 nm at maximum. The material for the photocathode that emits photoelectrons (on an incidence of light quanta) equivalent to that wavelength will be the material of choice as it will allow increasing the amount of electrons emitted and hence will be able to improve the certainty of the output signal [31].

The photons emitted from the NaI(Tl) crystal fall on the photocathode of the PMT to eject photoelectrons by the physical phenomenon of photoelectric effect. The emitted electrons are amplified through a series of dynodes placed in a special geometric pattern with high potential difference so that each dynode has greater voltage (100–300 keV) than the preceding one. When scintillation light strikes the photocathode, it releases electrons, which are accelerated by the effect of the high voltage on the first dynode to collide with it. Electrons emitted from the first dynode are accelerated to the second dynode to eject more electrons on collision. The third dynode accelerates the electrons from the second dynode toward its face; this multi-stage electron amplification continues until the electrons reach the last dynode. At the back end of the PMT, the anode of the PMT collects all the electrons that result from this cascade process. Figure 10.6 illustrates the process of photon conversion to electronic signal after interaction with the crystal.

10.2.4.2 Anode

The anode of the PMT is an electrode that collects the amplified electrons through the multistage dynodes and outputs the electron current to an external circuit. An adequate potential difference between the anode and the last dynodes can be applied to prevent space charge effects and obtain a large output current [32]. PMTs have a large electronic gain that can reach

10^6–10^8 in addition to low electric noise. However, the *quantum conversion efficiency* of PMT is low since, on average, for every ten scintillation photons that fall on the photocathode, there is approximately a release of two electrons, resulting in an efficiency of about 20–25% [29]. This in turn has an impact on intrinsic spatial resolution and energy resolution. The PMT is susceptible to variations in high-voltage power supply, and its performance is influenced by temperature, humidity, gravity, and magnetic field because of the high voltage applied on the dynodes (a limitation in design of PET/MRI scanners).

10.2.5 Preamplifier

The shape of the output signal from the PMT is a rapid rising peak with a slow decaying tail. The rapid peak denotes the decay time of the scintillation event within the crystal, and the decaying tail denotes the time taken by the electrons to traverse the PMT. The output signal of the PMT cannot be fed directly into the amplifier because of the impedance difference between the PMT and the amplifier. The preamplifier plays an important role in this regard. It matches the impedance between the PMT and the main amplifier so that it could be handled by the amplifier and other subsequent electronics. The function of the preamplifier is matching, shaping, and sometimes amplification of the signal [9].

Matching: The signal produced from the PMT has a high impedance value, and this requires matching with the other electronic circuit components, (i.e., amplifier).

Shaping: The signal that is to be fed into a main amplifier needs to have a certain pulse decrease time to allow proper pole-zero and baseline correction. The preamplifier works to shape the PMT signal using an resistor-capacitor circuit (RC) by increasing the time constant, which is then handled by the amplifier.

Amplification: The amplification element of the preamplifier varies in the amount of amplification according to the type of detector and the magnitude of the signal. In PMT electronic assembly, the preamplifier sometimes has no significant amplification gain since the PMT itself provides a considerable amplification through the multistage process of the dynodes. The output signal from the preamplifier is a slow decaying pulse that causes pulse pileup. However, it conveys information regarding the signal amplitude and timing of the scintillation event. This information requires more additional manipulation by an amplifier without introducing any type of distortion. The newly developed SiPM (silicon photomultiplier) photodetectors (discussed in a separate section of this chapter) provide similar amplification gain as that of PMTs; hence, preamplification requirements are less demanding in comparison to photodetectors with low gain properties.

10.2.6 Amplifier

The amplifier plays a major role in signal amplification and shaping; it is therefore called a shaping amplifier. Signal amplification is required to permit further processing by the rest of the detector electronics. However, the amplification factor varies greatly with application and typically is a factor of 100–5,000 [20]. Shaping of the signal is accomplished by eliminating the tail from the output signal and giving each signal its separate width and amplitude without overlapping with other signals. In summary, the functions of the amplifier are shaping the pulse and decreasing the resolving time and providing higher gain to drive PHAs, scalars, and so on. It also provides stability to maintain proportionality between pulse height and photon energy deposition in the crystal. The amplifier serves to increase the signal-to-noise ratio and maintain proper polarity of the output signal [33].

10.2.7 Pulse Height Analyzer

There are different probabilities for the interaction of the incident gamma radiations with the crystal. Some photons impart a fraction or all of their energy into the crystal, whereas other photons impart some of their energy and escape the crystal without further interactions. Another fraction of photons undergo more than one interaction, dissipating all their energies. Therefore, there are two general forms of scatter that serve to reduce the capability of the system to accurately determine the position and the energy of the incident

gamma radiations. One part results from scattering that takes place inside the patient body, and the other part results from scattering that occurs in the camera crystal. The latter is not significant and does not contribute to a great extent to the total fraction of scattered radiation and the shape of the pulse height spectrum. It is important in medium- and high-energy gamma photons (e.g., In-111 and ^{131}I) and in thick crystals. The former type of scattering dominates the spectrum and results in degraded image quality and contrast resolution. As a result and for other instrumental reasons (e.g., detector energy resolution), the output signal is not a sharp peak line on the spectrum; it is a distribution of pulse heights with one or more photo peaks representing the energies of the administered radionuclides. The output signal is measured in terms of voltage or "pulse height," and every pulse has amplitude proportional to the amount of energy deposited by the gamma ray interactions. A pulse height analyzer (PHA), as the name implies, is a device that that is able to measure the amplitude pulse heights and compare them to preset values stored within it. There are two types of PHA: single channel and multichannel.

10.2.7.1 Single-Channel Analyzer

The single-channel analyzer records events within a specified range of pulse amplitude using one channel at a time, applying lower and upper voltage discriminators. The output signal of the amplifier has a range of heights (voltages), and selection of the desired signals for counting is achieved by setting the lower discriminator to a level that diminishes all lower amplitudes, thereby allowing the upper values to be recorded.

10.2.7.2 Multichannel Analyzer

Acquisition studies that require more energies to be detected, as in dual-radionuclide acquisitions (e.g., parathyroid Tl-201–Tc-99m subtraction, meta-iodobenzylguanidine(MIBG)-131–Tc-99mDTPA [diethylenetriaminepentaacetate], and others) and radionuclides with more than one energy photo peak (e.g., Ga-67, In-111, and Tl-201), the proper choice for recording these energies separately and simultaneously is to use a multichannel analyzer (MCA). An MCA provides a means of rejecting the scatter region from the spectrum, allowing the acquired image to be less contaminated by scattered photons. However, the photo peak region will still contain a significant fraction of photons that have undergone small-angle scattering. The MCA allows an energy window to be set over the photo peak centerline to confine the accepted photons to a certain energy range. This range is chosen by lower and upper voltage discriminators. The former determines the threshold below which all pulse heights are rejected, and the latter determines the value at which no higher values are accepted. Values that fall between the lower and upper discriminator are adjusted by a window width and often are a percentage of the photo peak energy. For example, a 20% energy window is usually selected over the 140-keV photons emitted by Tc-99m. A 15% window is also used with an improvement in contrast and minimal loss in primary photons. Moreover, a 10% window is used at the expense of reducing sensitivity [34]. An asymmetric window is another way to reduce the effect of scattered photons as it can improve image contrast, spatial resolution, and clinical impression [35, 36].

A variety of scatter correction techniques has been devised to reduce the adverse effects of scattered radiation. For proper quantitation and absolute measures of tracer concentrations, images must be corrected for scatter and other image-degrading factors. A gamma camera with an MCA is necessary when energy-based scatter corrections are applied to the acquired data. Advances in semiconductor technology have motivated the development of gamma camera systems with significant improvement in energy resolution. This in turn improves the spatial contrast and signal-to-noise ratio, resulting in improved image quality. Chapter 15 has more details about the scatter phenomenon and its correction techniques.

10.3 Other Photodetectors

10.3.1 Position-Sensitive PMT

The position-sensitive PMT (PSPMT) is a modified version of the conventional PMT but with compact size and position determination capabilities, allowing

for an improvement in image spatial resolution. The PSPMT-based gamma camera shows the same advantages of a standard gamma camera with the additional possibility of utilizing scintillation arrays with a pixel dimension less than 1 mm, thus giving the ability to achieve submillimeter spatial resolution [37]. Several models have been developed since its introduction in 1985 [38]. Three different types can be found [39, 40]:

Proximity mesh dynode: This is the first generation and is based on the proximity mesh dynode, by which the charge is multiplied around the position of the light photon striking the photocathode. The charge shower has a wide intrinsic spread. This model can provide a large active area (e.g., 5 in.) and large number of dynodes (e.g., 256) but with large dead space.

Multichannel dynode: This is a multianode structure that minimizes cross talk between anodes and provides better localization measurements. This type has the following drawbacks: large dead zone, limited effective area, and limited number of dynodes.

Metal channel dynode: Combined with multichannel or crossed-plate anode techniques, this dynode can provides low cross talk and well-focused charge distribution, reducing the intrinsic spread to 0.5 mm FWHM [39]. For SPECT imaging, the use of a crossed-wired anode PSPMT is more suitable when coupled with a flat crystal because of continuous position linearity requirements. However, this configurations may not allow the best performance of the PSPMT; thus, to utilize the full potential of its intrinsic characteristics, a multicrystal array is needed to attain high detection efficiency, narrow light spread function, and reasonable light output [41].

A PSPMT is relatively more expensive than the conventional type, and most of its use is in preclinical small-animal SPECT and PET scanners and portable and compact miniaturized gamma cameras, and it is of interest in producing high-resolution breast scanners [42, 43]. This type of diagnostic examination requires compact and flexible systems to fit geometric requirements imposed by the female breast. The technologic advances in the development of a compact flat-panel PSPMT with less dead space allowed manufacture of a portable gamma camera with a large detection area and high imaging performance with better spatial resolution [44]. It has become possible that an array of 256 crystal elements can be coupled directly to one PMT, and the crystals can be read out individually [45].

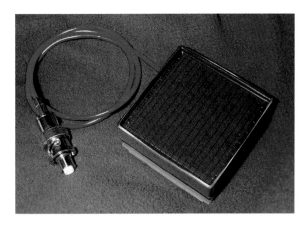

Fig. 10.7 Hamamatsu H8500 flat-panel position-sensitive photomultiplier tube (PSPMT). (From [100]. © 2006 IEEE with permission)

The Hamamatsu H8500 flat-panel PSPMT is shown in Fig. 10.7.

10.3.2 Avalanche Photodiode

An interesting trend is the development of semiconductor photodetectors to replace the bulky and significantly large volumetric shape of the PMT. One of the major drawbacks of PMTs is their sensitivity to magnetic fields. As the electrons are accelerated within the PMT by the effect of high potential applied between photocathode and dynodes and between successive dynodes, any source that influences this process would be an undesired component of noise leading to tube performance degradation. A magnetic field more than 10 mT is able to alter the gain and energy resolution of a PMT [46]. One of the earliest solutions was to use long cables of fiber optics. The better alternative was then to use semiconductor photodetectors. Efforts have been made to develop semiconductor detectors with better detection efficiency and intrinsic spatial resolution, providing a reliable and robust performance compared to PMTs or PSPMTs. Among these developments are the avalanche photodiodes (APDs), which can be produced in small dimensions, providing an improvement of spatial resolution in addition to reduced detector volume, and thereby fit space requirements imposed by multimodality imaging scanners. They are also well suited for pixilated

detectors and crystals of longer wavelengths, such as mentioned for CsI(Tl) crystals. They have higher gain than silicon photodiodes and better timing characteristics, on the order of 1 ns [47].

In comparison to the PMT, the APD is sensitive to temperature variations, can be operated in a lower voltage than a PMT, and is stable in the presence of high magnetic fields, like that encountered in MRI [48]. Thus, the APD was suitable in PET inserts incorporated into MRI machines, providing compact and simultaneous hybrid PET/MRI imaging systems. The semiconductor junction is operated at a high reverse bias, and the output signal is proportional to the initial number of light photons. They are characterized by low gain and relatively higher quantum efficiency.

The *position-sensitive APD (PSAPD)* is similar to the APD but with fewer readout requirements. The back surface is connected to a resistive layer that allows for multiple contacts to be fabricated. Position information can then be obtained by the charge sharing among electrodes that enables the determination of position of interaction [49]. Consequently, this structure allows for simple and compact detector assembly and enables use of significantly fewer readout channels, resulting in lower manufacturing costs. The alignment of the detector with the crystal array in this design is not as important as is the case in the individual APD array. This type of photodetector has an attractive interest in small-animal scanners, including depth of interaction encoding, to improve scanner spatial resolution and sensitivity [50–52]. This type also has applications in high-resolution small-animal imaging systems. For example, it has been coupled to a CsI(Tl) scintillator in a multipinhole small-animal SPECT system with significant improvement in detection efficiency and spatial resolution on the order of 1 mm [53].

10.3.3 Silicon Photomultiplier

The Geiger-mode APD or silicon photomultiplier (SiPM) is a densely packed matrix of small APDs (20×20–100×100 μm^2) joint together on common silicon substrate and work in limited Geiger discharge mode. Each cell is an independent Geiger mode detector, voltage biased, and discharges when it interacts

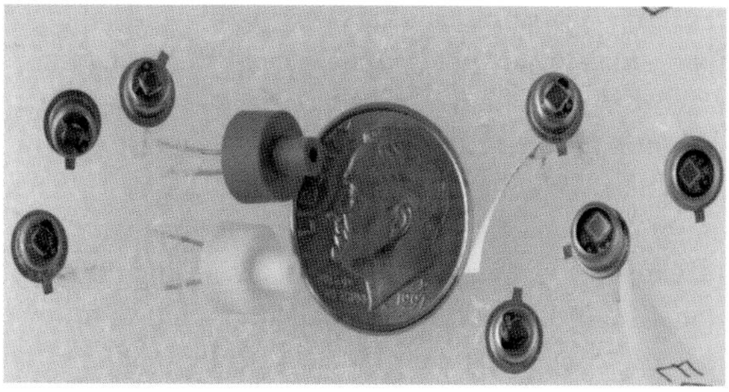

Fig. 10.8 Silicon photomultipliers (SiPMs) from different manufacturers. (From [101]). © IEEE with permission)

with an incident photon. The scintillation light causes a breakdown discharge for triggering a cell resulting in a fast single photoelectron pulse of very high gain $10^5–10^7$. SiPM produces a standard signal when any of the cells goes to breakdown. When many cells are fired at the same time, the output is the sum of the standard pulses [54]. Characteristics of SiPM are low noise factor, photon detection efficiency equivalent to the standard PMT, and low bias voltage. The higher gain feature provided by SiPM detector marginalizes the electronic noise in contrast to the standard APDs, which generally have a gain of 100–200. However, the dead space around each pixel and the finite probability of photons to produce avalanche breakdown reduce the detection efficiency of the SiPM, making it significantly lower than for the APD [55]. An SiPM is an interesting alternative to the conventional PMT in terms of compactness, same level of electronic gain, suitability for PET inserts in magnetic resonance systems and in detector design based on depth encoding information [56, 57]. Figure 10.8 shows SiPMs from different manufacturers.

10.4 Semiconductors

Instead of detecting the scintillation light on multiple stages, semiconductor detectors provide a detection means by which the incident radiation is converted to an electronic signal once it interacts with the detector material. The standard gamma camera, however, relies on converting the incident photon to a scintillation light, which is then amplified through a multistage

process in the vacuum of the PMT to yield an amplified signal that afterward is used in the calculation of event position and energy.

The use of semiconductor material in the field of radiation detection and measurements has been established for many years in different areas of science and engineering. The most commonly used are silicon (Si) and germanium (Ge). The atomic number of the former is 14, while for the latter it is 32; incorporating them in a radiation detector necessitates cooling to liquid nitrogen temperatures to avoid electronic noise generated from excessive thermal effects [58]. To fabricate a gamma camera based on a semiconductor detector, there has been efforts to search for other materials of high detection efficiency and amenable for operation in a room temperature environment.

Better alternatives of interest in the design of gamma ray detection systems are cadmium telluride (CdTe) and cadmium zinc telluride (CdZnTe), which can be considered promising materials for radiation detectors with good energy resolution, high detection efficiency, and room temperature operation. Several advantages can be obtained when designing a gamma camera based on semiconductor detectors. One is system portability as they enable construction of a compact structure free from the PMT and its bulky volume. A semiconductor camera also provides improved image contrast due to its better energy resolution compared to a sodium iodide crystal. Besides this last feature, high spatial resolution images can be obtained owing to the pixilated structure that can be implemented in the detector design [59].

More than one commercial SPECT system has been released to the market making use of semiconductor technology for improving imaging quality and diagnostic accuracy. D-SPECT (Spectrum Dynamics) is a CZT-based semiconductor camera commercialized for imaging cardiac patients. The system consists of nine collimated detector columns arranged in a curved configuration to conform to the shape of the left side of a patient's chest. Each individual detector, which consists of 1,024 (16 × 64) 5-mm thick CZT elements (2.46 × 2.46 mm), is allowed to translate and rotate independently so that a large number of viewing angles can be achieved for the region of interest [60]. The improved energy resolution (5.5% at 140 keV) also allows simultaneous application of a dual-isotope protocol with better identification of lesion defect and reduction of photon cross talk [61, 62]. Another design has been introduced by GE Healthcare (Discovery NM 530c) that utilizes an array of pixilated (CZT) semiconductor detectors in fixed positions (without motion) that allow acquisition of cardiac projections in a simultaneous manner. Preliminary evaluations of the system demonstrated an improvement in image spatial resolution, energy resolution, and sensitivity as opposed to a conventional gamma camera design [63]. An additional feature was brought about by combining this system with CT in an integrated SPECT/CT (Discovery NM 530c with the LightSpeed VCT or Discovery NM/CT 570c) system.

A semiconductor camera made of CZT is relatively expensive; thus, most of the current commercial versions are confined to handheld, miniaturized imaging systems or intraoperative small probes. Scintimammography is one of the diagnostic procedures that requires a dedicated device able to match the position and geometry of the breast. Small and deep lesions are a challenging task and require characteristics better than provided by a standard gamma camera. The sensitivity of the test is limited by the lesion size, particularly for those less than 10 mm [64].

The difficulty in detecting small and deep pathologic breast lesions by conventional imaging systems lies in their limited detection efficiency and relatively poor spatial resolution. However, earlier detection of a breast lesion has better diagnostic and prognostic implications. This in turn should be met by instruments with high performance characteristics that provide better lesion detectability. A breast imager based on semiconductor materials such as CZT can provide better spatial and energy resolution, leading to improved lesion contrast. This can be achieved using a narrow energy window, reducing the adverse effects of scattered photons on image quality. Another property of the semiconductor camera is its compactness, portability, and smaller dimensions, which fit well with breast imaging [65–67].

10.5 SPECT/CT

Nuclear imaging using SPECT or PET techniques have well-known capabilities in extracting functional and metabolic information for many human diseases. The anatomical details provided by CT and MRI enjoy better structural description for human organs by resolving capabilities that are significantly higher than that provided by nuclear SPECT and PET machines. They have the advantages of providing a resolution in the submillimeter range, precise statistical characteristics, and better tissue contrast, especially in the presence and use of contrast media [68]. However, it lacks the property of describing the functional status of a disease. This is important in following up cancer patients postsurgically and in the presence of fibrotic or necrotic lesions after chemo- or radiotherapy [69].

The early work of Hasegawa and colleagues opened a gate to many applications in the field of diagnostic radiology and nuclear medicine by coupling two imaging techniques into one operating device: The SPECT camera has been merged to x-ray computed tomography (CT) in the same device to provide an inherent anatomolecular imaging modality able to depict morphological as well as functional changes in one imaging session. While this process of image coregistration can be accomplished by fusing images obtained from two separate modalities, it has been demonstrated that inline SPECT or PET and CT image acquisition would be more advantageous.

The advantages provided by CT to functional imaging are not singular. It enables the reading physicians to precisely localize pathological lesions detected on functional images with great confidence. The other advantage is the improvement in performing attenuation correction. Again, although this can be performed by radionuclide transmission sources, the CT-based attenuation correction has been shown to outperform radionuclide-based transmission scanning by providing fast and significantly less-noisy attenuation maps.

Another benefit provided by CT is the capability of deriving dosimetric measurements from the fused images due to accurate outlining of the region of interest and thus better volumetric assessment. In the field of nuclear cardiology, SPECT/CT systems are of particular importance due to the continuous debate about attenuation correction [70, 71] and other degrading factors that reduce diagnostic quality and quantitative accuracy, such as partial volume effects [72]. Apart from attenuation correction, calculation of calcium scoring is also possible with the CT portion of the machine in addition to performing noninvasive coronary angiography.

In some instances, the addition of CT data to the functional images provides a guiding tool for image-based biopsy and thus can play a role in patient management; it also can be of synergistic effect in radiotherapy treatment planning, targeted treatment with brachytherapy, or intensity-modulated radiation therapy [73]. However, this has become more attractive with PET imaging than SPECT derived data.

The image of the year for 2006 was an SPECT/CT image showing both the coronary arteries and blood flow to the heart. This took place at the 53rd annual meeting of the Society of Nuclear Medicine in San Diego, California. The images clearly depicted the anatomical correlation of the blood flow defects to the corresponding artery. SPECT/CT devices also are of interest in preclinical and molecular imaging research with similar benefits as those provided to the clinical arena in addition to increased flexibility in performing longitudinal research studies.

On the research level, a tremendous improvement in the spatial resolution of micro-CT systems has enabled the investigators to look at minute structural changes that were not possible to see with conventional systems. Advances in micro-CT systems has revealed images of 10 μm and far better, permitting subcellular dimensions to be imaged [74].

10.5.1 Levels of Integration

Transmission scanning has been defined as "a useful adjunct to conventional emission scanning for accurately keying isotope deposition to radiographic anatomy" [75]. This article was published by Edward and coworkers in the mid-1960s when they realized the importance of combining functional data with their anatomical templates, although they used a simple approach to obtain the transmission scanning. Investigators assigned this as the first demonstration of the feasibility of hybrid imaging [76]. They used an Am-241 source located at the center hole of a collimated detector; the other detector was adjusted to acquire the emission and transmission data. This early functional/anatomical study is a clear sign of the early recognition of combining the two types of images to strengthen each other and to overcome their inherent weaknesses. However, despite this interesting beginning, it was not pursued, and both imaging modalities were almost developed independently until the early 1990s. Before this time, there was some interest

and research efforts to use radioactive transmission sources for attenuation correction [77, 78]. The approaches and different levels of integrating structural imaging with the functional data were as follows:

1. The *primitive level* of integrating functional and structural images is evidenced by the human brain. This is the traditional way that diagnosticians used to correlate two images acquired from separate imaging modalities. However, human spatial perception and differences in image textures acquired from two different modalities represent a challenge for the reading physicians to mentally correlate the two data sets. This can be more problematic in small-size lesions and in identifying the spatial extent and spread of a disease.

2. The second level of image coregistration was brought to the clinic by software algorithms. They are relatively simple to apply to rigid structures such as the brain, where images acquired by CT or MRI can be merged to functional images acquired and processed on a separate SPECT or PET machine. This successful implementation is due to brain rigidity, and variations in the position of internal structures are less likely to occur compared to lung or abdominal image fusion. In a review [79], localization of brain structures was less challenging compared to whole-body applications, and image fusion may be required for only a subgroup of patients. Moreover, in a wide comparison of various available software tools for retrospective registration of PET/MRI and PET/CT, an accuracy of 2–3 mm was consistently achieved, which was below the voxel dimension of PET [80] and SPECT as well.

3. Use of intrinsic landmarks or extrinsic markers to accurately fuse the two data sets has been implemented with some impractical drawbacks placed on its feasibility in the clinical routine, added technical complexity to the diagnostic procedures, or inaccurate image correlation. This could arise from variations that may exist between imaging sessions, fixation strategy, or perhaps inability to correlate internal organs with external markers [69]. Furthermore, automatic registration for internal landmarks could also be affected by the limited spatial resolution of nuclear images with precise selection of anatomical landmarks; therefore, accurate alignment is not guaranteed. These apparent shortcomings of

image coregistration, particularly in nonrigid body structures, have motivated the development of nonlinear 3D image fusion algorithms able to improve the accuracy of alignment.

4. Ideally, one would like to acquire the structural as well as the functional data in a simultaneous manner in the same spatial and temporal domain. This can be achieved when the detector systems can be incorporated into each other, achieving concurrent image acquisition. This multimodality design has been realized in hybrid PET/MRI systems with substantial modification to the PET detector system using APDs instead of the conventional PMTs, as mentioned in this chapter (see [81]).

5. The other alternative is to modify the detector technology so that a single detector system can record the two signals with adequate distinction for each individual electronic pulse. However, x-ray detector systems are energy integrators and do not allow individual events to be discriminated according to their energies. This is in great part due to the high fluence of the x-ray source compared to nuclear photon emission and owing to beam polychromaticity [82]. In other words, the significant differences in photon rates pose challenges to implement multimodality imaging using a "conventional" detector for both x-ray and radionuclide processes; this requires a detector that can switch between pulse-mode SPECT/PET acquisition and charge integration mode [83]. Nevertheless, it has been proposed to simultaneously acquire trimodality images, namely SPECT/PET/CT, with great complexities placed on detector design [84]. Moreover, an emerging technology is evolving to record both types of data in a single counting and energy integrator modes.

6. The other strategy is to place the two detector systems side by side such that images can be acquired in a sequential manner. This is the way all clinical SPECT/CT as well PET/CT scanners are presently manufactured and operated. Therefore, one can simply deduce that the higher the level of integration, the more demands placed on the technologic complexity. The range of multimodality imaging has been extended to include functional only, structural only, or a combination of functional and structural imaging modalities to yield a variety of integrated or hybrid diagnostic options [85] SPECT/CT is among the best

dual-modality approaches that drew the attention of many researchers in the field, and its technical value has been proven in a significant number of clinical conditions, leading to a change in patient management. Although other multimodality imaging approaches have been or are being developed, they are aimed most of the time toward preclinical imaging, and their clinical counterparts are yet to be determined.

10.5.2 Early and Recent SPECT/CT Systems

As mentioned, the work of SPECT/CT was launched and pioneered by Hasegawa and colleagues at the University of California, San Francisco, by designing the first prototype imaging system able to acquire both single-photon emitters and x-ray transmission scanning in one imaging session. The detector material was a high-purity germanium (HPGe) designed for simultaneous acquisition of functional and anatomical information. The system was a small-bore SPECT/CT system with some technical limitations for direct application in the clinical setting. The same group then developed a clinical prototype SPECT/CT system using a GE 9800 CT scanner and GE X/RT as the SPECT component mounted in tandem with data acquired sequentially using the same imaging table.

The industry recognized the potential of combining the two imaging techniques, and the first commercial SPECT/CT system was released by GE Healthcare. The transmission component of the scanner was a one-slice CT scanner providing a slice thickness of 10 mm. The transmission x-ray source was mounted on a slip-ring gantry of the Millennium VG gamma camera (GE Healthcare). The x-ray detector system was similar to third-generation CT scanners and was designed to move along with the gamma camera detector system. The time required for one-slice acquisition was about 14 s, and contiguous slices were taken by moving the patient in the axial direction [86].

Coincidence detection was also available since the crystal thickness was thicker than used in regular SPECT systems (16.5 mm). The voltage of the x-ray tube was 140 kVp, and tube current was 2.5 mA, leading to a significant reduction of the x-ray absorbed dose when compared to standard diagnostic CT machines. With these characteristics, the system was not able to reveal useful diagnostic information but satisfied the requirements of attenuation correction. The CT subsystem could cover the heart in 13–17 slices in a period of 5 min.

The same manufacturer released another SPECT/CT version (GE Infinia Hawkeye-4) that provided a four-slice low-dose CT with fewer demands on room space requirements. The slice thickness of this system was fixed to 5 mm. The system was able to provide adequate attenuation correction and lesion localization with emphasis placed on limited spatial resolution when compared to fully diagnostic CT machines. Furthermore, the volumetric dose index in the acquisition of a head protocol was found to be 8 mGy, in comparison to 42 mGy as measured by DST, which is a 16-slice diagnostic CT used in PET/CT scanners [87]. Other vendors have SPECT/CT systems that are able to provide diagnosticians high-quality and fully diagnostic CT information; thereby, the utility of the CT portion of the hybrid SPECT/CT scanner is no longer concerned with attenuation correction and lesion localization, but its clinical benefits have been extended to other areas of cardiac imaging, such as calculation of calcium scoring and coronary CT angiography. Different SPECT/CT models are shown in Fig. 10.9.

The tube voltage and current are important parameters that determine image quality and levels of the absorbed dose. Vendors vary in their CT specification, such that the tube voltage can be 90–140, 110–130, 120, or 120–140 kVp. Also, the tube current could be as low as 1–2.5 mA or higher, such as 5–80, 20–354, or 20–500 mA. The number of slices has also been increased to 6, 16, 64, or even more, as can be found in the Philips BrightView XCT using a flat-panel CT in which the number of slices is 140 and slice thickness is 1 mm. However, the slice thickness can be lower than 1 mm, in some SPECT/CT scanners reaching a value of 0.6 mm. An important feature of the currently available commercial designs is the high-speed acquisitions using spiral CT generation by which the rotation time can be even less than 0.5 s. This allows for scanning the heart region in one full rotation, minimizing problems of temporal coverage associated with older CT models. Also, it can help reduce the likelihood of patient motion and enhance patient throughput.

One of the disadvantages provided by fully diagnostic CT acquisition is the increased absorbed dose to the subject under examination. As discussed by Kauffman and Di Carli [88], cardiac imaging using hybrid functional and anatomical SPECT/CT is challenged by the high radiation dose to the patients. However, recent approaches to minimize high levels of absorbed doses have been implemented, such as low-dose CT angiography and a reduced amount of injected activity into the patient.

10.5.3 Temporal Mismatch

Another problem also of concern is the differences that arise from temporal data sampling. The CT scan is

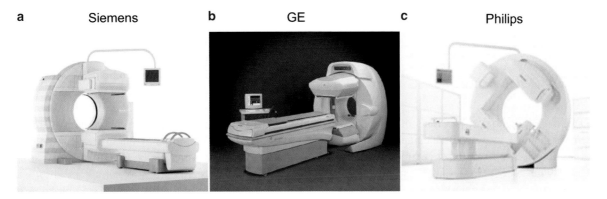

Fig. 10.9 (**a**) The Siemens Symbia single-photon emission computed tomography/computed tomography (SPECT/CT) scanner. (**b**) Millennium VG Hawkeye SPECT/CT scanner. (**c**) BrightView XCT, which integrates the SPECT system with flat detector x-ray CT

acquired in a relatively short duration compared to emission acquisition. This actually is a problem especially in the thoracic region as the lung and heart are moving organs and not fixed in one spatial position. The emission images are a temporal average of the organ motion over the respiratory or cardiac cycles. This phenomenon has its undesired consequences in corrupting the attenuation correction and leading to misregistration errors and false interpretation results.

One of the potential applications of SPECT/CT systems is their utility in cardiac imaging, for which better attenuation correction can be performed. However, due to the mentioned limitation, there are recommendations to check the acquired emission/transmission data for possible artifacts [89]. This issue of data misalignment between CT and radionuclide emission scanning has also been found in cardiac PET studies as well as in lung FDG examinations.

Kennedy et al. [90] have recently shown that 23% of the patient studied using cardiac SPECT/CT had a misregistration errors of significant effects and 16% were in the direction of the most severe artifacts [91]. A comparable percentage was also found in Rb-82 cardiac PET/CT scanning with magnitudes of 24.6% and 29.0% in adenosine stress and rest studies, respectively [92]. Misregistration errors resulted in false-positive results in 40% of patients undergoing dipyridamole stress and rest Rb-82 cardiac PET/CT [93]. Another study demonstrated 42% errors in cardiac SPECT/CT images, concluding that careful inspection of attenuation correction maps and registration are needed to avoid reconstruction artifacts due to misregistration [94]. Nonetheless, manual intervention as well as quality control software programs are possible ways to realign the images and improve the correction and imaging task [95].

10.5.4 Other Artifacts

One of the potential applications of SPECT/CT systems is their use in skeletal scintigraphy. Gnanasegaran et al. [96] discussed the most common artifacts associated with bone SPECT/CT. These are SPECT/CT misregistration, respiratory artifacts due to lung motion, arms up or down, metal or contrast agent artifacts, patient size and noise, together with limitations arising from CT scanners. Factors that affect

SPECT image quality could be potentially a candidate to cause undesired errors in the coregistered images. The center of rotation and alignment of the two imaging modalities is a pertinent factor in the accuracy and reliability of attenuation correction and image alignment. The existence of a patient's arms in the field of view could also introduce attenuation or truncation artifacts. Metals and high-density materials have the capability of altering the attenuation coefficients and serve to enhance beam hardening effects.

10.5.5 SPECT/CT Applications

The utility of SPECT/CT systems is expanding in many areas of research and clinical practice. In addition to attenuation correction, other image degrading factors can also be accounted for from the use of the CT images. A model-based approach to derive Compton probabilities or transmission-based scatter correction can be applied using CT images to correct for scattered photons, as shown by Willowson et al. [94]. In the same report, the effect of partial volume also was accounted for using the CT data, and all corrections revealed an accurate tracer estimate of 1% with a precision of $\pm7\%$. In brain studies, correction for partial volume is critical, and reliable and quantitative outcome cannot be obtained without considerations placed on the phenomenon. The binding potential of the striatum can be underestimated by 50% in the absence of partial volume correction. However, in the presence of anatomically guided partial volume correction, substantial improvement can be obtained [97, 98]. In a porcine model, Da Silva et al. [73] showed that an attenuation correction alone for myocardial perfusion Tc-99m-labeled sestamibi cannot yield higher quantitative accuracy without proper correction for partial volume. The combined corrections, however, resulted in higher absolute activity concentrations within a range of 10%. CT data provided an accurate template for modeling the subject anatomy and for accurate definition of the myocardial boundaries (further discussion can be found in Chap. 15).

SPECT/CT systems are also helpful in absorbed dose estimation since the CT images are able to provide a highly accurate assessment of tumor volume. This is an important step in dose calculation schemes required in radioimmunotherapy and other dose estimation disciplines. As SPECT data can provide important functional information about drug distribution, residence time, and patient follow-up, the additive value of CT can enhance the quantitative accuracy of the measurements for subsequent accurate dose estimates. In the case of pure beta emitters and attempts to image radiotracer distribution based on bremsstrahlung radiation, x-ray CT provides a good anatomical template to delineate and distinguish various tissue uptakes [99].

10.6 Conclusions

The gamma camera is a device with multicompartments. Each of these elements plays a role in the photon detection task and determination of tracer biodistribution. Digital technology and multihead systems were key factors that enhanced and motivated the performance of the gamma camera. Implementations of new camera design with different geometry, fast acquisition protocols, and reconstruction algorithms provide relatively new features for the current and future generations of the gamma camera. Semiconductor systems with room temperature materials and good performance characteristics are of interest among some manufacturers and medical users. Use of new photodetectors would help to enhance the diagnostic quality of nuclear medicine images. They also provide compactness, portability, and better imaging features. The addition of CT as a structural imaging modality to SPECT systems has found numerous applications in many areas of clinical practice as well as in the research setting.

References

1. Patton DD (2003) The birth of nuclear medicine instrumentation: Blumgart and Yens, 1925. J Nucl Med 44(8):1362–1365
2. Graham LS, Kereiakes JG, Harris C, Cohen MB (1989) Nuclear medicine from Becquerel to the present. Radiographics 9(6):1189–1202
3. Anger H (1985) Scintillation camera. Rev Sci Instrum 29:27–33
4. Chandra R (1998) Nuclear medicine physics: the basics, 5th edn. Williams &Wilkins, London
5. Vesel J, Petrillo M (2005) Improved gamma camera performance using event positioning method based on distance dependent weighting. IEEE Nucl Sci Symp Conf Rec 5:2445–2448
6. Kulberg GH, Muehllehner G, van Dijk N (1972) Improved resolution of the Anger scintillation camera through the use of threshold preamplifiers. J Nucl Med 13 (2):169–171
7. Ricard M (2004) Imaging of gamma emitters using scintillation cameras. Nucl Instrum Meth Phys Res A 527(1–2): 124–129, In: Proceedings of the 2nd international conference on imaging technologies in biomedical sciences
8. Joung J, Miyaoka RS, Kohlmyer S, Lewellen TK (2000) Implementation of ML based positioning algorithms for scintillation cameras. IEEE Trans Nucl Sci 47(3):1104–1111
9. Cherry SR, Sorenson JA, Phelps ME (2003) Physics in nuclear medicine. Saunders, Philadelphia
10. Moore SC, Kouris K, Cullum I (1992) Collimator design for single photon emission tomography. Eur J Nucl Med 19(2):138–150
11. Lau YH, Hutton BF, Beekman FJ (2001) Choice of collimator for cardiac SPET when resolution compensation is included in iterative reconstruction. Eur J Nucl Med 28 (1):39–47
12. Murphy PH (1987) Acceptance testing and quality control of gamma cameras, including SPECT. J Nucl Med 28 (7):1221–1227
13. Inoue Y, Shirouzu I, Machida T, Yoshizawa Y, Akita F, Doi I, Watadani T, Noda M, Yoshikawa K, Ohtomo K (2003) Physical characteristics of low and medium energy collimators for 123I imaging and simultaneous dual-isotope imaging. Nucl Med Commun 24(11):1195–1202
14. Accorsi R (2008) Brain single-photon emission CT physics principles. Am J Neuroradiol 29(7):1247–1256
15. Peremans K, Cornelissen B, Van Den Bossche B, Audenaert K, Van de Wiele C (2005) A review of small animal imaging planar and pinhole SPECT gamma camera imaging. Vet Radiol Ultrasound 46(2):162–170
16. Wong TZ, Turkington TG, Polascik TJ, Coleman RE (2005) ProstaScint (capromab pendetide) imaging using hybrid gamma camera-CT technology. AJR Am J Roentgenol 184:676–680
17. Kupinski MA, Barrett HH (2005) Small-animal SPECT imaging. Spinger Science + Business Media, New York
18. Giokaris N, Loudos G, Maintas D, Karabarbounis A, Lembesi M, Spanoudaki V, Stiliaris E, Boukis S et al (2005) Partially slotted crystals for a high-resolution g-camera based on a position sensitive photomultiplier. Nucl Instrum Meth Phys Res A 550:305–312
19. Giokaris N, Loudo G, Maintas D, Karabarbounis A, Lembesi M et al (2006) Comparison of CsI(Tl) and CsI(Na) partially slotted crystals for high-resolution SPECT imaging. Nucl Instrum Meth Phys Res A 569:185–187
20. Knoll GF (2000) Radiation detection and measurements, 3rd edn. Wiley, New York
21. Patt BE, Iwanczyk JS, Rossington TC, Wang NW, Tornai MP, Hoffman EJ (1998) High resolution CsI(Tl)/Si-PIN detector development for breast imaging. IEEE Trans Nucl Sci 45(4):2126–2131
22. Garcia EV, Faber TL (2009) Advances in nuclear cardiology instrumentation: clinical potential of SPECT and PET. Curr Cardiovasc Imag Rep 2(3):230–237

23. Walrand S, Jamar F, de Jong M, Pauwels S (2005) Evaluation of novel whole-body high-resolution rodent SPECT (Linoview) based on direct acquisition of linogram projections. J Nucl Med 46:1872–1880

24. Del Guerra A, Di Domenico G, Scandola M, Zavattini G (1998) YAP-PET: first results of a small animal positron emission tomograph based on YAP:Ce finger crystals. IEEE Trans Nucl Sci 45:3105–3108

25. Pani R, Bennati P, Betti M, Cinti MN, Pellegrini R (2006) Lanthanum scintillation crystals for gamma ray imaging. Nucl Instr Meth A 567:294–297

26. Bennati P, Betti M, Cencelli O, Cinti MN, Cusanno F, DeNotaristefani F, Garibaldi F, Karimian A, Mattiolo M et al (2004) Imaging performances of LaCl3:Ce scintillation crystals in SPECT. IEEE Nucl Sci Symp Conf Rec 4: 2283–2287

27. Pani R, Pellegrini R, Cinti MN, Bennati P, Betti M, Vittorini F (2007) LaBr3(Ce) crystal: the latest advance for scintillation cameras. Nucl Instrum Meth A 572 (1):268–269

28. Groch MW, Erwin WD (2001) Single-photon emission computed tomography in the year instrumentation and quality control. J Nucl Med Technol 29:12–18

29. Madsen M (2007) Recent advances in SPECT imaging. J Nucl Med 48(4):661–673

30. Sayeram S, Tsui BMW, De Zhao X, Frey EC (2003) Performance evaluation of three different SPECT systems used in In-111 ProstaScint® SPECT imaging. IEEE Nucl Sci Symp Conf Rec 5:3129–3133

31. Harbert JC, Eckelman WC, Neumann RD (1996) Nuclear medicine: diagnosis and therapy. Thieme Medical, New York

32. http://sales.hamamatsu.com/assets/pdf/catsandguides/PMT_handbook_v3aE.pdf. Accessed 20 Jan 2010

33. Boyd C, Dalrymple G (1974) Basic science principles of nuclear medicine. Mosby, London

34. Buvat I, De Sousa MC, Di Paola M, Ricard M, Lumbroso J, Aubert B (1988) Impact of scatter correction in planar scintimammography: a phantom study. J Nucl Med 39 (9):1590–1596

35. Graham LS, LaFontaine RL, Stein MA (1986) Effects of asymmetric photopeak windows on flood field uniformity and spatial resolution of scintillation cameras. J Nucl Med 27:706–713

36. Collier BD, Palmer DW, Knobel J, Isitman AT, Hellman RS, Zielonka JS (1984) Gamma camera energy windows for Tc-99m bone scintigraphy: effect of asymmetry on contrast resolution. Radiology 151(2):495–497

37. Pani R (2004) Recent advances and future perspectives of position sensitive PMT. Nucl Instrum Meth Phys Res B 213:197–205

38. Kume H, Suzuki S, Takeuchi J, Oba K (1985) Newly developed photomultiplier tubes with position sensitivity capability. IEEE Trans Nucl Sci NS-32(1):448

39. Pichler BJ, Ziegler SI (2004) Photodetectors. In: Wernick M, Aarsvold J (eds) Emission tomography: the fundamentals of PET and SPECT. Elsevier Academic Press, San Diego

40. Del Guerra A, Belcari N, Bisogni MG, Llosá G, Marcatili S, Moehrs S (2009) Advances in position-sensitive photo-detectors for PET applications. Nucl Instrum Meth Phys Res A 604(1–2):319–322

41. Dornebos P, van Eijk CW (1995) In: Proceedings of the international conference on inorganic scintillators and their applications. Delft University of Technology, Delft, The Netherlands, 28 August–1 September 1995

42. Loudos GK, Nikita KS, Uzunoglu NK, Giokaris ND, Papanicolas CN, Archimandritis SC et al (2003) In: SCINT95, Proceedings of the international conference on inorganic scintillators and their applications. Improving spatial resolution in SPECT with the combination of PSPMT based detector and iterative reconstruction algorithms. Comput Med Imaging Graph 27(4):307–313

43. Del Guerra A, Di Domenico G, Scandola M, Zavattini G (1998) High spatial resolution small animal YAPPET. Nucl Instrum Meth Phys Res A 409:537–541

44. Pani R, Pellegrini R, Cinti MN, Trotta C, Trotta G, Scafe R, Betti M et al (2003) A novel compact gamma camera based on flat panel PMT. Nucl Instrum Meth Phys Res A 513:36–41

45. Renker D (2007) New trends on photodetectors. Nucl Instrum Meth Phys Res A 571:1–6

46. Lecomte R (2009) Novel detector technology for clinical PET. Eur J Nucl Med Mol Imaging 36(Suppl 1):S69–S85

47. Lewellen TK (2008) Recent developments in PET detector technology. Phys Med Biol 53(17):R287–R317

48. Pichler B, Lorenz E, Mirzoyan R, Pimpl W, Roder F, Schwaiger M, Ziegler SI (1997) Performance test of a LSO-APD PET module in a 9.4 tesla magnet. IEEE Nucl Sci Symp 2:1237–1239

49. Shah KS, Farrell R, Grazioso R, Harmon ES, Karplus E (2002) Position-sensitive avalanche photodiodes for gamma-ray imaging. Nucl Sci IEEE Trans Nucl Sci 49 (4):1687–1692

50. Yang Y, Wu Y, Qi J, St. James S, Huini Du A, Dokhale P, Shah K et al (2008) A prototype PET scanner with DOI-encoding detectors. J Nucl Med 49:1132–1140

51. Burr KC, Ivam A, Castleberry DE, LeBlanc JW, Shah KS, Farrell R (2004) Evaluation of a prototype small-animal PET detector with depth-of-interaction encoding. IEEE Trans Nucl Sci 51:1791–1798

52. Yang Y, Dokhale PA, Silverman RW, Shah KS, McClish MA, Farrell R, Entine G, Cherry SR (2006) Depth of interaction resolution measurements for a high resolution PET detector using position sensitive avalanche photodiodes. Phys Med Biol 51:2131–2142

53. Funk T, Després P, Barber WC, Shah KS, Hasegawa BH (2006) Multipinhole small animal SPECT system with submillimeter spatial resolution. Med Phys 33(5):1259–1268

54. Renker D (2006) Geiger-mode avalanche photodiodes, history, properties and problems. Nucl Instrum Meth Phys Res A 567:48–56

55. Otte N, Dolgoshein B, Hose J, Klemin S, Lorenz E, Mirzoyan R et al (2006) The SiPM – a new photon detector for PET, nuclear physics B. In: Proceedings of the 9th topical seminar on innovative particle and radiation detectors, vol 150, pp 417–420

56. Schaart DR, van Dam HT, Seifert S, Vinke R, Dendooven P, Löhner H, Beekman FJ (2009) A novel, SiPM-array-

based, monolithic scintillator detector for PET. Phys Med Biol 54:3501

57. Maas MC, Schaart DR, van der Laan DJ, Bruyndonckx P, Lemaître C, Beekman FJ, van Eijk CW (2009) Monolithic scintillator PET detectors with intrinsic depth-of-interaction correction. Phys Med Biol 54(7):1893–1908

58. Wagennar DJ (2004) CdTe and CdZnTe semiconductor detectors for nuclear medicine imaging. In: Wernick MN, Aarsvold JN (eds) Emission tomography. The fundamentals of PET and SPECT. Elsevier, San Diego

59. Mori I, Takayama T, Motomura N (2001) The CdTe detector module and its imaging performance. Ann Nucl Med 15(6):487–494

60. Gambhir SS, Berman DS, Ziffer J, Nagler M, Sandler M, Patton J, Hutton B, Sharir T, Haim SB, Haim SB (2009) A novel high-sensitivity rapid-acquisition single-photon cardiac imaging camera. J Nucl Med 50(4):635–643

61. Berman DS, Kang X, Tamarappoo B, Wolak A, Hayes SW, Nakazato R, Thomson LE, Kite F, Cohen I, Slomka PJ, Einstein AJ, Friedman JD (2009) Stress thallium-201/rest technetium-99m sequential dual isotope high-speed myocardial perfusion imaging. JACC Cardiovasc Imaging 2(3):273–282

62. Erlandsson K, Kacperski K, van Gramberg D, Hutton BF (2009) Performance evaluation of D-SPECT: a novel SPECT system for nuclear cardiology. Phys Med Biol 54:2635–2649

63. Keidar Z, Kagna O, Frenkel A, Israel O (2009) A novel ultrafast cardiac scanner for myocardial perfusion imaging (MPI): comparison with a standard dual-head camera. J Nucl Med 50(Suppl 2):478

64. Taillefer R (2005) Clinical applications of 99mTc-sestamibi scintimammography. Semin Nucl Med 35:100–115

65. Mueller B, O'Connor MK, Blevis I, Rhodes DJ, Smith R, Collins DA, Phillips SW (2003) Evaluation of a small cadmium zinc telluride detector for scintimammography. J Nucl Med 44(4):602–609

66. Pani R, Pellegrini R, Cinti MN, Bennati P, Betti M, Casali V et al (2006) Recent advances and future perspectives of gamma imagers for scintimammography. Nucl Instrum Meth A 569:296–300

67. Blevis Ira M, O'Conner MK, Keidar Z, Pansky A et al (2006) CZT for scintimammography. Phys Med 21(Suppl 1):56–59

68. Stout DB, Zaidi H (2008) Preclinical multimodality imaging in vivo. PET Clin 3(3):251–273

69. Keidar Z, Israel O, Krausz Y (2003) SPECT/CT in tumor imaging: technical aspects and clinical applications. Semin Nucl Med 33(3):205–218

70. Garcia EV (2007) SPECT attenuation correction: an essential tool to realize nuclear cardiology's manifest destiny. J Nucl Cardiol 14:16–24

71. Germano G, Slomka PJ, Berman DS (2007) Attenuation correction in cardiac SPECT: the boy who cried wolf? J Nucl Cardiol 14:25–35

72. Da Silva AJ, Tang HR, Wong KH, Wu MC, Dae MW, Hasegawa BH (2001) Absolute quantification of regional myocardial uptake of 99mTc-sestamibi with SPECT: experimental validation in a porcine model. J Nucl Med 42(5):772–779

73. Ellis RJ, Kim EY, Conant R et al (2001) Radioimmuno-guided imaging of prostate cancer foci with histopathological correlation. Int J Radiat Oncol Biol Phys 49:1281–1286

74. Ritman EL (2007) Small-animal CT – its difference from, and impact on, clinical CT. Nucl Instrum Meth Phys Res A 580(2):968–970

75. Kuhl DE, Hale J, Eaton WL (1966) Transmission scanning: a useful adjunct to conventional emission scanning for accurately keying isotope deposition to radiographic anatomy. Radiology 87(2):278–284

76. Patton JA, Townsend DW, Hutton BF (2009) Hybrid imaging technology: from dreams and vision to clinical devices. Semin Nucl Med 39(4):247–263

77. Bailey DL, Hutton BF, Walker PJ (1987) Improved SPECT using emission and transmission tomography. J Nucl Med 28:844–851

78. Tsui BM, Gullberg GT, Edgerton ER et al (1989) Correction of nonuniform attenuation in cardiac SPECT imaging. J Nucl Med 30:497–507

79. Slomka PJ, Baum RP (2009) Multimodality image registration with software: state-of-the-art. Eur J Nucl Med Mol Imaging 36(Suppl 1):S44–S55

80. West J, Fitzpatrick JM, Wang MY, Dawant BM, Maurer CR, Kessler RM et al (1997) Comparison and evaluation of retrospective intermodality brain image registration techniques. J Comput Assist Tomogr 21(4):554–566

81. Beyer T, Pichler B (2009) A decade of combined imaging: from a PET attached to a CT to a PET inside an MR. Eur J Nucl Med Mol Imaging 36:S1–S144

82. Seibert JA, Boone JM (2005) X-ray imaging physics for nuclear medicine technologists. Part 2: X-ray interactions and image formation. J Nucl Med Technol 33(1):3–18

83. Darambara DG (2006) State-of-the-art radiation detectors for medical imaging: demands and trends. Nucl Instrum Meth Phys Res A 569(2):153–158

84. Saoudi A, Lecomte R (1999) A novel APD-based detector module for multi-modality PET/SPECT/CT scanners. IEEE Trans Nucl Sci 46(3):479–484

85. Cherry SR (2009) Multimodality imaging: beyond PET/CT and SPECT/CT. Semin Nucl Med 39(5):348–353

86. Bocher M, Balan A, Krausz Y, Shrem Y, Lonn A, Wilk M, Chisin R (2000) Gamma camera-mounted anatomical X-ray tomography: technology, system characteristics and first images. Eur J Nucl Med 27(6):619–627

87. Hamann M, Aldridge M, Dickson J, Endozo R, Lozhkin K, Hutton BF (2008) Evaluation of a low-dose/slow-rotating SPECT-CT system. Phys Med Biol 53:2495–2508

88. Kaufmann PA, Di Carli MF (2009) Hybrid SPECT/CT and PET/CT imaging: the next step in noninvasive cardiac imaging. Semin Nucl Med 39(5):341–347

89. Goetze S, Wahl RL (2007) Prevalence of misregistration between SPECT and CT for attenuation-corrected myocardial perfusion SPECT. J Nucl Cardiol 14(2):200–206

90. Kennedy JA, Israel O, Frenkel A (2009) Directions and magnitudes of misregistration of CT attenuation-corrected myocardial perfusion studies: incidence, impact on image quality, and guidance for reregistration. Nucl Med 50 (9):1471–1478

91. Kennedy JA, Israel O, Frenkel A (2009) Directions and magnitudes of misregistration of CT attenuation-corrected

myocardial perfusion studies: incidence, impact on image quality, and guidance for reregistration. J Nucl Med 50 (9):1471–1478

92. Schuster DM, Halkar RK, Esteves FP, Garcia EV, Cooke CD, Syed MA, Bowman FD, Votaw JR (2008) Investigation of emission-transmission misalignment artifacts on rubidium-82 cardiac PET with adenosine pharmacologic stress. Mol Imaging Biol 10(4):201–208

93. Gould KL, Pan T, Loghin C, Johnson NP, Guha A, Sdringola S (2007) Frequent diagnostic errors in cardiac PET/CT due to misregistration of CT attenuation and emission PET images: a definitive analysis of causes, consequences, and corrections. J Nucl Med 48:1112–1121

94. Willowson K, Bailey DL, Baldock C (2008) Quantitative SPECT reconstruction using CT-derived corrections. Phys Med Biol 53(12):3099–3112

95. Chen J, Caputlu-Wilson SF, Shi H, Galt JR, Faber TL, Garcia EV (2006) Automated quality control of emission-transmission misalignment for attenuation correction in myocardial perfusion imaging with SPECT-CT systems. J Nucl Cardiol 13(1):43–49

96. Gnanasegaran G, Barwick T, Adamson K, Mohan H, Sharp D, Fogelman I (2009) SPECT/CT in benign and malignant bone disease: when the ordinary turns into the extraordinary. Semin Nucl Med 39(6):431–442

97. Soret M, Koulibaly PM, Darcourt J, Hapdey S, Buvat I (2003) Quantitative accuracy of dopaminergic neurotransmission imaging with 123I SPECT. J Nucl Med 44(7):1184–1193

98. Vanzi E, De Cristofaro MT, Ramat S, Sotgia B, Mascalchi M, Formiconi AR (2007) A direct ROI quantification method for inherent PVE correction: accuracy assessment in striatal SPECT measurements. Eur J Nucl Med Mol Imaging 34(9):1480–1489

99. D'Asseler Y (2009) Advances in SPECT imaging with respect to radionuclide therapy. Q J Nucl Med Mol Imaging 53:343–347

100. Riboldi S, Seidel J, Green M, Monaldo J, Kakareka J, Pohida T (2003) Investigation of signal readout methods for the Hamamatsu R8500 flat panel PSPMT. *Nuclear Science Symposium Conference Record, 2003 IEEE* 4:2452–2456

101. Xie Q, Chien-Min Kao, Byrum K, Drake G, Vaniachine A, Wagner RG, Rykalin V, Chin-Tu Chen (2006) Characterization of Silicon Photomultipliers for PET Imaging. *Nuclear Science Symposium Conference Record, 2006. IEEE* 2:1199–1203

Positron Emission Tomography (PET): Basic Principles

11

Magdy M. Khalil

Contents

11.1 Introduction

Single-photon emission computed tomography (SPECT) and positron emission tomography (PET) are three-dimensional (3D) techniques provided by nuclear imaging to functionally map radiotracer uptake distributed in the human body. SPECT systems have been described previously; PET imaging is the main topic of the present chapter. The radiopharmaceuticals of PET provide more insights into the metabolic and molecular processes of the disease. This in turn has made PET a molecular imaging technique that examines biochemical processes that take place at the molecular level [1].

PET has become a potential "multipurpose" imaging technique in biomedical, clinical, and research arenas. Clinical indications for PET are numerous and include many diseases for which tumor imaging occupies the most important and abundant patients. Thus, it has a well-defined and established role in oncology and diagnosing many types of cancer in patients besides staging and assessment of response to therapy. Another important role of PET lies in its ability to diagnose some neurologic and psychiatric disorders in addition to noninvasive quantitation of cerebral blood flow, metabolism, and receptor binding [2]. Further, PET has a significant role in evaluating patients with coronary artery disease and detection of tissue viability, together with its ability to provide an absolute measure of myocardial blood flow. PET by nature is "molecular" since its radioligands are acceptable and familiar to living tissues; therefore, it is considered an indispensible tool in molecular imaging research. It has several quantitative features as it can determine with acceptable accuracy the amount of tracer transported to or deposited in tissues. In comparison to other imaging modalities, PET has

M.M. Khalil
Biological Imaging Centre, MRC/CSC, Imperial College London, Hammersmith Campus, Du Cane Road, W12 0NN, London, UK
e-mail: magdy.khalil@imperial.ac.uk or magdy_khalil@hotmail.com

M.M. Khalil (ed.), *Basic Sciences of Nuclear Medicine*, DOI: 10.1007/978-3-540-85962-8_11,
© Springer-Verlag Berlin Heidelberg 2011

significantly higher detection sensitivity such that tracers with low concentrations, in the nano or pico range, can be detected.

PET imaging has moved from a useful research tool mainly in neurology (and cardiology) to more specific tasks in oncology and has become a potential clinical diagnostic modality. The instrumental aspects were a cornerstone in the development of PET imaging and its introduction into the clinic. Furthermore, advances in PET technology are moving forward and are not only confined to clinical whole-body scanners but also are expanding to include organ-dedicated instruments such as positron emission mammography and dedicated brain and prostate scanners in addition to small-animal imaging systems [3]. Now, more attention is paid to the hybrid PET/CT (computed tomographic) systems, by which the functional information obtained by PET imaging and morphologic data obtained from diagnostic CT are merged into a fused image to reveal a more accurate and confident anatomolecular diagnosis [4]. This instrumental marriage has resulted in a significant improvement of patient diagnosis, disease staging, and therapy monitoring. Moreover, it has had a positive impact on patient comfort, throughput, and more importantly clinical outcome that has been proven to outperform both techniques used separately [5].

In the next few years, PET/MRI (magnetic resonance imaging) will prove its clinical usefulness, and efforts will determine whether it will complement, replace, or combine PET/CT devices in the routine practice of patient diagnosis [6]. The technologic advances in merging the anatomical structures with PET metabolic information besides developments in tracer chemistry will definitely improve the radiologic capability of disease detection, and the diagnostic "world" will be based on the molecular aspects rather than the traditional methods of detection.

11.1.1 History

In 1928, Paul Dirac predicted the existence of he positron, and he shared the Nobel Prize with Erwin Schrödinger in 1933. In 1932, Carl Anderson observed positrons in cosmic rays and shared the Nobel Prize in 1936 with Victor Hess. From the beginning, one could expect that the electron antiparticle known as a positron would receive much interest or at least provide important applications as those who discovered it were awarded well-ranked and recognized scientific prizes. The positron is one of the antimatter physical particles that has a short lifetime and decays quickly by combining with a surrounding electron to release two 511-keV photons in a back-to-back collision process. These two photons are the two arms by which the physics of PET imaging is rotating.

11.1.2 Positron Physics

There are several positron emitters that are of particular clinical interest. Fluorine-18 is the most widely used positron emitter for many reasons. It has well-defined radiochemistry, and labeling with various biomolecules is continuously advancing to suit specific target tissues (see Chap. 5). It has a half-life (109.8 min) that allows radiochemists to synthesize labeled compounds in a reasonable time and permits other imaging logistics, such as injection, patient preparation, and imaging over several time points on either a static or dynamic basis, to be carried out. The physical characteristics of fluorine are also desirable for production of high-resolution PET images. The maximum energy of the decay of F-18 is 0.650 MeV with a small positron range. Other positron emitters, such as oxygen-15 (2.03 min), nitrogen-13 (9.97 min), carbon-11 (20.3 min), and others, have documented clinical utility in PET imaging (see Table 11.1).

The physics of PET imaging is based on positron emission, in which nuclei of an excess amount of protons exhibit nuclear transition by emitting a positron particle whose half-life is short. The positron travels a short distance based on its kinetic energy and then annihilates by combining with an electron present in the surrounding medium to give two opposing 511-keV photons with an angular distribution of 0.5° full width at half maximum (FWHM) at 180°. Before annihilation takes place, the positron forms a new configuration with an electron called positronium, which is a hydrogen-like atom with a short lifetime of about 10^{-7} s [7]. Because of this unique emission process, a single detector system does not provide appropriate geometry for detection of the two photons as in SPECT imaging; hence, two detectors in coincidence are the most convenient way to detect the two

Table 11.1 Physical properties of clinically useful PET radionuclides (From [142])

Radionuclide	Half-life	Maximum energy (MeV)	Average kinetic energy (MeV)	Resolution (mm)		
				FWHM	FWTM	Effective range = 2.355 × rms
Carbon-11	20.3 min	0.96	0.386	0.102	1.03	0.92
Nitrogen-13	9.97 min	1.19	0.492	0.104	1.05	1.4
Oxygen-15	122 s	1.72	0.735	0.188	1.86	2.4
Fluorine-18	109.8 min	0.64	0.250	0.282	2.53	0.54
Copper-64	12.7 h	0.65	0.278	0.501	4.14	0.55
Gallium-68	68.1 min	1.83	0.783	0.58	4.83	2.8
Rubidium-82	1.27 min	3.3	1.475	1.27	10.5	6.1

rms: root mean square
FWTM full width at tenth maximum
FWHM full width at half maximum

events concurrently. Therefore, any two photons that will reach two opposing detectors (in coincidence) will be recorded as long as their incidences on the detector fall within a predefined timing window (2τ). The line that connects the two detectors in space is called the *tube* or *line of response* (LOR). The LOR does not necessarily indicate the path along which annihilation took place since one or both photons may have undergone a scattering interaction before reaching the detectors or both may have originated from different annihilating sites. Accordingly, there are different types of events that can describe the coincidence events detected by a PET scanner. These are true, scatter, and random coincidences and are discussed further in this chapter.

Positron Range

A physical phenomenon reduces the resolution capability of the scanner to record events exactly as emitted from their true original locations (Fig. 11.1). Once the positron is emitted from the nucleus, it undergoes an annihilation with an electron to produce the clinically useful 511-keV photons. However, before this interaction takes place, the positron travels a distance before collision occurs. This distance is a function of the kinetic energy of the emitted positrons being higher in positron emitters with high maximum β^+ energy, such as O-15, Ga-68, and Rb-82 nuclei (maximum energy 1.72, 1.83, and 3.3 MeV, respectively) [8] (Table 11.1). Besides the kinetic energy of the released positron, the surrounding medium contributes to the

spatial blurring caused by the positron range. In tissues with low density (e.g., lung tissue), the resolution degradation is more pronounced than in tissues with high density (e.g., compact bone) (see Fig. 11.2). Together with the radionuclide maximum energy and the density of the medium, the relative influence of the positron range on the final resolution of the reconstructed image depends on the spatial resolution of the system [9, 10].

The distribution of the positron trajectories was found not to follow a normal Gaussian-like distribution and the cusp-shaped pattern was found in a number of simulation studies [8, 9]. The effect of positron range on resolution loss is thus recommended to be measured using the positron root mean square range in the medium of interest or the full width at 20% of maximum [9]. The characteristic shape of the positron distribution preserves some high frequencies, and the long tail estimated by full width at tenth maximum (FWTM) causes severe resolution degradation [8].

Acollinearity

Acollinearity is another physical phenomenon that is related to the conservation of momentum of the annihilated positron-electron pair. The conservation of mass and energy requires that the two photons are released in 180°; however, some residual kinetic energy remains to reduce this angular measure, on average, by $\pm 0.25°$ FWHM as shown in Fig. 11.1. This in turn leads to a LOR that does not exactly pass through the annihilation site, resulting in event

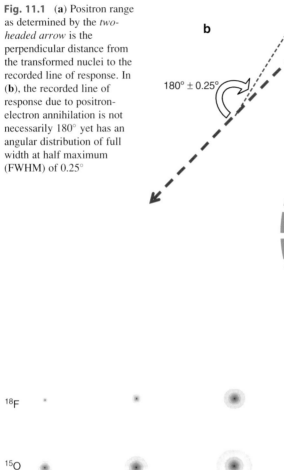

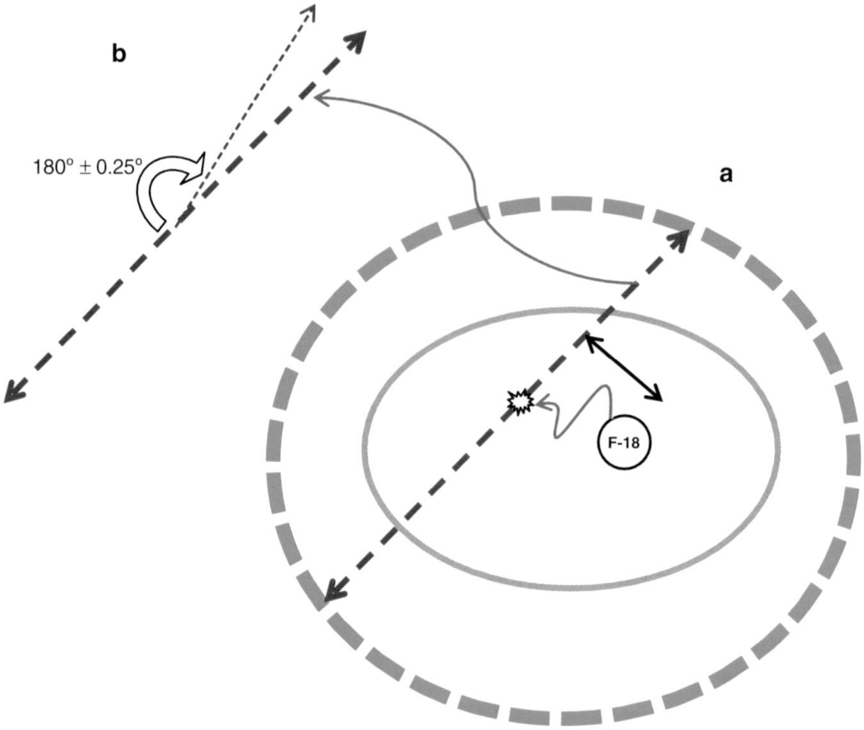

Fig. 11.1 (**a**) Positron range as determined by the *two-headed arrow* is the perpendicular distance from the transformed nuclei to the recorded line of response. In (**b**), the recorded line of response due to positron-electron annihilation is not necessarily 180° yet has an angular distribution of full width at half maximum (FWHM) of 0.25°

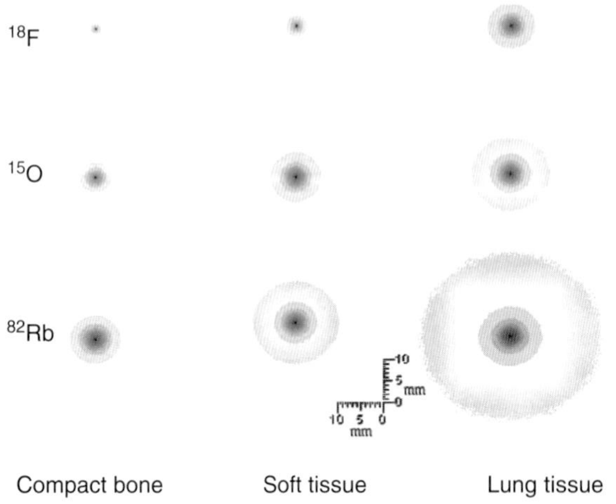

Fig. 11.2 Monte Carlo-calculated distribution of annihilation events around a positron source inserted in different human tissues (compact bone, soft tissue, and lung tissue). The spread of the distribution is larger for positron emitters of high maximum kinetic energy in tissues with low density. (From [9] with permission from Springer + Business media)

mm = 1.76 mm. The constant 0.0022 is derived from the geometry of the ray and can be calculated as 0.5 tan 0.25°. For a 15-cm detector diameter, resolution loss would be 0.33 mm, approximately five to six times less than a clinical whole-body scanner. Corrections for acollinearity and positron range are discussed in the spatial resolution section.

11.2 PET Scanners: Geometry and Components

A number of different geometries have been implemented in the design of PET scanners. Starting from the simple geometry of two opposing detectors as in the conventional dual-head gamma camera to more sophisticated full-ring scanners, performance characteristics vary from one system to another and are superior in the latter design. However, full-ring scanners are more expensive. Other system design geometries are partial ring and polygonal (hexagonal, octagonal, …). Figures 11.3 and 11.4 illustrate different geometries used in clinical PET systems.

Hybrid PET/SPECT Camera. As mentioned, the process of positron-electron annihilation and the

mispositioning and spatial resolution loss. Unlike the positron range, the acollinearity resolution effects are a function of the detector diameter; thus, a PET scanner of with an 80-cm diameter would suffer a resolution degradation of $0.0022 \times D$ or 0.0022×800

Fig. 11.3 Different geometries used in positron emission tomographic (PET) scanners. (**a**) A dual-head gamma camera with coincidence circuitry and sufficient crystal thickness of about 2.5 cm. (**b**) Partial-ring detector geometry that requires rotation around the patient for data sampling. (**c**) Full-ring detector geometry

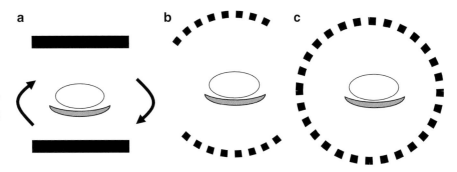

release of two antiparallel photons impose geometric constraints on PET detector design. This requires that the detector pair must be in an opposite direction to determine the path traversed by annihilation photons to reach the detectors. Anger proposed the use of two opposing gamma cameras at 180° and electronic collimation of the 511-keV photons to record coincident events [11]. This has been employed in longitudinal tomography using a dual camera without a rotating system. Further developments resulted in the design of two large field-of-view gamma cameras with a thicker crystals mounted on a rotating gantry [12].

Several limitations faced the early dual opposing detector design in providing a convenient measure of activity distribution inside human subjects, such as low sensitivity, poor count rate capability, and lack of a radionuclide to provide sufficient count statistics over the time course of the study. These limitations were attributed mainly to the use of NaI(Tl) crystal, old-fashioned system electronics, and the inherent open design. NaI(Tl) crystals have a low stopping power against 511-keV photons and a slow decay time. The open design, however, allows for more single events and random coincidences to be accepted, especially from regions outside the field of view, resulting in a low signal-to-noise ratio and reduced image contrast [13].

This system is today named as hybrid SPECT/PET camera and is able to provide dual functionality in imaging single-photon radiopharmaceuticals and positron-labeled compounds by switching between SPECT and coincidence detection mode (Fig. 11.3a). Using appropriate collimators for 511 keV, this type of imaging system was also used to image patients injected with dual tracers to look at two different metabolic or functional processes that happen simultaneously [14–16].

Modifications must be made on the conventional gamma camera to operate in the coincidence mode [17]. Coincidence triggering is the basic electronic element that needs to be incorporated in the detector electronics. The count rate capability must be high enough since collimators are unmounted, and the system sensitivity is larger. Crystal thickness (e.g., 16–25 mm) should be larger than that normally used in SPECT systems to provide a sufficient interaction depth to stop a significant portion of the incident photons, thus improving the detection efficiency. Dual- and triple-coincidence gamma cameras have been manufactured, and owing to some performance limitations, such as spatial resolution, sensitivity, and count rate performance, they are not attractive coincidence PET scanners when compared to the full-ring design [18–20].

Partial Ring. In PET systems with partial detector rings, the detectors are packed in two opposing detector banks arranged in a circular system that continuously rotates to capture a complete data set necessary for image reconstruction [21] (Fig. 11.3b). For example, the ECAT ART (Siemens/CTI, Inc., Knoxville, TN) consists of two opposing detectors, each of 3×11 crystal blocks arranged in axial and tangential direction. The banks are slightly asymmetrically opposed to increase the effective transaxial field of view. The block material is bismuth germanate (BGO) and is segmented into $6.75 \times 6.75 \times 20$ mm³ and coupled to four photomultiplier tubes (PMTs). There are three blocks in the axial dimension, giving a 16.2-cm axial field of view and 24 crystal rings with 242 possible planes of response [21]. The partial ring design was used in prototyping the first PET/CT scanner in which the PET electronics were placed at the rear portion of the CT gantry housing but with different operation consoles [22].

Fig. 11.4 Another set of positron emission tomographic (PET) scanners that was proposed in the literature and implemented in practice. (**a**) and (**b**) Hexagonal designs using flat- or curved-plate detector arrays, respectively. (**c**) Discrete crystals arranged in modular style in which modules are adjoined side-to-side

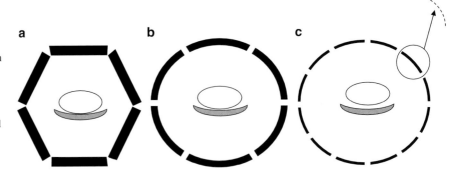

Hexagonal geometry. Other systems were also implemented that were based on arrays of six- or eight-sided geometry. The former design is shown in Fig. 11.4a, b and has more than one variant, such that the detector assembly can be a single continuous scintillation detector or curved-plate design. However, the number of detectors can be larger, with flat modules and discrete crystal structure (Fig. 11.4c).

The hexagonal design has some good features as it is relatively simple and uses fewer PMTs than used in a full-ring block detector design. The number of PMTs may vary from 180 or 288 as in NaI(Tl)-based detector to an even larger number (e.g., 420) as in discrete GSO (gadolinium oxyorthosilicate) or LYSO (Cerium doped lutetium yttrium orthosilicate) modular detectors [23–27]. Further, it has a relatively large axial field of view that can reach 25 cm, such as that found, for example, in the curved-plate NaI(Tl) design [25].

The use of a large continuous crystal allows only 3D data acquisitions; to some extent, the large axial field of view can compensate for the lower sensitivity of the NaI(Tl) crystal. However, such a detector design and the use of Anger logic position circuitry led to an increase in the system dead time. Limiting the light signal to a finite number of PMTs and optimizing the light guide for light spread were proposed to mitigate these effects [28]. One of the disadvantages of hexagonal geometry is the intercrystal dead space left by adjoining the detector modules, a reason that could cause some reduction of the system sensitivity and confound the reconstruction process.

A hectagonal or eight-sided detector system can be found in the HRRT system (High Resolution Research Tomograph, Siemens Medical Solutions), a dedicated brain PET scanner that uses two types of scintillation crystals to indentify the depth of interaction (DOI) of the 511-keV photons. The system achieves a spatial resolution of 2.3–3.2 mm in the transaxial direction and a resolution of 2.5–3.4 mm in the axial direction, together with a point source system sensitivity of 6% and National Electrical Manufacturers Association (NEMA) NU-2001 line source sensitivity of 3%. The transaxial and axial extents are 31 and 25 cm, respectively [29].

Cylindrical design. The most efficient geometries that found wide acceptance among manufacturers and PET users are those that depend on circular or ring design. The advantage provided by full-ring scanners is their detection efficiency and count rate capabilities. This in turn provides better system spatial resolution by realizing the statistical requirements imposed by image reconstruction [30]. The ring design is the most widely used system geometry and is preferred among manufacturers in clinical and preclinical PET scanners.

11.2.1 PET/CT

The introduction of PET/CT in the early years of this century was attractive for many practitioners as well as some manufacturers; now, almost all PET scanners are purchased as hybrid PET/CT systems. As mentioned in the level of integration (chapter 10), the current generation of hybrid PET/CT systems is configured side-by-side such that the CT component is placed in the front portion of the scanner while the PET component is placed at the back end mounted using the same housing over the two gantries or gantries with separate

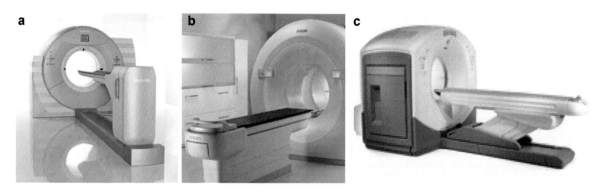

Fig. 11.5 State-of-the-art positron emission tomographic/computed tomographic (PET/CT) scanners. (**a**) Biograph mCT, Siemens Medical Solutions. (**b**) Gemini TF Big Bore system, Philips Company. (**c**) Discovery PET/CT 600, GE Healthcare

covers and in all cases using the same imaging table. The axial length traversed by the imaging table varies among manufacturers, and as the bed travels axially there is more chance for bed deflection, resulting in misalignment errors. A number of approaches were therefore undertaken by scanner manufacturers to take into account this deflection of the imaging bed.

Moving from a single to more CT slices (e.g., 4, 6, 8, 16, 64, and beyond) offered a great opportunity to enhance the diagnostic speed and possibility of performing cardiac CT as well as angiography. The addition of spiral CT technology was remarkable and significantly reduced the acquisition times by many-fold together with the advantage of acquiring a large number of thin slices. In this type of data acquisition, the imaging table moves forward in a simultaneous motion with rotation of the x-ray source in a spiral path. The delay between interscans can thus be eliminated (a feature of older CT generations), while the z-axis is kept variable across projections. Data interpolation is then used to account for these angular inconsistencies. These fully diagnostic CT systems, when combined with state-of-the art PET machines, have made a "one-stop-shop" diagnosis a clinical reality. The radiation dose delivered to the patient using multislice CT systems has been considered, and solutions such as beam modulations and optimized acquisition protocols have been used. Low-dose attenuation correction using low tube current is another way to reduce patient dose as long as diagnostic CT is not required. The two major advantages provided by the CT are attenuation correction and anatomical localization of the PET images; both features have significantly improved the diagnostic performance of the nuclear

scans. State-of-the-art PET/CT systems are shown in Fig. 11.5.

There have been several attempts to improve the performance characteristics of PET scanners in terms of spatial resolution, system sensitivity, coincidence timing resolution, and energy resolution while keeping the cost of the device reasonably affordable. These requirements are as follows [31]:

1. High detection sensitivity for the 511-keV photons to improve the detection or areas of low tracer concentration, enhance the statistical quality of dynamic images, and to reduce the injected dose
2. High resolving capabilities to achieve the maximal spatial resolution for volume elements
3. High-energy resolution to minimize the contribution of scattered events
4. Low dead time to improve count rate performance and high timing resolution to improve random rejections and for time-of-flight (TOF) applications
5. Low cost

Achieving such requirements in one practical tomograph is difficult from physical and engineering perspectives as well as financial issues. Some performance parameters are traded off while maintaining the quality of others. For instance, reducing the detector diameter is advantageous for improving count sensitivity, while it is not in favor of spatial resolution due to the DOI errors. Small-animal scanners have better angular coverage owing to smaller ring diameter but suffer from depth of interaction. Another factor that is affected by ring diameter is photon acollinearity, which increases and decreases in a linear fashion with the ring diameter. Extension of the axial extent of the PET scanner can be used to improve scanner sensitivity, but this comes with increased cost and degradation of spatial resolution in the axial direction.

11.2.2 Scintillation Crystals

The type and composition of the scintillation crystal are of considerable importance in the detection efficiency of 511-keV photons. The function of the crystal is to convert the energy received by the incident photons into light quanta that are proportional to the imparted energy. Two major interactions occur when the photon deposits its energy in the crystal: photoelectric and Compton scattering. The electrons released from either photoelectric or Compton processes undergo several interactions within the scintillator material and excite other electrons, which in turn decay to emanate the scintillation light [32].

Crystal with a high probability of photoelectric effect, or photofraction, is preferred since all energy is imparted on the crystal and at one site. However, Compton interactions reveal more than one interaction site and hence degrade the spatial resolution as well as the energy spectrum by broadening the photo peak width. Figure 11.6 shows the dependence of the photoelectric effect on the atomic number of various types of scintillation crystals.

The light emitted by the crystal is viewed and detected by photodetectors, where light photons are converted into an electronic signal for determination of event attributes such as energy and position. Many types of the scintillator material have been proposed and implemented to improve the detection performance of PET scanners. Crystals that are able to provide high photon detection efficiency, short decay time, and better energy resolution are highly preferred. Other optical properties, such as an emission wavelength that matches the photocathode of the PMT, transparency, and good refractive index, are also important factors to ensure maximum transfer of the scintillation light to the PMT. Other manufacturing requirements, such as mechanical flexibility, hygroscopic properties, ease of handling and fabrication into small crystal elements, cost, and availability, are all of concern in the selection of the scintillator material [33, 34]. The following is a list of the major

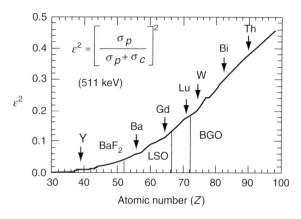

Fig. 11.6 The probability that both 511-keV photons interact via the photoelectric effect as a function of Z_{eff}. There is an increasing trend in the photofraction probability with the effective atomic number. (From [144] with permission from William Moses, Lawrence Berkeley Lab, USA)

properties of the scintillation crystals that can significantly improve the scanner performance:

1. Crystals with *high density and high effective atomic number* Z_{eff} have good intrinsic efficiency. Photoelectric effect is strongly related but Compton scattering is linearly related to the atomic number of the material for photons (>100 keV). Crystals with high ρZ_{eff}^4 have good stopping capabilities for 511-keV photons [35]. The density and effective atomic number also determine the attenuation length when crystals of smaller attenuation length are desired as they serve to reduce resolution degradation caused by parallax errors.

2. Crystals should have high *light output* since event positioning and energy resolution are related to the amount of light quanta released from the crystal. A sufficient amount of scintillation light can release a significant number of photoelectrons from the photocathode and thus provide better accuracy in signal measurements and improve energy resolution. The small size of the crystal elements in the block detector design requires a scintillator that can produce high light output so that position encoding can be done with good precision. There are a number of factors responsible for the statistics of light emanating from the scintillator, such as homogeneous distribution of the activation centers, nonproportional response of the crystal, and variation in crystal luminosity [33].

3. Crystals with *short decay constants* or "fast scintillators" serve to improve the timing of the coincidence detection and thus reduce the dead time and random fractions. Scintillators with a short decay constant help to improve the count rate performance, especially for scanners operating in 3D mode and for clinical studies in which short-lived radionuclides with high activities are used [36]. Another advantage gained by such crystals is their recent introduction in TOF applications, which require high efficiency and fast scintillators, leading to an improvement in the signal-to-noise ratio.

4. Although the selection of the scintillator material is important and can potentially affect the performance of the scanner, one should realize that the overall system performance is a function of many components of the imaging system, such as electronic circuitry and acquisition and reconstruction parameters, together with the correction and computational techniques [37]. This has been noted in PET scanners upgraded using better electronic circuitry or when new scintillation crystals were introduced in scanners not equipped with appropriate electronic components [38, 39].

11.2.2.1 NaI(Tl)

NaI(Tl) has been extensively used in many nuclear medicine devices, especially in the design of the gamma camera. In the early 1970s, it was the most commonly used crystal in PET scanners even though it was an inefficient scintillator for 511-keV photons. The detection efficiency of NaI(Tl) crystal to Tc-99m energy and other relatively low-energy gamma emitters is reasonably good, and it remains the scintillator of choice in many SPECT cameras. In comparison to other types of scintillation crystals, it has better energy resolution, poor timing resolution, high dead time, and low stopping power. The low density and moderately low atomic number are responsible for the poor detection efficiency of NaI(Tl) crystal for 511-keV photons. Another limitation of NaI(Tl) crystal is its hygroscopic properties, and careful handling to avoid humidity effects must be taken into account; hermetic sealing is required. This in turn led to difficulty in producing small-size elements suitable for block detector design.

11.2.2.2 BGO

The BGO type of crystals has a better detection efficiency and high probability of photoelectric interaction (40%) for 511-keV photons. It contains the bismuth element (Bi), which has a large atomic number ($Z = 83$) and its ionic form (Bi^{3+}) is the intrinsic luminescence center in the crystal [33]. The density of the crystal is approximately two times greater than for NaI(Tl), and the attenuation coefficient is three times larger (Table 11.2). These properties have allowed BGO to replace NaI(Tl) crystal, and it was the scintillator of choice for many years, until the end of 1990s. However, the low light yield [~15–20% relative to NaI(Tl)] and poor energy resolution and response time have made it inferior to the other new scintillators, which showed a better response time and better light output, such as GSO, LSO (Cerium-doped Lutetium Orthosilicate) , or LYSO. As mentioned, better response time allows a significant reduction of system dead time and works to minimize the amount of random coincidences that contaminate the prompt events. Moreover, it allows a reduction of pulse pile-up in 3D mode, in which system sensitivity is high, thereby resulting in better count rate performance. The first small-animal PET scanner designed specifically to image rodents was made of BGO-based block detectors and was developed in the mid-1990s [40]. When compared to NaI(Tl), both the nonhygroscopic nature of BGO and its high detection efficiency have permitted manufacturing a more compact detector assembly and narrower crystals that improved significantly the system resolution and sensitivity.

11.2.2.3 Gadolinium Oxyorthosilicate

Cerium-doped GSO has good properties that have made it applicable in recent PET scanners (Allegro and Gemini-GXL, Philips Company). Also, it has some applications in small-animal scanners and in combination with LSO in systems equipped with parallax error correction. The density of this scintillator is comparable to BGO and LSO crystals, and it is roughly twice as dense as NaI(Tl). The effective Z is intermediate between NaI(Tl) and both BGO and LSO. The decay constant (60 ns) is slightly higher than LSO but significantly lower than BGO and NaI(Tl) crystals. An evaluation of a pixilated GSO Anger

Table 11.2 Properties of scintillation crystals used in positron emission tomographic (PET) scanners

	NaI(Tl)	BGO	GSO:Ce	LSO:Ce	LYSO:Ce	LaBr$_3$	BaF$_2$
Density (gm/cm^3)	3.67	7.13	6.7	7.4	7.1	5.3	4.89
Effective atomic number (Z)	51	74	59	66	64	47	54
Linear attenuation coefficient (1/cm)	0.34	0.92	0.62	0.87	0.86	0.47	0.44
Light yield (% NaI[Tl])	100	15	30	75	75	160	5
Decay time (ns)	230	300	65–60	40	41	16	0.8
Emission maximum (nm)	410	480	440	420	420	370	220
Hygroscopic	Yes	No	No	No	No	Yes	Slightly
Photoelectric effect (%)	17	40	25	32	33	13	12
Refractive Index	1.85	2.15	1.85	1.82	1.81	1.88	1.56

NaI(Tl) Thallium-activated sodium iodide crystal
BGO Bismuth germanate oxyorthosilicate
GSO:Ce Cerium-doped gadolinium oxyorthosilicate
LSO:Ce Cerium-doped Lutetium orthosilicate
LYSO:Ce Cerium-doped lutetium yttrium orthosilicate
LaBr3:Ce Cerium-doped lanthanum bromide
BaF2 Barium fluoride

logic-based scanner using NEMA NU 2-2001 procedures revealed acceptable results in terms of energy resolution, sensitivity, and better image quality provided that a patient study can be performed in a time course of half an hour, including transmission measurements [24]. That system also demonstrated a better count rate capability in 3D mode served by the fast decay constant of the GSO crystal and optimizing the light spread detected by PMTs [28]. GSO is not hygroscopic, absent intrinsic radioactivity, has good stability versus temperature, and has a good uniform light output but is not simple to manufacture, and a special fabrication procedure is followed to avoid cracking during crystal design. Another disadvantage is its susceptibility to magnetic field effects, rendering it an unsuitable scintillator for PET/MR hybrid systems [41].

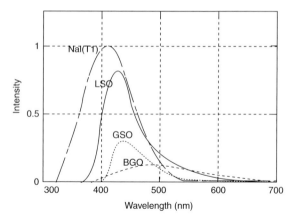

Fig. 11.7 LSO is ranked second among other different scintillation crystals in the amount of light yield produced, data normalized to NaI(Tl) crystal. Further, the peak emission wavelength does match the bialkali material of the photocathode of photomultiplier tubes (PMTs). (From [145] © IEEE with permission)

11.2.2.4 LSO/LYSO

Unlike BGO, which has no activator, LSO is a cerium-activated scintillator and has a large ρZ_{eff}^4, but this is lower than BGO. It has good characteristics for dealing with 511-keV photons: The effective Z is 66, density (7.4), and $\mu = 0.87$ cm^{-1}; thus, it is an efficient scintillator for stopping the annihilation coincidence photons. LYSO is similar to LSO and is produced such that some lutetium is replaced by yttrium atoms.

LSO scintillators are characterized by their fast response, represented by short decay time, achieving excellent timing resolution. These properties have made LSO/LYSO an attractive scintillator for PET scanners, in particular for TOF applications, and with its high light output, there is no compromise in detector efficiency [42] (see Figs. 11.6 and 11.7). The light output is approximately three or five times higher than BGO when using an avalanche photodiode (APD) or

PMT, respectively. Because of the statistical nature of the detection process, an LSO-based PET scanner should enjoy better energy resolution (~12%), better event positioning, and a short coincidence timing window. The last is instrumental in establishing the noise level resulting from random events [43].

LSO is nonhygroscopic and mechanically rugged, and simple fabrication is relatively possible to produce small and discrete versions of the crystal [34]. However, it has a number of limitations, such as inhomogeneity of light production, high melting point (>2,000°C), and cost higher than other crystal types [GSO, BGO, and NaI(Tl)]. Another limitation of LSO scintillation crystals is their Lu-176 content, which emits low-level radioactivity; yet, this has been found not to affect the extrinsic 511-keV coincidence detection but can affect precise measurements of system sensitivity and scatter fraction using low-level radiation.

LSO crystals are found in many PET systems, such as high-resolution dedicated brain scanners [44] and hybrid multimodality imaging, such as PET/CT, PET/SPECT, and PET/MRI systems. Other special-purpose systems have also been designed using LSO crystals, such as breast PET scanners and small-animal imaging systems [45, 46].

One decade ago, the acquisition of whole-body fluorodeoxyglucose-F18 (FDG) studies could take about 1 h, including measurements of transmission data [47]. However, these days the same scan can be acquired in significantly shorter time. This significant reduction in the acquisition time is due to many reasons; one is related to the introduction of efficient and fast scintillators in the scanner design (in addition to other factors such as CT-based attenuation correction, fast electronic circuitry and computer processors).

11.2.3 Crystal Photodetector: Light Readout

In the conventional gamma camera, the scintillation crystal is a continuous large slab of NaI(Tl) viewed from its back surface by an array of PMTs that collect the scintillation light produced from interaction of the emitted photons with the detector material (Fig. 11.8a). In one of the earliest PET detector designs, the PMT is coupled to a single crystal; thus, the cross section of the crystal defines the LOR and

intrinsic spatial resolution [48]. Following this procedure in building up a full multiring scanner is neither efficient nor cost-effective as one needs a significantly large number of PMTs and crystal material along with electronic channels to implement such a design. Earlier efforts in coupling the scintillation detector to PMTs included four crystals per one or two PMTs. However, this strategy was advanced by using more crystal elements per PMTs. It was a turning point when the block detector concept was introduced in the design of the PET scanners, which is a cost-effective technique in coupling the PMT to the scintillation detectors and has also led to an improvement in spatial resolution [49].

In block detector design, as shown in Fig. 11.8b, c, the scintillation block is segmented into an array of small crystals by cutting into precise and well-defined dimensions in the transaxial and axial directions. The cutting process leaves a space between the small crystals; therefore, a reflective material is used to optically separate between the neighboring crystals, defining a path for the light to travel to the PMTs and to maximize light collection efficiency (Fig. 11.9a). The depth of cutting is empirically implemented so that the light is distributed in a spatially linear fashion among the exposed array of PMTs [48]. In this pseudodiscrete design, a greater depth of cutting is found at the block periphery rather than at the center. The advantage of the block detector design is improved spatial resolution by segmenting the scintillation crystal into smaller elements viewed by a finite number of PMTs (usually 4), thus minimizing the high cost required if each crystal element is coupled to a single PMT.

In the original design developed by Casey and Nutt, the block was cut into a 4×8 crystal array, each $5.6 \times 13.5 \times 30$ mm^3, using BGO detector material. The crystal block was glued to four square PMTs, each 25 mm, through a Lucite light guide [49]. Now, the crystal dimensions vary among PET scanners using different types of scintillation materials. In commercial clinical PET/CT scanners, the crystal dimension varies from one system to another (e.g., 4×4, 6.4×6.4, etc.), while the crystal thickness ranges from 20 to 30 mm. Crystal size can be reduced to 1–2 mm in an array of larger elements, such as 20×20 or 13×13, based on design specifications. However, this arrangement is most common in small-animal micro-PET scanners.

Fig. 11.8 (**a**) Light readout by continuous-based scintillation detector. (**b**) Block detector showing crystal segmentation. (**c**) Photograph of block detector coupled to four photomultiplier tubes (PMTs). (Image courtesy of Siemens Medical Solutions)

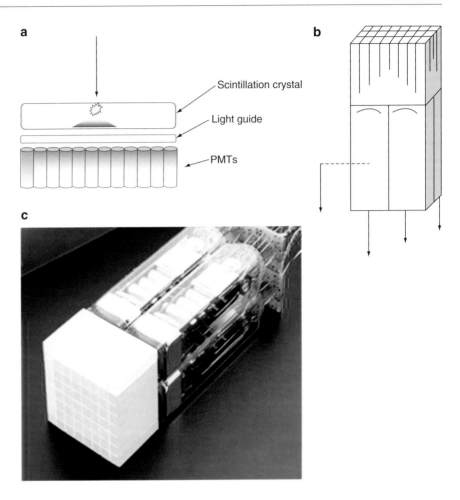

Fig. 11.9 (**a**) Crystal segmentation in block detector design. It allows defining a path for incident photons and improved collection efficiency. (**b**) Discrete crystal design, a useful approach in high-resolution PET but with some limitations (see the text). (**c**) Anger logic positioning

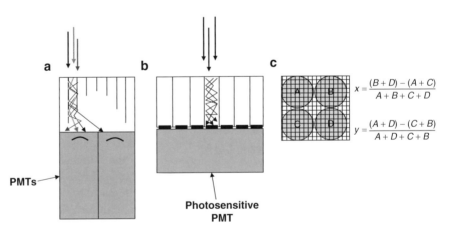

Another choice is an assembly of *discrete individual* scintillation crystals that are packed together yet optically separated by reflective material to confine the light spread to those crystals that receive the scintillation light (Fig. 11.9b). This finger-like array of discrete crystals provides an improvement in spatial resolution. It can be read out by a position-sensitive or multichannel photodetector or individual and separate readout channels [50]. Use of semiconductor readout devices has also been implemented in the last design, in which discrete crystals are read out by an array of elements of APD [51]. APDs can be produced in dimensions (individual elements or array) similar to discrete crystal dimensions and therefore can overcome size limitations encountered in fabricating small PMTs (smaller than 10 mm) [52, 53]. They have been successfully introduced as light photodetectors in encoding the position of the light signal and offer a compact volume that is useful in PET/MRI systems and small-animal scanners, including SPECT and PET imagers.

Discrete detector design has a number of limitations, especially when an individual crystal is read out by a single readout channel. Crystal fraction and packing must match with the size of the available photodetectors [50]. Further, it requires extensive use of electronic readout channels and thus is an expensive and cost-ineffective approach. PET systems based on discrete crystal design are more common in research and small-animal scanners [50, 52]. Alternatively, discrete crystal design can be used in a modular structure in which the crystal sets are mapped by an array of PMTs with a continuous light guide adjoining the detector modules, as can be found, for example, in the Allegro system (Philips Company). Table 11.3 shows the various approaches used to couple the PMT and the crystal in PET scanners.

In the block detector, four PMTs are often used to read out the light emitted from the scintillation material. The centroid Anger logic is used to identify the individual crystals from which light photons were emitted (Fig. 11.9c). Another approach that improved the encoding ratio but suffers from increased dead time is the quadrant-sharing approach, in which the PMT is shared among four block detectors; the encoding ratio of 16:1 in the conventional block detector design is increased by three to four times based on the PMT size and the crystal dimensions [54] (Fig. 11.10). This design was initially proposed to improve the spatial resolution of the PET scanner without increasing the cost and to reduce the high price of the scanner by lowering the number of PMTs decoding the scintillation detector [55]. However, dead time effects and pulse pileup can be treated using recent progress in signal-processing electronics employing event recovery methods [56, 57].

11.3 Events Detected by a PET Scanner

Singles: PET detectors receive a large amount of events. A small fraction of these events are detected as in coincidence, while the remaining are singles that

Table 11.3 Summary of various approaches implemented to couple the photomultiplier tubes (PMTs) and scintillation crystals in clinical positron emission tomographic (PET) scanners

		Scintillation crystals	
		Continuous	Discrete
PMTs	2 × 2	–	Conventional block detector design (e.g., many partial- and full-ring scanners)
	Array	Large crystal coupled to an array of PMTs (e.g., curve plate, C-PET)	Discrete crystals arranged in large flat module, PIXELAR Technology (e.g., Allegro and Gemini-TF)

Fig. 11.10 Quadrant light sharing (**a**) Frontal view. (**b**) Lateral view

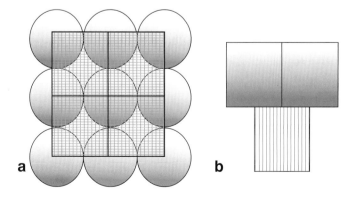

constitute a large fraction of the detected count rate. Singles can be detected from the coincidence field of view as well as from activity lying outside the field of view. They are a problem in 3D data acquisition, for which the axial extent of data acquisition is larger and extends over the area examined [58].

11.3.1 True Coincidences

True coincidences are those photons emitted from a single nuclei and detected by the detectors without interactions in the surrounding medium (Fig. 11.11a). They are the most preferred type of events not actually achievable in practice without contamination with other events (scatter and randoms).

11.3.2 Random Coincidences

Random or accidental coincidences are undesired types of events that occur as a result of detecting two coincident events from two different locations by which their detection timing falls within the coincidence timing window of the system (Fig. 11.11b). Because these two photons are unrelated, they have nearly equal probability to occur between most decaying nuclei in the field of view, resulting in a high background image. True coincidences increase in linear proportion to the object activity; however, random coincidences are estimated to equal the product of count rates of the two detectors multiplied by the timing window (2τ):

$$R_{ij} = 2\tau\, S_a S_b$$

where S_a and S_b are the single-photon event rate of detectors a and b, respectively. Thus, they are approximately proportional to the square of the singles count rate. Random coincidences add false information regarding position and serve to reduce image contrast and quantitative accuracy as well. They are large in areas with high count rates, such as the abdomen and pelvis, especially if bladder activity is high. A longer coincidence timing window increases the chance of accepting more random events, but a shorter timing window reduces the number of true events. Consequently, selection of coincidence time is a trade-off between sensitivity of the scanner and reduction of undesired events such as randoms [59]. In fully 3D acquisition mode, the random events are greater than for 2D acquisition (with use of septa) since the former provides a larger axial field of view relative to the field of the true events.

The formula can be used in estimating the random events in the acquired images if the activity in the field of view remains constant during the time course of the

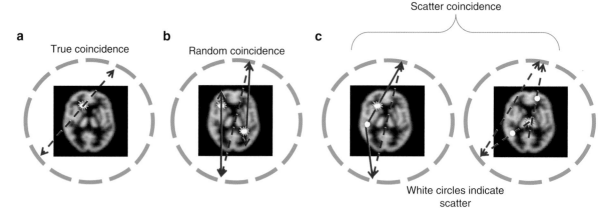

Fig. 11.11 Three different types of coincidences that take place during PET imaging. (**a**) True coincidence occurs due to decay of a single nuclei and emission of two antiparallel 511-keV photons and without undergoing any further interactions. (**b**) Random coincidence occurs due to decay of two unrelated nuclei such that their detection by two opposing detector pairs is within the acceptance timing window. (**c**) Scatter events take place when one or two of the 511-keV photons undergo Compton interaction during their travel to the detector pair and again with detection time within the specified limit; however, single-photon scattering is more abundant than two-photon scattering

Fig. 11.12 Scatter fractions simulated for different crystals as a function of energy threshold using a cylinder (70 cm long) of diameters 20 cm (O), 27 cm (■), and 35 cm (▲) in a typical 3D scanner. Data simulated using a scanner of diameter 85 cm and 18 cm axial field of view. The *gray band* is the energy range threshold used for each scintillator. (From [54] with kind permission from IOP Publishing and the corresponding authors)

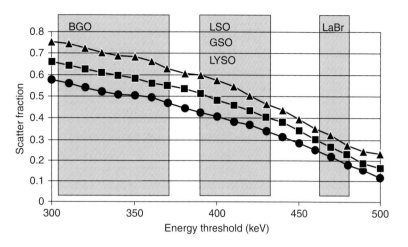

study. However, in some situations in which the tracer undergoes some dynamic or fast metabolic processes, this method may not be precise enough. Another approach that is frequently applied is the delayed window subtraction method. This method is based on measuring the random coincidences in a delayed acceptance window; then, data are corrected on the fly by subtraction or saved for further analysis [60]. The variance estimate in data collected by the delayed window is high, and applying it directly on the prompts window will add noise to the reconstructed images. A variance reduction technique can be used to suppress such a problem to yield a better signal estimate [61].

11.3.3 Scatter Coincidences

Another undesired type of events is scattered coincidence, which results from deflection of one or both annihilation photons from their true LOR, resulting in a false recorded event regarding position of the annihilated nuclei and energy of the 511-keV photons (Fig. 11.11c). Further, scatter coincidences are a function of the activity distribution, source size, and composition of the surrounding media. Scatter events cause a loss of image contrast and degrade the quantitative accuracy of the measurements. Energy resolution plays an important role in controlling the amount of scattered photons in the acquired data. PET systems with better energy resolution have a greater capability to reject scattered photons. For a scanner with good energy resolution, such as those with LSO/LYSO or GSO detector material, the lower energy bound can be

set at a threshold greater than 400 keV, and a significant amount of photons with large-angle scattering can be rejected. For a scanner with less energy resolution (e.g., BGO), the energy width is set wider, and the lower bound may go to 300 keV, which results in projection data contaminated by large proportion of scattered events. Figure 11.12 shows the scatter fraction for a number of scintillators used in commercial PET scanners as a function of the lower energy discriminator and different object sizes.

The contribution of multiple coincidences is also another possible type of events that result from three or more photons detected in the coincidence timing window, leading to detector confusion regarding where the annihilation photons are located.

The detection system does not discriminate between the various types of the coincidences, and they are automatically recorded as long as their detection time falls within the specified timing limits of the scanner. These events (true, random, and scatter coincidences) are collectively called *prompts,* bearing in mind that the most useful type is the true coincidence.

11.4 Scanner Performance

11.4.1 System Sensitivity

For a given activity distribution inside a human body and fixed acquisition time, the signal-to-noise ratio and image quality are substantially influenced by the sensitivity of the PET scanner. This can be noted in dynamic studies in which short time intervals require a detection system with high sensitivity to collect the maximum amount of information. This is particularly important in areas of poor count uptake or in short half-life positron emitters (e.g., Rb-82 or O-15). PET systems with high detection efficiency allow for better counting statistics and have a positive impact on image quality in terms of signal-to-noise ratio, spatial resolution, and other subsequent quantitative analysis.

The sensitivity of PET scanners can be classified into two major components: geometric and intrinsic efficiency. The former is related to the detector geometric design and how its elements are packed closely together so that fewer photons can escape without undergoing an interaction [33]. In other words, the angular coverage obtained by the detector surface area should be large enough when exposed to the emitted radiations. The ring-packing fraction can be defined as the ratio of the true detection area to the total circumferential ring area [62]. For example, the packing fraction of the Advance GE scanner was calculated to be 0.844 in comparison to a nonsegmented solid annulus detector using the SimSET simulation software [63]. The other component is the intrinsic efficiency of the detector, which is related to the type and composition of the scintillation material and is determined by scintillator density and its effective atomic number Z_{eff}. Other factors that influence the overall system sensitivity are energy and time window settings.

Geometric efficiency can be increased by reducing the diameter of the detector ring or extending the field of view in the axial direction. Reducing the system diameter will expose the detector more efficiently to the annihilation photons by increasing the solid angle, but this comes at the cost of spatial resolution loss caused by parallax DOI error. This phenomenon is of importance when attempts are made to improve the spatial resolution of small-animal scanners in which the scanner diameter is significantly small (10–15 cm) when compared to a clinical whole-body PET scanner (70–90 cm).

Dedicated PET scanners for brain imaging enjoy better solid-angle coverage for the emitted 511-keV photons, and hence an improvement in sensitivity can be realized, but again this is accomplished at the cost of increased radial resolution errors. This last limitation has been treated by designing dedicated brain scanners that include DOI correction utilizing two scintillation layers or what is called a "phosphowich" design, in which LSO crystals are stacked to GSO or LYSO and differences in light decay are exploited to

discriminate between events based on pulse shape discrimination [64]. See the discussion of DOI further in this chapter.

The other way is to increase the axial extent of the scanner, an issue that is more related to the cost of the scanner as one needs to add more detector material, including scintillation crystals, readout channels, and additional electronic circuitry. In 3D acquisition, an increase in the axial extent by 30% can lead to an increase in the volume sensitivity by approximately 80% [65, 66].

Simulation studies showed that an improvement in photon detection sensitivity can be achieved by manyfold using box-shaped geometry, especially when applied in small-animal scanners using APD and Cadmium zinc telluride (CZT) detector configurations. Other advantages of such a design are its simplicity and the possibility of the detector approaching to the object being imaged, improving the geometric efficiency [67]. Another approach consists of a rotating panel system of five large-area LSO detectors with a large axial field of view (53 cm), achieving a system sensitivity of 2% of F-18 line source and spatial resolution of less than 5 mm [68]. Nevertheless, these last approaches are not the typical commercial designs provided by PET scanner manufacturers.

The *intrinsic efficiency*, however, is a matter of crystal type and thickness. The crystal density and effective atomic number determine the linear attenuation coefficient, that is, the ability of the detector material to attenuate incident radiations. One can therefore estimate the coincidence detector intrinsic efficiency using the formula $(1-e^{-ul})^2$. A 3-cm thick BGO crystal can stop approximately 87% of the incident photon and thereby is considered an efficient scintillator material, whereas the same crystal thickness for NaI(Tl) can stop about 40% of incident 511-keV photons. Increasing the LSO crystal thickness from 2 to 3 cm would lead to an increase by 40% of the detector intrinsic efficiency [66]. However, these values are altered when an energy threshold is varied or the timing window of the system is changed. Increasing the crystal thickness is also not an advantage as it enhances DOI errors. Increasing the crystal thickness could lead to more crystal penetration, especially for photons that are radially shifted from the center field of view; this results in event mispositioning and spatial resolution errors. For example, BaF_3 crystal is a fast scintillator, but unfortunately it has lower detection efficiency; thus,

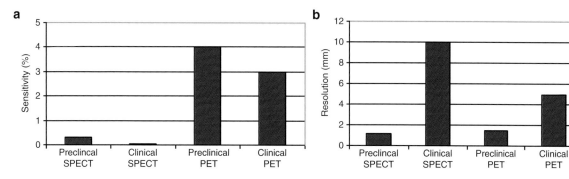

Fig. 11.13 Sensitivity and spatial resolution of clinical as well as preclinical scanners in single-photon emission computed tomographic (SPECT) and positron emission tomographic (PET) imaging. (Adapted from [143]). Note that some new scanners can achieve values better than shown in the graph

the crystal needs to be thicker (e.g., 45 mm) than normally used for BGO or other crystals of high detection efficiency. This was found to degrade the spatial resolution of the system as a function of source radial position [62]. For comparison, Fig. 11.13a shows the sensitivity of clinical PET and SPECT scanners together with their preclinical counterparts.

11.4.2 2D Versus 3D

In SPECT imaging, photon detection is performed by collimator holes, which define the path along which emitted photons are collected. In a similar manner, PET scanners are able to limit the emitted photons to be accepted through one or more planes using inter-plane septa or the 2D acquisition mode. To increase the sensitivity of the PET scanner, the interplane septa are removed (retracted) so that the coincidence field of view can be larger than that when septa are extended. Radiation shielding provided by septa was mandatory in early PET scanners to avoid many problems arising from high count rates, scatter, and random events. Brain studies were the first to exploit volumetric imaging provided by 3D acquisition [69]. However, the count rate arising from outside the field of view was problematic; this has been tackled by appropriate shielding at the axial end of the scanner [70]. In whole-body PET scanning, 3D acquisition has become the common mode of data acquisition, although there is some discussion surrounding the advantages of 3D over 2D imaging.

Advantages of 3D imaging are an increase in sensitivity by four to five times when compared to 2D

imaging, and fast scanning can be performed, avoiding patient discomfort and minimizing the likelihood of patient motion. An increase in patient throughput is an important outcome of 3D imaging and is demanded in busy and high-workload nuclear medicine departments. However, this increase in system sensitivity comes at the expense of increasing the accidental random coincidences, scatter events, and singles from activity outside the field of view. This increase in the singles count rate also leads to an increase in the system dead time and count losses.

3D PET imaging requires an improvement in scatter and random correction techniques and detectors with high count rate performance. Part of the problem can be solved by selecting an appropriate scintillation crystal coupled to electronics for high-speed signal processing. As mentioned, the emergence of fast scintillators such as LSO or LYSO has motivated the successful use of 3D imaging in the clinical setting with a significant reduction of imaging time [71]. Fast scintillators also provide a means of reducing system dead time and serve to improve the coincidence timing window, which are critical requirements imposed by 3D data acquisition.

11.4.3 Noise-Equivalent Count Rate

Count rate response is an important intrinsic performance measure of the PET scanner. From the statistical viewpoint and image quality requirements, higher counting rates are desired. This can be achieved by injecting higher doses or permitting longer acquisition times. Both ways have their own limitations since the former is restricted by radiation protection and safety issues while the latter is not preferable due to patient inconvenience, such as discomfort, high likelihood of motion, and lower throughput. However, if no restrictions are placed on the radioactivity to be injected, another problem would arise, which is the nonlinear system response represented by count rate saturation and dead time losses as the random rate increases in a quadratic fashion with the injected activity. Scatter fraction, as mentioned, is also nonnegligible, particularly in 3D imaging mode or in large patients. As a result, the response of the PET scanner versus the wide range of clinically relevant activity concentrations should be studied to determine the most operable range that allows for optimizing the injected dose.

A metric that allows accounting for factors that alter the observed count rate will be more likely an appropriate measure of the system count rate performance [60]. The noise-equivalent count rate (NECR) is the metric that reflects the ability of the scanner to measure true events while accounting for other interfering factors, such as dead time, scatter, and random events [72]. By plotting the NEC curve (see figure 11.14) the peak NEC that maximizes the ratio of true events with respect to other undesired events can be determined:

$$NEC = \frac{T^2}{S + T + kR}$$

where T, S, and R are the trues, scatter, and random rates, respectively; k is a constant that depends on the random estimate technique. It has a value of 2 when random correction is performed using online random subtraction (the estimate is noisy as in the delayed window subtraction method); otherwise, the value is 1 for the noise free estimate [73]. The NEC is a global measure of signal-to-noise ratio and does not reflect the regional count variation for a particular activity distribution.

The NEC can be used in acceptance testing procedures, comparing different protocols, imaging techniques, or acquisition modes (2D, 3D, or partial collimation) and as a figure of merit to optimize patient dose, but not as a direct or sole measure of lesion detectability, image quality, or overall system performance [74, 75].

To accommodate realistic conditions of clinical count rate measurements, the updated NEMA guidelines have replaced the 20×20 (diameter $\times$ length) phantom by a different one measuring 20×70 cm to account for the activity contributions arising from outside the field of view [73]. After calculating the trues, scatter, randoms, and NECRs and plotting them versus the activity concentrations, the peaks of true counting and NECRs are determined along with their corresponding activity concentrations. The peak NEC is the best estimate of the activity concentration that if met with an injected activity should reveal the best counting rate performance, better signal-to-noise ratio, and improved detectability.

11.4.4 Coincidence Timing Window

In the conventional gamma camera, the geometric angle of the collimator holes and septa determine the direction along which emitted photons are accepted. However, in PET imaging, an electronic timing window is used to determine the acceptance of the coincident events. The timing coincidence circuitry plays a significant role in the inclusion of coincidence events and in the rejection of other undesired events, such as randoms. The random rate is a function of the timing coincidence window; thus, a window width with a lower value allows a reduction of the random contribution to the total collected coincidences. This directly affects the count rate performance of the scanner such that the peak NECR can be increased by shortening the coincidence timing window. As stated, the fast new scintillators were key elements in designating scanners with a narrow timing window. An obvious application of these advances has been the production of TOF scanners [76].

To demonstrate the benefits of system timing resolution, a simulation study showed an apparent reduction of random rates as the coincidence timing window decreased, leading to an improvement in NECR measurements (see Fig. 11.14). The timing coincidence window can be a few nanoseconds (2–12 ns), as in many commercial PET scanners, to hundreds of picoseconds, as in systems equipped with TOF.

11.4.5 Time of Flight

Time of flight (TOF) is originally a biophysical phenomenon used by some mammals (e.g., bats) to determine the distance of objects. Similarly, in PET

a

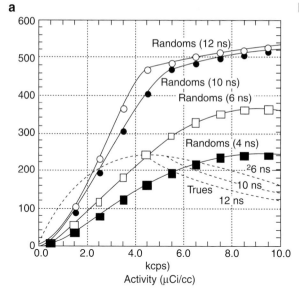

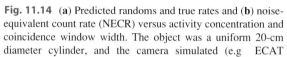

b

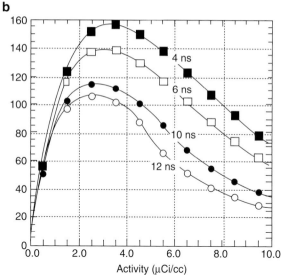

Fig. 11.14 (**a**) Predicted randoms and true rates and (**b**) noise-equivalent count rate (NECR) versus activity concentration and coincidence window width. The object was a uniform 20-cm diameter cylinder, and the camera simulated (e.g ECAT EXACT HR) has an 82 cm detector ring and 15 cm axial extent in 2D mode (with interplane septa). (From [76] © 2002 IEEE with permission)

imaging, TOF is a time-distance relationship through which the site of annihilation can be determined if the time difference of the arrival of the two coincident events can be measured. Incorporating the TOF information in the reconstruction process allows for precise localization of the emitted photons. It is simply demonstrated in Fig. 11.15. Without TOF, the annihilation site is equally likely to emanate from any point that lies along the LOR. In other words, TOF constrains this large distance (i.e., LOR) to a smaller value determined primarily by the time resolution capability of the scanner (see previous discussion). The simple formula $\Delta x = (1/2) c . \Delta t$ is used to define the distance that most probably confines the length along which annihilation took place. Δx is the error in position (positioning uncertainty), Δt is the error in the timing measurement, and c is the speed of light (3×10^8 m/s).

With an accurate measurement of the coincidence timing of the two 511-keV photons, the probability of the annihilation site could be assigned to a single point; thus, a 3D image can be obtained without reconstruction. In a PET scanner with timing resolution of $\Delta t = 6$ ns, the measurements of position error will extend along the whole diameter of the scanner because the calculated Δx would be 90 cm. Reducing the timing resolution, for instance, to 500 ps would

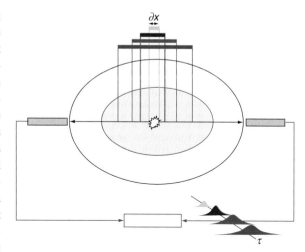

Fig. 11.15 Time of flight (TOF) can enhance the precision of localizing the positron emission along the line of response as a result of improving the timing resolution of the scanner. Scanners with relatively large coincidence window width have lower precision in event position determination (*blue* and *red bars*), while other systems manifested with better timing resolution serve to improve the probability of event localization, being best for systems with the lowest coincidence timing window (*black* and *green*)

allow reduction of the positioning uncertainty to 7.5 cm, a value that still cannot provide the full potential of using TOF in image reconstruction yet is able to reduce the statistical noise in the reconstructed image by limiting the propagation of noise to an area of smaller diameter represented by fewer reconstruction pixels in the image space [77, 78]. As a result, the gain obtained in image quality using TOF is therefore proportional to the object size and inversely proportional to the timing resolution of the system. Systems with TOF capability have the chance to improve the signal-to-noise ratio, reduce significantly the accidental random events, and are able to handle high count rates [78].

BaF$_2$ and CsF were used in the early generation of TOF systems, achieving a system timing resolution of 470–750 ps; use was mainly in research laboratories without commercial release of any practical tomograph [79]. Even though these scintillators are fast and provide excellent timing properties, they suffer from low photofraction and low light output, produce images with low spatial resolution, and have poor sensitivity compared to BGO-based scanners. The relatively recent introduction of LaBr$_3$ with its short decay time (16 ns), excellent energy resolution, and high light output has attracted some researchers to implement it in TOF applications, realizing a timing resolution of 460 ps with further improvement to 375 ps in a prototype TOF-based system [80, 81]. Moving from the research setting to the clinical arena with great effort made in detector technology, including new fast scintillators and data acquisition and reconstruction techniques, the first commercial TOF system was introduced in 2006 by Philips Company and had a timing resolution of 585 ps [27].

Experimental and patient evaluation studies reported fast convergence for high-contrast recovery coefficients with considerable benefits to small lesions and large patients [27]. Another feature of systems working with TOF is that it permits an injection of lower tracer activity into patients or reduces the imaging time while keeping the image properties fairly acceptable in comparison to non-TOF operating scanners [82].

11.4.6 Spatial Resolution

Spatial resolution is a crucial performance parameter of the PET imaging systems. Attempts are continuously carried out to improve the spatial resolution of PET images. Functional images acquired with poor spatial

resolution have several drawbacks, such as the likelihood of missing small metabolically active lesions, inaccurate quantitative measurements, and finally misdiagnosis. Factors affecting the resolution limits are detector size, positron range, and photon acollinearity in addition to other factors.

The spatial resolution of PET scanners is evaluated by measuring the FWHM of the point spread function. The FWHM can be parameterized as

$$ \text{FWHM} = \left(\sum_i^n R_i^2 \right)^{1/2} $$

By including as many parameters (i.e., n) as far as they affect image spatial resolution, this is most often written as

$$ \text{FWHM} \approx \sqrt{(d/2)^2 + b^2 + (0.0022D) + r^2} $$

where d is the detector width, b accounts for secondary components that contribute to spatial resolution loss in the photon detection process or spatial resolution loss due to block detector effect, the factor $(0.0022D)$ is the acollinearity associated with angular deviations from $180°$ and D is the detector ring diameter, and r^2 is a parameter related to positron range blurring effects.

The NEMA guidelines measure the spatial resolution of the PET scanner at different locations within the field of view using a small point source of ^{18}F, and the spatial resolution is determined by measuring the FWHM and FWTM of the resulting images. Image reconstruction is performed by filtered backprojection (FBP) with a ramp filter [73]. Figure 11.13b shows the spatial resolution of clinical and preclinical PET scanners in comparison to their SPECT counterparts.

Positron range is an unavoidable physical phenomenon, and some investigators suggested the use of a high magnetic field to reduce its impact on the resolution of the reconstructed images. However, this is an impractical approach due to the fact that PET/MRI is still not widely available and a limited magnetic field strength currently is applied in clinical PET/MRI scanners [83].

Fortunately, the most usable positron emitter, F-18, has a minimal positron range effect on the resolution of the reconstructed images. While efforts are often performed to improve scanner resolving capabilities, particularly for those of preclinical imaging and dedicated PET systems, an appropriate correction for the positron blurring effects would be essential to realize the full potential of the scanner spatial resolution. An intrinsic spatial resolution of 600 μm (0.6 mm, FWHM) has been achieved after successful fabrication of small-size LSO crystals (0.43 × 0.43 mm^2) for the purpose of developing high-resolution small-animal imaging systems [84, 85].

The incorporation of positron range effects in the system matrix of iterative reconstruction has been suggested and implemented to restore images degraded due to positron range [86, 87]. In radionuclides with a high positron range, it was found that the inclusion of positron range in the reconstruction process (i.e., maximum a posteriori (MAP)) was successful in restoring the spatial resolution of the images; however, long computation time was placed on data processing. The utility of iterative reconstruction in this regard lies in its ability to control the amount of noise in the Bayesian framework of MAP [87].

Deconvolution using the Fourier transform of the positron blurring effect was also proposed and was found useful in restoring the degraded images and improved activity quantitation, especially for positrons with high range, but this occurs at the cost of increased projection count uncertainty due to amplification of noise [88]. A residual correction method using a dual-matrix approach has been introduced to deal with the effects of positron range through the use of Monte Carlo simulation and a simplified system matrix. The method showed a trade-off between a complex system model and a simplified system matrix in terms of efficiency and model accuracy [89].

Acollinearity effects, as mentioned, are dependent on the detector diameter and hence are influential in PET systems with large transaxial dimension. Acollinearity resulting from positron-electron annihilation again can be included in the iterative scheme, and corrections can be obtained to reduce its effect. A reduction of ring diameter is necessary to geometrically control the phenomenon, and this will also improve the detection efficiency of the scanner; however, resolution measurements will be confounded by DOI errors. As a result, correction for the last phenomenon would serve to improve the resolution measurements and system sensitivity.

Detector size. A key instrumental factor that determines the intrinsic spatial resolution of the PET scanner is the crystal dimension *d*. For a point source located at mid-distance between two detectors in coincidence, the resultant FWHM is a convolution of the point spread function (PSF) of the two detectors and is equal to *d*/2. The geometrical response of these two opposing detectors is triangular at the center and worsens as the source moves closer to either of the detectors, yielding a trapezoidal shape as the object approaches the surface of the detector. This is in contrast with the gamma camera, for which distant objects exhibit lower spatial resolution than objects in close proximity to the detector surface.

Manufacturing small-size crystal arrays is technically challenging and costly. Small-crystal dimensions may also limit the amount of light that is received by the photodetector, thereby reducing energy and spatial resolution of the detected photons. However, the advent of new scintillators that showed better light output and improvements in cutting techniques have made the production of small-size crystals a successful process in improving detector resolution.

Most of the state-of-the-art PET/CT scanners use crystal sizes of 4–6 mm; however, in some dedicated brain scanners the crystal size is approximately 2 mm wide, such as in HRRT. Moreover, in small-animal imagers, the crystal dimension is typically 1–2 mm, with a recent development of a submillimeter version of LSO crystals as mentioned.

Detector size, positron range, and acollinearity are major factors that convolve to determine the fundamental resolution limit of the scanner. Another important resolution element that plays a significant role in the uniformity of the spatial resolution across the field of view is the DOI error or parallax error.

Parallax error. The geometric design of the block detectors and their arrangement in a circular fashion to form a closed ring has introduced another resolution-limiting element, parallax error. It results from the uncertainty of the depth of the interaction of the 511-keV photons within the crystal. This factor was described in the sensitivity section in the discussion about how PET scanners with small diameters can improve system sensitivity and how this will enhance image blurring, especially for events detected at the periphery. This degrading factor is also a concern in detector design with larger crystal thickness.

As the rays arising from the patient move away from the center field of view, there is a greater chance that rays detected in coincidence will produce a blurring error, affecting the resolution of the scanner. This blurring effect is shown in Fig. 11.16, in which photons arising from the center of the field of view do reach the detector pair in a direction normal to the crystal surface, while those photons shifted radially from the center fall on the detector pair with oblique angles, causing false determination of event position. As a result, data acquired without DOI correction suffer from an additional component of resolution degradation. It can reach 40% of the FWHM for a clinical system at 10 cm from the radius and increases linearly with further increase in the radial position of the annihilation site [90]. DOI errors also influence the spatial resolution of 3D imaging and thus place physical limits on increasing the axial extent of the PET scanner.

Approaches for depth encoding and parallax error correction are various and can be implemented using a bilayer (or more) of different scintillation crystals, applying two photodetectors, one at the entrance and one at the back side, or measuring the scintillation light distribution on position-sensitive photodetector array; or using a dual-ended photosensitive APD read-out scheme [91]. The former is implemented by using two scintillation crystals of different decay constants. Examples of commercially available scanners that use DOI correction are HRRT (LSO/LYSO, Siemens Medical solution) or the small-animal scanner eXplore (GE Healthcare), which uses LYSO/GSO stacked together, and the difference in their scintillation decay time is used to identify the DOI by analyzing the energy signal using pulse shape discrimination [92]. Proper correction for the phenomenon allows an opportunity for producing scanners with greater crystal thickness; hence, an improvement in system sensitivity can be realized.

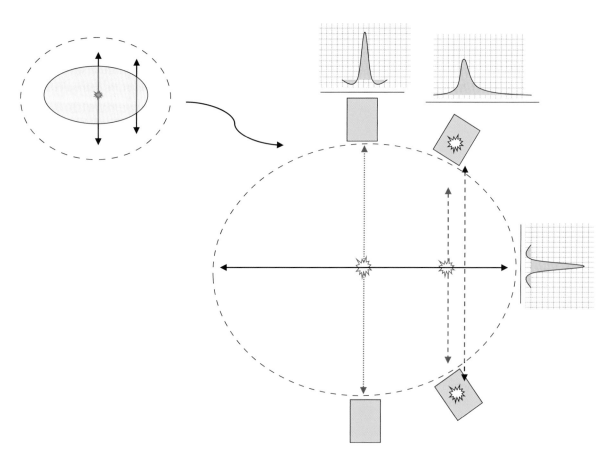

Fig. 11.16 Demonstrates the depth-of-interaction (DOI) error. Note that the intrinsic point spread function is broader and asymmetric when compared to a similar one from the center field of view

11.4.6.1 Other Factors

Data Sampling

Although PET scanners designed in cylindrical geometry provide better detection efficiency than other proposed geometries, they possess two fundamental problems regarding data sampling and spatial resolution. Events collected at the center of the field of view have the chance to fall perpendicularly on the detector pairs, with equal sampling intervals determined basically by the detector width. However, as the sampling moves radially toward the patient's periphery, the LORs are no longer equally spaced in comparison to rays arising from the center. The reconstruction algorithm, however, assumes a uniform sampling across the scanner field of view; therefore, a correction for such a problem is necessary. This correction is called *arc correction* and is of particular importance in objects with large dimensions for which the periphery is located a distance away from the center and in dedicated brain PET systems and small-animal scanners [93].

The discrete nature of the crystals in block detectors places physical limitations on the data-sampling regime and hence restrict the realization of the full potential of the resolving capabilities of the scanner. Linear and angular samplings are the two parameters that define the spatial resolution of the acquired images. The former is defined by the detector width, while the latter is determined by the number of detectors in the ring. Data undersampling is a reported resolution problem in the literature, and several data-sampling schemes were proposed to solve it. Wobbling motion of the detector array was implemented in some systems to compensate for information lost or the sampling inconsistency that occurs between the unevenly spaced LORs. Data interleaving between adjacent projection angles does help to reduce the effect of undersampling, and this occurs by interleaving the LORs of a given projection to the neighboring angle so that the resolution of the sampled data can reach the $d/2$ limits equivalent to the resolution of a detector pair in coincidence (Fig. 11.17). This interpolation process leads to increased linear sampling and reduction of angular sampling by a factor of 2 [10].

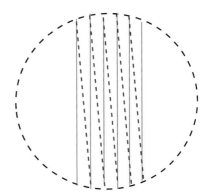

Fig. 11.17 Lines of response (*red lines*) for a given projection are interleaved to the adjacent projection angle (*blue lines*) so that linear sampling can reach the detector response $d/2$. This process yields an increment in the linear sampling by a factor of 2, while it reduces the angular intervals into half. For the purpose of reconstruction, the increased number of LORs mimic an additional detector inserted between the detector arrays

Reconstruction

The two major reconstruction methods in emission tomography are filtered backprojection and iterative reconstructions. As discussed in Chap. 13, FBP is an analytic approach that does not allow modeling the noise in the backprojection step during image reconstruction. However, iterative reconstructions outperform FBP in handling noise such that regions of low-activity concentrations can be reconstructed with better noise properties

Smoothing filters in FBP are essential to eliminate the drawbacks of the ramp filter and result in data with lower spatial resolution. In OSEM (Ordered Subset-Expectation Maximization), MLEM (Maximum Likelihood-Expectation Maximization) or iterative reconstruction, however, convergence depends on the size of the structure; thus, small lesions converge slower than other structures with large or different dimensions. This in turn produces metabolic information with variable resolution properties. At a high number of iterations, a postsmoothing filter is required to reduce the noise amplification during the iterative process and to improve visual quality. Consequently, the reconstruction algorithm and its parameters are influential in controlling the final spatial resolution of the reconstructed images. In FBP, a trade-off between noise and resolution should be maintained in selecting the cutoff frequency. However, the noise is signal dependent, and achieving a bias variance trade-off using this type of filtering is not particularly effective [94]. The number of subsets, number of iterations, and smoothing kernel in iterative reconstruction should also be optimized for a given detection task. Image restoration using Fourier filtering has been used to improve image spatial resolution; however, these filters produce different noise texture, require calculations of the system modulation transfer function, and its performance is based on the system resolution [95].

The most promising but technically challenging is to model the resolution elements in the system matrix of iterative reconstruction. Modeling the response function by measuring the system response for a large number of points across the transaxial and axial fields of view and incorporating this information in the system matrix can lead to an improvement of spatial resolution and noise properties of the reconstructed image [96]. The importance of improving the spatial resolution of the reconstructed images has several benefits, among which it serves to improve tracer quantitative accuracy, lesion contrast recovery, and reduction of partial volume effects (PVEs) [97, 98].

Another analytical approach modeling the effects of positron range, photon acollinearity, intercrystal scattering, and intercrystal penetration in Rb-82 myocardial perfusion images has been proposed such that individual analysis has been made for each of these effects and modeled in the reconstruction algorithm. An improvement in contrast, noise, and spatial resolution could be realized with an increase in the reconstruction time [99].

Partial volume. One of the practical consequences of the relatively low spatial resolution of PET scanners versus small structures is the PVE. This phenomenon has caught the attention of many researchers to develop correction techniques able to overcome bias in data measurements and to improve quantitative accuracy. As stated, the spatial resolution of a given scanner is determined by the FWHM of the point spread function. Tracer uptake or small structures that occupy an area smaller than the measured PSF would suffer from PVE provided that the measured value is less than thrice or twice the FWHM. This effect is a 3D problem and not only related to the size of the structures being measured but also involves

those voxels of the structure that contain signals from surrounding tissues or what is called the "spillover" effect. Count spillover from one tissue to another results from the fact that data are sampled by a discrete number of cells or "voxels," each of finite dimension, which causes imprecise distinction between tissue borders. The tissue fraction effect, on the other hand, reflects the underlying tissue heterogeneity (e.g., gray and white matter in the brain); therefore, coregistered anatomical information is particularly important in the correction procedure [100]. However, both effects sometimes are thought of as one phenomenon instead of two faces of the same coin. Data sampling is a digitized process and does not allow image voxels to realistically outline the actual activity distribution within different structures. As a result, the intensity of a particular voxel could be a mixture of counts measured from different and neighboring tissues. This process becomes more complicated if these tissues have different tracer uptake or different metabolic activities. An ideal correction method for PVE must therefore compensate for both effects together [101].

The PVE in PET imaging can be seen in a number of clinical situations, such as brain studies in which many cerebral structures are small in size and accurate quantitation requires a reliable correction of PVE. This is also important in oncologic FDG studies, in which small-size lesions suffer from biased quantitative accuracy demonstrated by altered standardized uptake value (SUV). In sequential studies in which response to therapy is assessed on a quantitative basis and tumor size is pursued with respect to its physical size, SUV values should be carefully interpreted unless an accurate technique has been applied to correct for PVE [102]. Another problem that is encountered in dealing with partial volume is when the lesion is located in or adjacent to a moving organ, such as the lung/heart or lung/liver interface.

In dynamic cardiac PET studies, the determination of myocardial blood flow necessitates correction for PVEs, which are represented by underestimation of myocardial wall thickness, inclusion of arterial or blood counts with the measurements of myocardial walls, and spillover that comes from neighboring walls or blood pool counts within the chamber. The inclusion of partial volume correction terms in the kinetic model has been implemented in many studies and was found successful in reducing the bias introduced in the measurements (see Chap. 17 for further discussion). Furthermore, a reconstruction-based partial volume correction using normalization and attenuation weighted OSEM was found to improve the spatial resolution and tracer kinetics outcome, leading to improved quantitative accuracy for brain PET imaging [103].

11.5 Data Corrections

PET images provide metabolic information about the tissue under investigation, and data obtained have several qualitative and quantitative features. The qualitative information is represented by images that reflect the spatial activity distribution within different biological tissues. The quantitative outcome, however, is numerical values on which one can reach more straightforward results and to some extent can reduce interobserver variability and increase reader confidence. Because of the importance of these measures that are taken from the PET images, system calibration and correction techniques are essential to satisfy the qualitative and quantitative tasks placed on the scanner.

NEMA acceptance testing is the first-line procedure recorded for scanner performance, and its measurements can be used as reference values for subsequent operations or calibrations needed for the scanner. NEMA-94 and NEMA-2001, in addition to the recent NEMA-2007, and the International Electrotechnical Commission (IEC) provide guidelines to those who are involved in accepting the machines as well those who are assigned to keep the device in a uniform mode of performance. Performance measures required by NEMA are spatial resolution, sensitivity, scatter fraction, count losses and random generation, image quality, accuracy of correction for scatter, dead time, randoms, and attenuation.

Daily performance tests are essential to check the stability of the system and to ensure day-to-day performance consistency. The scanner detectors are illuminated by a uniform source of activity (cylindrical phantom or rotating line source) to measure detector output regarding singles and coincidences, coincidence timing, dead time, and PMT gain and energy spectrum.

11.5.1 Normalization

In the gamma camera, a number of corrections are needed to verify that all PMTs have equal or nearly equal signal output when exposed to a uniform source of radiation. In a similar manner and to accurately measure the LORs in PET scanning with minimal electronic and geometric effects, a normalization test must be performed to account for variation in detector efficiency. This variability of detector sensitivity could arise from a number of sources, such as variations in solid angle and distance between detector pairs, electronic PMT drifts, and crystals with unequal efficiencies. Accurate normalization is essential to perform accurate quantification of data measurements, and improper normalization may result in artifacts, poor uniformity, and increased image noise.

One of the earliest methods devised to account for normalization was implemented by generating a normalization factor for each detector pair with respect to the averaged acquired counts across all LORs. This is a direct method, and its implementation is straightforward. However, it requires extended acquisition times to achieve adequate statistical accuracy. Also, it may produce biased results if the source does not have a uniform activity distribution or the scatter coincidences are dissimilar to real patient acquisition [104]. The situation is further complicated in 3D, for which the calibration procedure requires a low amount of activity to reduce dead time effects and normalization techniques able to account for scatter events as normalization factors are different for true and scatter coincidences. A number of source distributions have been used in detector normalization, such as uniform cylinder, planar source, and rotating line source. Iterative approaches have been proposed to treat the problem of normalization and methods based on scanner self-normalization [105–109].

Other approaches that account for system geometry and individual detector pair efficiency have been employed. One method is component-based normalization. Initially, it was suggested by dividing normalization factors into two major components, detector efficiency and spatial distortion [110]. This approach has resulted in a reduction of the total acquired counts and has been extended to normalize data acquired in fully 3D [111] and use of geometric means rather arithmetic means to calculate geometric factors.

Further modifications have been made by including crystal intrinsic efficiency as well as geometric factors such as the detector geometric profile and block detector interference [112, 113]. Other developments resulted in the inclusion of the time alignment factor and count-rate-dependent block profile [114, 115]. Systems operating in 2D and 3D modes are preferred to have separate normalization tests to account for geometric and different sensitivities that arise when septa are retracted or extended.

11.5.2 Dead Time

While a detector is busy handling and processing one event, it would not be able to process any further successive events during this time period. This phenomenon is called *dead time*. With the increased activity concentrations inside the object being investigated, particularly in 3D imaging mode, the probability of emitting a significant number of consecutive or simultaneous photons is relatively high when viewed and compared to lower-activity concentrations and when compared to 2D imaging. At high rates, the likelihood of pulse pileup is therefore increased because there is a higher chance that events that reach the detector are so close in time and thus the output signal would be their sum rather than an individual signal for each event. This process might lead to events whose amplitudes are greater than the upper energy threshold or signal amplitudes that fall within the energy window. The former events will be rejected while the latter will be accepted with false determination of position and energy [116]. As a result, the count rate performance of PET scanners toward increased activity concentrations is not a linear relation, especially at high activities, for which count losses and pulse pileup start to dominate. Ignoring dead time as a degrading factor of the acquired data results in loss of spatial resolution and signal-to-noise ratio and reduced quantitative accuracy.

The loss in effective sensitivity of the scanner (a quantitative performance parameter that combines between absolute sensitivity and NECR) showed the necessity of employing fast scintillators with high-performance electronics to realize the full potential of using septaless-volumetric 3D imaging over a wide dynamic range [117]. Hardware components that contribute to dead time in the event detection chain are front-end electronics, coincidence processing stage, and coincidence data transfer with more burden placed on the front end electronics component due to the increased signal multiplexing [116].

Because of these significant count rate increases, saturation in 3D imaging occurs at a lower activity level than if the scanner is operated in 2D mode. Fast scintillators coupled to electronics of high-speed signal processing serve to handle a large amount of data and are able to reduce dead time effects. Note the decay constant of BGO and NaI(Tl) versus GSO and LSO in Table 11.2. However, the specific tomograph construction and the associated electronic assembly together with the administered dose are the factors that determine the overall system count rate performance [118]. For instance, a significant improvement of the peak NECR was not realized when the LSO crystal was investigated in the PET scanner originally designed with electronics that match the BGO crystal until additional modifications were carried out on the coincidence timing window and some other electronic circuitry [119].

PET systems based on Anger logic large scintillation crystals tend to have limited count rate capability versus those scanners designed by block detector. Furthermore, the quadrant-sharing design presented also has higher dead time values when compared to the standard block design as the event readout is implemented by nine rather than four PMTs. Engineering approaches to improve count rate performance and to reduce pulse pileup have been developed, as have methods based on computer software [56, 57, 120]. Mathematical models for dead time have been proposed and classified mainly into paralyzable and nonparalyzable. The count rate response of the PET scanner can be modeled using these two different models, and determination of model parameters could then help to correct for count losses observed on the measured count rates.

11.5.3 Attenuation Correction

Attenuation correction is an important issue in SPECT and PET imaging and is discussed in Chap. 14. In our context here, however, one should list the advantage provided by x-ray CT over that given by radionuclide transmission imaging, which has been used for many years in clinical practice and research arena. The former technique is able to improve the statistical noise of the attenuation map to a significant degree, reducing noise propagation from the transmission data to the radionuclide distribution within tissues. The CT attenuation map is performed in a short time course as compared to radionuclide transmission scanning and thus provides an efficient mechanism for attenuation correction. This allows minimization of patient movement during the imaging session and leads to higher patient throughput. However, radionuclide transmission scanning has the same temporal characteristic of the emission acquisition; therefore, problems associated with high-speed CT scanning are absent. On the other hand, problems of source decay, maintenance, and replacement are not applicable to the x-ray transmission source, which is an additional advantage provided by CT transmission scanning. In PET imaging, radionuclide transmission using positron emitters (e.g., Ga68/Ge68) or single-photon emitters (Cs-137) were used to provide an attenuation map for the 511-keV emission images.

Because of the kinetic properties of the chest region due to respiration, it is the most frequent area where image fusion fails to register the two data sets. Respiratory motion is a problem in PET scanning based on CT attenuation correction, and several approaches were adopted to account for such a temporal mismatch. Different breathing protocols, respiratory gating (4D PET/CT), correlated dynamic PET techniques, list mode data-based techniques, modeling of the respiratory motion in iterative reconstruction, cine or averaged CT scanning, and other methods were proposed to resolve or mitigate this source of imaging artifacts.

Respiratory motion serves to blur the emission images and degrade the quantitative accuracy of radiotracer uptake. The degree of degradation depends on lesion size, location, and patient breathing pattern. This problem is more critical in pathological lesions that lie in a region that is near to a tissue interface, more specifically in the lower base of the right lung. In this particular site, diaphragmatic motion may develop cold artifacts in patients scheduled for PET/CT scanning. Further, a metastatic liver lesion might be misinterpreted and localized in lung tissue, misleading the diagnostic process. In cardiac PET studies, it has also been found that fast CT scanning may result in significantly altered FDG uptake within the myocardium, with it higher in myocardial segments located in close proximity to the lung-heart interface (i.e., anterior and lateral wall) (see Chap. 10 in the section on SPECT/CT).

CT-based attenuation correction has another drawback that should be discussed. The x-ray beam is polychromatic, meaning that it has a range of energies released from the tube, and the resulting spectrum depends on the tube voltage. This heterogeneity of the energy spectrum produces what is called a *beam-hardening effect*. As the rays pass through the different tissues toward the detector, there is a preferential occurrence for the low-energy photons to be absorbed in a greater amount than high-energy photons. This phenomenon is due to the fact that the probability of the photoelectric effect at low photon energies is higher, leading to an increase of the mean photon energy of the radiation beam. In turn, this causes some kind of heterogeneity for determination of the Hounsfield numbers of the same tissue. Therefore, attempts to correct beam hardening have been implemented in commercial CT scanners.

The fact that the CT numbers are derived from the effective x-ray energy requires a conversion step so that the calculated attenuation coefficients reflect the attenuation properties of the emission SPECT or PET radionuclides [121]. Methods developed to solve this problem have been segmentation, scaling, bilinear transformation, hybrid methods [122, 123], and others, whereas initial efforts have used single- or dual-energy CT to generate a transmission data set. Scaling techniques are used to convert the attenuation coefficients into the corresponding values of the radionuclide energy using a global attenuation coefficient ratio. An essential problem with this approach is the differences of photoelectric and Compton probabilities that occur as a result of energy differences, in particular for μ values generated by CT in bone structures, which are dominated by the photoelectric effect, while at higher energies the Compton effect dominates, resulting in large errors of the estimated attenuation coefficients for bone structures.

Segmentation is a process of classifying patient tissues based on their anatomical borders and outline from neighboring regions and hence provides a chance to separate and assign each individual segment its corresponding attenuation coefficient. These areas of the human body are typically air, bone, and soft tissue. The assumption that each anatomical region is homogeneous and has one μ value may be invalid in some

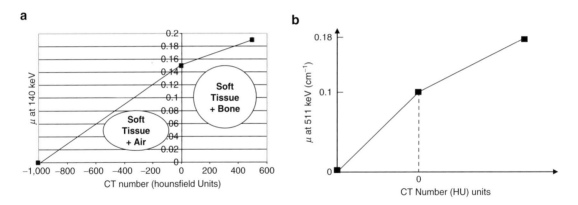

Fig. 11.18 Bilinear transformation curve used in computed tomographic (CT)-based attenuation correction in (**a**) single-photon emission computed tomography (SPECT) and in (**b**) positron emission tomography (PET)

anatomical regions, such as lung tissues, where investigators found a variability of tissue density that may reach 30% [124].

Bilinear transformation is a common method used in many commercial hybrid scanners and is based on experimental phantom measurements containing different concentrations of tissue-equivalent materials that could mimic biological tissue. These are air, water, and K_2HPO_4 bone-equivalent solutions prepared in clinically relevant concentrations. The linear attenuation coefficient of these materials, which are known, are plotted versus the CT numbers obtained from phantom studies acquired using the CT machine. The resulting plot is used as a calibration curve in estimating the attenuation map from the CT information obtained from a patient scan. The calibration curve has generally two distinct zones such that CT numbers below zero are combinations of air and soft tissue, while values greater than zero are combinations of bone and soft tissue [125, 126] (Fig. 11.18). However, the piecewise linear conversion method can be confounded by beam-hardening effects and in the presence of metallic implants or contrast agents, for which tissues of contrast uptake must be identified and properly corrected.

The CT images are characterized by high-resolution properties, and to use the same image as an attenuation map for images acquired with larger pixel dimensions (i.e., emission images), a pixel-matching procedure is performed by downsampling the CT images into larger pixel sizes. The pixel size of the CT images is commonly built on a matrix of 512×512, while the emission images are often 64×64 or 128×128. The

attenuation correction factors can then be included in the forward step of iterative reconstructions, as can be seen in attenuation-weighted OSEM reconstruction, yielding emission data of superior signal-to-noise ratio. Further, the CT images must be aligned with the emission image before correction to verify that an accurate attenuation correction and image correlation would be implemented. For the purpose of reducing dose levels delivered to the patient, a low-current CT scan can be performed for the sake of attenuation correction without compromising the accuracy of the attenuation factors.

11.5.4 Scatter Correction

As described in this chapter, one of the undesired effects that contaminate the total coincidence counts is scattered radiation. Many factors contribute to determine the proportion of scatter in clinical studies, such as the distribution of activity within the patient studied, composition and shape of the attenuating structures, as well as detector characteristics such as geometry of the imaging system, system energy resolution, and the pulse height window setting [127–131].

In 3D PET, the absence of septal collimation results in the acceptance of a large amount of scattered events, which can reach 50% or even more. Scattered events could arise from areas that lie out of plane and from regions located outside the field of view; both are important to account for in the correction scheme. Consequences of scattered events are increased image noise, reduced lesion contrast, and reduced quantitative accuracy. Accurate measures of SUV and reliable estimates of tracer kinetic parameters necessitate proper scatter correction. Many scatter correction approaches have been suggested and implemented in PET imaging, and some are similar to those used in SPECT imaging. Use of two, three, or more energy windows was proposed and implemented such that more than an energy window is used to record scattered and unscattered coincidences. The following are some correction methods used in research and clinical PET studies.

1. The dual-energy window (DEW) method is one of the simplest energy-based techniques that found application in both SPECT and PET scatter correction. One approach in the dual-energy method is to use two contiguous energy windows, one photo peak and another for scatter; both are assumed to have scattered as well as unscattered coincidences. Phantom measurements are used to generate scaling parameters of ratio measures of scattered and unscattered events in both energy windows. A scaled subtraction of the two energy windows is then performed to yield an estimate of the scatter distribution in the acquired patient data, which is then smoothed and subtracted from the data of the photo peak window [132].

2. An alternative approach to DEW is to use two overlapping energy windows, namely, a higher and a standard window, such that both have the same upper energy level, which is greater than 511 keV. The lower discriminator level for the higher-energy window is set at 511 keV, whereas the corresponding one for the standard window is positioned at energy below 511 keV. These energy settings allow for the calculation of the scattered coincidences by subtracting the data of the higher-energy window from that of the standard window, considering that the true unscattered estimate can be obtained from the higher-energy window. Subtraction results yield information about the distribution of scattered coincidences, which is then smoothed and subtracted from the standard energy window. Since this method seeks to measure the true unscattered events and utilize them in the estimation task, it is therefore called the estimation of trues method [131].

3. Another type of scatter correction is carried out by deconvolution or convolution subtraction. This type of correction technique has a number of variants in terms of whether the correction is applied on projection data or image space, the scatter response function (*srf*) used in the correction, and whether it is modeled as stationary or nonstationary [133–135].

(a) *In convolution subtraction*, the estimation task uses the photo peak data to extract the scatter component based on the assumption that the measured data are a combination of two components, which are scattered and unscattered events, in addition to a noise term [134]. Other components could also be included to account for different sources of photon scatter. Mckee et al. [135] used a Gaussian function to model the scatter response function in the backprojection space, assuming that the system is shift invariant with no considerations placed on the source position and the scatter object. The article published by Bailey and Meikle [134] showed that the scatter estimate can be computed by convolving the unscattered component with a *scatter function,* and the result is scaled by a *scatter fraction* and subtracted from the measured data. Because the unscattered component is unknown in advance, the convolution process can be carried out iteratively using the measured data as a first approximation of the unscattered component [134]. The two major requirements needed to execute deconvolution subtraction are the scatter function and the scatter fraction; the former defines the scatter distribution and the latter accounts for the magnitude of scatter. In the same study, the scatter function was modeled as monoexponential using a line source inserted in a cylindrical water phantom, while Mckee et al. used a point source to model the scatter function. The scatter function can also be estimated using Monte Carlo simulations.

(b) *In nonstationary assumptions*, the *srf* is considered to depend on the source position, object size, and detection angle. However, systems modeled as stationary are considered independent of such factors. In the former, nonstationary scatter correction kernels are generated based on phantom measurements for a line source at different locations within the field of view. The scatter kernels are then used to remove the scatter components in the image using the integral transform method [136]. Another approach uses a dual-exponential scatter kernel to remove the scatter effects of the object under investigation and scattered photons in the gantry and detectors [137].

Deconvolution filtering is a subclass in which the modulation transfer function of the system is used to restore the spatial resolution and to some extent scatter coincidences. This method has extensively been used in planar and SPECT imaging, and its drawback again stems from the shift invariance assumptions placed on using a single system point spread function.

4. Another approach that integrates the information of the reconstructed radioactivity distribution and transmission measurements into the scatter correction process has been implemented. It is called the model-based technique and relies on the physics of Compton scattering, such as photon energy, probability of the scattering angle, and attenuation properties of the scattering medium. Monte Carlo simulation demonstrated that most scattered photons that are detected in the photo peak window are single-scatter photons, and their percentage is within a range of 75–80%. This has made some investigators think of correcting the scatter based on single-scattered photons, and the distribution of multiple scatter can then be obtained by integral transformation of the single-scatter estimate [138].

For a given LOR, photon scatter is simulated through selected points distributed over the emission image and determined by the attenuation coefficients obtained from the transmission map. Using the emission image in the estimation procedure may produce a bias scatter estimate; however, this can be mitigated by incorporating the scatter estimate in the iterative reconstruction [139].

5. The single-scatter simulation approach has been pursued, and faster implementation was applied with advances in using the iterative reconstruction for the simulation images, as well as the iteration of the scatter calculation [140]. Further, extension of the algorithm was used in the TOF application, for which it can explicitly model the TOF of the annihilation photon pair along their individual scattered paths to produce an estimate of the scatter distribution for each time offset bin of the measured TOF.

However, this takes place with increased computation times [141].

Monte Carlo simulation has several features and capabilities in elucidating and characterizing the scattered versus unscattered photons in terms of magnitude and spatial distribution. Monte Carlo simulation is an efficient procedure to follow the history of photons from birth to death (emission of the positron, annihilation process, traveling distance before scattering, scattering interaction with the detector, or escaping from the gantry, etc.) and is able to account for other physical interactions as well as detector characteristics. This large numerical capability must be met by computers with high computation performance and fast processors to make its application feasible in practice. It is considered a gold standard for evaluating scatter correction techniques and can be used as a tool in the correction algorithm [129, 130]. More challenging is the development of Monte Carlo-based scatter correction techniques in 3D PET imaging that might be available in the near future in clinical workstations.

11.6 Conclusion

Positron emission tomography is an invaluable piece of medical technology that has demonstrated successful results in patient diagnosis and biomedical research. Scanner performance has changed significantly in the last decade due to the incorporation of new scintillators with better detection capabilities. Digital-processing technology, including fast electronics and high computation power, along with robust correction algorithms were milestones in the development of a new generation of PET scanners showing better performance characteristics. The new advances in these technologies have resulted in a reduction of the acquisition time, reduction of the injected dose, and an increase in scanner throughput. Diagnostic confidence and better clinical outcome were also remarkable. TOF adds benefits to the detectability of small lesions, imaging obese patients, and reduction of the injected dose. Fully diagnostic CT devices have been coupled to state-of-the-art PET scanners in hybrid PET/CT systems, leading to a significant change in image quality, data interpretation, and patient management.

References

1. Phelps MR (2000) PET: the merging of biology and imaging into molecular imaging. J Nucl Med 41(4):661–681
2. Tai YF, Piccini P (2004) Applications of positron emission tomography (PET) in neurology. J Neurol Neurosurg Psychiatry 75:669–676
3. Pichler BJ, Wehrl HF, Judenhofer MS (2008) Latest advances in molecular imaging instrumentation. J Nucl Med 49(Suppl 2):5S–23S
4. Blodgett TM, Meltzer CC, Townsend DW (2007) PET/CT: form and function. Radiology 242(2):360–385
5. Hany TF, Steinert HC, Goerres GW, Buck A, von Schulthess GK (2002) PET diagnostic accuracy: improvement with in-line PET-CT system: initial results. Radiology 225:575–581
6. Zaidi H, Mawlawi O, Orton CG (2007) Point/counterpoint. Simultaneous PET/MR will replace PET/CT as the molecular multimodality imaging platform of choice. Med Phys 34:1525–1528
7. Podgorsak EB (2005) Radiation physics for medical physicists. Springer, Berlin
8. Levin CS, Hoffman EJ (1999) Calculation of positron range and its effect on the fundamental limit of positron emission tomography system spatial resolution. Phys Med Biol 44:781–799, Corrigendum: Phys Med Biol 2000; 45:559
9. Sanchez-Crespo A, Andreo P, Larsson SA (2004) Positron flight in human tissues and its influence on PET image spatial resolution. Eur J Nucl Med Mol Imaging 31:44–51
10. Cherry SR, Sorenson JA, Phelps ME (2003) Physics in nuclear medicine. Saunders, Philadelphia
11. Anger HO (1958) Scintillation camera. Rev Sci Instrum 29:27–33
12. Budinger TF (1998) PET instrumentation: what are the limits? Semin Nucl Med 28(3):247–267
13. Ruhlmann J, Oehr P, Biersack H-J (2000) PET in oncology. Springer, Berlin
14. Peschina W, Conca A, König P, Fritzsche H, Beraus W (2001) Low frequency rTMS as an add-on antidepressive strategy: heterogeneous impact on 99mTc-HMPAO and 18 F-FDG uptake as measured simultaneously with the double isotope SPECT technique. Pilot study. Nucl Med Commun 22(8):867–873
15. Sandler MP, Videlefsky S, Delbeke D, Patton JA, Meyerowitz C, Martin WH, Ohana I (1995) Evaluation of myocardial ischemia using a rest metabolism/stress perfusion protocol with fluorine-18 deoxyglucose/technetium-99m MIBI and dual-isotope simultaneous-acquisition single-photon emission computed tomography. J Am Coll Cardiol 26:870–878
16. Laymon CM, Turkington TG (2006) Characterization of septal penetration in 511 keV SPECT. Nucl Med Commun 27(11):901–909
17. Turkington TG (2001) Introduction to PET instrumentation. J Nucl Med Technol 29(1):4–11, Erratum: J Nucl Med Technol 2002, 30(2):63
18. Lonneux M, Delval D, Bausart R, Moens R, Willockx R, Van Mael P, Declerck P, Jamar F, Zreik H, Pauwels S (1998) Can dual-headed 18F-FDG SPET imaging reliably supersede PET in clinical oncology? A comparative study in lung and gastrointestinal tract cancer. Nucl Med Commun 19(11):1047–1054
19. Bergmann H, Dobrozemsky G, Minear G, Nicoletti R, Samal M (2005) An inter-laboratory comparison study of image quality of PET scanners using the NEMA NU 2-2001 procedure for assessment of image quality. Phys Med Biol 50(10):2193–2207
20. Kadrmas DJ, Christian PE (2002) Comparative evaluation of lesion detectability for 6 PET imaging platforms using a highly reproducible whole-body phantom with (22)Na lesions and localization ROC analysis. J Nucl Med 43 (11):1545–1554
21. Bailey DL, Young H, Bloomfield PM et al (1997) ECAT ART: a continuously rotating PET camera-performance characteristics, initial clinical studies and installation considerations in a nuclear medicine department. Eur J Nucl Med 24:6–15
22. Beyer T, Townsend DW, Brun T et al (2000) A combined PET/CT scanner for clinical oncology. J Nucl Med 41:1369–1379
23. Karp JS, Muehllehner G, Mankoff DA et al (1990) Continuous-slice PENN-PET: a positron tomograph with volume imaging capability. J Nucl Med 31:617–627
24. Surti S, Karp JS (2004) Imaging characteristics of a 3-dimensional GSO whole-body PET camera. J Nucl Med 45:1040–1049
25. Adam LE, Karp JS, Daube-Whitherspoon ME, Smith RJ (2001) Performance of a whole-body PET scanner using curve-plate NaI(Tl) detectors. J Nucl Med 42:1821–1830
26. Karp JS, Surti S, Daube-Witherspoon ME et al (2003) Performance of a brain PET camera based on Anger-logic gadolinium oxyorthosilicate detectors. J Nucl Med 44:1340–1349
27. Surti S, Kuhn A, Werner ME, Perkins AE, Kolthammer J, Karp JS (2007) Performance of Philips Gemini TF PET/CT scanner with special consideration for its time-of-flight imaging capabilities. J Nucl Med 48(3):471–480
28. Surti S, Karp JS, Freifelder R, Liu F (2000) Optimizing the performance of a PET detector using discrete GSO crystals on a continuous lightguide. IEEE Trans Nucl Sci 47:1030–1036
29. de Jong HW, van Velden FH, Kloet RW, Buijs FL, Boellaard R, Lammertsma AA (2007) Performance evaluation of the ECAT HRRT: an LSO-LYSO double layer high resolution, high sensitivity scanner. Phys Med Biol 52:1505–1526
30. Phelps ME (2002) Molecular imaging with positron emission tomography. Annu Rev Nucl Part Sci 52:303–338
31. Lewellen TK (2008) Recent developments in PET detector technology. Phys Med Biol 53(17):R287–R317
32. Knoll GF (2000) Radiation detection and measurement, 3rd edn. Wiley, New Work
33. Humm JL, Rosenfeld A, Del Guerra A (2003) From PET detectors to PET scanners. Eur J Nucl Med Mol Imaging 30(11):1574–1597
34. Melcher CL (2000) Scintillation crystals for PET. J Nucl Med 41:1051–1055

35. van Eijk CW (2002) Inorganic scintillators in medical imaging. Phys Med Biol 47(8):R85–R106

36. Surti S, Karp JS (2005) A count-rate model for PET scanners using pixelated Anger-logic detectors with different scintillators. Phys Med Biol 50(23):5697–5715

37. Karp JS (2002) Is LSO the future of PET? against. Eur J Nucl Med Mol Imaging 29:1525–1528

38. Teräs M, Tolvanen T, Johansson JJ, Williams JJ, Knuuti J (2007) Performance of the new generation of whole-body PET/CT scanners: discovery STE and discovery VCT. Eur J Nucl Med Mol Imaging 34(10):1683–1692

39. Martínez MJ, Bercier Y, Schwaiger M, Ziegler SI (2006) PET/CT Biograph Sensation 16. Performance improvement using faster electronics. Nuklearmedizin 45 (3):126–133

40. Bloomfield PM et al (1995) The design and physical characteristics of a small animal positron emission tomograph. Phys Med Biol 40:1105–1126

41. Yamamoto S, Kuroda K, Senda M (2003) Scintillator selection for MR-compatible gamma detectors. IEEE Trans Nucl Sci 50:1683–1685

42. Cherry S (2006) The 2006 Henry N. Wagner lecture: of mice and men (and positrons) – advances in PET imaging technology. J Nucl Med 47(11):1735–1745

43. Nutt R (2002) For: is LSO the future of PET? Eur J Nucl Med Mol Imaging 29(11):1523–1525

44. Wienhard K et al (2002) The ECAT HRRT: performance and first clinical application of the new high resolution research tomograph. IEEE Trans Nucl Sci 49:104–110

45. Doshi NK, Shao Y, Silverman RW, Cherry SR (2000) Design and evaluation of an LSO PET detector for breast cancer imaging. Med Phys 27(7):1535–1543

46. Cherry SR et al (1997) MicroPET: a high resolution PET scanner for imaging small animals. IEEE Trans Nucl Sci 44:1161–1166

47. Lonneux M, Borbath I, Bol A, Coppens A, Sibomana M, Bausart R, Defrise M, Pauwels S, Michel C (1999) Attenuation correction in whole-body FDG oncological studies: the role of statistical reconstruction. Eur J Nucl Med 26 (6):591–598

48. Zanzonico P (2004) Positron emission tomography: a review of basic principles, scanner design and performance, and current systems. Semin Nucl Med 34:87–111

49. Casey ME, Nutt R (1986) A multicrystal two dimensional BGO detector system for positron emission tomography. IEEE Trans Nucl Sci 33(1):460–463

50. Tai YC, Laforest R (2005) Instrumentation aspects of animal PET. Annu Rev Biomed Eng 7:255–285

51. Pichler BJ, Swann BK, Rochelle J, Nutt RE, Cherry SR, Siegel SB (2004) Lutetium oxyorthosilicate block detector readout by avalanche photodiode arrays for high resolution animal PET. Phys Med Biol 49(18):4305–4319

52. Surti S, Karp JS, Kinahan PE (2004) PET instrumentation. Radiol Clin North Am 42(6):1003–1016

53. Ziegler SI, Pichler BJ, Boening G, Rafecas M, Pimpl W, Lorenz E, Schmitz N, Schwaiger M (2001) A prototype high-resolution animal positron tomograph with avalanche photodiode arrays and LSO crystals. Eur J Nucl Med 28 (2):136–143

54. Muehllehner G, Karp JS (2006) Positron emission tomography. Phys Med Biol 51(13):R117–R137, 2006

55. Wong W, Uribe J, Hicks K, Hu G (1995) An analog decoding BGO block detector using circular photomultipliers. IEEE Trans Nucl Sci 42:1095–1101

56. Wong WH, Li H, Uribe J, Baghaei H, Wang Y, Yokoyama S (2001) Feasibility of a high-speed gamma-camera design using the high-yield-pileup-event-recovery method. J Nucl Med 42(4):624–632

57. Liu J, Li H, Wang Y, Kim S, Zhang Y, Liu S, Baghaei H, Ramirez R, Wong W (2007) Real time digital implementation of the high-yield-pileup-event-recover (HYPER) method. IEEE Nucl Sci Symp Conf Rec 4230–4232

58. Bailey DL (2006) Data acquisition and performance characterization in PET. In: Bailey DL, Townsend DW, Valk PE, Maisey MN (eds) Positron emission tomography: basic sciences. Springer, London

59. Meikle SR, Badawi RD (2006) Quantitative techniques in PET. In: Bailey DL, Townsend DW, Valk PE, Maisey MN (eds) Positron emission tomography: basic sciences. Springer, London

60. Lewellen T, Karp J (2004) PET systems. In: Wernick M, Aarsvold J (eds) Emission tomography: the fundamentals of PET and SPECT. Elsevier Academic, San Diego

61. Badawi RD, Miller MP, Bailey DL, Marsden PK (1999) Randoms variance reduction in 3D PET. Phys Med Biol 44 (4):941–954

62. Wong WH (1988) PET camera performance design evaluation for BGO and BaF2 scintillators (non-time-of-flight). J Nucl Med 29(3):338–347

63. Schmitz RE, Kinahan PE, Harrison RL, Stearns CW, Lewellen TK (2005) Simulation of count rate performance for a PET scanner with different degrees of partial collimation. IEEE Nucl Sci Symp Conf Rec 23–29 Oct. 2005, 2506–2509

64. Schmand M et al (1998) Performance results of a new DOI detector block for a high resolution PET-LSO research tomograph HRRT. IEEE Trans Nucl Sci 45:3000–3006

65. Townsend DW (2008) Positron emission tomography/ computed tomography. Semin Nucl Med 38(3):152–166, Review

66. Townsend DW (2008) Multimodality imaging of structure and function. Phys Med Biol 53(4):R1–R39

67. Habte F, Foudray AMK, Olcott PD et al (2007) Effects of system geometry and other physical factors on photon sensitivity of high-resolution positron emission tomography. Phys Med Biol 52:3759–3772

68. Conti M, Bendriem B, Casey M, Eriksson L, Jackoby B, Jones WF, Michel C (2005) Performance of a high sensitivity PET scanner based on LSO panel detectors. Nucl Sci Symp Conf Rec 5:2501–2505

69. Dhawan V, Kazumata K, Robeson W, Belakhlef A, Margouleff C, Chaly T, Nakamura T, Dahl R, Margouleff D, Eidelberg D (1998) Quantitative brain PET. Comparison of 2D and 3D acquisitions on the GE advance scanner. Clin Positron Imaging 1:135–144

70. Bailey DL, Miller MP, Spinks TJ, Bloomfield PM, Livieratos L, Young HE, Jones T (1998) Experience with fully 3D PET and implications for future high-resolution 3D tomographs. Phys Med Biol 43(4):777–786

71. Everaert H, Vanhove C, Lahoutte T, Muylle K, Caveliers V, Bossuyt A, Franken PR (2003) Optimal dose of 18F-

FDG required for whole-body PET using an LSO PET camera. Eur J Nucl Med Mol Imaging 30 (12):1615–1619

72. Strother SC, Casey ME, Hoffman EJ (1990) Measuring PET scanner sensitivity: relating count rates to image signal-to-noise ratios using noise equivalent counts. IEEE Trans Nucl Sci 37:783–788

73. Daube-Witherspoon ME, Karp JS, Casey ME et al (2002) PET performance measurements using the NEMA NU 2–2001 standard. J Nucl Med 43:1398–1409

74. Badawi RD, Dahlbom M (2005) NEC: some coincidences are more equivalent than others. J Nucl Med 46(11):1767–1768

75. Lartizien C, Comtat C, Kinahan PE et al (2002) Optimization of the injected dose based on noise equivalent count rates for 2- and 3-dimensional whole-body PET. J Nucl Med 43:1268–1278

76. Moses WW (2002) Advantages of improved timing accuracy in PET cameras using LSO scintillator. IEEE Nucl Sci Symp Conf Rec 3:1670–1675

77. Budinger TF (1983) Time-of-flight positron emission tomography: status relative to conventional PET. J Nucl Med 24:73–78

78. Moses WW (2003) Time of flight in PET revisited. IEEE Trans Nucl Sci NS-50:1325–1330

79. Conti M (2009) State of the art and challenges of time-of-flight. PET Phys Med 25(1):1–11

80. Kyba CCM, Wiener RI, Newcomer FM, Perkins AE, Kulp RR, Werner ME, Surti S, Dressnandt N, Van Berg R, Karp JS (2008) Evaluation of local PMT triggering electronics for a TOF-PET scanner. IEEE Nuclear Science Symposium and Medical Imaging Conf. Record (Dresden, Germany, 2008) Sellin P (ed)

81. Daube-Witherspoon ME, Surti S, Perkins A, Kyba CC, Wiener R, Werner ME, Kulp R, Karp JS (2010) The imaging performance of a LaBr3-based PET scanner. Phys Med Biol 55(1):45–64

82. Karp JS, Surti S, Dube-Witherspoon ME, Muehllehner G (2008) Benefit of time-of-flight in PET: experimental and clinical results. J Nucl Med 49:462–470

83. Rahmim A, Zaidi H (2008) PET versus SPECT: strengths, limitations and challenges. Nucl Med Commun 29(3):193–207

84. Stickel JR, Qi J, Cherry SR (2007) Fabrication and characterization of a 0.5-mm lutetium oxyorthosilicate detector array for high-resolution PET applications. J Nucl Med 48:115–121

85. Stickel JR, Cherry SR (2005) High-resolution PET detector design: modeling components of intrinsic spatial resolution. Phys Med Biol 50:179–195

86. Palmer MR, Zhu X, Parker JA (2005) Modeling and simulation of positron range effects for high resolution PET imaging. IEEE Trans Nucl Sci 52:1391–1395

87. Ruangma A, Bai B, Lewis JS, Sun X, Michael JW, Leahy R, Laforest R (2006) Three-dimensional maximum a posteriori (MAP) imaging with radiopharmaceutical labeled with three Cu radionuclides. Nucl Med Biol 33:217–226

88. Derenzo SE (1986) Mathematical removal of positron range blurring in high resolution tomography. IEEE Trans Nucl Sci 33(1):565–569

89. Fu L, Qi J (2010) A residual correction method for high-resolution PET reconstruction with application to on-the-fly Monte Carlo based model of positron range. Med Phys 37(2):704–713

90. Levin CS, Zaidi H (2007) Current trends in preclinical PET system design. PET Clin 2:125–160

91. Yang Y, Wu Y, Qi J, St James S, Du H, Dokhale PA, Shah KS, Farrell R, Cherry SR (40) A prototype PET scanner with DOI-encoding detectors. J Nucl Med 49(7):1132

92. Wang Y, Seidel J, Tsui BMW, Vaquero JJ, Pomper MG (2006) Performance evaluation of the GE Healthcare eXplore VISTA dual-ring small-animal PET scanner. J Nucl Med 47:1891–1900

93. Fahey FH (2002) Data acquisition in PET imaging. J Nucl Med Technol 30(2):39–49

94. Qi J, Leahy RM (2006) Iterative reconstruction techniques in emission computed tomography. Phys Med Biol 51(15):R541–R578

95. Links JM, Leal JP, Mueller-Gaertner HW, Wagner HN Jr (1992) Improved positron emission tomography quantification by Fourier-based restoration filtering. Eur J Nucl Med 19(11):925–932

96. Panin VY, Kehren F, Michel C, Casey M (2006) Fully 3-D PET reconstruction with system matrix derived from point source measurements. IEEE Trans Med Imaging 25:907–921

97. Varrone A, Sjöholm N, Eriksson L, Gulyás B, Halldin C, Farde L (2009) Advancement in PET quantification using 3D-OP-OSEM point spread function reconstruction with the HRRT. Eur J Nucl Med Mol Imaging 36(10):1639–1650

98. Sureau FC, Reader AJ, Comtat C, Leroy C, Ribeiro MJ, Buvat I et al (2008) Impact of image-space resolution modeling for studies with the high-resolution research tomograph. J Nucl Med 49:1000–1008

99. Rahmim A, Tang J, Lodge MA, Lashkari S, Ay MR, Lautamäki R, Tsui BM, Bengel FM (2008) Analytic system matrix resolution modeling in PET: an application to Rb-82 cardiac imaging. Phys Med Biol 53(21):5947–5965

100. Aston JA, Cunningham VJ, Asselin MC, Hammers A, Evans AC, Gunn RN (2002) Positron emission tomography partial volume correction: estimation and algorithms. J Cereb Blood Flow Metab 22(8):1019–1034

101. Soret M, Bacharach SL, Buvat I (2007) Partial-volume effect in PET tumor imaging. J Nucl Med 48(6):932–945

102. Boellaard R, Krak NC, Hoekstra OS, Lammertsma AA (2004) Effects of noise, image resolution, and ROI definition on the accuracy of standard uptake values: a simulation study. J Nucl Med 45(9):1519–1527

103. Mourik JE, Lubberink M, van Velden FH, Kloet RW, van Berckel BN, Lammertsma AA, Boellaard R (2010) In vivo validation of reconstruction-based resolution recovery for human brain studies. J Cereb Blood Flow Metab 30(2):381–389

104. Ollinger JM (1995) Detector efficiency and compton scatter in fully 3D PET. IEEE Trans Nucl Sci 42:1168–1173

105. Badawi RD, Marsden PK (1999) Self-normalization of emission data in 3D PET. IEEE Trans Nucl Sci 46:709–712

106. Zhang Y, Li H, Baghaei H, Liu S, Ramirez R, An A, Wang C, Wong W (2008) A new self-normalization method for PET. J Nucl Med 49(Suppl 1):62

107. Bai B, Li Q, Holdsworth CH, Asma E, Tai YC, Chatziioannou A, Leahy RM (2002) Model-based normalization for iterative 3D PET image reconstruction. Phys Med Biol 47(15):2773–2784

108. Hermansen F, Spinks TJ, Camici PG, Lammertsma AA (1997) Calculation of single detector efficiencies and extension of the normalization sinogram in PET. Phys Med Biol 42:1143–1154

109. Ishikawa A, Kitamura K, Mizuta T, Tanaka K, Amano M (2004) Self normalization for continuous 3D whole body emission data in 3D PET. IEEE Trans Nucl Sci 6:3634–3637

110. Hoffman EJ, Guerrero TM, Germano G, Digby WM, Dahlbom M (1989) PET system calibrations and corrections for quantitative and spatially accurate images IEEE Trans Nucl Sci 36:1108–1112

111. Defrise M, Townsend D, Bailey D, Geissbuhler A, Michel C, Jones T (1991) A normalization technique for 3D. PET data. Phys Med Biol 36:939–952

112. Casey ME, Gadagkar H, Newport D (1995) A component based method for normalization in volume PET. In: Proceedings of the 3rd International Meeting Fully Three-Dimensional Image Reconstruction in Radiology and Nuclear Medicine. Aix-les-Bains, France, pp 67–71

113. Kinahan PE, Townsend DW, Bailey DL, Sashin D, Jadali F, Mintun MA (1995) Efficiency normalization technique for 3D PET data. In: Proceeding of the IEEE Nuclear Science Symposium and Medical Imaging Conference Recording, vol 2, pp 21–28

114. Badawi RD, Marsden PK (1999) Developments in component-based normalization for 3D PET. Phys Med Biol 44:571–594

115. Badawi RD, Ferreira NC, Kohlmyer SG, Dahlbom M, Marsden PK, Lewellen TK (2000) A comparison of normalization effects on three whole-body cylindrical 3D PET systems. Phys Med Biol 45:3253–3266

116. Germano G, Hoffman EJ (1990) A study of data loss and mispositioning due to pileup in 2-D detectors in PET. IEEE Trans Nucl Sci 37(2):671–675

117. Bailey DL, Meikle SR, Jones T (1997) Effective sensitivity in 3D PET: the impact of detector dead time on 3D system performance. IEEE Trans Nucl Sci NS–44:1180–1185

118. Spinks TJ, Bloomfield PM (2002) A comparison of count rate performance for ^{15}O-water blood flow studies in the CTI HR + and Accel tomographs in 3D mode. Nuclear Science Symposium Conference Record, 2002 IEEE vol 3, 10–16 November 2002, pp 1457–1460

119. Moisan C, Rogers JG, Douglas JL (1997) A count-rate model for PET and its application to an LSO HR plus scanner. IEEE Trans Nucl Sci 44:1219–1224

120. Wong WH, Li H (1998) A scintillation detector signal processing technique with active pileup prevention for extending scintillation count rates. IEEE Trans Nucl Sci 45(3):838–842

121. Blankespoor SC, Xu X, Kaiki BKJK, Tang HR, Cann CE et al (1996) Attenuation correction of SPECT using x-ray CT on an emission-transmission CT system: myocardial perfusion assessment. IEEE Trans Nucl Sci 43:2263–2274

122. Kinahan PE, Townsend DW, Beyer T, Sashin D (1998) Attenuation correction for a combined 3D PET/CT scanner. Med Phys 25:2046–2053

123. Burger C, Goerres G, Schoenes S, Buck A, Lonn AHR, Von Schulthess GK (2002) PET attenuation coefficients from CT images: experimental evaluation of the transformation of CT into PET 511-keV attenuation coefficients. Eur J Nucl Med Mol Imaging 29:922–927

124. Bénard F, Smith RJ, Hustinx R, Karp JS, Alavi A (1999) Clinical evaluation of processing techniques for attenuation correction with 137Cs in whole-body PET imaging. J Nucl Med 40(8):1257–1263

125. Bai C, Shao L, Da Silva AJ et al (2003) A generalized model for the conversion from CT numbers to linear attenuation coefficients. IEEE Trans Nucl Sci 50:1510–1515

126. Seo Y, Mari C, Hasegawa BH (2008) Technological development and advances in single-photon emission computed tomography/computed tomography. Semin Nucl Med 38(3):177–198

127. Thompson CJ (1993) The problem of scatter correction in positron volume imaging. IEEE Trans Med Imaging MI-12:124–132

128. Lercher MJ, Wienhard K (1994) Scatter correction in 3D PET. IEEE Trans Med Imaging 13:649–657

129. Adam L-E, Belleman ME, Brix G, Lorenz WJ (1996) Monte Carlo based analysis of PET scatter components. J Nucl Med 37:2024–2029

130. Zaidi H, Koral KF (2004) Scatter modelling and compensation in emission tomography. Eur J Nucl Med Mol Imaging 31(5):761–782

131. Bailey DL (1998) Quantitative procedures in 3D PET. In: Bendriem B, Townsend DW (eds) The theory and practice of 3D PET. Kluwer Academic, Dordrecht, pp 55–109

132. Grootoonk S, Spinks TJ, Sashin D, Spyrou NM, Jones T (1996) Correction for scatter in 3D brain PET using a dual energy window method. Phys Med Biol 41:2757–2774

133. Bentourkia M, Lecomte R (1999) Energy dependence of nonstationary scatter subtraction-restoration in high resolution PET. IEEE Trans Med Imaging 18:66–73

134. Bailey DL, Meikle SR (1994) A convolution-subtraction scatter correction method for 3D PET. Phys Med Biol 39:411–424

135. McKee BA, Gurvey AT, Harvey PJ, Howse DC (1992) A deconvolution scatter correction for a 3-D PET system. IEEE Trans Med Imaging 11(4):560–569

136. Bergström M, Eriksson L, Bohm C, Blomqvist G, Litton J (1983) Correction for scattered radiation in a ring detector positron camera by integral transformation of the projections. J Comput Assist Tomogr 7(1):42–50

137. Lubberink M, Kosugi T, Schneider H, Ohba H, Bergström M (2004) Non-stationary convolution subtraction scatter correction with a dual-exponential scatter kernel for the Hamamatsu SHR-7700 animal PET scanner. Phys Med Biol 49(5):833–842

138. Ollinger JM (1996) Model-based scatter correction for fully 3D PET. Phys Med Biol 41:153–176

139. Watson CC (2000) New, faster, image-based scatter correction for 3D PET. IEEE Trans Nucl Sci 47:1587–1594

140. Watson CC, Casey ME, Michel C, Bendriem B (2004) Advances in scatter correction for 3D PET/CT. IEEE Nucl Sci Symp Conf Rec 5:3008–3012

141. Watson C (2007) Extension of single scatter simulation to scatter correction of time-of-flight PET. IEEE Trans Nucl Sci 54(5):1679–1686
142. Lecomte R (2009) Eur J Nucl Med Mol Imaging 36 (Suppl 1):S69–S85
143. Jansen FP, Vanderheyden JL (2007) Nucl Med Biol 34:733–735
144. Moses WW, Derenzo SE (1996) Proceedings of SCINT '95 (Edited by P. Dorenbos and C. W. E. v. Eijk), Delft, The Netherlands, pp. 9–16. (LBNL-37720). With permission from William Moses, Lawrence Berkeley Lab, USA).
145. Melcher CL, Schweitzer JS (1992) Ceruim-doped lutetium orthosilicate: A fast, efficient new scintillator. IEEE Trans Nucl Sci 39:502–505

Part IV

Image Analysis, Reconstruction and Quantitation in Nuclear Medicine

Fundamentals of Image Processing in Nuclear Medicine

12

C. David Cooke, Tracy L. Faber, and James R. Galt

Contents

12.1 Learning Objectives

The purpose of this chapter is to introduce the reader to the fundamentals of image processing in Nuclear Medicine. It is not meant as a comprehensive guide, but more as an overview and introduction to those topics important to understanding the various forms of image processing. At the conclusion of this chapter, it is hoped that the reader will be able to briefly describe the following:

1. The history of imaging in Nuclear Medicine.
2. The components and processes necessary for generating an image.
3. Spatial resolution and how to calculate it.
4. Image interpolation.
5. How images are converted to color and displayed.
6. Image filtering and its effect on images, as well as have a working knowledge of the two most common filters in Nuclear Medicine.
7. The Fourier Transform and its use in nuclear medicine.
8. The process of analyzing regions of interest.
9. Different ways of segmenting images to extract useful information.
10. Different ways of generating and displaying three-dimensional images.
11. The principles of image registration.
12. The importance of image normalization.

12.2 Introduction

Most Nuclear Medicine procedures are, by their very nature, image-oriented. As early as 1950, printed images of the Thyroid, using I-131, could be obtained

C.D. Cooke (✉), T.L. Faber, and J.R. Galt
Emory University School of Medicine, Atlanta, GA, USA

M.M. Khalil (ed.), *Basic Sciences of Nuclear Medicine*, DOI: 10.1007/978-3-540-85962-8_12,
© Springer-Verlag Berlin Heidelberg 2011

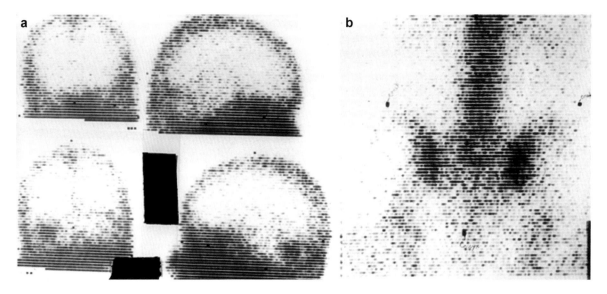

Fig. 12.1 Early rectilinear scans. (**a**) Brain perfusion scan (note defect in bottom left and bottom right images). (**b**) Bone scan (three markers can be seen delineating the left and right iliac crests and the coccyx) (Images courtesy of Naomi Alazraki, MD, Emory University and VA Medical Center, Atlanta, GA)

using the rectilinear scanner developed by Benedict Cassen [1] (see Fig. 12.1). In 1958, the Anger scintillation camera [2], developed by Hal Anger, could be used to image an entire organ at one time; and by 1963, Kuhl and Edwards were using the Anger camera to produce tomographic images [3]. It has been over 50 years since Hal Anger's initial developments, and the traditional gamma camera remains largely unchanged, though now, most have better electronics resulting in increased sensitivity, spatial resolution, energy resolution, and stability. Space will not permit for a detailed history of the gamma camera; however, those who are interested might enjoy the article by Ronald Jaszczak [4].

Today, Nuclear Medicine images are acquired and stored on computers, making the data easily accessible and readily available for further processing and quantification. The goal of this chapter is to familiarize the reader with the basic fundamental techniques of image processing, and specifically, those techniques most useful in Nuclear Medicine.

12.3 Image Presentation

12.3.1 Analog and Digital Images

The scintillation camera was first developed by Hal Anger of the University of California at Berkley in the late 1950s and early 1960s [5], long before computers were in common use and even longer before computer displays that could adequately display a diagnostic image were invented. A major component of these early cameras was circuitry that could convert the output of the photomultiplier array into three voltages representing the x and y locations and the energy (z, the brightness of a scintillation is proportional to the incident photon's energy) of the scintillation photon. If the z voltage matched the voltages calibrated to define the energy window, the x and y locations were sent to an oscilloscope and a momentary flash would appear at a corresponding point on the screen. By placing a focusing lens between the oscilloscope screen and a piece of x-ray film the film was exposed one flash of light (corresponding to one scintillation event) at a time. This type of image is called an analog image, because the x and y locations of the oscilloscope flashes that exposed the film are continuous; they can occur anywhere on the screen. Very nice images could be created with these systems, but they also had some drawbacks. Like all film-based systems, they were subject to under- and overexposure if the technologist cut the exposure time too short or let it go too long. If the clinician wanted to monitor the activity over time, several pieces of film had to be exposed or a system for making several images on one piece of film had to be used.

The progress of computers over the years brought about the development of digital scintillation cameras where a computer is an integral part of the system that processes a scintillation event. Digital cameras provide images in the form of a computer matrix or a digital image. Each cell of this computer matrix is called a picture element or pixel, and represents the counts collected at a corresponding point on the camera face. The values of the pixels are often called pixel counts, because they represent the count of the number of scintillation events detected. The great benefit of a digital image is that it is available for computer processing and display. The exposure time is not a problem because the brightness of the image can be controlled when it is displayed. The pixel counts are also available for computerized analysis instead of being limited to the strictly visual interpretation common with analog images.

The image, or scintigram, is built over time by calculating the x and y location of each scintillation event and, if the energy is determined to be within the desired energy window, incrementing the corresponding pixel. If this is done in real time, the acquisition is said to be in frame mode. If, instead, a list of events and locations is kept it is said to be in list mode. An image is produced from a list mode acquisition after the acquisition is completed. List mode acquisition requires a great deal of more memory and disk space than frame mode, because all scintillation events (regardless of energy) are recorded and more information is kept per event. Regardless of how the image is formed it still needs to be displayed. Scintigram formation is illustrated in Fig. 12.2 and scintigram display is illustrated in Fig. 12.3.

Images are displayed by coding the pixel values to the brightness, or color, of the pixels in the image displays. Usually, scintigrams are displayed in a grayscale format, where black is equal to zero counts and white is equal to the brightest pixel in the image. At times, this is inadequate to capture the dynamic range of an image. It is possible to rescale the image so that a pixel count well below the image maximum but better matching the area of clinical interest is scaled to white. An example of this would be a bone scan that includes the bladder as shown in Fig. 12.4.

Another benefit of digital imaging in nuclear medicine is the ability to acquire images in different formats (Fig. 12.5). Static scintigrams are formed when the scintillation camera acquires a single image from a single location. Dynamic scintigrams are a sequence of static images acquired by defining phases, where each image is acquired for a specific period of time.

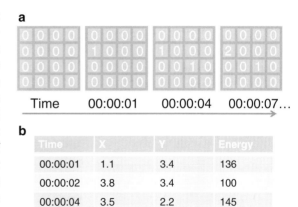

Time   00:00:01   00:00:04   00:00:07…

b

Time	X	Y	Energy
00:00:01	1.1	3.4	136
00:00:02	3.8	3.4	100
00:00:04	3.5	2.2	145
00:00:07	1.4	3.1	142
…			

Fig. 12.2 (a) In frame mode acquisition, each pixel in the image is incremented as scintillations are counted at a particular point on the camera face. This panel shows how pixels are incremented as photons with the desired energy are detected and localized by the camera. (b) In list mode, the same scintillation events are placed into a list and the image is formed from the list after acquisition. Note that if this is a ^{99m}Tc image the second entry may be excluded from the image because of its energy

Gated scintigrams of the heart (often called multigated or MUGA scans, but officially known as equilibrium radionuclide angiography or ERNA) are formed as a sequence of static images that each represent a segment of the heart's EKG R-to-R interval. These images are built up over many heart beats. Whole body images are made by using the scintillation camera to scan from the patient from head to foot (or vice versa) and building an image that appears to be one long image made with a very large camera.

Tomograms represent slices through the body and are reconstructed from projection data. SPECT images are traditionally made by acquiring static images in an arc around the patient of at least 180° and reconstructing tomograms from these projections. While it is possible to construct projections from a PET acquisition, such a display has little value and is not needed for reconstruction.

12.3.2 Image Math

At times, it may be desirable to perform basic mathematical functions on scintigrams and tomograms. Since these images are made up of pixels and those

Fig. 12.3 A scintigram is a matrix or array of individual pixels, where each pixel has a numeric value related to the number of scintillation events detected in that location. The image is displayed by coding the brightness, or color, of each pixel of the display to the pixel counts

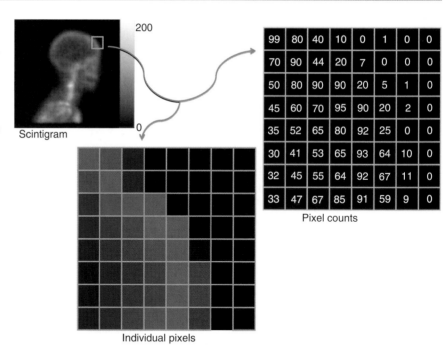

99	80	40	10	0	1	0	0
70	90	44	20	7	0	0	0
50	80	90	90	20	5	1	0
45	60	70	95	90	20	2	0
35	52	65	80	92	25	0	0
30	41	53	65	93	64	10	0
32	45	55	64	92	67	11	0
33	47	67	85	91	59	9	0

Pixel counts

Individual pixels

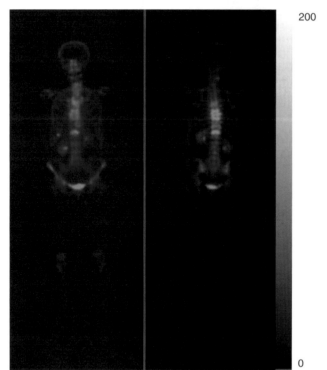

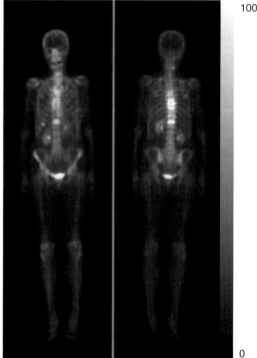

Fig. 12.4 Some scintigrams, such as the bone scan shown here may contain areas of dynamic range well outside of the range of pixel counts in the area of clinical interest. This may be due to high organ uptake in a different organ or, as is the case here, the extraction and excretion of the tracer into the bladder. If the image is displayed scaled from zero to the image maximum, the organ of clinical interest (for example, the bones in the left hand panel) may have too little contrast to be read. By reducing the maximum pixel of the display, it is possible to increase the displayed contrast in the area of clinical interest as shown by the right hand panel. The process of adjusting the displayed brightness and range to suit the scintigram is called windowing

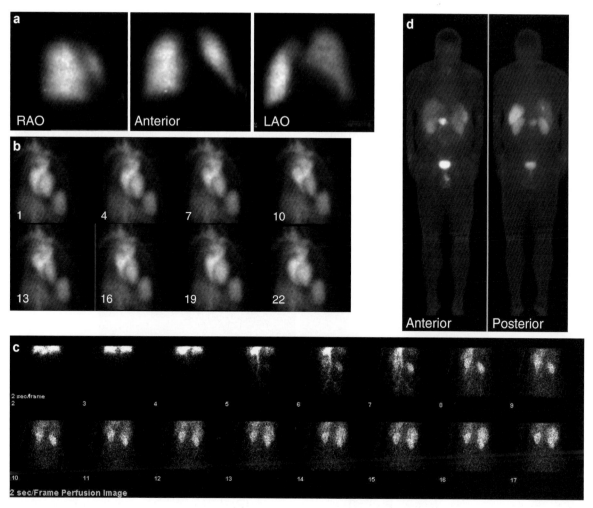

Fig. 12.5 Planar scintigrams may be acquired in different formats. (**a**) Static scintigrams are formed when the scintillation camera acquires a single image from a single location. The technologist manually moves and positions the camera at each desired position. Three views taken in the ^{99m}Tc MAA perfusion lung scan are shown here. (**b**) Gated scintigrams of the heart are acquired over several minutes and show the beating of the heart over an "average" cycle. Each frame of the image represents one segment of the heart's R to R interval. In this example, 8 of the 24 frames that were acquired are shown. The sequence shows the cardiac blood pool starting at diastole, proceeding to systole, and ending back at diastole. (**c**) Dynamic scintigrams allow the clinician to follow a process over time. The example shows the uptake phase of a ^{99m}Tc renogram. Beginning immediately after injection, each of the images in the sequence represents 2 s. The progress of the tracer can be followed as it appears in the blood stream and begins to appear in the kidneys. (**d**) Whole-body scans are acquired by scanning the length of a patient's body with a large field of view scintillation camera. An image is formed that appears to have been made with a single very large scintillation camera. This example shows the uptake of ^{111}In OctreoScan in a patient with an islet cell tumor in the pancreas and metastasis in the liver. (The authors would like to acknowledge Raghuveer K. Halkar, MD, Emory University, Atlanta, GA, for his assistance with this figure.)

pixels define a pixel count at a specific location in space, it is possible to add, subtract, multiply, or divide images by a constant or to perform the operation between two images. Addition of images may be used to reduce the number of images in a dynamic image set by summing frames within a phase, a process known as reframing. This is used in renal imaging, for example, to reduce the number and improve the displayed quality of the frames of the dynamic image, where the original images appear to be very noisy on display but are preferable for extraction of the renogram curves. Subtraction of two images may be used to highlight the difference between two images as in ^{99m}Tc sestamibi – ^{123}I subtraction scintigraphy for hyperparathyroidism where subtraction of the ^{123}I scintigram removes the thyroid gland from the images, making it easier to locate abnormal parathyroid tissue [6] (Fig. 12.6). Prior to subtraction, the two images must be carefully normalized, so that the thyroid glands have the same pixel count values in both scintigrams. This is done by determining a constant that is multiplied by each pixel in the ^{123}I scintigram to give the same pixel counts (on average) as in the ^{99m}Tc sestamibi scintigram. Thus when the images

are subtracted, only the areas that represent different activity levels are left.

12.3.3 Matrix Size and Spatial Resolution

Digital images are, as the name implies, discrete representations of the objects that were imaged. This discrete nature can be quantified in terms of Matrix Size and Spatial Resolution. The spatial resolution can actually be broken down into two separate categories: (1) the inherent resolution of the actual imaging device (both with and without a collimator) and (2) the resolution or size of each individual pixel in the image.

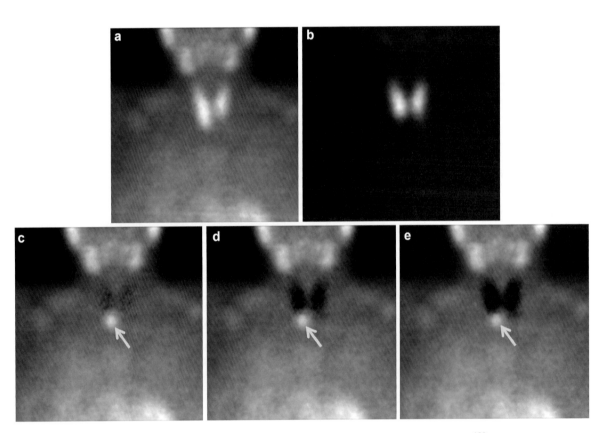

Fig. 12.6 ^{99m}Tc sestamibi – ^{123}I scintigraphy illustrates how one image may be subtracted from the other. While ^{99m}Tc sestamibi (**a**) localizes in both thyroid and parathyroid tissue, ^{123}I (**b**) only localizes in the thyroid tissue. The ^{123}I scintigram is normalized to have the same counts over the thyroid gland as the ^{99m}Tc sestamibi scintigram and subtracted from that image resulting in subtraction scintigram (**c**, **d**, and **e**), making abnormal parathyroid tissue more conspicuous (*arrow*). In the subtraction scintigram labeled C, the ^{123}I scintigram, which has many times fewer counts in the thyroid than the ^{99m}Tc sestamibi scintigram, has been normalized to match the pixel count level of the ^{99m}Tc sestamibi image. In (**d**) and (**e**) it has been normalized to have progressively more counts. (The authors would like to acknowledge Raghuveer K. Halkar, MD, Emory University, Atlanta, GA, for his assistance with this figure.)

12.3.3.1 Matrix Size

Before we delve into calculating Spatial Resolution, we need to briefly cover image matrices. As mentioned above, an image is made up of a collection of discrete picture elements or pixels. These images (collections of pixels) are most often arranged in a square grid or pattern whose size is given as the number of pixels across the face of the image (columns) by the number of pixels down the face of the image (rows); this is also referred to as the image matrix size. For instance, an image that has 64 rows by 64 columns (4,096 total pixels) would be said to have a matrix size of 64 × 64 pixels. Knowing the matrix size of an image is important when calculating the spatial resolution of an imaging system.

12.3.3.2 Spatial Resolution

The spatial resolution of an imaging system can be measured with (extrinsic) and/or without (intrinsic) a collimator, by placing a point source on the face of the camera and acquiring an image. The spatial resolution is then calculated by extracting the counts and location of a row of pixels (called a profile) in this image that go through the point source and measuring the width of the point source profile at half the height of the point source profile (see Fig. 12.7). This number is called the Full Width at Half Maximum (FWHM) and is a direct measure of the spatial resolution of the imaging system. As an example, Fig. 12.7 shows a profile drawn through a point source whose maximum count is 2,908. At half this height (1,454) the width of the

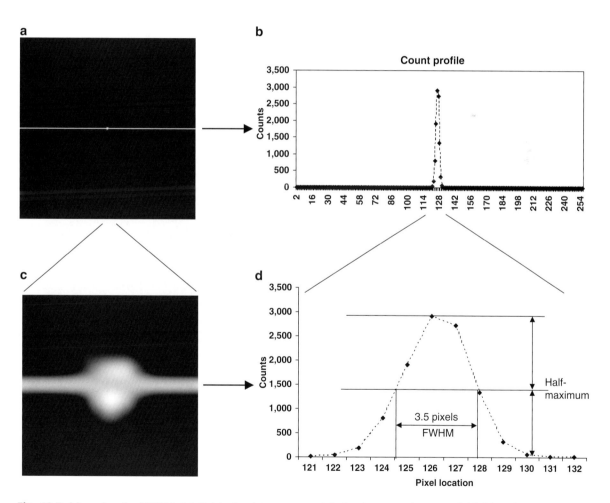

Fig. 12.7 Measuring the FWHM. (**a**) Original point source acquired in a 256 × 256 matrix, (**b**) Plot of counts vs. pixel location for the original image, (**c**) 12 × 12 pixel zoom of original point source image, and (**d**) Plot of counts vs. pixel location for the 12 center pixels showing how the FWHM is calculated

profile is 3.5 pixels, so the spatial resolution of this imaging device is 3.5 pixels. To convert this to mm, we need to know the matrix size of the image and the field-of-view of the camera. For this example, the point source was acquired on a camera with a field-of-view of 532 mm, and the acquired image has a matrix size of 256 × 256 pixels. Putting all of this together, the resultant spatial resolution is:

$$\text{Spatial resolution} = 3.5 \text{ pixels} * (532 \text{ mm}/256 \text{ pixels})$$
$$= 7.27 \text{ mm}$$

The second part of the above equation, (532 mm/ 256 pixels) is the answer to the second category of the resolution question, the resolution or size of each individual pixel in an image. In the above case, each pixel in this image is 2.08 mm, and is specific for this camera size and this image matrix size. If we had acquired the image in a 128 × 128 pixel matrix, instead of a 256 × 256 pixel matrix then the pixel size would have been 4.16 mm (532 mm/128 pixels). Likewise, if we had used a different camera, with a different field-of-view, this would have also affected the pixel size.

Before we leave this topic, let's explore, briefly, why the FWHM is a measure of the resolution of the imaging system. Another way to refer to the resolution of the imaging system would be to indicate its "resolving" power, or its ability to resolve two different point sources. In other words, how close can two point sources be and the system still be able to distinguish the two point sources. If you look at Fig. 12.8, you will see an example of two point sources spaced generously apart (10 pixels, panel A). As the point sources are moved closer together, the counts begin to overlap (5 pixels, panel B). At the point where half of each profile overlaps each other, we can no longer resolve the two different point sources; for all practical purposes, it looks like one big point source (3 pixels, panel C). You will notice that this happens when the two point sources are spaced exactly one FWHM apart (FWHM = 3.5 pixels for this particular camera), which is why, this number is often used as the resolution of the imaging

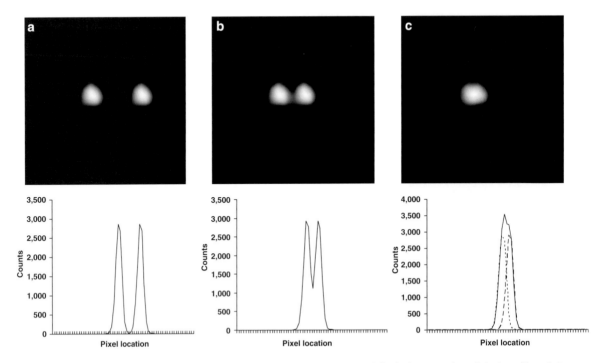

Fig. 12.8 Explanation of FWHM as resolution or resolving power. (**a**) Two-point sources spaced 10 pixels apart. (**b**) Same two-point sources spaced 5 pixels apart. (**c**) Same two-point sources spaced 3 pixels apart; the original profiles of the two separate point sources are seen as dashed lines

system (the point at which two point sources can no longer be resolved) [7, 8].

12.4 Image Interpolation

Another aspect of images and matrix size is changing the size of the image; for instance, you might want to make an image smaller or larger for display purposes. This is usually accomplished by interpolating the original image pixels and making them smaller or larger; in most instances, we are generally interested in making the images larger. As an example, if you were to display a 64 × 64 pixel image on a typical 19″ computer screen whose resolution is 1,280 × 1,024, the image would only take up 1/320th of the screen and would measure approximately inch square. To make the image easier to see, we could zoom or interpolate the image to a larger matrix size, say 256 × 256, which would result in an image size 1/20th of the screen or approximately 3 square in. There are many ways to interpolate an image; we will take a look at three of the more popular methods: Nearest Neighbor (or Pixel Replication), Bilinear Interpolation, and Bicubic Interpolation. An important point to remember is that regardless of the interpolation method used, you can never add more detail

or information to an image than what was there to begin with.

12.4.1 Nearest Neighbor

Nearest neighbor interpolation is the process of copying pixels to make an image larger, and is only useful when your final image size is an integer multiple of the original image size. In our previous example, we could have used the nearest neighbor method to interpolate our 64 × 64 image into a 256 × 256 image by replicating each original image pixel 4 times in the new image. Let's illustrate this with a much simpler example. Suppose we have a 2 × 2 image that we want to interpolate to a 4 × 4 image (effectively doubling its size). Figure 12.9a shows our original 2 × 2 image with 4 pixels whose values range from 3–13, and Fig. 12.9b shows our resultant 4 × 4 image with the nearest neighbor interpolation. The advantage of this technique is that it can be done very quickly on any computer and all of the original image data is preserved; however, the results are not always visually pleasing (typically, the resultant images will look blocky). The main disadvantage of this technique is that you can only interpolate images by integer multiples of the original image size. Figure 12.9d shows a central

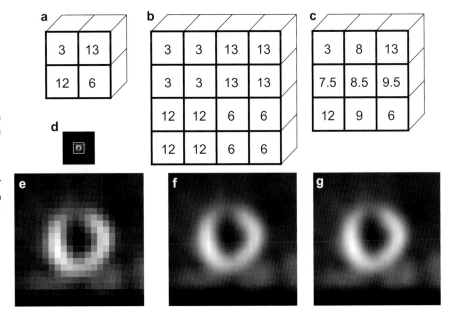

Fig. 12.9 Example of image interpolation. (**a**) Original 2 × 2 image with 4 pixels, (**b**) Nearest neighbor interpolation to 4 × 4 image, (**c**) Bilinear interpolation to 3 × 3 image, (**d**) original 64 × 64 central short-axis slice from a SPECT myocardial perfusion scan, (**e**) nearest neighbor interpolation of central 21 × 21 pixels of original image (shown as white box in (**d**)) to 256 × 256, (**f**) bilinear interpolation of same area as (**e**), and (**g**) bicubic interpolation of same area as (**e**)

64×64 pixel short-axis slice from a myocardial perfusion scan, with a white box around the central 21×21 pixels. Figure 12.9e shows a nearest neighbor interpolation of this central 21×21 pixel region zoomed to a 252×252 pixel region ($12 \times$ the original size); notice how blocky the resultant image is.

12.4.2 Bilinear Interpolation

Bilinear interpolation fills in the missing pixels by linearly interpolating between the four neighboring pixels (the closest 2×2 neighborhood). As an example, we can use linear interpolation to zoom the original 2×2 pixel image shown in Fig. 12.9a to a 3×3 pixel image. Using bilinear interpolation (linear interpolation applied separately in the x and then the y directions), the resultant image is shown in Fig. 12.9c. Notice how each edge pixel value is halfway between the pixel values on either side (both in the x and y directions – this is a special case for the pixels on the edge of the image), and the very center pixel (8.5) is the average of the four corner or neighbor pixels $((3 + 13 + 12 + 6)/4 = 8.5)$. The main advantage of this method over the nearest neighbor method is that the resultant image does not need to be an integer multiple of the original image and it produces an image that is more visually pleasing (not as blocky); however, it does take more computing power. Figure 12.9f shows a bilinear interpolation of the same central 21×21 pixel region zoomed to a 252×252 pixel region. Note that this image still contains some slight blockiness.

12.4.3 Bicubic Interpolation

Bicubic interpolation has shown improvement over bilinear interpolation by considering the nearest 4×4 neighborhood of pixels (instead of the nearest 2×2 neighborhood) and using a weighted average of these 16 pixels to calculate the value of the new pixel. In this technique, closer pixels are weighted higher than further pixels and the result is a sharper image than can be achieved with bilinear interpolation. The disadvantage is that it takes even more computing power to calculate. Figure 12.9g shows a bicubic

interpolation of the same central 21×21 pixel region zoomed to a 252×252 pixel region. Note how smooth this interpolation is (there is no apparent blockiness).

12.5 Image Display and Lookup Tables

12.5.1 Pseudocolor Displays

In medical imaging, images are usually displayed by assigning a color to each pixel value consisting of red, green, and blue (R, G, and B) intensities. This type of display is called a pseudocolor display. The mapping from pixel value to color is called a lookup table (LUT) or video lookup table (VLT). The number of entries in the lookup table; that is, its length, determines the number of colors that can be displayed, and while historically this has been limited to 256, in theory, it may be much larger. In fact, the number of entries in the lookup table should be equal to the maximum value in the image, so that entries exist for every possible pixel value. However, it is always possible to scale the image prior to display, so that the lookup table size is more a matter of hardware considerations.

The depth of the lookup table is split into three portions, one each for the red, green, and blue values of the color to be assigned. In most cases, each of these portions is one byte, so the total depth of the lookup table is three bytes. Again, this is more a consideration of the hardware and software used for display and may not be user selectable. Note, however, that the size of the R, G, and B entries determines the range of possible values for those colors. That is, if each entry is one byte long, then only the values of 0–255 can be used. Note that this allows 2^{24} possible colors to be placed in the lookup table (256^3); however, as noted above, the number that can be placed there at one time is a function of the length of the lookup table rather than its width. Figure 12.10 shows how the LUT works to define a color that will be used to display each pixel.

Pseudocolor displays are very flexible, because the color mapping associated with the LUT can be interactively changed. A completely new LUT can be loaded almost instantaneously so that the image may be viewed in color, or using a gray scale, without

Fig. 12.10 Graphic explanation of pseudocolor displays. Each pixel value in the image is used as an index into the video lookup table (LUT). *Red* (R), *green* (G), and *blue* (B) color values are obtained from the LUT at that index entry. These values are then used to display that pixel

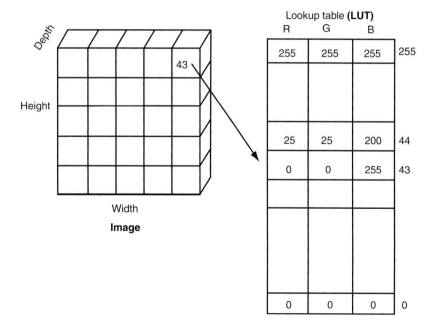

modifying the image data itself. The most common operation for changing a LUT is that of modifying the lower bound or upper bound. The lower and upper bounds are the pixel values at which the LUT changes from its first to its second color or from its next-to-maximum to maximum color. Generally, if the LUT has 256 entries, then the default lower bound is 0, and the upper bound is 255. (The lower bound is also called the level, and the difference between the upper and lower bounds may be called the window.) However, if the lower bound is changed to 10, then the LUT will be compressed, so that the value that was originally at 0 will be placed at all values between 0 and 10, the value at 255 will remain the same, and the other colors that originally ranged from 0 to 255 will be compressed, using interpolation, between those values. Raising the lower bound acts as a type of background subtraction, because low values are now displayed using the same color as "0," so that these low intensity regions seem to disappear. Lowering the upper bound tends to enhance lower values, because smaller pixel values are now displayed using the portions of the color map that used to be assigned to the higher intensity pixel values. Figure 12.11 shows how modifying the color tables changes the display of a bone scan.

Some particular lookup tables are important to understand. The gray scale contains the same R, G, and B values for each entry, so the "colors" are all gray. They range from black (R,G,B = 0) at the first entry, to white (R,G,B = 255) at the top entry, so that background colors are dim and high pixel values are near white. The reverse gray scale ranges from 255 at the first entry to 0 at the top entry, so that background colors are white, while high pixel values are black. Discrete lookup tables change to different colors in the space of a single entry, and are often scaled so that these color changes occur every 10%. In this way, a quantitative assessment of the pixel values can be obtained – a green value may be associated with pixel values equal to 50–60% of the maximum in the image, for example. However, discrete lookup tables, and indeed, any color table that changes hue in the space of a few pixel values can result in what are called false contours. Two pixel values that are very similar in value may end up being assigned very different colors. This leads the eye to believe that there are hard boundaries between the two pixel values when in fact, there is very little difference between them.

12.5.2 True Color Displays

A second type of display requires that each pixel value in the image contain values for red, green, and blue colors. This is typically not the case for any medical

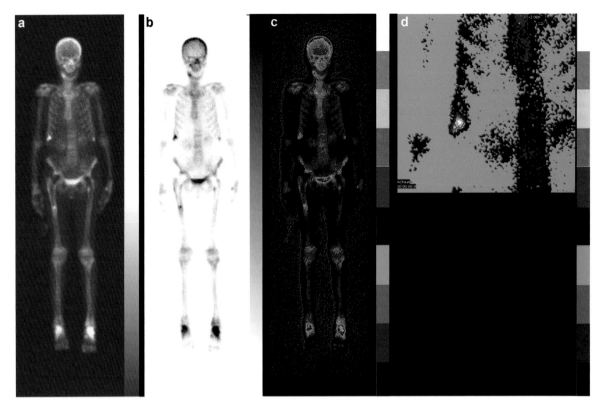

Fig. 12.11 Bone scan displayed using different lookup tables (LUT). (**a**) Grayscale mapping, with bright shades of gray (*white*) indicating large counts. (**b**) Reverse gray scale, where dark shades of gray indicate large counts. This LUT has been modified so that its lower bound is greater than 0, giving the image the appearance of having fewer counts in the background.

(**c**) Ten-step color scale, so that at every 10% of maximum counts, the color changes dramatically. When a portion of the image is zoomed (**d**), the rapid changes from about 50–100% of maximum counts in the hot region of the right rib cage can be appreciated

image; however, such displays can be generated and are frequently used for 3D graphics. In these images, the data has three "planes," each associated with the red, green, and blue values used for display. Again, these planes are usually one byte in width, so that the R, G, and B values can range from 0 to 255. No lookup table needs to be used to translate the image into a display; rather, the three planes already encode the colors. Note that in true color displays with byte-sized planes, 2^{24} colors can be displayed at one time all in the same image. This color resolution is necessary in three-dimensional graphics, since many more colors are necessary to give the display realism. However, given that nuclear medicine images really have only one value per pixel, true color displays are not generally needed for displaying slices.

12.6 Image Filtering

Image filtering can be thought of as a mathematical process applied to an image for various reasons, such as removing noise or enhancing features. This process can occur before, during, or after the image reconstruction process, and in most Nuclear Medicine procedures, it is employed to remove noise. It is a very necessary process for SPECT reconstruction, as shown in Fig. 12.12.

Because filtering is a mathematical process, it is much easier to convert images into the math "world" (better known as frequency space) for filtering, rather than converting the filters into the image world. This process of converting images into the math world, or frequency space, is accomplished using the Fourier

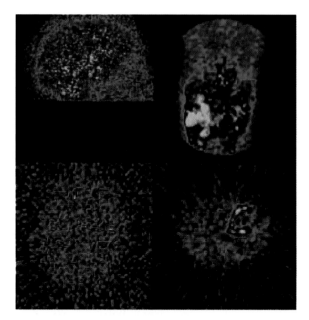

Fig. 12.12 *Top left panel* shows one frame from a Brain Perfusion SPECT acquisition, bottom left shows the same SPECT acquisition reconstructed with no filtering applied. *Top right* shows one frame from a Myocardial Perfusion SPECT acquisition, *bottom right* shows the same SPECT acquisition reconstructed with no filtering applied

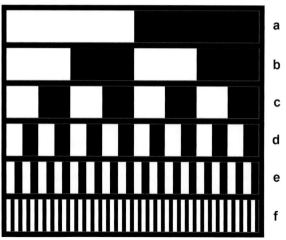

Fig. 12.13 Panels **a–f** show increasing numbers of cycles/pixel for a 64 pixel image (image was zoomed for display purposes). (**a**) 0.015625 cycles/pixel (1 cycle/64 pixels), (**b**) 0.03125 cycles/pixel (2 cycles/64 pixels), (**c**) 0.0625 cycles/pixel (4 cycles/64 pixels), (**d**) 0.125 cycles/pixel (8 cycles/64 pixels), (**e**) 0.25 cycles/pixel (16 cycles/64 pixels), and (**f**) 0.5 cycles/pixel (32 cycles/64 pixels)

Transform, and is covered in the next section. However, it would be good to take a step back and examine how image objects and properties relate to this new math world called frequency space.

12.6.1 Frequency Space

From Collins Essential English Dictionary [9], frequency is defined as the number of times that an event occurs within a given period. For instance, a clock pendulum that swings back and forth every second would have a frequency of one cycle (one back and forth swing) per second, or 1 Hz. Similarly (though overly simplified), since a digital image is made up of pixels, there are a finite number of these elements that can be turned on and off. Let's take the example of an image that has 64 pixels across the image. If we turn half of the pixels (32 pixels) on and then the remaining half of the pixels off, this would translate into a frequency of 1 cycle (pixels on, then off) per 64 pixels or 0.015625 cycles/pixel

(Fig. 12.13a). If this process were halved such that 16 pixels were on, then off, then on, then off, this would translate into a frequency of 2 cycles/64 pixels or 1 cycle/32 pixels or 0.03125 cycles/pixel (Fig. 12.13b). If we continue this process of halving the number of pixels that are on or off (Fig. 12.13c–e), we eventually get to the point where every other pixel is on and off, which translates into a frequency of 1 cycle/2 pixels or 0.5 cycles/pixel (Fig. 12.13f). This special case represents the maximum frequency (on/off cycles) that can be represented in a digital image, and is called the Nyquist Frequency (named after the Swedish-American engineer Harry Nyquist).

Up to this point, we have been using cycles/pixel as the unit of measure for frequency, but other units may also be used. As just noted, the maximum frequency that can be displayed in a digital image is 0.5 cycles/pixel, which can also be represented as a percentage or fraction of the Nyquist frequency. Thus 0.5 cycles/pixel = 1 × Nyquist frequency = 100% of the Nyquist frequency (note that when using units of percent or fraction of the Nyquist frequency, the maximum frequency is now greater than 0.5). In addition, if the physical size of the detector is taken into consideration, then the units of frequency can be converted into cycles/cm using the following formulas:

$$\text{freq(cycles/cm)} = \text{freq(cycles/pixel)}$$
$$*(\# \text{ pixels})/(\text{size of detector in cm})$$

or

$$\text{freq(cycles/cm)} = \text{freq (\% of Nyquist)}$$
$$*0.5 \text{ cycles/pixel}$$
$$*(\# \text{ pixels})/(\text{size of detector in cm})$$

For instance, in our above example, if the field of view was 40 cm, then the Nyquist frequency would be 0.5 cycles/pixel × 64 pixels/40 cm = 0.8 cycles/cm (note that when using units of cycles/cm, the maximum frequency can again be greater than 0.5).

Now that we know what a frequency is, the next obvious question is how do frequencies relate to image objects?

12.6.2 Spatial Domain Versus Frequency Domain

If we look again at Fig. 12.13, we notice that as more pixels are turned on and off (more cycles), the corresponding frequency also increases (from 0.015625 to 0.5 cycles/pixel). Following this line of reasoning, low frequencies correspond to the slowly varying portions of images, while high frequencies correspond to quickly varying portions of images. This means that "edges" (points in an image with an abrupt change in intensity such as going from black to white, or white to black) contain numerous high frequency components. In addition, image noise (spurious bright and dark pixels scattered randomly throughout the image) also contains numerous high frequencies; this makes sense if you stop and think about it. Randomly distributed bright and dark pixels will have very abrupt edges when compared with their neighbors, and as mentioned before, it's these edges that contribute to the high frequency components. However, real edges in images (such as boundaries between myocardium and background) also contribute high-frequency components. So, filtering is always a balance between removing as much noise as possible while preserving as much resolution and detail as possible.

12.6.3 Fourier Transform

12.6.3.1 Types of Filters

Generally speaking, all filters fall into one of three classes: (1) Low-Pass filters (filters that pass low frequencies), (2) High-Pass filters (filters that pass high frequencies), and (3) Band-Pass filters (filters that pass a narrow range of frequencies). From the previous section, we learned that noise in Nuclear Medicine images is almost always a high-frequency component; therefore, the goal of most of the filtering we do in Nuclear Medicine is to reduce this noise, which means we mostly employ low-pass filters. The one exception to this is the ramp back-projection filter, a High-Pass filter used in the Filtered Back-Projection process (this topic is covered in a later chapter in this book). Band-Pass filters are a special class of filters, and since they are not generally used in Nuclear Medicine, we will not discuss them here.

There are many Low-Pass filters that we could discuss, including Metz, Weiner, Hanning (or Hann), and Butterworth. Because of space constraints, we shall focus on two of the more popular filters, Hanning and Butterworth.

Hanning Filters

In years past, the most common filter in Nuclear Medicine was the Hanning filter. It is a relatively simple filter with one parameter defining its characteristics, the cutoff frequency. The mathematical definition of the Hanning Filter is as follows:

$$w(f) = 0.5 + 0.5 \cos\left(\frac{\pi f}{f_m}\right) \quad \text{if } |f| < f_m$$

where f = spatial frequencies of the image; f_m = cutoff frequency.

By definition, this filter is defined to be 0 at all frequencies greater than the cutoff frequency, completely removing them from the image. Figure 12.14 shows three different Hanning filters with cutoff frequencies of 0.4 cycles/cm, 0.6 cycles/cm, and 0.822 cycles/cm. Note how the filter rolls quickly toward the cutoff frequency and is 0 for all frequencies above the cutoff frequency. This figure also shows

Fig. 12.14 Hanning filter with three different cutoff frequencies shown, 0.4 cycles/cm, 0.6 cycles/cm, and 0.822 cycles/cm. Note how changing the critical frequency effectively shifts the Hanning filter up and down the Frequency axis of the plot

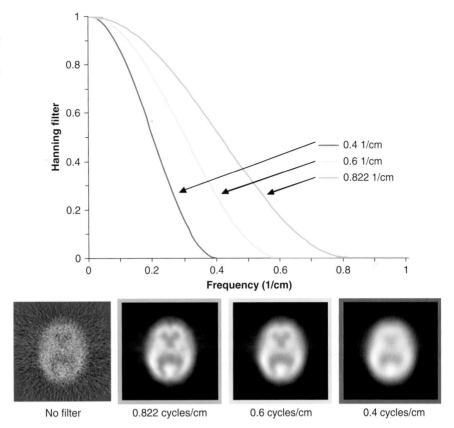

No filter   0.822 cycles/cm   0.6 cycles/cm   0.4 cycles/cm

a typical brain SPECT study filtered with these three filters. Because the Hanning filter rolls-off to 0 so quickly, it is a very good smoothing filter (it very effectively removes high-frequency components, including noise and edge detail); however, it tends not to preserve image resolution.

Butterworth Filters

Sometime in the 1990s, the popularity of the Butterworth filter started gaining momentum. Today, it seems to be the filter of choice in Nuclear Medicine. Perhaps, it is because the Butterworth Filter is so versatile, it can be constructed in such a way that mimics the properties of a Hanning filter, but it can also do a lot more.

There are two parameters that define the Butterworth filter; they are (1) Critical Frequency and (2) Power Factor (sometimes called Order). Notice that the first parameter is called the "critical frequency" instead of the "cutoff frequency" as it was for the Hanning filter. This is because the critical frequency is the point at which the Butterworth filter starts its roll-off toward 0, rather than being defined as 0, as in the Hanning filter. In fact, mathematically, the Butterworth filter never reaches 0, it merely approaches 0. Unfortunately, there is some confusion as to the correct name of the second parameter (what I have called power factor). Mathematically, the power factor = 2 × order, though there are some manufacturers who do not follow this rule. The only real way to determine if the Butterworth filter, as implemented in your particular equipment, is using the power factor or order is to examine the equation that was actually implemented. Here is the equation for the Butterworth filter using power factor:

$$w(f) = \frac{1}{\sqrt{1 + \left(\frac{f}{f_c}\right)^p}}$$

where f = spatial frequencies of the image; f_c = critical frequency; p = power factor.

In the case where a manufacturer has implemented the Butterworth filter using order instead of power factor, then the equation would look like this (note that p has been replaced with $2n$, where n is the order):

$$w(f) = \frac{1}{\sqrt{1 + \left(\frac{f}{f_c}\right)^{2n}}}$$

In practice, the critical frequency of the Butterworth filter behaves much like the cutoff frequency of the Hanning filter, in that, as the critical frequency is changed, the effect is to shift the resultant Butterworth filter up and down the Frequency-axis, as shown in Fig. 12.15. The power factor effectually changes the steepness of the Butterworth filter's roll-off toward 0, as shown in Fig. 12.16. Because of this versatility (the ability to change not only the frequency of the roll-off, but also the steepness of the roll-off), the Butterworth filter can be used to more effectively remove noise while still preserving resolution. Note how the noise in the Brain images at the bottom of Fig. 12.16 is affected

by the change in power factor (increasing the power factor effectively reduces the higher frequency components, such as noise), but the detail in the interior structures is preserved.

12.6.3.2 Fourier Transform in Filter Application

In this section, we shall examine the process of actually applying a filter to an image. As mentioned in the previous section, filtering usually takes place in the mathematical world of frequency space, because filter implementation and application is easier. The complete filtering process is shown in Fig. 12.17 and goes something like this: an image is converted to frequency space, the filter is applied, and the resulting image is converted back to image space. The process of converting an image into frequency space is accomplished using the Fourier transform [10–14]. This mathematical operator is nondestructive, completely reversible, and can be computed fairly quickly for images whose dimensions are a power of 2 (using the

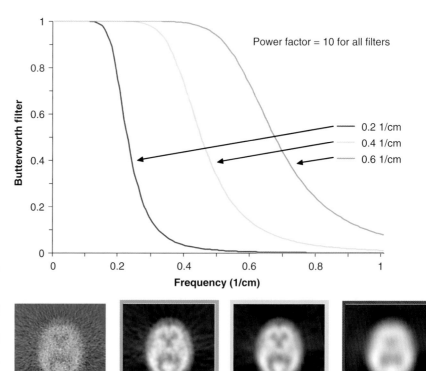

Fig. 12.15 Butterworth filter with three different critical frequencies and a constant power factor of 10: 0.6 cycles/cm, 0.4 cycles/cm, and 0.2 cycles/cm. Note how changing the critical frequency (like changing the cutoff frequency of the Hanning filter) effectually shifts the filter up and down the Frequency axis of the plot

Fig. 12.16 Butterworth filter with three different power factors and a constant critical frequency of 0.4 cycles/cm: PF = 20, PF = 5, and PF = 2. Note how increasing the power factor increases the steepness of the filter's roll-off toward 0

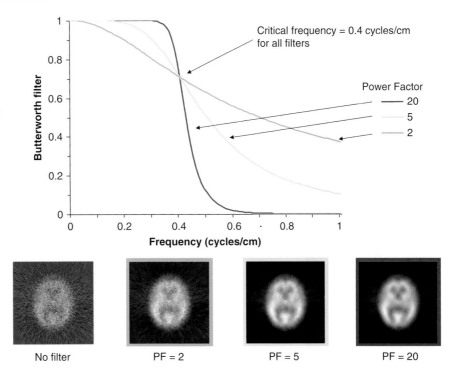

No filter   PF = 2   PF = 5   PF = 20

FFT or Fast Fourier Transform). The frequency information that is returned by the Fourier Transform can also be viewed as a series of sine or cosine waves. For instance, the square wave shown in Fig. 12.18, panel A has frequency components that are shown in panel B. These components can also be shown as a series of sine waves, as seen in panel C. If one were to do a point-by-point addition of all of the sine waves, the resultant waveform would be equal to the square wave shown in panel A. Another term for each of these individual sine waves, or frequencies, is harmonics. The lowest frequency is referred to as the first harmonic, the second lowest frequency as the second harmonic, and so on. In reality, the first harmonic is the best "fit" of a sine wave to the original data. As one adds more harmonics, the "fit" becomes more and more like the original curve. There are several different ways to display this frequency information to the user, we will be showing the information in graph style, where each point on the x-axis represents a specific frequency, and the height of each point represents how much of that frequency is in the image (as in Fig. 12.18b. Let's illustrate this with several examples.

Figure 12.19a shows an image consisting of eight increasing frequencies, ranging from .0039 cycles/

pixel to 0.5 cycles/pixel. Panel B shows the corresponding graph of these eight frequencies (also referred to as the input frequency spectrum or just input spectrum). Panel C shows a graphical representation of a uniform filter; note that this graph uses the same units as the input frequency spectrum. In frequency space, filtering is simply the multiplication of the input frequency spectrum, point-by-point, with the filter. In other words, every frequency point in the input spectrum is multiplied by its corresponding point in the filter graph. For this example, since the uniform filter has a value of "1" for each frequency, each input frequency is multiplied by 1 and copied to the output frequency spectrum graph (see panel D). We can now convert this filtered output frequency spectrum into an image by running the inverse of the Fourier transform; the resultant image is seen in panel E. Since the output spectrum is identical to the input spectrum, it is not surprising that the filtered image (output image) is identical to the input image.

We can now add what we learned about different filters in the previous section to the filtering process. Figure 12.20, panels A and B show the same input image and spectrum as Fig. 12.19. However, the filter in Fig. 12.20c is now that of a Hanning filter with

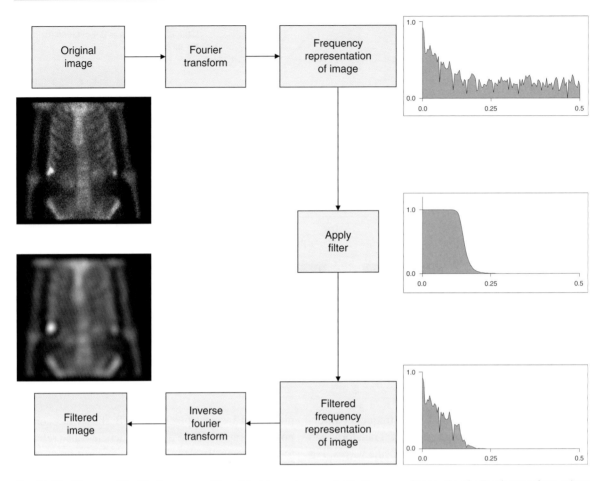

Fig. 12.17 Diagram of the filtering process. The original image is converted to Frequency Space using the Fourier transform, where an image filter is applied. The resultant frequency spectrum is converted back to image space using the inverse Fourier Transform

a cutoff value of 0.5 Nyquist. The output spectrum in Panel D shows the results of multiplying the input spectrum by this filter, and the corresponding image is shown in panel E. Note that because of this filter's sharp roll-off, the frequency at 0.5 Nyquist is completely removed from the image, and the other frequencies have been somewhat reduced. Figure 12.21 shows an additional example using a Butterworth filter with a critical frequency of 0.03125 Nyquist and an order of 5. Note that this filter has completely removed the frequency at 0.5 Nyquist, and has all but completely removed the frequencies at 0.125 and 0.25 Nyquist as seen in the output spectrum and the resultant filtered image.

As a final example of filtering, let's look at a real case involving a Planar Bone Scan (Fig. 12.22). In Panel A you can see the original image. Panel B

shows the input spectrum of the Bone scan (note the rather continuous nature of the input spectrum, indicating that frequencies of all values are present). Panel C shows a Butterworth filter with a critical frequency of 0.125 Nyquist and a Power Factor of 20. The resultant spectrum (Panel D) and image (Panel E) show the results of this filter.

12.6.3.3 Fourier Transform in Curve Fitting

We can use the "fitting" property of the Fourier Transform to our advantage when looking at various physiologic phenomena. For instance, when calculating an ejection fraction, the time-volume curve generally looks much like a time-shifted sine wave (see Fig. 12.23). We can use the first harmonic of the

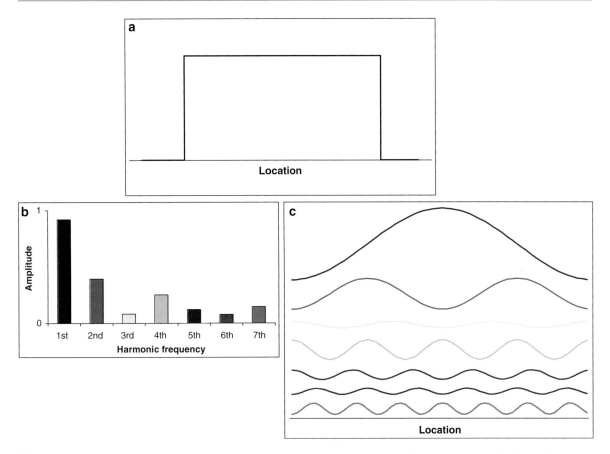

Fig. 12.18 Decomposition of square wave into frequency components using the Fourier transform. (**a**) Original square wave. (**b**) Fourier transform frequency spectrum of the square wave shown in (**a**). (**c**) Another way of showing the Fourier Transform spectrum as sine waves

Fourier Transform of the time–volume curve to actually "fit" this time–volume curve to a sine wave. This is of particular interest when there are few time points or where the data is particularly noisy [15]. As you can see in Fig. 12.23, the first harmonic of the Fourier Transform is much smoother than the curve of the original eight points. In addition, recent research has shown that the temporal resolution of an 8 or 16-frame study is equivalent to a 64-frame study, when the original study has been "fitted" to the first, second, or third harmonics of a Fourier Transform [16].

There are at least two exciting Cardiology applications of fitting time-volume curves using the Fourier Transform: (1) Determination of Wall Thickening and (2) Phase Analysis. Though space will not permit a detailed treatment of these two applications, we shall describe them briefly below.

12.6.3.4 Fourier Transform in the Determination of Wall Thickening

It has been shown that if the size of an object being measured is less than or equal to twice the resolution of the imaging equipment (twice the FWHM), then the counts in the object increase linearly with its thickness [17]. This property of linear count increases can be used to measure the "thickening" of the myocardial wall in myocardial perfusion gated SPECT studies [18]. A typical SPECT system has an intrinsic resolution of about 10 mm, and the average end-diastolic width of the walls of the left ventricle are about 1 cm [19]; this falls into the category of the object size being less than twice the FWHM of the imaging system. If we extract the counts of the left-ventricular myocardium from a myocardial perfusion gated SPECT

Fig. 12.19 Example of filtering. (**a**) Original image with eight frequencies. (**b**) FFT spectrum of original image. (**c**) Unity filter (one everywhere). (**d**) FFT spectrum after application of filter. (**e**) Filtered image

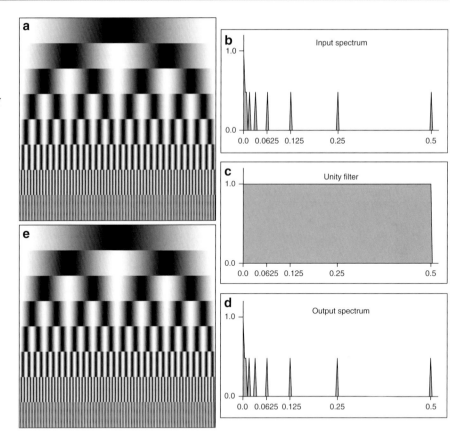

study, and look at the counts of each point in the myocardium as it goes through the cardiac cycle, we will get a series of time-count curves similar to the curve shown in Fig. 12.23. If we fit each of these curves using the first harmonic of the Fourier Transform (also shown in Fig. 12.23), then we can estimate the percentage of thickening of the myocardium between end-systole and end-diastole. Assuming that the counts are linearly proportional to thickness, then the percentage of increase of counts from end-diastole to end-systole should be linearly proportional to the increase in wall thickness. For example, if the amplitude of the sine wave is 13, and the DC component is 135, then the percentage thickening could be calculated as (2 × amplitude)/(DC − amplitude) and would be 21%. Though this number could be calculated directly from the counts extracted from the myocardium, it is less affected by noise or number of acquired frames/cardiac cycle if the Fourier Transform is used. By calculating this percentage thickening for every point in the myocardium, we can come up with a global assessment of how the myocardium is thickening throughout the cardiac cycle. This assessment can be important, as areas that are not thickening (which implies impaired function) may be an independent indicator of dead or dying myocardial tissue. It can also be used to rule-out false positives. For instance, an area of the myocardium that does not exhibit many counts at stress and at rest (compared to the surrounding tissue) would normally be viewed as dead myocardial tissue. However, if this same area is seen to "thicken," i.e., there are count changes between end-diastole and end-systole, then the count reductions are probably due to some kind of artifact (Breast or Diaphragm attenuation), and the tissue is more than likely alive and well [20].

12.6.3.5 Fourier Transform in the Calculation of Phase Analysis

Another benefit of using the Fourier Transform is that we can also measure the onset of thickening (or onset of mechanical contraction); this is sometimes referred

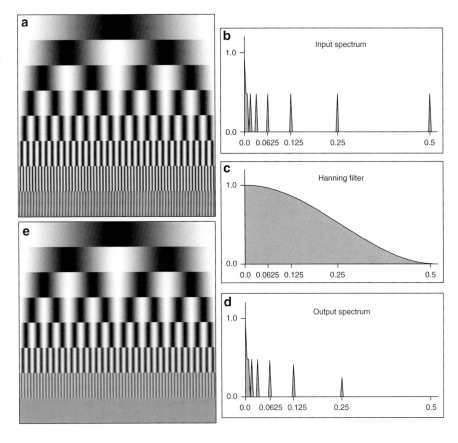

to as Phase Analysis. If we again look at Fig. 12.23, the point at which the thickening curve crosses the DC component of the Fourier Transform is known as the phase shift or just phase of the curve. A sine wave with no phase shift would have started at the DC crossing point, which would be a phase of 0. As the sine wave is shifted to the right, the phase increases indicating a delay in the contraction of the ventricle. If we calculate this phase shift for every point in the myocardium (much like we calculate the percentage thickening for every point in the myocardium) we can use this distribution of phases to diagnose various cardiac conditions. There are several ways to look at this distribution of phases, two of which are most common: (1) as a histogram and (2) as an image. Figure 12.24 shows the output screen of a normal Multiple Gated Acquisition (MUGA) study. Notice that the phase image is all one color and the histogram is very narrow, both indicating that all sections of the ventricle are essentially contracting at the same time. Figure 12.25 shows the output screen of a MUGA for a patient with an apical aneurysm. Notice that the

phase image is no longer a single color and the histogram has broadened a little. More recently, phase analysis information extracted from gated SPECT or PET studies [15, 21, 22] has proven useful in evaluating patients being considered for Cardiac Resynchronization Therapy (CRT) [23–26]. Figure 12.26 shows the normalized phase polar maps and histograms from two different studies, a normal study (top) and an abnormal study (bottom). Note how the normal study has a tall, narrow, well-defined peak, indicating that the left ventricle is very synchronous. In contrast, notice how the abnormal study has a very broad diffuse distribution, indicating that the left ventricle is severely dyssynchronous.

12.7 Region of Interest Analysis

Generally, quantitative measures from nuclear medicine images are obtained only from certain important regions; these are called regions of interest (ROIs).

Fig. 12.21 Example of Butterworth filter (**a**) Original image with eight frequencies. (**b**) FFT spectrum of original image. (**c**) Butterworth filter, critical frequency = 0.03125 Nyquist, Power Factor = 5. (**d**) FFT spectrum after application of filter. (**e**) Filtered image

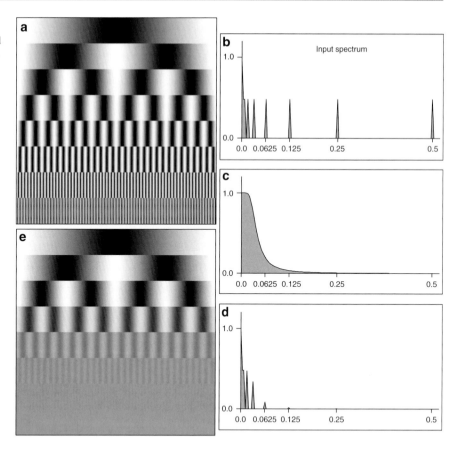

If the region is 3-dimensional (3D), the term "volume of interest" is sometimes used (VOI). A ROI can be, for example, a tumor in an oncologic image, the kidney in a renal image, or the myocardium in a cardiac image. Measurements may be taken from the count values within the region; for example, the mean and maximum count values can be computed. They may also be taken from the shape of the boundary of the ROI; for example, the number of pixels within it, or its size may be determined. Obtaining an appropriate, or accurate, ROI is one of the most basic steps in image quantitation. In some cases, geometric ROIs, such as an oval or circle, may be appropriate. It is always possible to interactively trace the region of interest, and this is still probably the most common approach. An expert user can use his or her knowledge of the expected shape of the organ along with the appearance of the image to obtain a good boundary. These two approaches are shown in Fig. 12.27. However, interactive processes are associated with significant inter

and intraobserver variability, they are time consuming, and there are not always experts available to perform the task. For that reason, automatic methods may be helpful, if only to aid the user in performing the interactive tracing.

12.7.1 Background Subtraction

In planar images, counts through the entire body are acquired, from soft tissue both in front of and behind the organ of interest. Accurate quantification of the counts within the organ may be obtained only if these counts can be eliminated from the organ ROI; this is called background subtraction. The most common approach for background subtraction is to find a region in the image that is near to, but not in the organ ROI, with no obvious additional high-count structures.

Fig. 12.22 Example of Butterworth filter with planar bone scan. (**a**) Original planar bone scan. (**b**) FFT spectrum of original image. (**c**) Butterworth filter.125 Nyquist, Power Factor = 20. (**d**) FFT spectrum after application of filter. (**e**) Filtered image

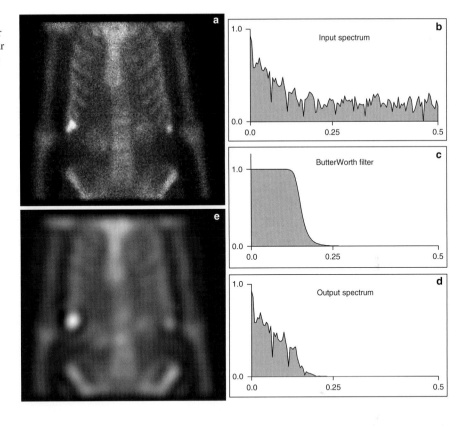

Fig. 12.23 Example of Fourier curve fitting. Eight time points from a midventricular gated short-axis slice are shown in the *dotted lines*. The result of fitting these eight points to the first harmonic of the FFT are shown in the *dark solid line*. The *light solid line* shows the DC component (or average) of the FFT

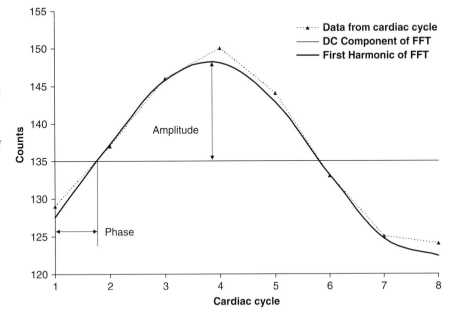

A background region can be drawn interactively or automatically in this area. The mean counts per pixel are determined, and this value is subtracted from every value in the image. More complicated background regions can be drawn as well; for example, an oval shell, or doughnut, can be used to surround the

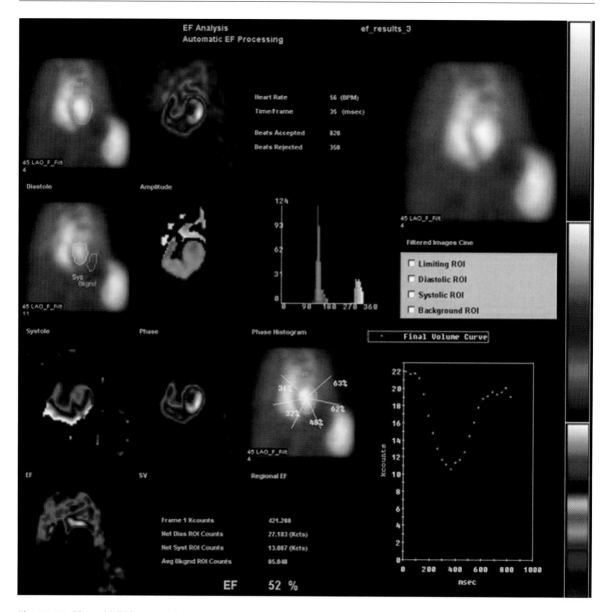

Fig. 12.24 Normal MUGA example

kidney in renal images. In this case, when the background region extends from one side of the organ ROI to the other, values within the background may be interpolated from the edge values to account for a varying background. The resulting 2-D map of background values is then subtracted pixel by pixel from the organ ROI. An example of this is shown in Fig. 12.28; there, the background was automatically generated in a renal processing program.

12.7.2 Time Activity Curves

In much of nuclear imaging, the changes in radiotracer concentration over time due to mechanical or physiological processes can be more important than visualization of anatomy. The primary tool for analyzing these changes are Time Activity Curves (sometimes abbreviated as TACs), which represent the counts in a

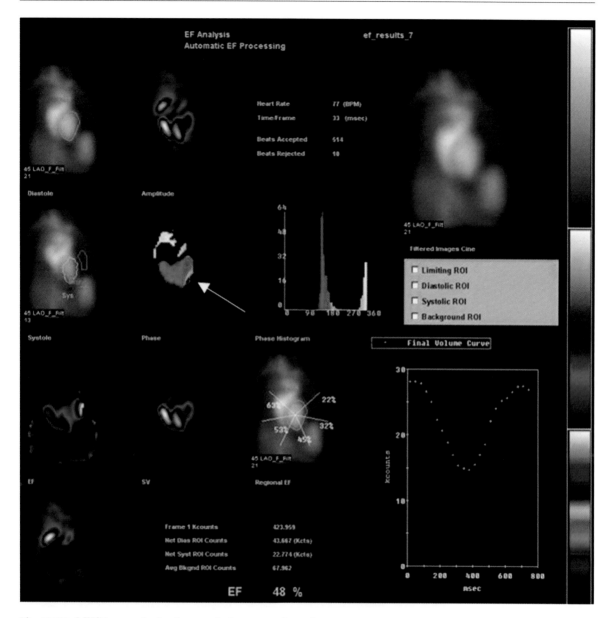

Fig. 12.25 MUGA example showing an apical aneurysm (*arrow*)

region of interest of a dynamic image graphed over time. Examples of widely used time activity curve analysis include estimation of filling and clearance of radiotracer from the kidneys in renograms and of left ventricular volume changes of gated blood pool studies of the heart.

Renogram curves are time activity curves of a radiopharmaceutical as it transits the kidney. Used for the diagnoses of renovascular disease, the curves are used to evaluate the kidney uptake and washout of

radiopharmaceuticals with key factors being the time to the peak height of the curve after injection (Tmax), the time it takes for the activity in the kidney to fall to 50% of its peak value and the relative uptake values between the left and right kidneys (T1/2) [27]. Since Tmax is much shorter than T1/2, the dynamic renogram is usually acquired in two phases with 1–3 s frames from the first 60 s and 1–3 min intervals for the remainder of the study. The rapid frame rate of the first phase allows the evaluation of the rapid uptake of the

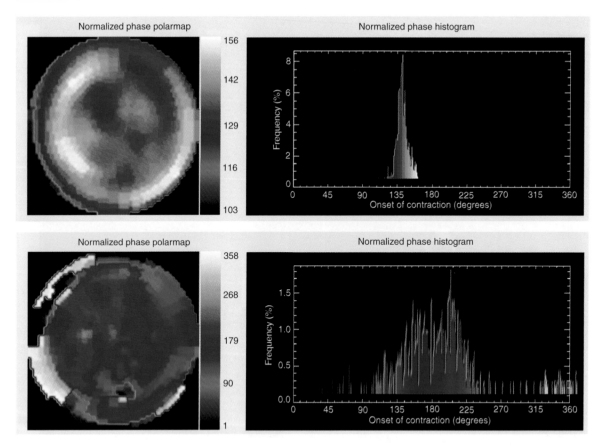

Fig. 12.26 Examples of phase analysis from gated myocardial perfusion SPECT studies. *Top*: normalized phase polar map and histogram from a Normal study, note how tall and narrow the histogram is, indicating that the ventricle is very synchronous. *Bottom*: normalized phase polar map and histogram from an abnormal study, note how spread out the histogram is, indicating severe myocardial dyssynchrony

Fig. 12.27 Examples of a geometric region of interest (*left*) and a free-hand drawn region of interest (*right*) placed around the left ventricle in a radionuclide ventriculogram, or MUGA study

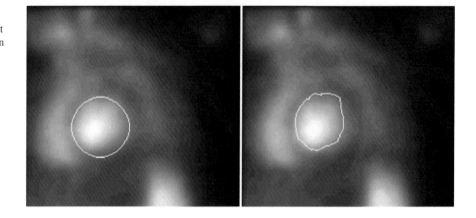

radiopharmaceutical as the kidney clears it from the blood. The second phase uses longer frames to evaluate the washout of the radiopharmaceutical from the kidney. The key ROIs are those placed over the kidneys and background (which may be elliptical around the whole kidney or crescent shaped as described earlier),

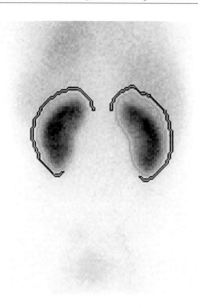

Fig. 12.28 An example of automatic ROIs placed on a renal image. The kidney ROIs are determined by a complex algorithm using expected location, image intensities, and edge detection in polar coordinates. Note the rather crescent-shaped background regions placed at the lateral edge of each kidney. Their shapes are based on the detected kidney ROIs, and are a single pixel thick

but ROIs over the bladder and aorta may also provide useful information [28, 29]. The generation and analysis of renogram curves is shown in Fig. 12.29.

Gated blood pool studies (equilibrium radionuclide angiography) of the heart provide a great deal of information about regional heart motion and other factors, but the single most important calculation is that of the ejection fraction calculated from a time activity curve of the left ventricle [27]. The EKG R-to-R interval is usually divided into 24 time segments, each with a corresponding scintigram representing the distribution of blood (which has been labeled with a radiopharmaceutical) at that time in the cardiac cycle. ROIs are drawn over the left ventricle of the heart at end diastole (and preferably at each of the intervals) [30] and counts are extracted. Displayed as a curve, the graph represents the change in volume of the left ventricle at that time in the heart's cycle. The assumption is made that the counts extracted from the ROI are proportional to the volume of blood in the ventricle. To improve the accuracy of this assumption, counts from the ROI that may originate in front of or behind the heart are estimated using a background ROI drawn over an area near the heart but not over areas of significant blood pool. The counts

per pixel in the background ROI are calculated, and subtracted from the counts in the volume curve. Selection of a proper background ROI is critical to the calculation as oversubtracting background can falsely elevate the ejection fraction as shown in Fig. 12.30.

Regardless of how time activity curves are generated, there are a number of techniques that maybe used to analyze the data they contain. If the frames are acquired very quickly or there is little activity in the ROI, it may be necessary to use curve-smoothing algorithms to reduce the noise in the curve. If the underlying processes behind the changes in activity represented by the time activity curve are understood, curve fitting techniques may be used to glean further information from the curve.

12.8 Image Segmentation

12.8.1 Thresholding

It may be possible to find a pixel value above which everything is in the region of interest, and below which everything is background. Such a pixel value is called a threshold. Thresholds can be set interactively, but a few methods for obtaining them automatically have been proposed. In some cases, setting a single threshold at a known percentage of the maximum pixel intensity may suffice. Multiple thresholds, for example, one every 10%, can be used to create isocontours; this may give the user an idea of which threshold is the correct one to define the ROI. These approaches are shown in Fig. 12.31.

Another simple approach is to use a histogram of pixel values, so that a graph of number of pixels vs. pixel value is obtained. In some images, for example, brain images, the histogram will be bimodal. A high peak will exist at low pixel values, indicating background pixels; a second peak will occur at higher pixel values, indicating brain pixels. The valley between the two peaks can be used as a threshold to separate brain from background. In other images, where more than one structure is higher in intensity, it may be possible for the user to select which structure is that which is important. The result of thresholding is an image where all areas above the threshold are set to 1, and all areas below are set to 0. An example of this type of approach on a single slice of a brain perfusion image is

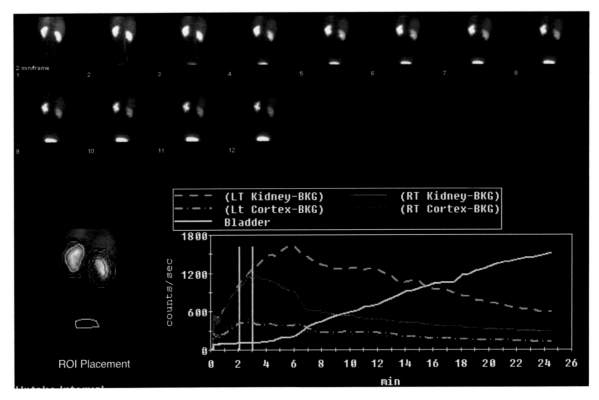

Fig. 12.29 ^{99m}Tc MAG3 renogram curves for each kidney are extracted from ROIs placed over the kidney, the renal cortex (along the outside rim of the kidney), and background. An ROI is also placed over the bladder. This image shows the clearance phase of the renogram, and each frame represents a 2 min interval. The uptake phase of this renogram is shown in Fig. 12.5. With 2 s per frame, counts from the uptake phase are shown in the first 30 s of the curve in this figure. Counts extracted from the kidney ROIs are background corrected before plotting. Counts extracted from the bladder ROI increase throughout the study as the tracer is cleared from the blood by the kidneys. (The authors would like to acknowledge Raghuveer K. Halkar, MD, Emory University, Atlanta, GA, for his assistance with this figure.)

shown in Fig. 12.32. Finding the boundary of the region containing 1s can be performed using the edge tracking method described below, for example.

While most thresholding operations are too simplistic to be widely applicable in defining ROIs, they are often used as an important step in a more complicated processing algorithm. One application where thresholding is particularly important is tumor delineation [31–33]. Again, additional processing is usually applied; however, given that there is rarely any a priori information about tumor shape or location, image intensity is often the most important factor in defining its boundaries.

12.8.2 Edge Detection

Edges of structures in images are generally defined points of quick intensity changes, or high intensity gradients. A portion of the image that falls rapidly from a high value to a low value is often taken to be the edge of a structure. High-pass filtering, or image sharpening, brings out these regions of changing intensity. However, in a complete image slice, there are usually many edges not associated with the region of interest. Conversely, some edges of the ROI may not actually have strong intensity changes associated with them, particularly, if there are low pixel values associated with some physiological process or abnormality. Some method of following the correct boundary is necessary. The problem is, given a potential point on the boundary, or seed, to successively follow the contour and create a closed boundary. This is generally posed as a search algorithm; that is, finding the best contour given some specific constraints that act as a cost function that is to be optimized. Moving from the seed pixel onward, a boundary "cost" is accumulated

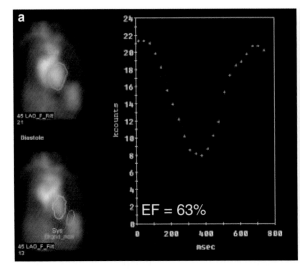
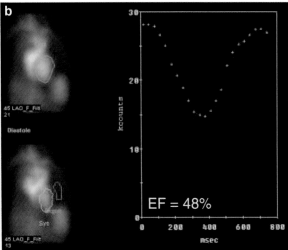

Fig. 12.30 Gated blood pool volume curves are extracted from ROIs drawn over the blood pool of the left ventricle of the ERNA study shown in Fig. 12.5. The volume curve represents background corrected counts at each of the 24 frames or segments of the cardiac cycle. Care must be taken in the placement of the background ROI, since the counts from this region are used to estimate the nonblood pool counts in ventricular ROI. In panel (**a**) the background ROI is placed in a standard location, but overlaps the spleen which has an unusually high concentration of activity. The resulting oversubtraction of background gives an artifactually high estimate of the ejection fraction (EF). In panel (**b**) the background ROI is placed in a more appropriate location for this patient and a much lower EF is calculated. (The authors would like to acknowledge Raghuveer K. Halkar, MD, Emory University, Atlanta, GA, for his assistance with this figure.)

Fig. 12.31 Example of threshold-based regions of interest placed in the same study as Fig. 12.1. A single threshold of 50% (*left*) creates multiple regions of interest; however, the user can indicate which is important. Use of multiple thresholds (*right*) provides isocontours that allow the user to choose more accurately the correct threshold to outline the heart

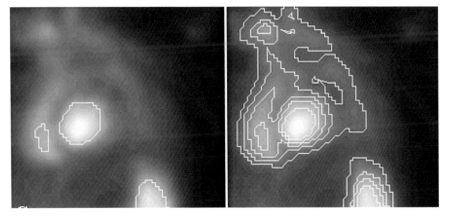

associated with the possible neighboring pixels that may be chosen as the next boundary point. Typical cost functions might include edge magnitude and direction, curvature of a segment, or closeness to a known average contour. One sophisticated approach is described generally for 2D medical image boundary detection [34]; however, note that edge following in 3D becomes much more complicated, and is infrequently used.

12.8.3 Model-Based Approaches

If the expected shape of the region of interest is known, then it may be possible to locate the ROI by fitting a model of the object to the image. This model may be obtained, for example, by hand tracing numerous training images and finding the average shape of the ROI. The model may be as simple as a new image

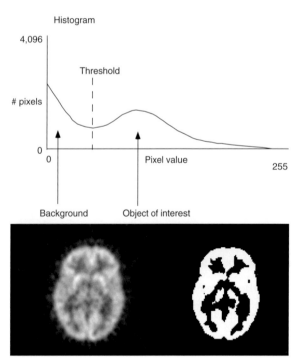

Fig. 12.32 A histogram of image intensities in a slice of a PET FDG brain image (*top*) shows a bimodal distribution. One peak occurs in the background pixel intensities, and another is seen in the gray matter pixel intensities. Choosing a pixel intensity between these two peaks allows the background to be separated from the object of interest, in this case, the gray matter. The original image and the result of the thresholding are seen at the bottom of the figure

containing nothing but this average shape with its values set to the average values obtained from the training set. In one simple approach, registration techniques may be used to fit the model to the new image containing the object. The model is shifted, rotated, and scaled over all possible locations in the new image, and a measure of the match is computed at each. It may even be nonlinearly warped to match the new image. A common metric for evaluating the goodness of the match is the sum of the squared differences between the template and the image. This difference should be small when the model matches well with the image. In a second more complicated approach, the boundaries of the model may be iteratively adapted so that it better fits the object of interest. Constraints on the boundary may be used so that they do not stretch too far beyond the original model and that they maintain a smooth surface. In fact, fitting of the model may also be posed as a registration problem. At any rate, the goal of fitting the model to the image

in this manner is to be able to use the boundaries of the transformed model as the boundaries of the ROI in the new image. This approach is becoming more and more common in 3D, as it is able to encode complicated 3D shapes as well as variances in image intensities. When shape is included, the model may be called an active shape model; when it includes image intensity, it may be called an active appearance model.

Most model-based approaches have focused on the brain and heart [35–39]. Often, they were developed as part of a first step in finding abnormal regions of perfusion or metabolism. The model is used to segment a set of normal studies, and then normal ranges within the model ROIs are determined. When a test subject is segmented with the model, the values within the model ROIs can be compared to the normal values in order to automatically determine any regions of hypometabolism or hypoperfusion. Figure 12.33 shows how this approach has been used in quantitation of brain FDG images.

12.8.4 Application-Specific Approaches

Most automatic quantitative programs use very application-specific techniques to isolate the region of interest. This is simply because encoding more specific information into the boundary detection algorithm tends to make it more accurate and more robust. One very common method for automated boundary detection in cardiac imaging, for example, is to perform the operation in polar (for 2D), spherical, or cylindrical (for 3D) coordinates. In this approach, the origin of the coordinate system is placed inside the region of interest. This may be done interactively or automatically. Searching along rays that extend from this origin at set angles, points of high intensity or of high gradient are determined. High-intensity points might be used when searching for the midmyocardium in perfusion images, while high-gradient points might be used when searching for the edge of the ventricular chamber in blood pool images. Because the radius of the boundary should not change greatly between neighboring rays, the search can be constrained, and the boundary can be forced to be smooth. Searches can be limited by placing constraints on how far the ray can extend, and filtering the radii after the boundary detection can further enforce smoothness constraints.

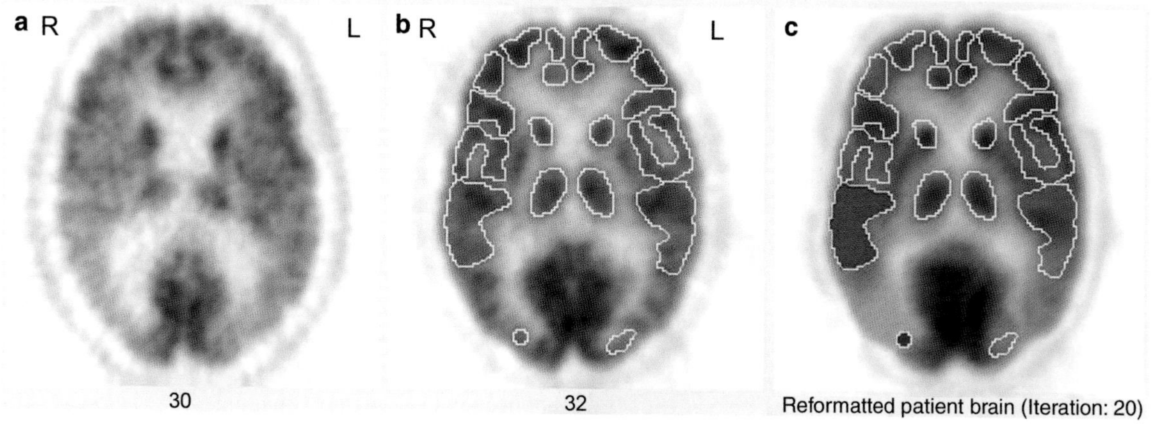

Fig. 12.33 An example of a model-based approach for defining ROIs on a PET FDG image of the brain. (**a**) One slice of a patient's FDG brain image. (**b**) One slice of the "standard," or model, normal FDG image. Regions of interest have already been defined on this standard. (**c**) The patient's image is aligned to the standard, and the ROIs from the standard can then be placed over the patient's brain

This sort of approach is used frequently in organs that are primarily convex, such as the kidney, the brain surface, and the heart [40, 41]. In addition, note that this approach provides a simple way to find the boundary of a thresholded object, given that the object is mostly convex. Figure 12.28 shows an example of how this approach has been applied to find kidney ROIs as a first step in quantitation of renal function [42].

12.9 Three Dimensional Displays

12.9.1 Surface Rendering

Three-dimensional graphics techniques can be used to display both the structure and function of organs visualized in nuclear medicine. If the organ of interest has been accurately segmented using edge detection techniques, then the resulting boundaries can be used to create a 3D surface onto which information about detected counts can be overlaid. The 3D surface may be generated by connecting points of the detected boundaries into triangles, or in some cases, quadrilaterals. Various algorithms exist to perform such triangulations. If the result of edge detection is a set of points, the theoretically most efficient triangularization is called a "Delauney" triangularization [43]. If the result of the edge detection is a binary image,

perhaps obtained by thresholding, then an efficient algorithm for generating the triangles of the surface, such as the marching cubes algorithm, can be used [44]. However, if a systematic approach has been used for the edge detection, often a standard triangularization will be sufficient. For example, if the boundary can be divided into the same number of points in each slice of the organ, then connecting the points into triangles is simple. Color can be assigned to each vertex of the triangles in numerous ways. In brain imaging, perfusion or metabolism may be estimated by sampling perpendicularly to the detected surface at each triangle vertex and determining the count value just inside of it. The LV epicardial surface can be color coded with the maximum values obtained at the middle of the myocardium; this is straightforward if both epicardial surface detection and midmyocardial maximum count determination are done using the same spherical coordinate system, for example. Once a set of triangles with vertex colors has been generated, standard software programs are used to display them. Such displays can routinely be rotated in real time and viewed from any angle with current computer power. Sophisticated effects, including highlights, reflection, and transparency may be easily applied. The mathematics behind these effects, as well as a much more detailed discussion of surface rendering can be found in the book by Foley and Van Dam [45]. Such displays have the advantage of showing the actual size and shape of the organ, and the extent and location of

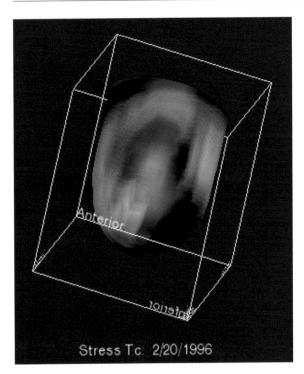

Stress Tc: 2/20/1996

Fig. 12.34 A surface-rendered 3D display created from a SPECT myocardial perfusion study. Once the epicardial and endocardial surfaces have been detected (i.e., a myocardial ROI has been defined), the x, y, and z values of the epicardial surface can be connected into a triangle mesh. The colors used to shade each triangle are based on the maximum values of the perfusion image between the epicardial and endocardial surface at each epicardial point

any defect. Some studies have shown that the 3D models displaying left ventricular perfusion are more accurate for evaluating the size and location of perfusion defects than polar maps [46] or slice-by-slice displays [47]. Figure 12.34 shows a typical surface rendering of the left ventricle, color coded for myocardial perfusion.

12.9.2 Maximum Intensity Projection

A second approach to creating 3D displays from cardiac images generates the myocardial boundaries directly from image voxels without explicit boundary detection. The most useful technique employed in nuclear medicine is maximum intensity projection (MIP) developed by Wallis et al. [48]. Maximum intensity projection involves rotating the 3D tomographic

volume into a desired viewing angle and extracting the maximum pixel along each row and column of the rotated volume onto a 2D image plane. To enhance the 3D effect of the image, the volume can be depth-weighted, so that pixels extracted from the front of the volume are scaled more highly than those extracted from the rear of the volume, even if their original intensities were equal. This emphasizes structures in the front of the volume. Since the maximum pixel is always extracted, this type of volume rendering is very useful in blood-pool imaging [49] as well as other hot-spot imaging procedures. Although not directly applicable to cold-spot imaging, a variation of this technique has been successfully applied to liver-spleen imaging and brain perfusion imaging [50]. This variation consists of blurring the original image using a 3D filter and subtracting the blurred image from the original image. The resultant dataset is then rendered using MIP as described above.

12.9.3 Volume Rendering

While maximum intensity projection techniques may be considered a simple type of volume rendering, generally, the term implies a much more complicated algorithm. Like maximum intensity projection, however, volume rendering techniques do not need explicit boundary detection or creation of geometric surfaces. While volume rendering techniques are more useful when used with CT data, it is useful to understand the methods given the current interest in combined PET/CT and SPECT/CT scanners. Volume rendering is a 3D graphics technique first described by Drebin et al. [51] which provides very realistic-appearing visualizations. For a volume of data, such as a stack of 2D tomographic slices, one assigns to every pixel value a transparency, a color, and a reflectivity. The visual process is then simulated by recreating the physical process of light traveling through or bouncing off the pixels that it encounters as it travels through the volume. For any given volume of data, the main problems involve the correct assignment of the pixel properties. Selecting a pixel intensity threshold above which everything is opaque, and below which everything is transparent, for example, will provide a 3D image with hard surfaces at that threshold. In nuclear medicine, the use of such a threshold often results in normal pixels being assigned a value of 1, and abnormal pixels being assigned a value of 0, so that the 3D display depicts a "hole" in the surface. Such techniques have been used primarily in brain images; however, they have also been applied to cardiac images. Unfortunately, very few medical images are accurately segmented with such simplistic threshold techniques, and note that the size of the abnormality, or hole, is completely dependent on choosing the right threshold. CT images are in fact probably the best adapted to this simple method of assigning pixel properties, since Hounsfield units are related to the electron density of particular tissues, and thus, bone can be made opaque and white, while muscle tissue can be made translucent and red, for example. In fact, a basic 3D display method similar to volume rendering was described quite early for use in CT images by Hoehne et al. [52]. While volume rendering of bone in CT images is generally quite robust, most 3D displays of soft tissue generated from CT require large amounts of preprocessing to remove unwanted structures or improve the segmentation. The accuracy of this preprocessing is generally related to the quality of the images, and user intervention may be required to produce a useable 3D display. In addition, large amounts of memory and processing power are required for volume rendering of large datasets. Nevertheless, the realism, high resolution, and flexibility of volume renderings give them an advantage over surface renderings in many cases; this can be appreciated in Fig. 12.35.

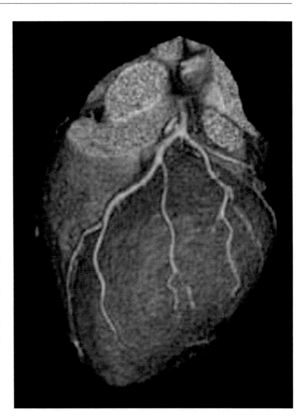

Fig. 12.35 A cardiac CT study may be volume rendered by assigning colors and transparencies to the Hounsfield units within it, and then reproducing the effect of light being transmitted and reflected from it. In this case, sophisticated segmentation and additional user interaction must be used to eliminate noncardiac structures from the CT prior to 3D rendering

12.10 Principles of Image Registration

As mentioned above in the model-based approach for segmentation, alignment of a presegmented model with a specific patient's image can be used to find regions or volumes of interest in the new image. In addition, alignment (also called registration or fusion) is often used with nuclear medicine for other important purposes. Low-resolution nuclear medicine images are aligned with higher-resolution anatomic images of the same patient to help identify the exact location of a hot or cold spot in the nuclear image. In this application, it may be sufficient to transform the test image using only linear transformations. Also, in order to use many quantitative programs, the patient's specific nuclear image must be put into a standard space. More and more, this standardization implies that the test image is being aligned to a standard, or atlas, image. In this application, frequently, a nonlinear warping transformation is needed.

Registration is generally posed as an iterative optimization problem. The differences between two images are to be minimized over some transformation. Thus, two separate pieces of software are needed: one to measure the difference, or cost function, and a second to determine how to change the image with respect to the standard to reduce this difference function at each iteration.

While there are many options for computing the cost function, a very popular approach is called the mutual information criterion [53, 54]. Mutual information can be described as the joint histogram between the two images. When two images are perfectly aligned, the joint histogram should ideally exist only along the line of identity. As the images are moved away from each other, the joint histogram also spreads out. Mutual information is a measure of the spread of the joint histogram. An example of this can be seen in Fig. 12.36.

For linear registration, that is, registration that includes only translation, scale, and rotation, generally closed form optimization methods are used to iteratively find the transformation that optimizes mutual information between two images. One such method is the Newton–Raphson method, which finds the roots of the derivative of the cost function, which occur at function minima. Woods et al. used this method in early work aligning PET brain images to MRI, and an example is shown in Fig. 12.37.

For nonlinear registration, or warping, the challenge is to find a good match between the images while making sure that the warping is smooth. This can be achieved by adding a regularizer, or smoothness constraint. For example, the warping can be constrained to be elastic, so that small deformations are easily achieved, but larger movements are "penalized," as they require more "force," similar to any elastic deformation. This is the approach taken by

Bajcsy et al. in early work aligning MR brain images [55]. Other constraints based on the known physical properties of the objects being aligned may be used to help find a good solution to the warping problem. For example, it is possible to constrain all deformations to be volume-preserving, so that pixels can change shape but must keep their original volumes, as suggested by Haber et al. [56]. Minimization of these more complicated functions may be attained by posing them as Euler-Lagrange equations, whose solution is a local optimum. An example of warping a brain image to match an atlas was shown in Fig. 12.33.

However, nonlinear warping has some major drawbacks. First, it can be quite time-consuming, especially for large images. One additional source of computational complexity is the nonlinear interpolation required. For example, a method such as thin plate splines may be required to interpolate multiple unevenly spaced points to new, unevenly spaced pixel locations [57]. Another problem is that if the proper constraints are not used in the warping algorithm, physically impossible deformations may occur. Parts of the image may "fold" onto one another, or more than one point may be mapped into a single location. Finally, it is very difficult to evaluate the

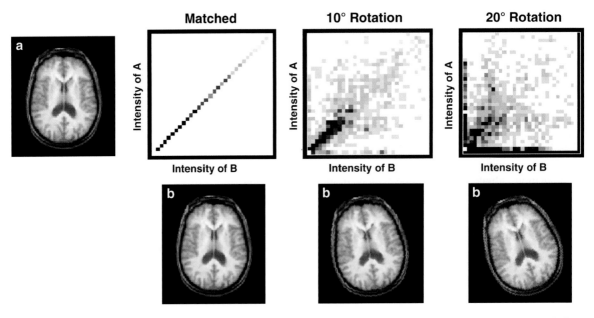

Fig. 12.36 Mutual information criteria for image registration. Image (**b**) is to be aligned with Image (**a**). At each rotation of (**b**) the joint histogram is created. When the images are in exact alignment, the joint histogram has values only on the line of

identity. As the images are rotated more and more out of alignment, the joint histogram becomes more diffuse. Mutual information is a measure of the spread of the joint histogram

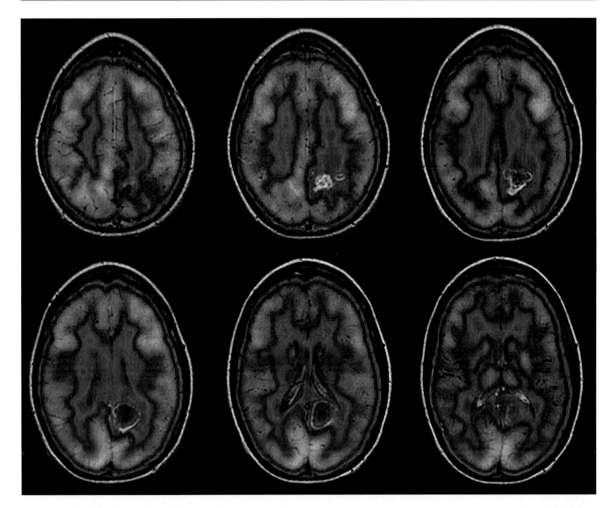

Fig. 12.37 An example of using linear registration to align a PET brain image to an MRI of the same patient. A function based on the ratio of the image pixel values was used as the difference measure, and this was minimized using a Newton–Raphson method. In this image, the PET is overlaid in color over the grayscale MRI

results of a warping algorithm. What may look like a reasonable deformation may not be accurate, as there is often no "ground truth." The user should be sure to accept nonlinear alignments only after careful assessment.

each pixel are relative (or related) to each other and the actual activity is being measured in the object; however, without additional processing, these counts are not absolute in nature. Furthermore, there may be some physiologic phenomena that occur that obscures the object of interest.

12.11 Image Normalization

As mentioned in the above section on Image Presentation, images that are acquired in Nuclear Medicine are generally constructed from the counts that are received at each individual pixel. This means that the counts in

12.11.1 Extraobject Activity

In Cardiac SPECT, it is not uncommon for the gallbladder or a loop of bowel to have more activity than the heart, thereby causing the heart to appear reduced in the images. Figure 12.38 shows a Cardiac SPECT study where a loop of bowel (seen in the bottom of the image) is much brighter than any of the pixels in the heart, thereby causing the counts in the heart to seem very low. To correct this problem, the study needs to be "normalized" to the counts in the myocardium, and not the counts in the entire image. This normalization (or scaling) process simply rescales the image such that the maximum displayed value is now equal to the maximum in the heart, instead of the maximum in the image

or volume. In this example, the maximum activity in the bowel was 839 counts and the maximum activity in the heart was 530 counts. Figure 12.39 shows the same image scaled to the maximum of the myocardium, instead of the maximum of the volume. Notice how the loop of bowel is now very bright but the myocardium looks much more normal. This phenomena can be seen in many different imaging scenarios, such as the bone scan shown previously (Fig. 12.4). Notice how hot the bladder is compared to the rest of the image in

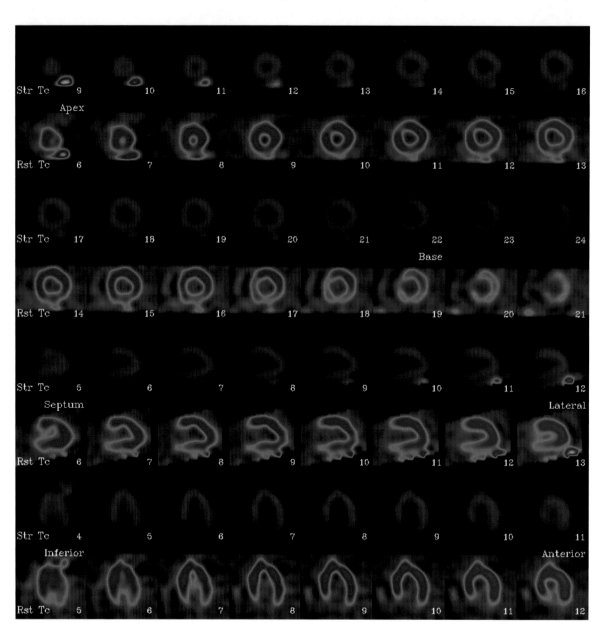

Fig. 12.38 Example of normalization, scaled to the maximum pixel in the volume

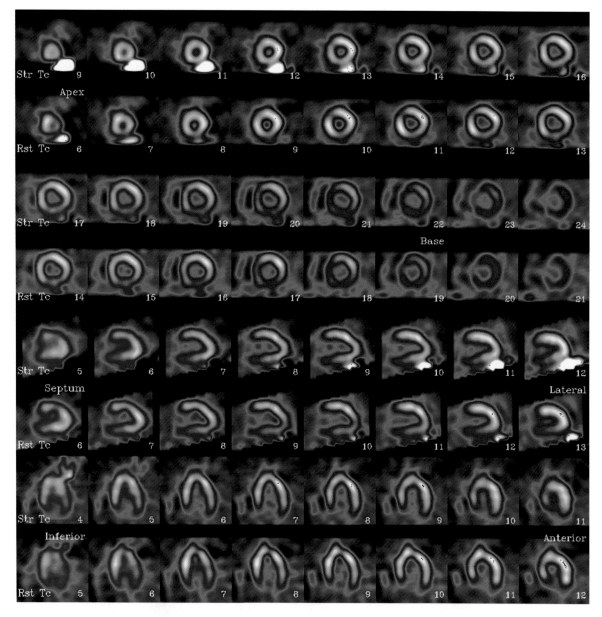

Fig. 12.39 Example of normalization, scaled to the maximum activity in the myocardium

the left-hand image. There are several ways to correct for this: (a) masking out the hot bladder and renormalizing to the maximum count in the image, (b) drawing a region-of-interest around most of the image (but excluding the bladder) and renormalizing to the maximum count in the ROI and (c) using the color table to renormalize the image by setting a new maximum value for display. In this case, the display maximum was reset to 100 in the right-hand image, thereby allowing the clinical details in the image to be seen.

12.11.2 Absolute Normalization/ Quantification

Another area of interest and research over the years has been in the area of absolute quantification, or converting the relative counts from the image into absolute measures of activity. Briefly, this involves correcting the image for attenuation, scatter, and resolution as well as measuring the counts in the arterial blood supply and then some form of modeling to predict the activity in the target organ. As you can see, this can be a complicated problem, but it can have big rewards. For instance, in Cardiac SPECT, if a patient has balanced disease (equal disease in all of the coronary territories), then all of the heart will look "relatively" the same which could easily be interpreted as a normal scan. However, if we could get an absolute measure of the activity in the heart, then we would be able to tell that the activity was below normal and that the scan was actually abnormal, though in "relative" terms it looked normal [58–60].

12.11.3 Normalization for Database Quantification

Because of the "relative" nature of the counts acquired in Nuclear Medicine, one of the approaches to overcome this is to compare a patient's scan to a database of normal volunteers. This technique is used in many imaging scenarios such as Cardiac, Renal, Neuro, and others. In order for this technique to work correctly, the patient's scan needs to be normalized or scaled to the same range as the data in the normal database. For instance, Fig. 12.40a shows the average or mean counts for the male and female normal files for a typical 1 day ^{99m}Tc Sestamibi myocardial SPECT scan. In order to compare a patient's scan to this normal file, it must first be scaled into the same range as the normal file, using the same region of activity. For instance, if the normal file had a maximum count of 1,000, which occurred in the anterior wall, and the anterior wall of the patient's scan had a maximum count of 1,200, then the patient's scan would need to be multiplied by 0.83 before comparison to the normal file. Figure 12.40 shows an abnormal patient after comparison to the normal file, in which abnormal areas have been turned black (note the large anterior and inferior wall defects) [61–63].

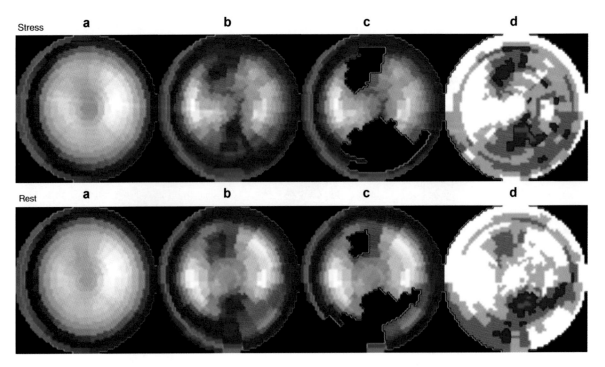

Fig. 12.40 Example of SPECT database comparison (**a**) Stress and rest female normal file for Tc-99m 1 day sestamibi. (**b**) Stress and rest raw polar maps (counts extracted from the stress and rest short-axis datasets). (**c**) Stress and rest blackout polar maps after comparison to the normal database; blacked-out areas show regions of significant hypoperfusion. (**d**) Stress and rest standard deviation polar maps, *darker areas* show regions that are more standard deviations from the normal file than lighter areas

12.12 Conclusion

Image processing is an integral part of the daily nuclear medicine routine and many physiological as well as functional parameters can be extracted from the different nuclear medicine procedures by various processing tools. Not only is image processing able to convey this desired information, but also a variety of display tools exist to assist in image interpretation and patient diagnosis. Hopefully, this overview has given you an appreciation for how difficult it would be to work with any kind of imaging modality without the use of computers. In fact, computers are a very necessary part of any imaging modality and will only become more important as we continue to push the envelope of imaging.

References

1. Cassen B, Curtis L, Reed CW (1949) A sensitive directional gamma ray detector. Technical Report #UCLA-49 (OSTI ID: 4434981), University of California, Los Angeles
2. Anger HO (1957) A new instrument for mapping gamma-ray emitters. Biology and Medicine Quarterly Report for October, November, December 1956, Report #UCRL-3653 (OSTI ID: 4354301), p. 51
3. Kuhl DE, Edwards RQ (1963) Image separation radioisotope scanning. Radiology 80:653–662
4. Jaszczak RJ (2006) The early years of single photon emission computed tomography (SPECT): an anthology of selected reminiscences. Phys Med Biol 51:R99–R115
5. Anger HO (1964) Scintillation camera with multichannel collimators. J Nucl Med 5:515–531
6. Gotway MB, Leung JW, Gooding GA, Litt HI, Reddy GP, Morita ET, Webb WR, Clark OH, Higgins CB (2002) Hyperfunctioning parathyroid tissue: spectrum of appearances on noninvasive imaging. AJR Am J Roentgenol 179:495–502
7. Hoffman EJ, Huang SC, Phelps ME (1979) Quantitation in positron emission computed tomography: 1. Effect of object size. J Comput Assist Tomogr 3:299–308
8. Demirkaya O, Al Mazrou R (2007) Performance test data analysis of scintillation cameras. IEEE Trans Nucl Sci 54:1506–1515
9. Anderson S (2005) Collins English dictionary, 7th edn. HarperCollins, Glasgow
10. Galt JR, Garcia EV, Nowak DJ (1986) Filtering in Frequency Space. J Nucl Med Technol 14:152–160
11. Hansen CL (2002) Digital image processing for clinicians, part I: basics of image formation. J Nucl Cardiol 9:343–349
12. Hansen CL (2002) Digital image processing for clinicians, part II: filtering. J Nucl Cardiol 9:429–437
13. Hansen CL (2002) Digital image processing for clinicians, part III: SPECT reconstruction. J Nucl Cardiol 9:542–549
14. Zubal IG, Wisniewski G (1997) Understanding Fourier space and filter selection. J Nucl Cardiol 4:234–243
15. Cooke CD, Garcia EV, Cullom SJ, Faber TL, Pettigrew RI (1994) Determining the accuracy of calculating systolic wall thickening using a fast Fourier transform approximation: A simulation study based on canine and patient data. J Nucl Med 35:1185–1192
16. Chen J, Faber TL, Cooke CD, Garcia EV (2008) Temporal resolution of multiharmonic phase analysis of ECG-gated myocardial perfusion SPECT studies. J Nucl Cardiol 15:383–391
17. Galt JR, Garcia EV, Robbins WL (1990) Effects of myocardial wall thickness on spect quantification. IEEE Trans Med Imaging 9:144–150
18. Faber TL, Cooke CD, Folks RD, Vansant JP, Nichols KJ, DePuey EG, Pettigrew RI, Garcia EV (1999) Left ventricular function and perfusion from gated SPECT perfusion images: an integrated method. J Nucl Med 40:650–659
19. Pflugfelder PW, Sechtem UP, White RD, Higgins CB (1988) Quantification of regional myocardial function by rapid cine MR imaging. Am J Roentgenol 150:523–529
20. DePuey EG, Rozanski A (1995) Using gated technetium-99m-sestamibi SPECT to characterize fixed myocardial defects as infarct or artifact. J Nucl Med 36:952–955
21. Chen J, Garcia EV, Folks RD, Cooke CD, Faber TL, Tauxe EL, Iskandrian AE (2005) Onset of left ventricular mechanical contraction as determined by phase analysis of ECG-gated myocardial perfusion SPECT imaging: development of a diagnostic tool for assessment of cardiac mechanical dyssynchrony. J Nucl Cardiol 12:687–695
22. Chen J, Henneman MM, Trimble MA, Bax JJ, Borges-Neto S, Iskandrian AE, Nichols KJ, Garcia EV (2008) Assessment of left ventricular mechanical dyssynchrony by phase analysis of ECG-gated SPECT myocardial perfusion imaging. J Nucl Cardiol 15:127–136
23. Henneman MM, Chen J, Dibbets-Schneider P, Stokkel MP, Bleeker GB, Ypenburg C, van der Wall EE, Schalij MJ, Garcia EV, Bax JJ (2007) Can LV dyssynchrony as assessed with phase analysis on gated myocardial perfusion SPECT predict response to CRT? J Nucl Med 48:1104–1111
24. Marsan NA, Henneman MM, Chen J, Ypenburg C, Dibbets P, Ghio S, Bleeker GB, Stokkel MP, van der Wall EE, Tavazzi L, Garcia EV, Bax JJ (2008) Left ventricular dyssynchrony assessed by two three-dimensional imaging modalities: phase analysis of gated myocardial perfusion SPECT and tri-plane tissue Doppler imaging. Eur J Nucl Med Mol Imaging 35:166–173
25. Henneman MM, Chen J, Ypenburg C, Dibbets P, Bleeker GB, Boersma E, Stokkel MP, van der Wall EE, Garcia EV, Bax JJ (2007) Phase analysis of gated myocardial perfusion single-photon emission computed tomography compared with tissue Doppler imaging for the assessment of left ventricular dyssynchrony. J Am Coll Cardiol 49:1708–1714
26. Trimble MA, Borges-Neto S, Honeycutt EF, Shaw LK, Pagnanelli R, Chen J, Iskandrian AE, Garcia EV, Velazquez EJ (2008) Evaluation of mechanical dyssynchrony and myocardial perfusion using phase analysis of gated SPECT imaging in patients with left ventricular dysfunction. J Nucl Cardiol 15:663–670

27. Taylor A, Schuster DM, Alazraki NP (2006) A clinician's guide to nuclear medicine, 2nd edn. Society of Nuclear Medicine, Reston

28. Taylor A Jr, Corrigan PL, Galt J, Garcia EV, Folks R, Jones M, Manatunga A, Eshima D (1995) Measuring technetium-99m-MAG3 clearance with an improved camera-based method. J Nucl Med 36:1689–1695

29. Taylor AT Jr, Fletcher JW, Nally JV Jr, Blaufox MD, Dubovsky EV, Fine EJ, Kahn D, Morton KA, Russell CD, Sfakianakis GN, Aurell M, Dondi M, Fommei E, Geyskes G, Granerus G, Oei HY (1998) Procedure guideline for diagnosis of renovascular hypertension. Society of Nuclear Medicine. J Nucl Med 39:1297–1302

30. Corbett JR, Akinboboye OO, Bacharach SL, Borer JS, Botvinick EH, DePuey EG, Ficaro EP, Hansen CL, Henzlova MJ, Van Kriekinge S (2006) Equilibrium radionuclide angiocardiography. J Nucl Cardiol 13:e56–e79

31. Erdi YE, Mawlawi O, Larson SM, Imbriaco M, Yeung H, Finn R, Humm JL (1997) Segmentation of lung lesion volume by adaptive positron emission tomography image thresholding. Cancer 80:2505–2509

32. Jentzen W, Freudenberg L, Eising EG, Heinze M, Brandau W, Bockisch A (2007) Segmentation of PET volumes by iterative image thresholding. J Nucl Med 48:108–114

33. Brambilla M, Matheoud R, Secco C, Loi G, Krengli M, Inglese E (2008) Threshold segmentation for PET target volume delineation in radiation treatment planning: the role of target-to-background ratio and target size. Med Phys 35:1207–1213

34. Mortensen E, Morse B, Barrett W, Udupa J (1992) Adaptive boundary detection using live-wire 2-dimensional dynamic-programming. In: Proceedings of the Computers in Cardiology, pp 635–638

35. Declerck J, Feldmar J, Goris ML, Betting F (1997) Automatic registration and alignment on a template of cardiac stress and rest reoriented SPECT images. IEEE Trans Med Imaging 16:727–737

36. Slomka PJ, Hurwitz GA, Stephenson J, Cradduck T (1995) Automated alignment and sizing of myocardial stress and rest scans to three-dimensional normal templates using an image registration algorithm (see comment). J Nucl Med 36:1115–1122

37. Mykkanen J, Tohka J, Luoma J, Ruotsalainen U (2005) Automatic extraction of brain surface and mid-sagittal plane from PET images applying deformable models. Comput Meth Programs Biomed 79:1–17

38. Minoshima S, Koeppe RA, Frey KA, Kuhl DE (1994) Anatomic standardization: linear scaling and nonlinear warping of functional brain images. J Nucl Med 35:1528–1537

39. Minoshima S, Frey KA, Koeppe RA, Foster NL, Kuhl DE (1995) A diagnostic approach in Alzheimer's disease using three-dimensional stereotactic surface projections of fluorine-18-FDG PET. J Nucl Med 36:1238–1248

40. Garcia EV, Cooke CD, Van Train KF, Folks RD, Peifer JW, DePuey EG, Maddahi J, Alazraki NP, Galt JR, Ezquerra NF, Ziffer JA, Areeda JS, Berman DS (1990) Technical aspects of myocardial SPECT imaging with technetium-99m sestamibi. Am J Cardiol 66:23E–31E

41. Germano G, Kavanagh PB, Waechter P, Areeda J, Van Kriekinge S, Sharir T, Lewin HC, Berman DS (2000) A new algorithm for the quantitation of myocardial perfusion SPECT. I: technical principles and reproducibility (see comment). J Nucl Med 41:712–719

42. Garcia E, Folks R, Pak S, Taylor A (2008) Automatic definition of renal regions-of-interests (ROIs) from MAG3 renograms in patients with suspected renal obstruction. J Nucl Med (Meeting Abstracts) 49:386P

43. Delaunay B (1934) Sur la sphere vide. A memoire de Georges Voronoi. Izv Akad Nauk SSSR, Otdelenie Matematicheskih i Estestvennyh Nauk 7:793–800

44. Lorensen WE, Cline HE (1987) Marching cubes: a high resolution 3D surface construction algorithm. SIGGRAPH Comput Graph 21:163–169

45. Foley JD, Phillips RL, Hughes JF, van Dam A, Feiner SK (1994) Introduction to computer graphics. Addison-Wesley, Longman

46. Cooke CD, Vansant JP, Krawczynska EG, Faber TL, Garcia EV (1997) Clinical validation of three-dimensional color-modulated displays of myocardial perfusion. J Nucl Cardiol 4:108–116

47. Santana CA, Garcia EV, Vansant JP, Krawczynska EG, Folks RD, Cooke CD, Faber TL (2000) Three-dimensional color-modulated display of myocardial SPECT perfusion distributions accurately assesses coronary artery disease. J Nucl Med 41:1941–1946

48. Wallis JW, Miller TR (1990) Volume rendering in three-dimensional display of SPECT images (see comments). J Nucl Med 31:1421–1428

49. Miller TR, Wallis JW, Sampathkumaran KS (1989) Three-dimensional display of gated cardiac blood-pool studies (see comments). J Nucl Med 30:2036–2041

50. Wallis JW, Miller TR (1991) Display of cold lesions in volume rendering of SPECT studies. J Nucl Med 32:985

51. Drebin RA, Carpenter L, Hanrahan P (1988) Volume rendering. In: Proceedings of the 15th annual conference on Computer graphics and interactive techniques. ACM

52. Hoehne KH, Delapaz RL, Bernstein R, Taylor RC (1987) Combined surface display and reformatting for the three-dimensional analysis of tomographic data. Invest Radiol 22:658–664

53. Viola P, Wells WM (1995) Alignment by maximization of mutual information. In: Proceedings of the Fifth International Conference on Computer Vision (ICCV 95), June 20–23, Massachusetts Institute of Technology, Cambridge, MA. IEEE Computer Society, Washington, DC, pp 16–23

54. Collignon A, Maes F, Delaere D, Vandermeulen D, Suetens P, Marchal G (1995) Automated multi-modality image registration based on information theory. Inform Process Med Imaging 3:263–274

55. Bajcsy R, Kovacic S (1989) Multiresolution Elastic Matching. Comput Vision Graph Image Processing 46:1–21

56. Haber E, Modersitzki J (2004) Numerical methods for volume preserving image registration. Inverse Prob 20:1621–1638

57. Bookstein FL (1989) Principal warps – thin-plate splines and the decomposition of deformations. IEEE Trans Pattern Anal Mach Intell 11:567–585

58. Kuhle WG, Porenta G, Huang SC, Buxton D, Gambhir SS, Hansen H, Phelps ME, Schelbert HR (1992) Quantification of regional myocardial blood flow using 13N-ammonia and reoriented dynamic positron emission tomographic imaging. Circulation 86:1004–1017

59. Hutchins GD, Schwaiger M, Rosenspire KC, Krivokapich J, Schelbert H, Kuhl DE (1990) Noninvasive quantification of regional blood flow in the human heart using N-13 ammonia and dynamic positron emission tomographic imaging. J Am Coll Cardiol 15:1032–1042

60. Kaufmann PA, Camici PG (2005) Myocardial blood flow measurement by PET: technical aspects and clinical applications. (erratum appears in J Nucl Med. 2005 46(2):291). J Nucl Med 46:75–88

61. Van Train KF, Areeda JS, Garcia EV, Cooke CD, Maddahi J, Kiat H, Germano G, Silagan G, Folks RD, Berman DS (1993) Quantitative same-day rest-stress technetium-99m-sestamibi SPECT: definition and validation of stress normal limits and criteria for abnormality. J Nucl Med 34:1494–1502

62. Van Train KF, Garcia EV, Maddahi J, Areeda JS, Cooke CD, Kiat H, Silagan G, Folks RD, Friedman J, Matzer L, Germano G, Bateman T, Ziffer JA, DePuey EG, Fink-Bennett D, Cloninger K, Berman DS (1994) Multicenter trial validation for quantitative analysis of same-day rest-stress technetium-99m-sestamibi myocardial tomograms. J Nucl Med 35:609–618

63. Santana CA, Folks RD, Garcia EV, Verdes L, Sanyal R, Hainer J, Di Carli MF, Esteves FP (2007) Quantitative (82) Rb PET/CT: development and validation of myocardial perfusion database. J Nucl Med 48:1122–1128

Emission Tomography and Image Reconstruction

13

Magdy M. Khalil

Contents

13.1 Introduction

In the early days of nuclear medicine, measurement of radioactivity administered into a human body was simply acquired by placing a Geiger counter over the desired region of interest. Further progress was undertaken using a rectilinear scanner. The breakthrough, as mentioned in Chap. 10, came from the development of the gamma camera and the use of the scintillation crystal coupled to photomultiplier tubes (PMTs). To this end, there was no available tool to measure the spatial extent of tracer distribution in three-dimensional (3D)

fashion, and all measurements were confined to two-dimensional (2D) planar imaging. The third dimension is important to fully depict radiopharmaceutical uptake, hence enabling the interpreting physician to make a confident decision. Another feature of 3D imaging is the ability to quantify tracer concentrations more accurately than with 2D imaging. Tracer uptake, residence time, and clearance rates are important dynamics of tracer biodistribution in diseased and healthy tissues, in which temporal sampling is particularly useful for studying tracer or organ kinetics. Adding the time dimension to 2D planar imaging is important in some scintigraphic studies, such as renal scintigraphy and planar equilibrium radionuclide angiocardiography (ERNA). In the former case, kidney function is studied through a time course of about half an hour, dividing the examination time into two phases (perfusion and function) such that the first minute is assigned to depict organ perfusion while the rest of the study is used to assess renal function. In planar ERNA, the time dimension is essential to make snapshots of different phases of the heart cycle through identification of the R-R signal during heart contraction. This helps to obtain valuable information about heart motion and to assess its functional parameters.

Many nuclear medicine procedures are performed by acquiring planar views of the area under investigation. However, planar images are manifested by poor image contrast and lack of quantitative accuracy. Nuclear examinations such as bone scintigraphy and thyroid, parathyroid, and lung scanning are among those studies for which planar imaging is commonly used; however, under many circumstances the 2D nature of the acquired data have shortcomings in their yield of accurate diagnostic results, especially when dense overlying structures obscure the inspection of tracer spread and accumulation. This directly

M.M. Khalil
Biological Imaging Centre, MRC/CSC, Imperial College London, Hammersmith Campus, Du Cane Road, W12 0NN London, UK
e-mail: magdy.khalil@imperial.ac.uk, magdy_khalil@hotmail.com

M.M. Khalil (ed.), *Basic Sciences of Nuclear Medicine*, DOI: 10.1007/978-3-540-85962-8_13,
© Springer-Verlag Berlin Heidelberg 2011

influences the interpretation results and may lead to an inconclusive diagnosis.

Many nuclear medicine procedures have been revolutionized by use of 3D imaging in terms of the amount of information that can be extracted and incorporated into the decision-making process. Among those are myocardial perfusions, brain, and bone imaging, for which tomographic acquisition provides a greater opportunity to visualize organs from different angular perspectives. This allows reading physicians to thoroughly investigate pathological lesions from many directions, especially when appropriate visualization tools are available on the viewing workstation. This in turn has had a positive impact on the diagnostic accuracy of many nuclear medicine examinations. For example, a tomographic bone scan is more sensitive than planar imaging and has been reported to improve the diagnostic accuracy for detecting malignant bone involvement [1].

13.2 SPECT and PET

There are two 3D techniques provided by nuclear imaging, single-photon emission computed tomography (SPECT) and positron emission tomography (PET). Both are noninvasive diagnostic modalities that are able to provide valuable metabolic and physiologic information about many pathophysiologic and functional disorders. A remarkable feature of SPECT and PET is their ability to improve contrast resolution manyfold compared to planar scintigraphic imaging. The two imaging modalities have proved useful as applications in molecular imaging research and translational medicine. In addition, attempts to derive quantitative parameters are more accurate than planar imaging. Furthermore, when the timing factor is added to the 3D imaging, the amount of information that can be obtained from analyzing the data is significantly high. Two examples are worth mentioning when SPECT or PET is used to collect tracer spatial distribution and its associated temporal component. One of these is gated myocardial perfusion tomographic imaging, in which the tracer distribution and heart function can be captured in one imaging session, providing an assessment of myocardial perfusion (or metabolic) parameters, such as defect extent and severity or tissue viability, in addition to the calculations of regional and global left ventricular function and ejection fraction. Another important area of application is the study of tracer distribution during the time course of tracer uptake and clearance from biological tissues. In these acquisition protocols, dynamic frames are collected over predefined timing intervals (or reframed in case of list mode acquisition) to record tracer flow, extraction, retention, and clearance from the tissue of interest. The recorded data are then presented to an appropriate mathematical model to obtain physiologically important parameters, such as transport rate constants and calculation of tissue metabolic activity or receptor density (see Chaps. 16 and 17).

The addition of temporal sampling to tomographic imaging has other utilities, such as recording the respiratory cycle to correct for lung motion on myocardial perfusion imaging and to correct for spatial coregistration errors arising from temporal mismatch between computed tomography (CT) and PET in lung bed positions during whole-body fluorodeoxyglucose-F18 (FDG) studies. The time information required for motion characterization in four-dimensional (4D) imaging can be obtained either prospectively or retrospectively using respiratory-gating or motion-tracking techniques [2].

The advances in hybrid imaging and introduction of PET/CT and SPECT/CT to the clinic have added another dimension to the diagnostic investigations; currently, hybrid modalities provide greater opportunity to study functional as well as morphological changes that occur at different stages of disease progression or regression. The characterizing aspects that distinguish these imaging methods from other imaging modalities are the underlying physical principals, the way data are acquired, image reconstruction and correction techniques, and finally image quantitation and display.

13.2.1 History

Emission and transmission CT rely on the fact that to obtain a 3D picture of the human body a set of multiple 2D projections is required for image reconstruction. This necessitates collection of a sufficient amount of information about the object under examination. Johann Radon (1887–1956) introduced the principles of data formation through what is called the radon transform, which describes an object in 3D space as a sum of line integrals. In 1917, Radon developed a solution for image reconstruction utilizing projection data sets and applied his technique to nonmedical applications, namely, gravitational problems. In 1956, the reconstruction technique developed by Radon found another application by Bracewell in the field of radioastronomy [3]. Allan Cormack, a few years later after Bracewell, independently and without knowledge about Radon's work, developed a method for calculating radiation absorption distributions in the human body based on transmission scanning. Kuhl and Edwards were the first to introduce the concept of emission tomography using backprojection in 1963, and about 10 years later, Godfrey Hounsfield, the inventor of CT, succeeded to practically implement the theory of image reconstruction in his first CT scanner. Shorty after the invention, Hounsfield and Cormack were recognized by sharing the Noble Prize in Medicine and Physiology in 1979. By analogy to PET imaging, CT scanning was focused on brain imaging; however, body examinations were introduced a few years later, and the first body images taken in the body prototype machine were of Hounsfield himself on December 20, 1974 [4].

One of the earlier works on tomography was to move the object while keeping the imaging system stationary. This was in the late 1960s and early 1970s, when investigators used transaxial tomography to image a patient setting on a rotatable chair placed in front of a stationary gamma camera. After the mid-1970s, a gamma camera detector was mounted on a rotated gantry to take multiple images around the patient under investigation [5].

13.2.2 Crossroads

SPECT and PET have some similarities and differences. SPECT imaging relies on the emission of single-photon emitters such as Tc-99m, I-123, In-111, Ga-67, and so on, while PET imaging uses positron emitters such as F-18, C-11, O-15, and N-13, either labeled or unlabeled to other compounds as in some SPECT diagnostic compounds. For example, the most commonly used single-photon and positron emitters are Tc-99m and F-18, respectively, and both can be labeled with many compounds to target a particular physiologic or biochemical disorder. When compared with PET compounds, SPECT tracers are widespread and commercially available from many vendors in addition to their long-term use in clinical experience. Most PET tracers necessitate an on-site cyclotron especially for short-lived positron emitters; thus, costs are relatively higher.

13.2.3 Resolution and Sensitivity

Other differences also arise between the two imaging modalities, such as spatial resolution and sensitivity (see Fig. 11.13 in Chap. 11). In general, clinical PET systems have better spatial resolution than SPECT; the former can provide an intrinsic spatial resolution of about 4–6 mm, and the latter can hardly achieve 10 mm full width at half maximum (FWHM; i.e., conventional designs). The resolution of PET images is determined by many factors, which differ from those that affect SPECT resolution. Detector size, positron range, photon acollinearity, and some instrumental factors contribute by different degrees to the spatial resolution of PET images, as discussed in Chap. 11. On the other hand, SPECT imaging uses multihole collimation to identify structures and to determine directionality of the emitted radiation. This type of data collection imposes constraints on the overall system sensitivity and spatial resolution. There is often a trade-off between sensitivity and spatial resolution in collimator design. For instance, collimators with high spatial resolution are designed with attempts to improve spatial resolution, but geometric efficiency is scarified and vice versa. Another aspect of this trade-off is realized in some other (divergent) collimator geometry, in which the spatial resolution is improved while keeping the sensitivity at the same level, but this comes with a reduced imaging field of view.

In PET imaging, there is also a trade-off of these performance parameters but not in a similar manner as the principles of photon detection in PET imaging obviate the need for such photon collimation, leading to increased system sensitivity. However, collimation also exists in PET imaging in a form of 2D and 3D acquisition modes by using collimating septa between scanner rings. This has a significant impact on the detection efficiency such that the sensitivity of the scanner in 3D mode is significantly higher (four to

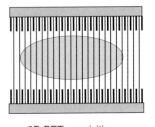 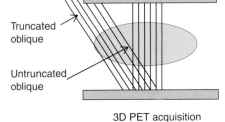 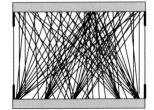

| 2D PET acquisition direct sinograms | 3D PET acquisition direct + oblique sinograms | 3D PET acquisition |

Fig. 13.1 Acquisition modes in positron emission tomographic (PET) scanning

six times) than that when the scanner is operated in 2D mode. In the last mode, collimator septa are placed between detector rings to confine the acquired projections to a set of 2D projection arrays. This facilitates image reconstruction so that any 2D reconstruction algorithms can be used, as is the case in 2D SPECT data reconstruction. In this way, image reconstruction is implemented in an independent slice-by-slice manner. Image reconstruction in 2D is a straightforward procedure, while in 3D some kind of data manipulation is required to utilize the increased system sensitivity in improving image quality. In septaless or 3D acquisition mode, however, the scanner sensitivity is not uniform across the axial field of view, and approaches to reconstruct images are either to use fully 3D reconstruction techniques or to rebin the data into a 2D projection array. Figure 13.1 shows the two acquisition modes offered by PET scanning.

13.2.4 Image Acquisition

Data sampling by gamma camera detector is implemented by computer digitization for the events detected on the scintillation crystal. The computer matrix varies according to system sensitivity, resolution, and data storage capacity. A lower matrix size, such as 64×64 and 128×128, is commonly used in emission tomography, while a higher matrix size (512×512) is used in x-ray CT. The photon density and spatial resolution provided by CT allows use of a higher matrix size. However, in nuclear PET and SPECT imaging, the relatively lower photon flux due to radioactive decay properties, restrictions on the injected dose, lower detection efficiency, acquisition time, and the expected spatial resolution all are underlying factors for reducing the matrix size.

In planar imaging, the patient is positioned in front of the detection system, and adequate time is given to form an image. The resulting image is a depiction of tracer distribution in two dimensions, x and y. The third dimension cannot be realized as the collected counts over a particular point of the detector matrix are a superimposition of tracer activities that lie along the accepted beam path. This manner of data acquisition does not allow for extracting valuable information about source depth. However, to solve such a problem additional information must be provided to obtain further details about tracer spatial distribution. Moving the detector to another position can produce another image for the given tracer distribution, and another angular view would again reveal information that was not present in the previous two views. This process can be repeated several times to complete an acquisition arc of at least 180°, which is the smallest angular arc that can be applied to reliably reconstruct an image. Let us go though some basic geometric and mathematical principles of this type of data acquisition.

In SPECT imaging, data acquisition is performed by a one-, two-, or three-head camera that is adjusted to rotate around the patient over small angular intervals to acquire an adequate set of 2D projections. The increased number of detector heads serves to improve study sensitivity and reduces the acquisition time. This is dissimilar to PET scanning, in which the circular ring design circumvents the patient in a 2π fashion; thus, detector rotation is not necessary. However, in the dual-detector coincidence gamma camera and partial-ring design, detector motion is required to satisfy angular requirements imposed by reconstruction algorithms. The detection process relies on annihilation photons (~180° apart) and coincidence circuitry to record events in an emission path, called

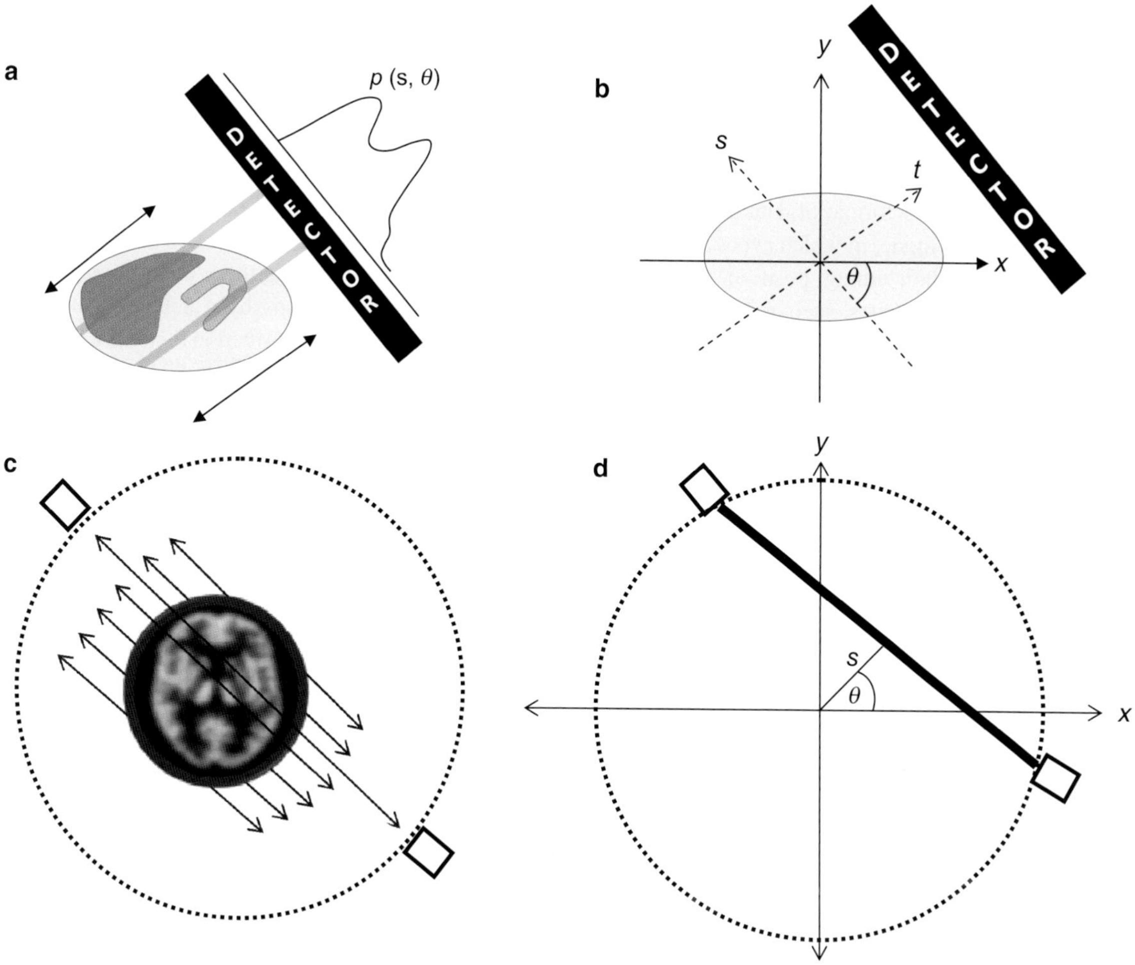

Fig. 13.2 (a) Projection profile for a one-dimensional (1D) row of the detector is displayed; a varying count intensity is evident. Any point on the profile is the line integral of all activity concentrations lying along the path of the ray. (b) The coordinate system (t, s) is defined so that s is parallel to the detector plane, while t is perpendicular on it. This coordinate system is used to define the projection profile $p(s, \theta)$ in relation to the stationary coordinate system (x, y). In (c, d) positron emission tomographic (PET) acquisition setting, similar projections are defined by sinogram variables s and θ, where both determine the location of the annihilation site on the sinogram

the tube or line of response (LOR). No physical collimation is required as in SPECT imaging.

Figure 13.2 shows one projection view for SPECT and PET cameras such that the former is positioned to acquire a cardiac study while the latter was chosen to image a brain patient. Suppose that we select one detector row (i.e., 1D) of the detector 2D matrix, and in 2D PET this corresponds to one projection angle acquired using a single ring. The activity distribution within a patient injected by myocardial tracer or FDG is defined by $f(x, y)$, where x and y are the coordinates of the tracer uptake inside the patient boundaries.

The counts collected over the elements of the projection row at an angle θ is denoted by the function $p(s, \theta)$, where θ is the angle subtended by the SPECT camera and the Cartesian x and y coordinates as shown in Fig. 13.2. This is also the same angle at which the PET camera was chosen to look at the brain study.

According to Radon, every projection bin of the 1D image is a result of count accumulation along the path traversed by the emitting radiations and falling perpendicular on the detector plane. However, in PET it is the line that connects a detector pair in coincidence. One can therefore consider the acquired counts at a given angle as a compressed version of the slice under investigation. At the end of data acquisition, we obtain a multiple number of projection angles; each is a compressed version of the object distribution viewed from different angles. In PET imaging, data format is mostly represented by rebinning the coincidence data in a sinogram. Another format of data acquisition and event storage is list mode, in which events are individually recorded for their timing, position, and possibly any other relevant attributes, such as energy.

The problem now is how to reconstruct or get a solution for the tracer concentration given the information provided by the set of projections. It is easy to understand that once we are able to reconstruct or find a solution for one transverse image, then it becomes possible to obtain the contiguous slices following the same steps. In the given examples, the function of the reconstruction algorithm is to find the best estimate of the tracer spatial distribution within the slices taken across the myocardium or the brain. Neglecting for photon scatter and detector response, one can write the measured projection as

$$p(s,\theta) = \int f(x,y)e^{-\int \mu(x,y)dt'} dt \qquad (13.1)$$

This is the attenuated radon transform, and solving the equation for $f(x, y)$ is the way to find estimates of tracer activity within the injected patient and hence image reconstruction. Here, s and t are elements of a coordinate system such that s is passing along the direction of the rays and perpendicular on the detector plane, while s is the axis parallel to the detector. In terms of x and y directions, s and t are defined as follows:

$$s = x\cos\theta + y\sin\theta$$

$$t = -x\sin\theta + y\cos\theta$$

By neglecting the exponential term, the resulting formula will be the Radon transform equation, which states that the acquired count over a particular projection bin $p(s, \theta)$ is the integration of tracer activity along the line that passes through the object studied and, in SPECT, falling perpendicular on the detector plane, while in PET it is the line that connects a coincident detector pair. The process that maps the tracer activity $f(x, y)$ onto the projection image $p(s, \theta)$ is defined as the x-ray transform.

In the case of SPECT, the exponential term of the formula denotes the amount of photon attenuation that extends from the site of emission $f(x, y)$ to the detector plane, demonstrated in Fig. 13.3, whereas in PET it refers to the amount of attenuation experienced by annihilation photons while traversing the corresponding patient thickness. Figure 13.4 shows how an attenuation correction problem in PET imaging can be solved by calculating the probability of detecting two coincident photons by a detector pair. It is noted that the attenuation correction factor is a function of the patient thickness and independent of the

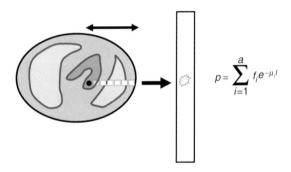

Fig. 13.3 Photon attenuation in single-photon emission computed tomography (SPECT)

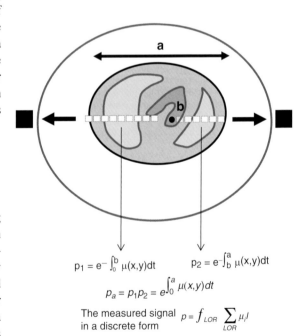

Fig. 13.4 Photon attenuation in positron emission tomography (PET)

emission site given a recorded LOR. By moving the exponential term to outside the integration, denoting the measured projection as I and the integration term as I_o, and rearranging the formula, we can obtain the attenuation correction factors (ACF) required to correct a measured LOR:

$$ACF = I_o/I$$

This is simply achievable in practice using a transmission source where I_o is the measurements performed while the patient is outside the field of view (i.e., blank scan), and I corresponds to the data taken when the patient is positioned inside the field of view (i.e., transmission scan).

Each LOR can be corrected for attenuation by multiplication with the corresponding correction factors, or the latter data can be reconstructed to obtain a spatial distribution of attenuation coefficients. In SPECT attenuation correction, the direct multiplication of the emission data by the correction factors is not applicable due to dependence of photon attenuation on the emission site, which is unknown. Instead, the logarithmic ratios of the initial and transmitted projections are reconstructed to obtain a spatial distribution of attenuation coefficients or what is known as an attenuation map.

The introduction of hybrid imaging such as SPECT/CT and PET/CT has allowed the use of CT images to correct the radionuclide emission data for photon attenuation. CT images provide low noise correction factors and faster scanning times, but corrected data may suffer from quantitative bias and correction artifacts. A CT scan also provides high-resolution anatomical images and with image coregistration serves to strength the confidence of lesion localization detected in radionuclide images. Radioactive sources provide more noise, less bias, and increased imaging time. Different methodologies have been devised to correct for the bias introduced by CT-based attenuation correction and methods to reduce noise propagation into radionuclide emission images when radioactive transmission scanning is used.

$$I = I_o e^{-\mu L}$$

where I and I_o are the transmitted and initial beam intensity, respectively. For an x-ray beam in CT, the rays traverse various body tissues of different attenuation properties due to their various compositions and effective Z number. Thus, the amount of attenuation that the beam encounters is equal to the total sum of all μ values that lie along the beam path.

Therefore, the measured transmission data for an x-ray beam of initial intensity I_o passing through a human body can be written as

$$p(s, \theta) = I_o e^{-\int \mu(x,y)dt}$$

Rearranging the formula and renaming the measured projection $p(s,\theta)$ as described, we obtain

$$ln\frac{I_o}{I} = \int \mu(x, y)dt$$

where $\mu(x, y)$ is the linear attenuation coefficient for a pixel located at position (x, y), and the integration is the line integral of attenuation coefficients along the transmission beam (see Fig. 13.5).

The reconstruction algorithm here does not try to find the activity distribution of the tracer, but it estimates the spatial distribution of attenuation coefficients using two pieces of information, the initial beam intensity I_o and the transmitted projection data. Note that this is the same equation used to derive the correction factors for PET emission data since it accounts for the total amount of photon attenuation experienced by the initial x-ray beam I_o while moving through the object. Actually, in real practice and data analysis of x-ray CT, determination of the distribution of attenuation coefficients is not simply performed by solving the equation stated here; several pre- and postprocessing steps are taken to correct for many variables and confounders that deviate the practical measurements from being consistent with the theoretical ideal conditions; for further details, see reference [6].

13.2.5 X-Ray CT

For a monoenergetic x-ray beam passing through an object of thickness L and linear attenuation coefficient μ, the transmitted radiation can be calculated from

13.2.6 Sinogram

Rebinning the acquired data in a single plot such that the projection bin represents the horizontal axis while

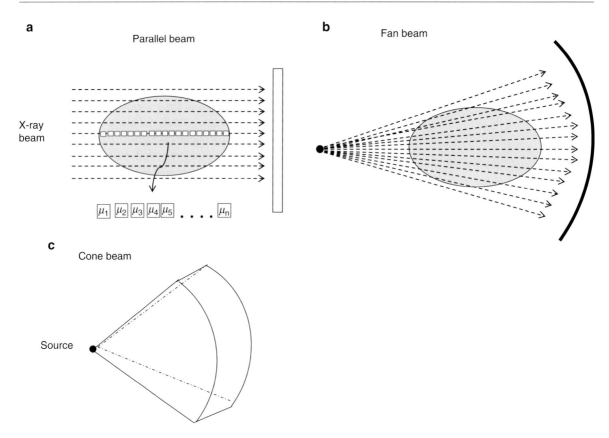

Fig. 13.5 In x-ray CT, different geometries have been used in image acquisition which in turn posed different requirements on image reconstructions. (**a**) image reconstruction is straightforwardly implemented using direct filtered backprojection (FBP). The other geometry is shown in (**b**) where image can be either reconstructed using rebining or direct FBP algorithm. (**c**) Cone beam: another design currently used in commercial CT scanners where image reconstruction is modified to adapt and account for beam geometry

the projection angle is placed on the vertical direction produces a sine wavelike pattern called a *sinogram*. Representing the acquired data in a sinogram has several benefits in terms of data processing, image reconstruction, and correction techniques. Also, it is useful in inspecting detector failure, in which a diagonal black line in a PET sinogram indicates an artifact in a single detector element, while a diagonal band could indicate a malfunction of a detector block [7]. It can also be used to correct for patient motion and for other correction techniques. Note that one selected pixel on the sinogram should indicate the total counts collected for a particular LOR regardless of any contamination from any other events (line-integral model). In SPECT, however, it is the integral of counts that lie along the emission path and falling perpendicular on the detector surface.

For a point source located at the center of the field of view, the resulting sinogram is just a vertical line that extends from the top to the bottom of the graph. Further, a horizontal line passing through the sinogram indicates a particular projection angle taken for a transverse slice. Figure 13.6 shows sinograms for an object having one and two hot spots on the transverse section. The figure clearly represents location (angle and position) and intensity of the two lesions. Figure 13.7 shows also how sinogram formation relies on the number of disintegrations collected from the positron source as opposed to conventional SPECT systems, in which detector rotation is necessary to build up a complete sinogram. This is one of the advantages provided by PET scanners based on circular design since all projections are acquired simultaneously and also possibly in 3D fashion. This

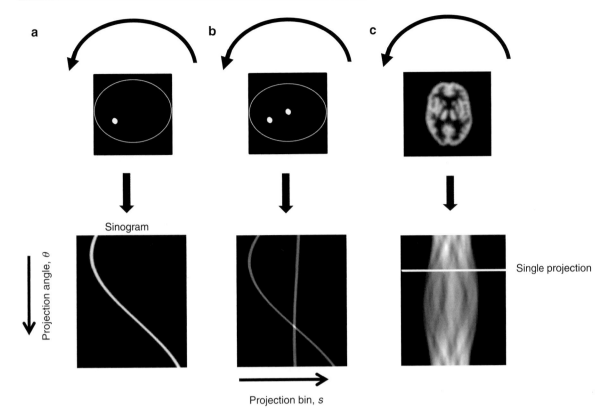

Fig. 13.6 Sinograms for different activity distributions. The sine wave pattern can be seen for a single hot lesion (**a**) and two hot lesions (**b**). The third sinogram (**c**) is more complicated due to its representation for many points in the projection profile, including all the angular views

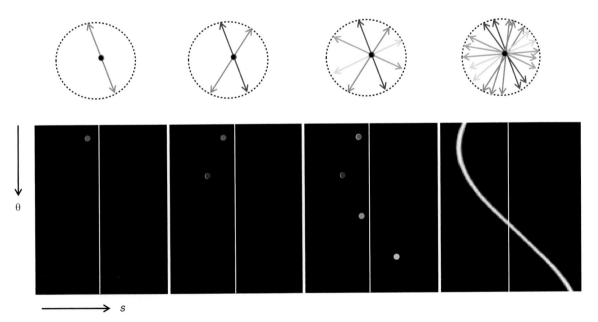

Fig. 13.7 The rebinning of the acquired events as the source decays into a sinogram that represents the projection bin on the horizontal axis, while the vertical axis denotes the projection angle. Note that each colored line of response (LOR) refers to a particular projection view; in other words, it points to a certain set of parallel LORs taken at a given angle

characteristic is absent in most conventional designs of the gamma camera, for which detector rotation is essential to accomplish the task. The sinogram of real clinical images such as shown in Fig. 13.6c is rather complicated as the object consists of a large number of points taken at multiple projection angles.

13.3 Image Reconstruction

13.3.1 Analytic Approaches

13.3.1.1 Simple Backprojection

As described, a collected count from a projection element according to the Radon transform is a line integral of tracer concentration along the emission path length. The task placed on the reconstruction algorithms is to find the spatial distribution of tracer activity within the body segment in question. One way to reconstruct an image from the raw data is to redistribute the collected counts (i.e., backproject) over the contributing individual pixels that lie along the path of the rays in the reconstruction matrix. Repeating this process for each projection element and for each acquired angle, one can obtain a picture of the tracer concentration as shown in Fig. 13.8. It can be seen that this method of image reconstruction cannot reveal useful information about tracer distribution due to the blurry appearance and substantially degraded signal-to-noise ratio.

Backprojection operation at point b can be represented as

The backprojected image f_{BP} at a particular point b is the result of summing all the corresponding projection bin values across all angular views taken during data acquisition. Here, s is the location of the projection bin on the detector. In PET geometry, the backprojection operation is performed for those LORs that connect detector pairs in coincidence. For obvious reasons, this process of count redistribution cannot determine the exact site where photon annihilation took place. Therefore, all pixels along the ray path are equally likely to get the same amount of counts. In PET systems with time of flight, calculation of the arrival of the two photons allows reduction of this LOR to a significantly smaller distance (based on system timing resolution) that, if included in image reconstruction, would result in an improvement of signal-to-noise ratio.

This is actually not the exact description of the backprojection operation since it is implemented on a grid of finite elements or computer matrix (and acquisition geometry), and thus it is possible that, for a given pixel, the backprojected ray can pass through a small part or intersect the pixel at its full length. Therefore, a number of backprojection methods have been developed to deal with this problem. Methods used in forward- and backprojection are pixel driven, ray driven, distance driven, distance weighted, matrix rotation, and others. Also, a combination of these methods, such as ray driven and pixel driven, can be used [8]. However, these methods differ in their computational efficiency, interpolation, and estimation accuracy. In iterative reconstruction, they should be carefully selected since several iterations may accumulate interpolation errors, introducing reconstruction artifacts.

Two clinical examples are shown in Fig. 13.9, one slice from a myocardial perfusion SPECT study and another one from brain-FDG PET study.

$$f_{BP} = \int_0^\pi p(x \cos \theta + y \sin \theta, \theta)d\theta$$

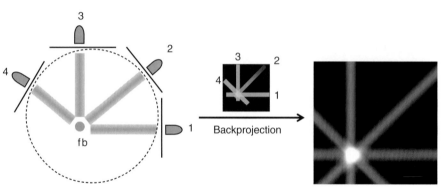

Fig. 13.8 Image reconstruction using simple backprojection

Fig. 13.9 The $1/r$ effect is shown where we can notice the overemphasis of lower frequencies in the backprojection images with an appearance of reduced higher frequencies across the images (brain and cardiac). The backprojection image is therefore a convolution of the underlying activity distribution with the $h(s)$ function. Analytic approaches remove this effect by deconvolving the acquired data with the blurring function, neglecting the noise component and leading to a tremendous increase in image noise. As a result, regularization using a smoothing function is required

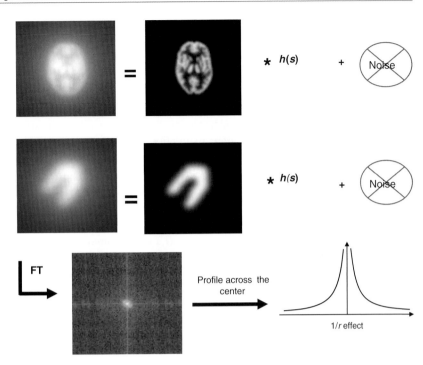

Fig. 13.10 Ideal versus realistic model of analytic image reconstruction

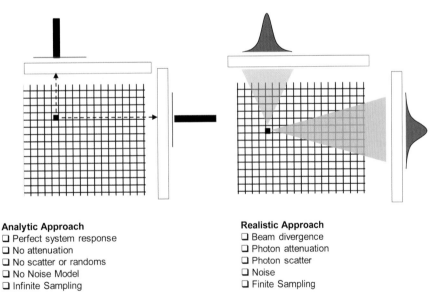

Analytic Approach
❏ Perfect system response
❏ No attenuation
❏ No scatter or randoms
❏ No Noise Model
❏ Infinite Sampling

Realistic Approach
❏ Beam divergence
❏ Photon attenuation
❏ Photon scatter
❏ Noise
❏ Finite Sampling

The characteristic blurring appearance of simple back-projection is clear in both studies, with most low-frequency components overexpressed with a remarkable reduction of high frequencies. This significant artifact is attributed to the fact that the sampling criteria do not match the model assumptions; hence, the reconstructed image is far from an accurate estimate of the tracer distribution. Simple backprojection assumes that data are collected with infinite linear and angular sampling, and the data collected are free from attenuation and scattered radiation in addition to shift-invariant and perfect system response (Fig. 13.10). Moreover, simple backprojection lacks a model for the inherent statistical noise associated with radioactive decay. These assumptions are violated in practice due to image digitization and the discrete angular intervals undertaken in image acquisition. Furthermore, the emitted photons undergo different types of interactions, resulting in photon loss or recoiling from the original path, and hence invalidate the absence of attenuation and scatter assumption in data formation. The measured projections are noisy due to the Poisson statistics of the radioactive decay process, and ignoring the noise component serves to alter the statistical properties of the reconstructed images and degrades image quality.

A profile drawn over the Fourier transform (FT) of the backprojected image shows a damping function that extends from the center of the spectrum (low-frequency region) toward the periphery (high-frequency region). This is referred to as the $1/r$ effect, in which the reconstructed image can be described as a convolution of the underlying activity distribution and a $1/r$ blurring function (Fig. 13.9). This situation can be written in the frequency domain as

$$F_{BP} = \frac{1}{\sqrt{{v_x}^2 + {v_y}^2}} F(v_x, v_y) = \frac{1}{v} F(v_x, v_y)$$

where the backprojected image F_{BP} is equal, in theory, to the original image $F(v_x, v_y)$ multiplied by the inverse of the function $h(s)$ in the frequency space. The latter function is defined as the system output to an ideal point source object and describes the system blurring effects on image formation. It is usually called the system spread function or point spread function (PSF). It is the key to solving the problem of back-projection by removing the blurring effect shown in Fig. 13.9 by either convolving the measured projections with the function $h(s)$ or multiplication in the frequency domain as described by the equation. Similarly, in 3D image reconstruction without data truncation, the backprojected image can be convolved with an appropriate 3D filter function to get an estimate of the original object distribution; alternatively, the measured projections are convolved with the 3D filter function. Before proceeding further to use this approach in image reconstruction, an important theorem that is central to many analytic reconstruction techniques should be discussed.

13.3.1.2 Fourier Reconstruction Theorem

Fourier analysis has a wide range of applications in many disciplines of science and engineering. This includes image and signal processing, filtering, image reconstruction, and many other biomedical applications. It has also been used in radioastronomy, electron microscopy, optical holography, magnetic resonance imaging (MRI), CT, and radionuclide SPECT and PET imaging [9]. Refer to Chap. 12, in which the FT is applied to a number of useful applications in nuclear medicine. In short, projection data and reconstructed slices can be represented in two different domains: spatial and frequency. The FT for a given input function can be represented by the sum of the sine and cosine waves with different amplitudes and phases.

Image reconstruction based on the FT is different from simple backprojection, and both can be combined to yield a variety of reconstruction approaches, as will be discussed further. The concept can easily be understood if we reversely assumed that we already have a transverse section of a patient thorax in which we can see the myocardium, and the 2D FT of this section has been calculated. The reconstruction theorem based on Fourier analysis states that a profile taken at a certain angle (θ) from the 2D FT of the transaxial section is equal to the 1D FT of the projection profile computed at the same angle. This is the underlying assumption of Fourier reconstruction theorem or the *central section* theorem, which relates the acquired projection data to the reconstructed image by the aid of Fourier transformation (Fig. 13.11).

Suppose the Fourier coefficients (intensity values in the frequency domain) are defined by the function $F(u, v)$, which is the 2D FT of the activity distribution $f(x, y)$ for a given cross-sectional slice; then, it can be proven that

$$F(v_x, v_y) = P(v, \theta)$$

where $P(v, \theta)$ is the FT of the projection $p(s, \theta)$, which is the function we have used to describe the counts collected over a 1D detector row.

Figure 13.12 summarizes the steps involved in Fourier reconstruction for a myocardial perfusion study, where the 1D FT of projection data is first calculated for all angular views, then data are collected

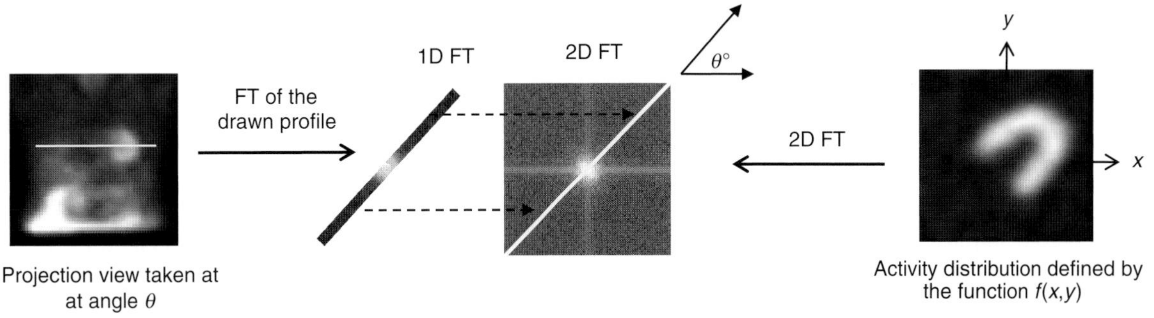

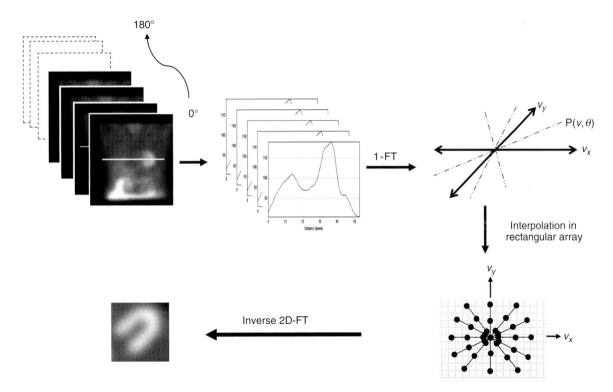

Fig. 13.11 The principle of two-dimensional (2D) Fourier reconstruction. The one-dimensional Fourier transform (1D-FT) of a horizontal profile drawn over a projection image at angle $\theta°$ is equal to the 2D-FT of the reconstructed image taken at the same angle

Fig. 13.12 Fourier transform reconstruction theorem states that the Fourier transform of a one-dimensional (1D) projection profile is equal to the two-dimensional (2D) Fourier transform of the corresponding activity distribution imaged at the same angle. This example shows a 1D profile taken across the patient's heart for all angles; then, the FT was calculated and interpolated in a rectangular array to obtain a 2D data set. Finally, the inverse Fourier transform is computed to generate the corresponding activity distribution represented here by the transaxial myocardial slice

in a 2D format and interpolated to account for gaps between views. Finally, inverse 2D FT is computed to yield a reconstructed myocardial image. Here, u and v are the spatial frequencies in the Fourier space and are defined in a square matrix; however, the polar sampling regime taken by the detector does not match the rectangular requirements, and therefore interpolation is required. Such a problem could be dealt with using standard interpolation methods or interpolation by gridding, taking into account that the accuracy of the results depends strongly on the interpolation method [10].

By analogy to 2D Fourier image reconstruction, a central plane through the FT of the 3D activity distribution is equal to the 2D FT of the 2D parallel projection data taken at the same orientation. However, the 3D transform of the object has different and more complex structure manifested by local sampling density when compared to 2D and thus requires special interpolation and weighting approaches [11].

The central section theorem and simple backprojection can be combined in different forms of image reconstruction utilizing the mathematical properties of FT and convolution theorem, which states that convolution in the spatial domain is equivalent to multiplication in the frequency domain. However, these methods differ in the order of reconstruction steps regarding whether convolution or backprojection is accomplished first and if convolution is implemented in the spatial or frequency domain, together with their computational efficiency.

Backprojection filtering (BPF) or filtering of the backprojection is one of these reconstruction approaches that combines Fourier reconstruction and backprojection in one procedure. BPF starts first by backprojecting the image into a reconstruction matrix, 2D FT is then computed, the result is multiplied by 2D ramp filter, and finally image reconstruction is performed by taking the inverse 2D FT. Image reconstruction can also be implemented by convolving the projection data with a convolution kernel, and then the product is simply backprojected to produce an image of the object activity distribution. However, the most computationally efficient and easy to implement is filtered backprojection, which has been extensively used in the routine practice of image reconstruction.

13.3.1.3 Filtered Backprojection

The most analytic approach that is used in SPECT and PET reconstruction is filtered backprojection. It has a historical dominance in many applications due to its speed and easy implementation in software reconstruction programs. It relies on filtering the projection data after Fourier transformation of all the acquired angular views; then, backprojection is carried out to give an estimate of the activity distribution. Data filtering is performed to eliminate the $1/r$ effect that works to blur the reconstructed images and is implemented in the Fourier space. Backprojection alone yields an image dominated by low-frequency components. By looking at the reconstructed brain and cardiac slices in Fig. 13.9, one can perceive the smoothing appearance of the images due to the prevalence of low frequencies with difficulty in identifying small details, a situation that results in a significant loss of signal-to-noise ratio. This problem can be tackled by using a ramp filter, which serves to suppress low frequencies and enhance high-frequency components of the projection data.

The ramp filter function $|v|$, as can be seen in Fig. 13.13, is a diagonal line that extends from the center in the frequency space to a sharp cutoff value.

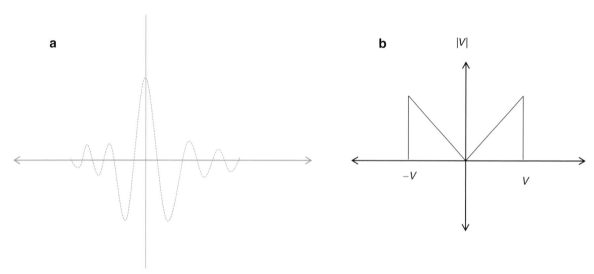

Fig. 13.13 Ramp filter in (**a**) spatial and (**b**) frequency domain

This significantly reduces the drawbacks of the backprojection step in image reconstruction. However, the sharp cutoff value has a disadvantage of producing count oscillations over regions of sharp contrast [12]. Further, it increases the image noise due to the enhancement of the high-frequency components. To overcome this problem, an additional filter function is often used with the ramp filter to roll off this sharp cutoff value and to suppress high frequencies to a certain level.

The steps involved in reconstructing one slice using filtered backprojection (FBP) are demonstrated in Fig. 13.14 and summarized as follows:

1. 1D FT is calculated for each projection profile.
2. The Fourier transformed projections are multiplied with the ramp filter (plus a smoothing filter) in the frequency domain.

3. The inverse FT of the product is computed.
4. The filtered data are backprojected to give an estimate of the activity distribution.

These steps can be written mathematically as

$$f(x,y) = \int_0^\pi p^F(s,\theta)d\theta = \int_0^\pi p^F(x\cos\theta + y\sin\theta,\theta)\,d\theta$$

The reconstructed image $f(x, y)$ is obtained by filtering the projection data in the frequency space (by multiplication with the ramp-smoothing function); then, the filtered data p^F are backprojected in the spatial domain to obtain the object activity distribution. 2D FBP is used in the reconstructions of the 2D PET (septa extended) and SPECT images acquired

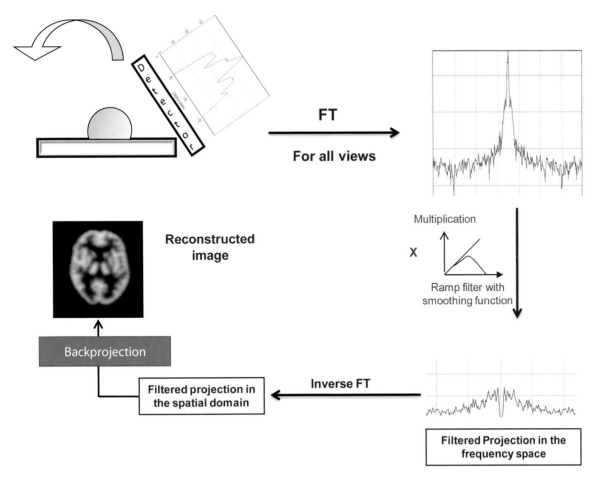

Fig. 13.14 Steps involved in filtered backprojection (FBP) image reconstruction. The projection profiles are Fourier transformed and are then multiplied by the ramp function to yield filtered data in the frequency domain. The inverse Fourier transform is then computed for the filtered data to move back to the spatial domain, and then backprojection is implemented. The filtration step can be performed prior to or after backprojection

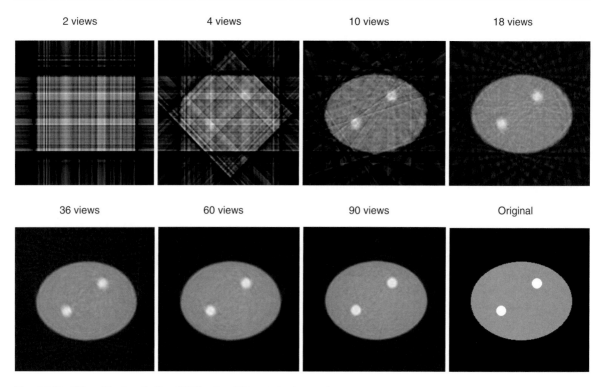

Fig. 13.15 Filtered backprojection (FBP) using different viewing angles

with parallel hole or fan beam collimators. An image reconstructed with FBP is demonstrated in Fig. 13.15 using different projection angles.

13.3.1.4 Filtering

As shown in Fig. 13.13, a ramp is a high-pass filter that does not permit low frequencies to appear in the image; therefore, it is used to overcome the problem of simple backprojection in image reconstruction. However, this filter has positive coefficients near the center and negative values at the periphery, as can be seen in Fig. 13.13a, in which the filter is plotted in the spatial domain. These characteristics of a ramp filter can introduce artifacts at regions that lie close to areas of high activity concentrations. This can be noted in the clinic in patients with full bladder activity undergoing bone SPECT imaging over the pelvic region. A severe cold artifact could be seen on the femoral head due to multiplying the ramp negative values with the projection counts. This could adversely affect the interpretation process and might be resolved by emptying the bladder and repeating the scan or

reconstructing the image using iterative techniques [13]. Another example can be seen in patients scheduled for whole-body FDG scanning and who have full bladder activity. This negative lobe effect introduced by a ramp filter can also cause a reduction of the inferior wall counts in myocardial perfusion SPECT studies if there are increased extracardiac activity concentrations in close proximity to the heart boundaries. This could result in an impression of diseased myocardial segments, causing false-positive results.

Another drawback of a ramp filer is its property of elevating the high-frequency components, thus increasing the noise level of the reconstructed images. An analytic solution for data acquired with noise is an ill-posed problem in which small perturbations (noise) in the input data cause a significant impact on the solution. Thus, a smoothing filter (regularization) is commonly used with a ramp filter to eliminate the noisy appearance of the ramp-filtered data and to improve image quality. Many filter functions were used with a ramp filter in several applications of nuclear medicine, such as Shep-Logan, parzen, hann, Hamming, and the commonly used Butterworth filter. Another class of filters has been proposed to correct for detector response function in image reconstruction, such as Metz and Wiener. Both filters rely on a system modulation transfer function taken at a certain depth and thus do not match the requirement of the shift-variant response imposed by the detector system. The inclusion of the detector response function in iterative reconstruction showed superior performance over other methods of image restoration.

A low cutoff value may smooth the image to a degree that does not permit perceiving small structures in the image, leading to blurred details and resolution loss. On the other hand, higher cutoff values serve to sharpen the image, but this occurs at the expense of increasing the amount of noise in the reconstructed images. The optimum cutoff value is therefore the value at which a fair suppression of noise is achieved while maintaining the resolution properties of the image. This trade-off task of the cutoff frequency is important to properly use a given filter function and to improve the image quality as much as possible. The cutoff value depends on factors such as the detector response function, spatial frequencies of the object, and count density of the image [14]. Better isotropic resolution properties are produced with 3D smoothing, and therefore it is preferred over 1D filters applied for individual slices. However, a 2D filter for the projection data may produce almost equal smoothing effects and is also computationally less intensive.

13.3.1.5 Summary of Analytic Image Reconstructions

Analytic approaches for image reconstruction in emission tomography seek to find an exact solution for tracer activity distribution. There are a number of assumptions that are invalid under the imaging conditions encountered in practice. Thus, the results provided by FBP are suboptimal to restore the true activity concentrations accumulated in target tissues. Images reconstructed with FBP need a number of corrections to improve the reconstruction results. As mentioned, effects of attenuation, scatter, and detector response are potential degrading factors that FBP does not account for in the reconstruction process. The correction for these effects is described in Chap. 14. Nevertheless, this reconstruction method has the advantages of being fast and easy to implement, and nuclear physicians have long-term experience

working with its outcome. Most image reconstruction in SPECT is implemented on a 2D slice-by-slice basis, so that at the end of image reconstruction one can obtain a complete set of transverse slices that, if stacked together, would represent the tracer distribution within the reconstructed volume. In PET image reconstruction, however, the same situation exists when data are acquired using 2D acquisition mode or the 3D data set are sorted into 2D projection arrays. Analytic image reconstruction can be summarized as follows:

1. Analytic reconstruction using FBP does not account for the inherent statistical variability associated with radioactive decay, and data collected are assumed to follow Radon transform, for which the object measured is approximated by line integrals. Regularization using linear filtering is necessary to control the propagation of noise into the reconstructed images. However, the noise is signal dependent, and filtering to achieve an optimal noise resolution trade-off is not an appropriate solution. Therefore, to solve the problem as accurately as possible, iterative refinement can be a better alternative.

2. Images reconstructed by FBP show streak artifacts as a result of the backprojection step along with the possibility of generating negative reconstruction values in regions of low count or poor tracer uptake. Both artifacts can be treated using iterative reconstruction techniques.

3. While many factors affect the PET LORs and serve to deviate the data to be approximated as line integrals when reconstructed by analytic image reconstruction, it remains an approximate reasonable approach in PET rather than SPECT [15]. Photon attenuation is an exact and straightforward procedure to implement in PET scanning, and the detector response function is not substantially degraded with source depth. In contrast, SPECT images suffer from photon attenuation in a more complicated way in addition to significant resolution loss as the source position increases.

4. The assumption of line integrals does not hold true for some imaging geometries, such as SPECT systems equipped with coded apertures and PET scanners based on hexagonal or octagonal detectors. In the former, analytical inversion of the acquired data is not a simple task and constitutes

a considerable challenge, while for the latter the gaps between detector modules (e.g., C-PET and HRRT) need to be filled before applying the analytic approach. Methods to account for the missed data were therefore developed, such as linear and bilinear interpolation or constraint Fourier space gap filling [16, 17].

5. In 3D data acquisition, coincidence events are allowed to be recorded among all scanner rings; accordingly, the collected data result in direct as well as oblique sinograms. For a point source located in a scanner operating in 2D mode, the in-plane system sensitivity does not depend on source location when compared to 3D imaging. In the latter scenario, the solid angle subtended by the scanner detectors differs from one position to another, especially when the source moves in the axial direction.

6. Another point that must be discussed is data truncation due to the fact that the axial extent of the PET scanner is limited. However, in the 3D situation, the oblique LORs are redundant in the sense that their statistical contribution to data reconstruction is unexploited. Direct 2D reconstruction uses LORs that arise from the direct planes to form an image, but this leads to scarifying a lot of useful coincident events recorded as oblique LORs. The incorporation of these events into image reconstruction serves to improve the statistical quality of the scan by increasing count sensitivity. Analytic FBP with using a Colsher filter can reconstruct the oblique projection if data are not truncated [18]. In the case of data truncation, however, the missed information due to the limited axial extent of the scanner can be estimated by reconstructing the direct planes of the 2D projections (they are adequate for data reconstruction) and then reprojecting the resulting images to get an estimate of the truncated oblique projections. This method is called 3D reconstruction by reprojection (3DRP) [19]. In other words, 3DRP estimates the missed information of the oblique sinogram in the forward projection step, assuming the scanner axis is extended beyond the practical limit of data acquisition. This step is important to satisfy the requirements of (axial) data shift invariance. Image reconstruction is then carried out using 3D FBP with a 2D Colsher filter. 3DRP is computationally demanding and was extensively used as a standard analytic 3D method of choice for volumetric PET imaging.

7. The other alternative to make use of the oblique LORs is to rebin the data so that the 3D data set is reduced to a 2D problem. A number of rebinning approaches have been developed to overcome the increased reconstruction times and to utilize the count sensitivity of the scanner, yet this occurs with some drawbacks placed on spatial resolution and image noise.

13.3.2 Rebinning Methods

For many reasons, 3D PET imaging was not the acquisition mode of choice; an important one is the lack of an acceptable reconstruction algorithm suited to provide clinically feasible reconstruction times. Another problem is the large amount of data that need to be processed along with extensive computational demands. An alternative way to handle this problem is to rearrange the oblique LORs into a direct array of parallel projections or a 2D data set. The latter allows for reconstruction times that are practically acceptable when compared to 3D reconstruction as the data can be reconstructed by any available 2D reconstruction algorithm. As mentioned, rebinning methods have been developed to benefit from the increased system sensitivity and to reduce computational speed requirements imposed by 3D reconstruction. Some of these rebinning approaches are as follows:

1. Single-slice rebinning (SSRB) is a simple geometric approach to reduce the 3D PET data into 2D parallel sinograms [20] (Fig. 13.16a). The method is implemented by rebinning an oblique sinogram that connects a two-detector pair into a parallel sinogram that lies midway between the two detectors. Although this method can simply be applied to rearrange the 3D information into direct planes consisting of parallel sinograms, it is valid when the oblique lines are close to the center of the field of view and in systems with small aperture size.

2. The geometric simplification provided by SSRB has been refined by the multislice rebinning (MSRB) method, in which the sinograms that lie across two detectors that connect an oblique LOR are incremented as shown in Fig. 13.16b. Stated another way, for each oblique LOR, the transverse slices intersected are identified, and the corresponding

Fig. 13.16 (**a**) Single-slice rebinning and (**b**) multislice rebinning

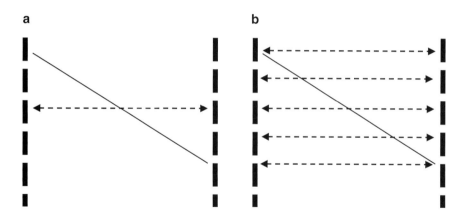

sinogram is incremented. Thus, it can be viewed as a backprojection on the *z*-direction [21]. This process depends on the number of sinograms to be incremented, and the increment varies with different oblique lines. However, axial blurring and amplification of noise are the drawbacks of MSRB.

3. By utilizing the properties of FT, the estimate of the FT of direct sinograms can be exactly and approximately derived in the frequency domain from the FT of the oblique sinograms using the frequency-distance relationship [22]. It is based on an acceptable equivalence between the Fourier transformed sinograms arising from direct and oblique LORs. This is called Fourier rebinning or FORE. It has significantly improved the computation time required to rearrange the 3D data sets into 2D direct sinograms with an order of magnitude gain in reconstruction times when compared to the 3DRP. FORE showed little differences compared to 3DRP, with good accuracy and stability in a noisy environment, but was less accurate in scanners with a large aperture [23, 24].

4. FORE has been used in time-of-flight applications [25] and extended to solve the problem of data truncation using an exact 3D rebinning approach; thus, it permits 3D reconstruction techniques to be applied [26].

5. Besides the reconstruction time gained from FORE, it can be combined with statistical iterative 2D image reconstruction techniques [27] to improve image quality when compared to FORE plus FBP or 3DRP and to exploit the incorporation of the imaging physics into the reconstruction model.

6. Several studies have shown that iterative techniques have the capabilities to improve image quality

and quantitative accuracy when compared to analytic techniques or hybrid approaches (rebinning + 2D reconstruction) with the drawback of increased computational burdens. However, this has been tackled using accelerating reconstruction algorithms implemented on fast computer systems.

13.3.3 Iterative Reconstructions

The task of the reconstruction algorithm is to solve $p = Af$ to find the best estimate of f. Here, p is the measured projection data, and A is a matrix that maps the tracer activity to the projection space. The presence of image noise does not allow finding a unique solution for the problem, or the solution might not exist or might not depend continuously on the data.

The better alternative to find a solution is to perform the task in an iterative manner. In this way, an initial estimate is assumed for the reconstructed image (solution), and the image is forward projected, simulating and accounting for all possible factors that work together to form the projection data. This initial estimate or guess can be a uniform image or FBP image and can be a zero image for additive-type algorithms. Many physical factors can be handled in the projection step to produce a projection image that is a close match to the acquired projections. Then, the measured and estimated projections are compared in such a way that allows derivation of a correction term. This last step allows the <u>algorithm</u> to modify the reconstructed slice through what is known as image update, and the process is controlled by the <u>cost function</u> or the objective likelihood function, as in the maximum likelihood

(ML) algorithm. It is clear that the initial estimate will be far from the solution; thus, the process is continued by repeating the same steps to reach the best estimate of the solution: convergence. This means that the algorithm will alternate through several steps of forward- and backprojection, in contrast to direct analytic methods, for which the estimated solution is obtained through a few predefined steps.

Most iterative techniques share the aforementioned idea and generally differ in the objective function, the optimization algorithm, and the computation cost [15]. The combined selection of the cost function and the optimization algorithm, as underlined above, is important in optimizing the iterative reconstruction technique. Both should not be confused and are distinguished in terms of their functionality as the first denotes the governing principle or the statistical basis on which the best estimate of the solution is determined, while the latter is the "driving" tool to achieve that estimate through a number of defined steps [28].

Iterative reconstructions have the advantages of incorporating corrections for image-degrading factors in the system matrix to handle an incomplete, noisy, and dynamic data set more efficiently than analytic reconstruction techniques. An important outcome of these advantages is that the final results enjoy better qualitative features in addition to more accurate estimation of tracer concentration improved image contrast, spatial resolution and better noise properties can be obtained from images reconstructed by iterative techniques when compared to analytic methods.

Iterative reconstruction can be statistical, such as ML or ordered subset (OS) expectation maximization (EM) algorithms, or nonstatistical, as in conventional algebraic reconstruction methods like algebraic reconstruction techniques (ARTs), steepest descent, simultaneous iterative reconstruction, and others. Another group of iterative methods based on FBP image reconstruction has also been proposed. Statistical methods can further be categorized into Gaussian or Poisson based on the noise model assumed. In Gaussian methods, the objective function can be weighted or nonweighted least square, while in Poisson-based models the objective function is the log likelihood function. The latter guarantees positivity constraint so that the pixel value is always in the positive direction, while in the Gaussian least square model, additional requirements are needed to maintain positivity.

Another possible classification for the statistical techniques is whether they consider prior information. The inclusion of prior information in image reconstruction allows driving the reconstructed images to the desired solution using penalty terms or prior function. This can be applied when Bayes's theorem is used in defining the objective function so that information regarding image distribution can be included in the reconstruction formula in advance. Morphological or patient anatomy, pixel smoothness, or nonnegativity constraints are different types of prior that can be used in Bayesian-based image reconstruction. The increased variance as the number of iterations increases is one of the noticeable but undesired features of statistical reconstruction techniques such as ML. Regularization using a smoothness penalty function can thus be applied to reduce image noise and to improve detectability of the reconstructed images.

13.3.3.1 System Matrix

A projection or system matrix (and also a transition matrix) is a key component in iterative techniques. It is based on the fact that the projection data are constructed by differential contributions of the object voxels being imaged. This transition from the image space to the projection space (Fig. 13.17) is the forward projection and is described in a matrix form as

$$P = Af$$

Unlike FBP, a system matrix in iterative reconstruction takes into account that each image voxel has a probability to contribute to a particular projection bin or sinogram. The system matrix A is the information reservoir that describes how the projection image is formed. It contains the coefficients a_{ij} that denote the probabilities of detecting a photon (or LOR) emitted from a particular site and detected in a particular bin. Many physical phenomena can therefore be incorporated as far as they significantly contribute to data formation. In other words, the image space is mapped to the projection space by the aid of the transition matrix that describes the probability of detecting a photon emitted from pixel j and measured in projection bin i such that

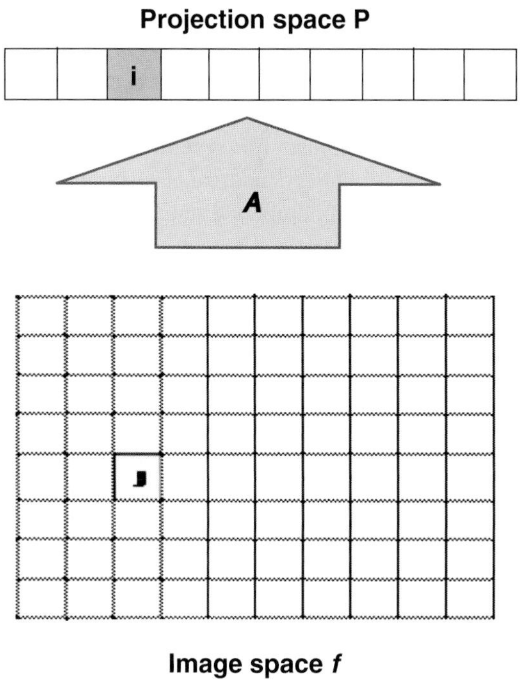

Projection space P

Image space _f_

Fig. 13.17 The system matrix maps the data from the image space to the projection space

$$p_i = \sum_j a_{ij} f_j$$

where f is the image vector representing the activity distribution indexed by pixel j, and p is the measured projection and indexed by pixel i. A is the transition matrix of elements and is equal to $i \times j$.

However, this is not only for a one-detector row at one angle but also for all the acquired views, including all the detector elements. The situation becomes more problematic in building up a transition matrix for 3D image reconstruction when the interslice plane (3D SPECT) or oblique LOR (3D PET) is considered. Overall, the size of the system matrix is a function of the type and dimension of the data acquisition, number of detectors, number of projection angles, and size of the reconstructed image [29].

The system matrix can be structured so that it can account for the imaging physics and detector characteristics. In the context of SPECT imaging, attenuation, scatter, and detector response are major degrading factors that can be incorporated in the iterative scheme. An accurate correction for these image-degrading elements can lead to a significant improvement in image quality and quantitative accuracy. In PET imaging, the system matrix can also be built to handle geometric components and many physical parameters of positron emission and detection. It can be decomposed into individual matrices so that each matrix can account for particular or combined physical effects [30]. The accuracy of the system matrix is essential to ensure that the sources of degrading effects are well addressed and to realize the benefits underlying the modeling procedure. Otherwise, oversimplification or inaccuracies of the system matrix would transfer the signal into noise due to inconsistencies that would arise as the estimated projection will no longer match the measured data [31, 32].

It can be calculated on the fly using efficient geometric operators, or it can be computed and stored prior to image reconstruction. Analytical derivation, Monte Carlo simulation, experimental measurements, or a combination of these techniques can be used to compute the system matrix. However, these estimation approaches vary in terms of their complexity, computational burdens, accuracy, and validity. To reduce storage capacity, the sparseness and intrinsic symmetry of the scanner is utilized to generate a compressed version of the probability matrix. Also, for efficient use of the 3D-PET matrix, it can be decomposed into individual matrices, such as geometric, attenuation, sensitivity, detector blurring, and physics of positron emission.

The inclusion of many effects that degrade image quality and contribute to image formation has expensive computational requirements. Attempts made to overcome these computational demands have been the development of accelerated image reconstruction approaches such as OSEM (ordered subset expectation maximization), the rescaled block iterative expectation maximization (RBI-EM) method [33], and the row action ML algorithm (RAMLA). Other approaches were to use an unmatched pair of projection–backprojection in the iterative scheme to accelerate the reconstruction process by not taking into account the effect of all degrading factors in both operations [34, 35]. Efficient algorithms that include dual-matrix and variance reduction techniques have significantly reduced the processing times of Monte Carlo-based statistical reconstructions to clinically feasible limits [35].

13.3.3.2 Maximum Likelihood Expectation Maximization

Maximum likelihood expectation maximization (MLEM) is a popular iterative reconstruction technique that gained wide acceptance in many SPECT and PET applications. The technique comprises two major steps:

1. Expectation
2. Maximization

The algorithm works to maximize the probability of the estimated slice activity given the measured projection data with the inclusion of count statistics. Stated another way, the ML algorithm seeks to find the best estimate of the reconstructed image f that with the highest likelihood can produce the acquired projection counts p. The probability function is derived from the Poisson statistics and is called the likelihood objective function:

$$L(p|f) = prob\ [p|f] = \prod_i e^{-q_i^k} \frac{(q_i^k)^{p_i}}{p_i!} \qquad (13.2)$$

where q_i^k is the estimated forward projection data and equal to $\sum a_{ij}f_j^k$, while the measured projection data are represented by p_i. The ML estimate can be calculated by Eq. 13.2 but it is more convenient and easier to work with the log of the likelihood function. The selection of Poisson function is appropriate since it maintains positivity of the pixel values and agrees with the statistics of photon detection. As a result, ML reconstruction has good noise properties and is superior to FBP, especially in areas of poor count statistics. One important issue in implementing the ML algorithm is that the input data (projections/sinograms) should be matched with the noise hypothesis of the ML model, and prior treatments or corrections for the acquired data would serve to alter the noise properties assumed by the algorithm. This can solved by either modifying the noise model (e.g., shifted Poisson) or feeding the data directly into the iterative process without a prior correction for any of the noise-disturbing elements.

Expectation maximization is the algorithm of choice to solve the likelihood function and works to estimate the projection data from knowledge of the system matrix and the current estimate of the image. The estimated and measured projection data are then compared by taking the ratio, which in turn is used to modify the current estimate of the slice. An image update takes place by multiplying that ratio with the current estimate to get a new image estimate "update." This process continues for several iterations until convergence is obtained and can be summarized as follows for iteration numbers k and $k + 1$:

1. The slice activity in the kth iteration is forward projected using the proposed imaging model to form a new projection image.
2. The ratio of the measured and estimated projection is calculated for each bin.
3. The result of the previous step is backprojected and normalized by dividing over the coefficients a_{ij} (see Eq. 13.3).

The new image f^{k+1} is produced by the multiplying the image in the kth iteration with the normalized backprojected data.

The equation used to define the MLEM reconstruction algorithm is [36]

$$f_j^{k+1} = \frac{f_j^k}{\sum_j a_{ij}} \left[\sum_i a_{ij} \frac{p_i}{q_i^k} \right] \qquad (13.3)$$

It tells us that the $(k + 1)^{th}$ iteration is equal to the immediate previous iteration k multiplied by a correction term. The correction term is a normalized backprojection of the ratio of the measured projection p_i and the estimated projection of the slice activity resulting from iteration k, or q_i^k.

The drawback of using the Poisson formula is that it makes the algorithm reach a solution (reconstructed image) that is statistically consistent with the proposed activity distribution of the acquired projections. The reconstructed images therefore tend to be noisy, especially at a high number of iterations. As the number of iterations increases and the algorithm approaches the solution, the log-likelihood of the function also increases but with image deterioration due to high variance estimate. This is one of the major drawbacks of the ML algorithm, which can be overcome using stopping criteria, postreconstruction smoothing filters, or regularization by Gaussian kernels: "the method of sieves" [37, 38]. This last approach is implemented by restricting the range of the optimization in least squares or ML to a subset of smooth functions on the parameter space.

Penalized likelihood and Bayesian algorithms are also applied to regularize the solution and reduce noise artifacts. In practice, however, noise reduction is accomplished mostly using postreconstruction smoothing filters. However, in analytic image reconstruction, regularization is implemented using linear filtering, compromising spatial resolution.

Convergence of the MLEM is slow, but guaranteed, and depends on the spatial frequency (object dependent) such that low-frequency regions converge faster than high-frequency regions. At a large number of iterations, however, resolution tends to be uniform across the reconstructed slice.

The second limitation of ML is the computation requirements since it converges slowly, and high-speed computer devices are needed to make it feasible in practice. However, new computer technology is continuously advancing to resolve this issue (Moore's law). The other alternative to ML estimation is the OS algorithm, which has gained wide acceptance in many areas of research and clinical practice as it provides a significant improvement in computation time by accelerating the reconstruction process.

13.3.3.3 Ordered Subset Expectation Maximization

The accelerated version of the ML algorithm is the OS. This type of algorithm is also called block iterative or row action as it relies on using a single datum or subset of data at each iteration. OSEM was derived by Hudson and Larkin to speed up the iteration process [39].

The underlying concept of OSEM reconstruction is that instead of using the whole data set to obtain an update for the reconstructed image, all projection data are divided into smaller groups of projections, or subsets, and thus the image update is implemented when one subset is used; this is called *subiteration*. However, full iteration takes place when the algorithm uses all the available subsets in the image reconstruction.

The number of projections is divided equally into subsets. For example, in SPECT acquisition of 72 projections, the data set can be divided into eight subsets, each with nine projections. The projections in each subset are not contiguous but are spread over the whole set of angular views such that the first subset includes the projection numbers 1, 9, 18, and so on, and the second subset would have the projection

numbers 2, 10, 19, and so on, and the same holds for the remaining subsets. The standard EM reconstruction of projection/backprojection is applied to each subset, one by one, so that the resulting reconstruction from subset 1 is the starting value for subset 2 and so on. In that example, a reduction of the reconstruction time by a factor of 8 can be achieved when using the OSEM technique as the rate of convergence is accelerated by a factor proportional to the number of subsets [39].

The properties of OSEM are similar to MLEM. Low-frequency regions converge faster than high-frequency regions. Thus, stopping iterations at an early stage may result in suboptimal results represented in a biased contrast; however, running a large number of iterations produces noisy images. Therefore, a trade-off between the number of iterations and detail recovery should be considered [40]. In regions of low tracer concentration, OSEM reconstruction might underestimate tracer activity concentration. This has been shown in a number of reports, including myocardial FDG studies and brain DatScan SPECT imaging [41, 42]. The spatially variant and object dependency convergence of iterative reconstruction is a limitation in determining the optimal number of iterations particularly with the increased noise as the iteration progresses. It is therefore of importance to optimize the reconstruction parameters, including the filtration step, given a particular detection task to exploit the full potential of the iterative technique in improving the observer performance or quantitative measurements [43].

Both 2D- and 3D-OSEM have found a number of successful applications in the reconstruction of SPECT and PET images, including corrections for many potentially degrading factors in addition to noise handling. These results have been exploited and commercialized in different software packages provided by scanner manufacturers. Attenuation-weighted OSEM reconstruction has been implemented in commercial PET scanners. Instead of precorrecting for photon attenuation before image reconstruction and presenting the data to the iterative technique in a Poisson-corrupted form, attenuation correction factors can be included in the system matrix to yield images with less noise and superior quality than data precorrected for attenuation. Not only attenuation but also other degrading factors, such as system response, has been incorporated into iterative OSEM and resulted in remarkable improvement of PET image quality and spatial resolution [44]. Also, it has become evident that including all corrections starting from random, dead time, normalization, geometric scatter, attenuation, and arc correction (the problem of unevenly spaced acquired projections) in the system matrix of iterative reconstruction allows preservation of the statistical nature of the raw data and satisfies the Poisson likelihood function of OSEM or MLEM, yielding an image with superior noise properties [45, 46].

13.3.3.4 Maximum A Posteriori

Maximum a posteriori (MAP) is a Bayesian reconstruction method that found several applications in SPECT and PET imaging [47]. It has a superior performance over analytic image reconstruction, especially when image-degrading factors are taken into account [48, 49]. However, in contrast to the ML mentioned here, MAP reconstruction uses prior knowledge to force the solution in the preferred or desired direction. According to Bayes's theorem, the probability of estimating an image provided the measured projection data is given by the posterior density function

$$prob\,[f|p] = \frac{prob\,[P|f]\,prob\,[f]}{prob\,[p]}$$

The first term of the nominator refers to the likelihood, while the second term denotes the distribution of the prior. The denominator is a constant (not a function of f) and can be dropped [43]. Note that in ML no preferences are placed on the reconstructed image; therefore, the objective function returns to the ML form once no information about the prior is assumed. The property given by MAP reconstruction to incorporate prior knowledge in the iterative procedure allows the associated noise elevation to be overcome as the number of iterations increases, as mentioned. This is implemented by penalizing the likelihood function by a prior term, driving the log-likelihood to the favored solution. The prior function is often selected to smooth the reconstructed images; however, this occurs with drawbacks of blurring sharp edges. Functions designed to smooth the image while being able to preserve edges have also been suggested. Another type of priors attempts to utilize morphological information

provided by anatomical imaging modalities such as CT and MRI and based on the assumption that tracer uptake within a given structure or organ is uniformly distributed. However, using MAP reconstruction with anatomical priors has a number of limitations that, if properly addressed, could significantly improve lesion detectability and image quality.

One of the commonly used is Gibbs distribution prior, which penalizes a given pixel based on differences with the neighboring pixels. It has the following mathematical representation:

$$P(x) = \frac{1}{Z} e^{-\beta U(x)}$$

$$U(x) = \frac{1}{2} \sum_{j=1}^{N} \sum_{k \in N_j} \psi\left(x_j - x_k\right)$$

where Z is a normalization constant, and β is a weighting parameter that determines the strength of the prior. $U(x)$ is the energy function and often contains potentials, $U(\cdot)$, defined on a pairwise cliques of neighboring pixels [49]. Prior functions based on absolute pixel differences have been devised as well as functions that use relative pixel differences. It is the selection and design of the potential function that allows penalization of the reconstructed images in favor of smoothing the images or preserving sharp edges, and this is implemented by increasing or decreasing the probability of the desired solution [50]. In the same vein, MAP-based reconstruction techniques produce an image with complex and object-dependent spatial resolution; this again can be controlled by the prior function. A nonuniform spatial resolution is obtained if a shift-invariant prior is used, whereas a uniform resolution comparable to postsmoothed ML (with a sufficient number of iterations) can be achieved with appropriate tuning of the prior [51, 52].

The availability of multimodality imaging devices such as SPECT/CT, PET/CT, and PET/MRI allows the introduction of morphological information in the iterative algorithm and thus has the potential to improve the quality of the diagnostic images. However, some problems could arise, such as image coregistration errors, identification of lesion location within the anatomical structures or segmentation errors, addition of lesion or organ boundaries or both, and selection of the penalty function and optimal prior strength [53];

ultimately, research efforts need to optimize the technique and prove an improved diagnostic confidence over other methods that do not rely on prior information. Furthermore, an underutilized application of MAP-type reconstruction is the unexploited feature of incorporating an anatomical prior to correct for the partial volume effect. There is an interest in improving the spatial resolution of PET images using resolution recovery approaches; however, investigations could also be directed to make use of the anatomical data provided by CT or MRI images to formulate feasible correction schemes in multimodality imaging practice [53–55].

13.4 Conclusions

Image reconstruction is a key element in conveying the diagnostic information given an activity distribution within different tissues. Analytic approaches are simple, fast, and easy to implement in research and clinical practice. However, they have some drawbacks that can be eliminated using iterative techniques. These provide improved image quality and quantitative accuracy, with some efforts to be done on optimizing the reconstruction parameters given a particular detection task. The system matrix of iterative reconstruction can be considered an information reservoir that allows the technique to reach the most accurate solution and thus should be optimally constructed.

References

1. Even-Sapir E (2005) Imaging of malignant bone involvement by morphologic, scintigraphic, and hybrid modalities. J Nucl Med 46(8):1356–1367
2. Li G, Citrin D, Camphausen K, Mueller B, Burman C, Mychalczak B, Miller RW, Song Y (2008) Advances in 4D medical imaging and 4D radiation therapy. Technol Cancer Res Treat 7(1):67–81
3. Bracewell RN (1956) Strip integration in radioastronomy. J Phys 9:198–217
4. Beckmann EC (2006) CT scanning the early days. Br J Radiol 79(937):5–8
5. Jaszczak RJ (2006) The early years of single photon emission computed tomography (SPECT): an anthology of selected reminiscences. Phys Med Biol 51:R99–R115
6. Hsieh J (2003) Computed tomography: principles, design, artifacts, and recent advances. SPIE. International Society for Optical Engineering, Bellingham
7. Zanzonico P (2008) Routine quality control of clinical nuclear medicine instrumentation: a brief review. J Nucl Med 49(7):1114–1131
8. Zeng G, Gullberg G (2000) Unmatched projector/backprojector pairs in an iterative reconstruction algorithm. IEEE Trans Med Imaging 19(5):548–555
9. Brooks RA, Di Chiro G (1976) Principles of computer assisted tomography (CAT) in radiographic and radioisotopic imaging. Phys Med Biol 21:689
10. Kinahan PE, Defrise M, Clackdoyle R (2004) Analytic image reconstruction methods. In: Wernick M, Aarsvold J (eds) Emission tomography: the fundamentals of PET and SPECT. Academic, San Diego
11. Matej S, Kazantsev IG (2006) Fourier-based reconstruction for Fully 3-D PET: optimization of interpolation parameters. IEEE Trans Med Imaging 25(7):845–854
12. Madsen MT, Park CH (1985) Enhancement of SPECT images by Fourier filtering the projection image set. J Nucl Med 26(4):395–402
13. Wells RG, Farncombe T, Chang E, Nicholson RL (2004) Reducing bladder artifacts in clinical pelvic SPECT images. J Nucl Med 45(8):1309–1314
14. Gilland DR, Tsui BM, McCartney WH, Perry JR, Berg J (1988) Determination of the optimum filter function for SPECT imaging. J Nucl Med 29(5):643–650
15. Qi J, Leahy RM (2006) Iterative reconstruction techniques in emission computed tomography. Phys Med Biol 51(15): R541–R578
16. van Velden FH, Kloet RW, van Berckel BN, Molthoff CF, Lammertsma AA, Boellaard R (2008) Gap filling strategies for 3-D-FBP reconstructions of high-resolution research tomography scans. IEEE Trans Med Imaging 27(7):934–942
17. Karp JS, Muehllehner G, Lewitt RM (1988) Constrained Fourier space method for compensation of missing data in emission computed tomography. IEEE Trans Med Imaging 7(1):21–25
18. Colsher JG (1980) Fully three-dimensional positron emission tomography. Phys Med Biol 25:103–115
19. Kinahan PE, Rogers JG (1990) Analytic three-dimensional image reconstruction using all detected events. IEEE Trans Nucl Sci NS-36:964–968
20. Daube-Witherspoon ME, Muehllehner G (1987) Treatment of axial data in three-dimensional PET. J Nucl Med 28 (11):1717–1724
21. Lewitt RM, Muehllehner G, Karp JS (1994) Three-dimensional reconstruction for PET by multi-slice rebinning and axial image filtering. Phys Med Biol 39:321–340
22. Defrise M, Kinahan PE, Townsend DW, Michel C, Sibomana M, Newport DF (1997) Exact and approximate rebinning algorithms for 3D PET data. IEEE Trans Med Imaging MI-16:145–158
23. Matej S, Karp JS, Lewitt RM, Becher AJ (1998) Performance of the Fourier rebinning algorithm for 3D PET with large acceptance angles. Phys Med Biol 43:787–797
24. Krzywinski M, Sossi V, Ruth TJ (1998) Comparison of FORE, OSEM and SAGE algorithms to 3DRP in 3D PET using phantom and human subject data. Nuclear Science Symposium, Conference Record. IEEE 1998 3:1546–1551

25. Defrise M, Casey ME, Michel C, Conti M (2005) Fourier rebinning of time-of-flight PET data. Phys Med Biol 50:2749–2763

26. Ben Bouallegue F, Crouzet F, Comtat C et al (2007) Exact and approximate Fourier rebinning algorithms for the solution of the data truncation problem in 3-D PET. IEEE Trans Med Imaging 26:1001–1009

27. Kinahan PE, Michel C, Defrise M, Townsend DW, Sibomana M, Lonneux M, Newport DF, Luketich JD (1996) Fast iterative image reconstruction of 3D PET data. In: IEEE nuclear science and medical imaging conference, Anaheim, pp 1918–1922

28. Lalush DS, Wernick MN (2004) Iterative image reconstruction. In: Wernick M, Aarsvold J (eds) Emission tomography: the fundamentals of PET and SPECT. Academic Press, San Diego

29. Loudos GK (2008) An efficient analytical calculation of probability matrix in 2D SPECT. Comput Med Imaging Graph 32(2):83–94

30. Qi J, Leahy R, Cherry S, Chatziioannou A, Farquhar T (1998) High-resolution 3-D Bayesian image reconstruction using the microPET small-animal scanner. Phys Med Biol 43:1001–1013

31. Qi J, Huesman RH (2005) Effect of errors in the system matrix on maximum a posteriori image reconstruction. Phys Med Biol 50(14):3297–3312

32. Ortuno J, Pedro Guerra-Gutierrez P, Rubio J, Kontaxakis G, Santos A (2006) 3D-OSEM iterative image reconstruction for high-resolution PET using precalculated system matrix. Nucl Instrum Meth Phys Res A 569:440–444

33. Byrne CL (1996) Block-iterative methods for image reconstruction from projections. IEEE Trans Imaging Process 5:792–794

34. Kamphuis C, Beekman FJ, Van Rijk PP, Viergever MA (1998) Dual matrix ordered subsets reconstruction for accelerated 3D scatter compensation in single-photon emission tomography. Eur J Nucl Med 25:8–18

35. De Wit TC, Xiao JB, Beekman FJ (2005) Monte Carlo-based statistical SPECT reconstruction: influence of number of photon tracks. IEEE Trans Nucl Sci 52:1365–1369

36. Lange K, Carson R (1984) EM reconstruction algorithms for emission and transmission tomography. J Comput Assist Tomogr 8:306–316

37. Snyder DL, Miller MI (1985) The use of sieves to stabilize images produced with the EM algorithm for emission tomography. IEEE Trans Nucl Sci 32:3864–3872

38. Snyder DL, Miller MI, Thomas LJ, Politte DG (1987) Noise and edge artifacts in maximum-likelihood reconstructions for emission tomography. IEEE Trans Med Imaging 6 (3):228–238

39. Hudson H, Larkin R (1994) Accelerated image reconstruction using ordered subsets of projection data. IEEE Trans Med Imaging MI-13:601–609

40. Seret A, Boellaard R, van der Weerdt A (2004) Number of iterations when comparing MLEM/OSEM with FBP. J Nucl Med 45(12):2125–2126

41. Dickson JC, Tossici-Bolt L, Sera T, Erlnadsson K, Tatsch K, Hutton B (2010) The impact of reconstruction method on the quantification of DaTSCAN images. Eur J Nucl Med Mol Imaging 37(1):23–35

42. van der Weerdt AP, Boellaard R, Knaapen P, Visser CA, Lammertsma AA, Visser FC (2004) Postinjection transmission scanning in myocardial 18F-FDG PET studies using both filtered backprojection and iterative reconstruction. J Nucl Med 45:169–175

43. Hutton B, Nuyts J, Zaidi H (2004) Iterative image reconstruction methods. In: Zaidi H (ed) Quantitative analysis in nuclear medicine imaging. Kluwer/Plenum, New York

44. Panin VY, Kehren F, Michel C, Casey M (2006) Fully 3-D PET reconstruction with system matrix derived from point source measurements. IEEE Trans Med Imaging 25:907–921

45. Kadrmas DJ (2004) LOR-OSEM: statistical PET reconstruction from raw line-of-response histograms. Phys Med Biol 49(20):4731–4744

46. Comtat C, Kinahan PE, Defrise M, Michel C, Townsend DW (1998) Fast reconstruction of 3D PET data with accurate statistical modeling. IEEE Trans Nucl Sci 45:1083–1089

47. Levitan E, Herman GT (1987) A maximum a posteriori probability expectation maximization algorithm for image reconstruction in emission tomography. IEEE Trans Med Imaging 6:185–192

48. Frese T, Rouze NC, Bouman CA, Sauer K, Hutchins GD (2003) Quantitative comparison of FBP, EM, and Bayesian reconstruction algorithms for the IndyPET scanner. IEEE Trans Med Imaging 22(2):258–276

49. Qi J (2003) Theoretical evaluation of the detectability of random lesions in Bayesian emission reconstruction. Inf Process Med Imaging 18:354–365

50. Qi J (2004) Analysis of lesion detectability in Bayesian emission reconstruction with nonstationary object variability. IEEE Trans Med Imaging 23(3):321–329

51. Fessler JA (1994) Penalized weighted least squares image reconstruction for PET. IEEE Trans Med Imaging 13:290–300

52. Fessler JA, Rogers WL (1996) Spatial resolution properties of penalized-likelihood image reconstruction: spatial-invariant tomographs. IEEE Trans Image Process 9: 1346–1358

53. Lehovich A, Gifford HC, Schneider PB, King MA (2007) Choosing anatomical-prior strength for MAP SPECT reconstruction to maximize lesion detectability. IEEE Nucl Sci Symp Conf Rec 6(1):4222–4225

54. Baete K, Nuyts J, Van Laere K, Van Paesschen W, Ceyssens S, De Ceuninck L, Gheysens O, Kelles A, Van den Eynden J, Suetens P, Dupont P (2004) Evaluation of anatomy based reconstruction for partial volume correction in brain FDG-PET. Neuroimage 23(1):305–317

55. Alessio AM, Kinahan PE (2006) Improved quantitation for PET/CT image reconstruction with system modeling and anatomical priors. Med Phys 33(11):4095–4103

Quantitative SPECT Imaging

14

Michael Ljungberg

Contents

14.1 Introduction

The scintillation camera is essentially a device that measures 2D images of a radionuclide distribution in vivo by detecting emitted photons. Due to the construction of the collimator, events in the image coming from photons emitted at different source depths will be superimposed and the source depth will not be resolved. The solution is to obtain the 3D information by measuring projections in different views around the patient and use a reconstruction algorithm. The method is called Single-Photon Emission Computed Tomography (SPECT). If the activity is not redistributed over the time of measurement then the assumption in any reconstruction method is that there exists one unique activity distribution for which a corresponding photon emission will result in the projections that are acquired by the system. Then the goal of any reconstruction process is to determine this distribution in 3D as accurate as possible.

14.2 Factors Degrading SPECT Imaging

In a reconstruction algorithm, such as the filtered backprojection or iterative MLEM/OSEM methods, the goal is thus to find an activity distribution (described by a set of consecutive 2D tomographic images representing different sections in the object) that matches the measured projection data. However, if the measured data suffers from physical effects, such as photon attenuation in the object or unwanted contribution to the projection data from photons scattered in the patient, then the reconstructed solution will not accurately describe the activity distribution [1]. Photon attenuation can actually result in false positive

M. Ljungberg
Department of Medical Radiation Physics, Clinical Sciences, Lund, Lund University, SE- 221 85, Lund, Sweden
e-mail: Michael.Ljungberg@med.lu.se

M.M. Khalil (ed.), *Basic Sciences of Nuclear Medicine*, DOI: 10.1007/978-3-540-85962-8_14,
© Springer-Verlag Berlin Heidelberg 2011

indications, especially in nonhomogeneous regions such as the thorax. It is therefore of importance to correct for these effects even if the actual numerical pixel values are of less importance.

The following examples that describe the major SPECT imaging degrading factors have been created by the use of the Monte Carlo program SIMIND [1, 2] and the NCAT anthropomorphic mathematical phantom [3, 4]. The Monte Carlo method allows for a simulation of the photons from emission in an object to the detection in a scintillation camera. During this process, it is possible to keep track of the interaction history of the photons and the formation of the image from these photons. The advantage of categorizing each event in the image based on origin, that is, from primary, scattered, or penetrated photons, is that it makes it possible to study the degradation in detail. Most of the examples in this chapter are based on activity distributions that mimic a myocardial perfusion study. Different photon energies have been simulated for visual purposes, but some of these energies may not be clinically relevant to the simulated radionuclide distribution.

14.2.1 Distance-Dependent Spatial Resolution

The commonly used parallel-hole collimator has the advantage of having a geometrical sensitivity that is independent of source-to-collimator distance of the source within the field of view (FOV). This means that the conversion factor (cps/MBq) remains constant within the FOV, which greatly simplifies the process of activity quantitation. The spatial resolution however depends on the distance to the collimator and the specification of the holes (diameter, shape, septum thickness, and length). In a clinical environment, it is common to have several types of collimators available, selected on the basis of the type of study and the energy of the photon. Examples are low-energy high-resolution (LEHR), low-energy general purpose (LEGP), medium-energy general purpose (MEGP), and high-energy general-purpose (HEGP) collimators. Because of the underlying design, even a parallel-hole LEHR collimator will limit the spatial resolution to be, at the best, about 10–15 mm for SPECT. This means

that although the correct number of counts are acquired by the camera, the position of each event are spread out over a large area (more pixels) if the source is located at a larger distance. This effect can be seen in Fig. 14.1, where profiles through images of three-point sources being located at different distances from the collimator surface are shown for both LEGP and LEHR collimators. The profiles show a larger value of the FWHM as the source moves away from the camera. This broadening is less pronounced for the LEHR collimator but with an expense of reduction in measured count rate.

The distance-dependent blurring of an image means that the cps/pixel will not reflect the MBq/ml in a particular voxel. This unwanted effect is often called the partial-volume effect. The spatial resolution also affects the image contrast and hence the ability to detect small lesions with moderate lesion-to-background activity ratios. In principle, however, very small lesions can be detected, but the lesion-to-background activity ratios in these cases need to be very high; however, the volume of a lesion can never be measured below the order of the spatial resolution of the system.

14.2.2 Photon Attenuation

Some of the photons, emitted from a radiopharmaceutical administered to a patient will interact within the patient and therefore not contribute to the image formation in the expected way. The basic interaction types for photon energies that are important to nuclear medicine applications are photoabsorption, Compton scattering, Rayleigh scattering, and pair production (rare since this interaction type can occur only for photons with energies above 1.022 MeV). Consider a fluence of photons impinging in a narrow-beam geometry on an object of the thickness x and the density . The number of photons, N, that pass through the object is given by

$$N = N_0 e^{-\frac{\mu}{\rho}\rho \cdot x} \quad (14.1)$$

where N_0 is the initial narrow-beam photon fluence and N is the photon fluence after passing through the object. The probability of each of the possible interactions can be described by differential attenuation coefficients, and, consequently, the sum of these differential

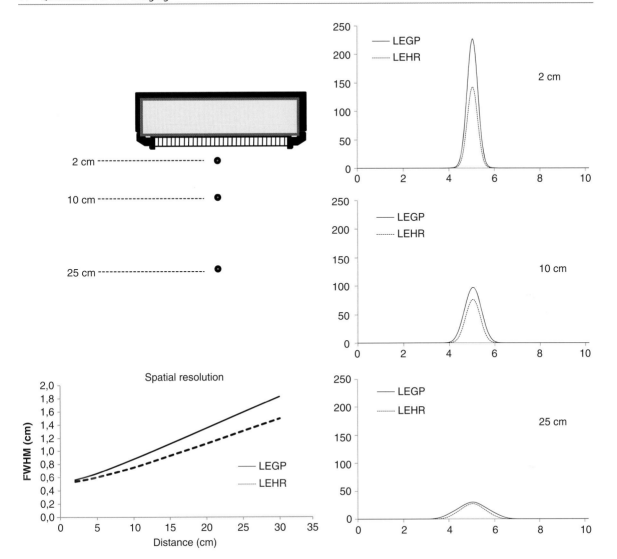

Fig. 14.1 Simulated point-spread function for a point source located at distances 2 cm (**a**), 10 cm, (**b**) and 25 cm (**c**) to the lower collimator surface. The images illustrate the importance of always keeping the camera as close as possible to the patient surface. The figure also shows that the magnitude of the degradation in spatial resolution for the two collimators also differs

coefficients describes the probability for any type of interaction. This sum of coefficients is the *linear* attenuation coefficient .

$$\mu = \tau_{photo} + \sigma_{inc} + \sigma_{coh} + \kappa_{pair} \qquad (14.2)$$

Photon attenuation depends on the photon energy (he), composition (Z), and the density () of the object and values are often tabulated as mass-attenuation coefficients, / (Fig. 14.2).

In a photo-absorption event, the energy of a photon is transferred to an electron in the interacting atom. This electron will, if the photon energy is high enough, liberate itself from the atom and leave the atom with a kinetic energy equal to the incoming photon energy minus the binding energy of the electron. When the vacancy in the electron shell is filled from an outer electron, the binding energy is emitted either as a characteristic x-ray photon or as an Auger electron. The probability for these occurrences depends on the atomic number of the material. Auger electron emission dominates for low-Z tissue-equivalent materials.

Figure 14.3 shows four frontal projections (Fig. 14.3a–d) of the NCAT phantom simulated for

Fig. 14.2 The relative
probability
for photoabsorptions,
Compton scattering, and
Rayleigh scatterings in the
energy range of 500 keV and
lower for tissue-equivalent
material (*upper*), bone-
equivalent material (*middle*),
and for NaI (*lower*). Note the
rapid decrease in probability
for photoabsorption in tissue.
Also note also that these data
are relative and that the
magnitude of the attenuation
is much larger for NaI(Tl) as
compared to water

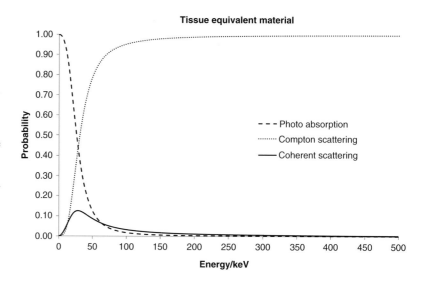

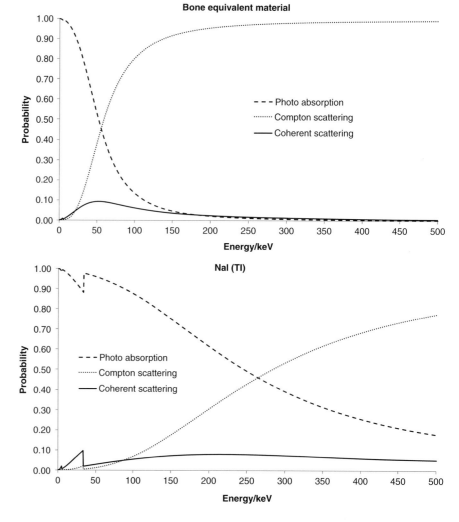

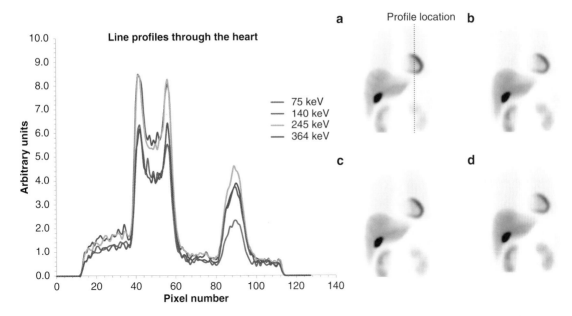

Fig. 14.3 Four frontal projections of the NCAT phantom showing the effect of photon attenuation in the cases of 75 keV (**a**), 140 keV (**b**), 245 keV (**c**), and 364 keV (**d**) photon emission, respectively. Vertical line profiles through the heart and part of the left kidney have been calculated and are compared in the *left* *diagram*. The *dotted line* in projection A indicates the location of the profiles. Note that imaging 75 keV and 364 keV photons result in about the same count rate. Also, note that these figures were simulated considering "only" photon attenuation

four different photon energies (75, 140, 245, and 364 keV, respectively). The effect of attenuation is shown as a decreased count level in the heart region and especially in the left kidney, a diminished uptake can be seen. The registered count rate also depends on the attenuation in the crystal. Imaging high photon energies that experience less attenuation in the phantom does not always reflect a high count rate because of the increased probability for the photon to travel through the crystal without any interaction and related contribution to the image formation.

14.2.3 Photon Scatter

The problem with photon scatter has its origin in the limitation of the scintillation camera to accurately measure the energy imparted in the NaI(Tl) crystal. The processes of converting the imparted energy to visible light photons and to guide these photons to the photomultipliers to achieve measurable signals are inherently a stochastic procedure. Therefore, the measured signal will have a statistical error even if the imparted energy always remains the same. For new NaI(Tl) crystals, this statistical error is about 8–10% (FWHM) for an absorbed energy of 140 keV. This relatively large error implies that an energy discriminator needs to cover about twice that width (16–20%) in order to maintain a reasonable counting statistics. Some of the photons that have been scattered in the patient with a small deflection angle (small loss of energy) will therefore have a possibility to be detected within such a large energy window and thus contribute to the image formation, but these photons carry wrong spatial information about the decay location in the object. The effect when registering scattered events will result in a degraded image contrast and a potential problem if aiming to quantify regional activity uptakes (Fig. 14.4).

The energy hν′ of a scattered photon is directly related to the deflection angle according to the Compton equation.

$$hv' = \frac{hv}{1 + \frac{hv}{m_o c^2}(1 - \cos\theta)} \qquad (14.3)$$

Fig. 14.4 The upper diagram (**a**) shows the true imparted energy in the NaI(Tl) crystal from 140 keV photons. Note the sharp peak that occurs because the full absorption from 140.5 keV photons will be within the same energy channel. The middle diagram (**b**) shows simulated data corresponding to a measured energy spectrum. The peaks have been broader due to the poor energy resolution of the camera. Because of this inaccuracy in the energy measure, some photons that have been scattered in the phantom are detected within the energy window. Diagram (**b**) also display curves that represent events from primary unattenuated photons and events from photons scattered in the object. Note that a substantial fraction of scattered photons will contaminate the images acquired within the energy window. Note that in the acquired image, it is not possible to distinguish these events from the primary events. Diagram (**c**) shows corresponding data for ^{201}Tl

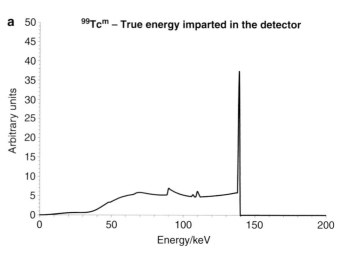

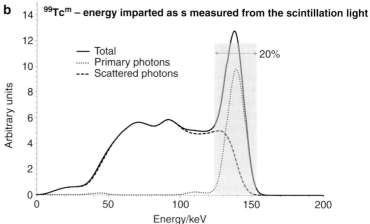

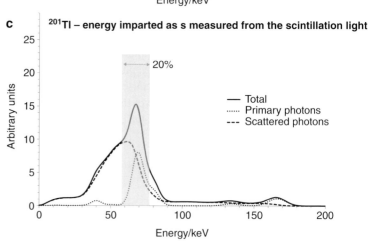

For higher photon energies, the scattering angles tend to peak in the forward directions, but at moderate photon energies (100 keV), the distribution is relatively symmetrical with a slightly lower probability for $\pm 90°$ scattering angles. The differential cross section, as described by the Klein-Nishina relation

$$\frac{\mathrm{d}\sigma}{\mathrm{d}\Omega} = \left(\frac{r_o^2}{2}\right)\left(\frac{h\upsilon}{h\upsilon'}\right)^2\left(\frac{h\upsilon}{h\upsilon'} + \frac{h\upsilon'}{h\upsilon} - 1 + \cos^2\theta\right) \quad (14.4)$$

which determined the probability for a photon being scattered by an angle into a solid angle d relative to the incoming photon trajectory. Equation 14.4 has been derived assuming that the electron is not bounded to the nucleus and in rest. When the photon energy decreases, the effect of the binding to the nucleus slightly changes the cross sections.

Since the contribution of scatter in a SPECT projection is a consequence of photon interactions in the object, the amount of scatter (sometimes defined as the scatter-to-total fraction) depends on photon energy, source depth and distribution, and on tissue composition in addition to camera-based parameters, such as, energy resolution and energy window settings. Figure 14.5 shows the dependencies on the scatter-to-total fraction as function of these parameters.

From Fig. 14.5a, it can be seen that the scatter-to-total fraction increases with increasing source depth but levels out at or above moderate source depth (>20 cm). This is because, although scattering increases with depth, the scattered photons will also be more attenuated compared to the primary photons with higher energies. The degradation in image quality, due to Compton scattering, is also a function of the energy

resolution (and thus related energy window setting) but, as can be seen from Fig. 14.4b and c, the dependence of these two parameters is very moderate. Thus, even for new crystals, the scatter-to-total fraction in a scintillation camera images remains quite high (30–50%). When reviewing tabulated cross sections for Compton scattering [5], one can see that the relative number of Compton scattering interactions increases with increasing photon energy, as can be seen in Fig. 14.2. It is therefore somewhat contradictory that scatter problem in SPECT is larger for photons of low energies (Fig. 14.4d). The reason for this is that a fixed energy window centered on the photo-peak energy is used. For an initial high photon energy, the relative loss of energy to a secondary electron in a Compton scattering is quite large which results in a scattered photon of significantly lower energy as when compared to using the energy window discriminator in the lower part of the energy distribution. For a lower initial photon energy, the relative loss of energy in a Compton scattering is small which implies that even for a large scattering angle, there is a good chance that a scattered photon in that energy range will be detected within the fixed energy window.

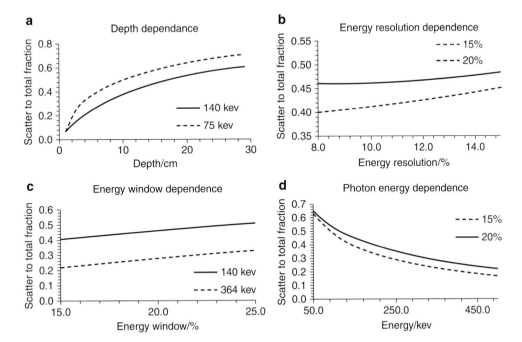

Fig. 14.5 The four diagrams show the scatter-to-total dependence on (**a**) the source depth, (**b**) the energy resolution, (**c**) the energy window setting, and (**d**) the photon energy. Two energy windows of 15% and 20% have been used when appropriate. The data have been simulated using a cylindrical water phantom of 11 cm radius and 20 cm length. The point source is located in center of the phantom for the results in graph (**b**–**d**)

14.2.4 Collimator Penetration

As mentioned above, the purpose of the collimator is to select only those photons emitted in a direction mainly determined by the axial direction of the collimator hole and to reject all photons emitted in other directions. However, because of the exponential characteristics of the photon attenuation, there will always be a finite probability for a photon to penetrate the collimator walls and thus interact in the crystal further away from the positions defined by the location of the hole. When constructing a collimator, the selection of the thickness of the walls is therefore a compromise between spatial resolution and system sensitivity and the chance for septum penetration.

To illustrate this effect, consider the simulated images shown in Fig. 14.6. Image (a) shows a simulation with 140 keV (^{99m}Tc) and a LEHR collimator and where a good image quality has been obtained. The second image (b) shows a simulation with photons of 364 keV (^{131}I) but still using a LEHR collimator. The image is completely deteriorated due to septum penetration and is, in practice, useless. The third image (c) shows the same simulation with 364 keV photons but now with a HEGP collimator. Because of the thicker septa (1.8 mm instead of 0.2 mm), the penetration effects have been reduced and a useful image quality has been obtained. The last image (Fig. 14.6d) shows a simulation with photon emission from a complete decay of ^{131}I including also the higher photon energies of 637 keV (7.3%) and 723 keV (1.8%). Even though the abundance of these photons is numerically of small magnitudes, the high photon energies make the photons penetrate the walls even when using a HEGP collimator [6] and contribute significantly to the image

formation. The degradation in image quality from these high-energy photons can be clearly seen in Fig. 14.6d.

The problem with septum penetration can be reduced by either using a collimator with thicker septa [7] of better attenuating properties, such as tungsten, or the effect can be included in some kind of correction method. If the septum penetration can be modeled, then this effect can be included as a collimator-response function in the forward projection step on an iterative reconstruction method.

14.2.5 Physiologic and Patient Motions

When acquiring data with a SPECT camera, one should always remember that the acquisition is made using a "camera shutter" that is open during the whole acquisition time. This means that if the patient is moving, this will result in degradation in the spatial resolution and in some cases, cause artifacts. Even if the patient is carefully strapped and remains very still, some movements cannot be avoided and these are the respiratory movements and the motion of the heart [8].

The respiratory movements due to breathing make a spatial change that depends on the organ. Since the frequency of the breathing is different as compared to the frequency of the cardiac motion, the respiratory movement will also have an effect on the quality of cardiac imaging even if gated SPECT is applied. The motion is complicated with translations in axial or superior/inferior direction causing a blurred image with a potential reduction of counts in anterior and inferior walls. In tumor detection, the form of the

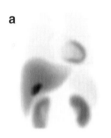 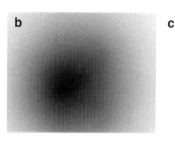 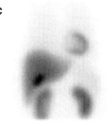 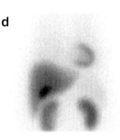

Fig. 14.6 The left image (**a**) shows 140 keV photons impinging on a camera with a LEHR collimator. Next image (**b**) shows 364 keV photons on a camera with the same collimator optimized for 140 keV. Image (**c**) represents an acquisition of 364 keV photons with a dedicated high-energy collimator and image (**d**) is the case where the complete ^{131}I decay has been simulated including also the high-energy photons in the decay

tumor may change to a more elongated or elliptical shape because of breathing and the result is also a lower image contrast. This has been seen in lung studies with PET and ^{18}F-DG.

14.2.6 Image Noise

Because of the randomness of a photon history, an acquired SPECT image will be affected by statistical errors and related image noise. The noise distribution of scintillation camera image follows the Poisson distribution where the variance of a measure in a region-of-interest is the sum of the counts. This implies that in order to get a good image quality, a sufficient long acquisition time together with a high administered activity should be used. The image noise also depends on the selection of matrix size. Changing from 64 64 to 128 128 in matrix size will increase the variance in a projection pixel by a factor of four. Also note that reconstruction is usually made slice by slice which means that the slice thickness (and consequently the acquired number of counts) is half for a 128 128 as compared to a 64 64. The mean counts per voxel in a reconstructed SPECT image will therefore be reduced by a factor of eight. It is thus not always an advantage to increase the matrix size. The time per projection and the number of projections are also of importance. These factors need to be optimized for each study since noise due to improper acquisition parameters can propagate through the reconstruction process and create artifacts in the final image.

14.2.7 Other SPECT Degradation Factors

It is essential that the scintillation camera is well tuned and calibrated. This is especially true for SPECT since deficiencies can result in visible artifacts. For example, nonuniformities in a planar image can be of less importance and sometimes hard to detect, but when reconstructing data from a SPECT camera with non-uniformity regions, artifacts appearing as distinct rings in the image can be seen. The center-of-rotation (COR), that is, the alignment of the electronic center

used in the reconstruction algorithm to the mechanic center of the camera orbit is also important to tune. A small error in COR results in degradation of spatial resolution and if larger shift occurs, then ring artifact can appear. It is also important to calibrate the pixel size carefully when performing correction for attenuation and other quantitative measures. A wrong value can result in either under- or overcorrection due to errors in the parameter x in Eqn 1. Other factors that can influence the accuracy in a SPECT study are the selection of acquisition parameters and the noise related to these. The most important selection here is the number of projections and the matrix size. There is a relation between the expected spatial resolution in an image and the number of samples (angles and pixels) as determined by the Nyquist frequency and the number of angular intervals.

Reaching this frequency limit may, in some cases, be difficult depending on the activity administered to the patient and the time required for the acquisition. Generally, there is a trade-off between image quality (the combination of spatial resolution, image contrast, and noise level) and realistic acquisition times and levels of administered activity. Often, image processing including low-pass filtering are required but here, one needs to remember that by using postacquisition image filtering, one sacrifices some extent of the spatial resolution. In some investigations, where high administered activities are used, limitations in the camera's count rate performance can lead to unexpected results. Dead time problems and pulse pile-up effects can change the system sensitivity (cps/MBq) and calibration factors for scatter correction methods, but also significant mis-positioning of events due to unwanted contribution of scintillation light from earlier events may occur, because the position of an event is calculated from the centroid of the emitted scintillation light. In this context, it should be remembered that calibrations made for low-count rates might thus not be relevant in high-count rate imaging.

Since data is collected for a relatively long time interval, it is important that the patient remains at the same position. Some movements such as cardiac motion and breathing can, however, not be avoided. Accounting for cardiac motion can be made by gated SPECT where the cardiac cycle is divided into a number of separate time-frame acquisitions based on the ECG information and especially the R-R interval. It has been a standard procedure for many years to collect information by this technique and display sep-arately reconstructed images of the different time intervals in a cine-mode display. The factor that ham-pers the image quality the most is noise because of the limited amount of collected count for 8 or 6 frame gated SPECT. Spatial and temporal filtering is a pre-requisite here for a reasonable image quality. In addi-tion, often the number of projections and the number of time frames per cardiac cycle is reduced in order to increase time per projection for a given total acquisi-tion time.

As a summary of this subsection, Fig. 14.7 shows how the image is degraded by the different factors discussed above. The upper row is the frontal projec-tions and the lower is corresponding reconstructed transversal image selected at a location through the heart. Reconstructions were made with an iterative

OSEM algorithm without any corrections. Simulation was made using 64 angle projections and a 360-degree rotation mode. The matrix size was 128 128 and 6 iterations and 16 subsets were used in the reconstruc-tion. The first set of images (a) represents no motion of the heart and breathing and an acquisition with a perfect system. Note that the reconstructed image still shows some degradation in spatial resolution due to the finite sampling in projection angles, matrix size, and of the forward projection algorithm. The second column (b) shows the blurring due to respiration and heart motion. When determining the expected image quality reachable in clinical studies based on phantom experiments, it is important to keep this motion in mind since physical phantoms are most often static. In addition, the third column (c) includes degradation in the spatial resolution caused by the characteristics

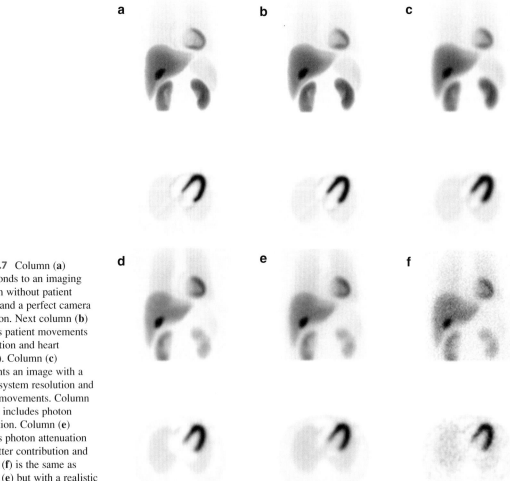

Fig. 14.7 Column (**a**) corresponds to an imaging situation without patient motion and a perfect camera resolution. Next column (**b**) includes patient movements (respiration and heart beating). Column (**c**) represents an image with a typical system resolution and patient movements. Column (**d**) also includes photon attenuation. Column (**e**) includes photon attenuation and scatter contribution and column (**f**) is the same as column (**e**) but with a realistic noise level added

of the LEHR collimator. The forth column (d) includes attenuation of primary photons but no scatter contribution. This mimics a system with perfect energy resolution and a corresponding narrow energy window. The fifth column (e) also includes the presence of scatter due to the limited energy resolutions. The last column (f) has the same images as in column (e) but with a realistic noise level added.

14.3 Correction Algorithms

The objective of a reconstruction method is to obtain a source distribution, described as transversal images, that matches the measured projections as accurate as possible. However, if the measured data are affected by photon attenuation, scatter, and collimator blurring the reconstructed images will be more or less wrong. It is therefore important that these physical effects are compensated for even if the numerical values in the final image are of less importance in order to obtain a diagnostic high-quality image with better sensitivity and specificity.

14.3.1 Attenuation Correction Methods

When using filtered backprojection (FBP) method to reconstruct images, an attenuation correction needs to be applied either prior to the reconstruction step or after. As a preprocessing method, the conjugate-view method can be applied if opposite projection data are available. The main advantage is that the source depth dependence x in Equation 14.1 is cancelled out when combining opposite projections by a geometrical-mean operator on a pixel-by-pixel basis. Let p_{ant} and P_{post} be the counts in opposite projections and P_{air} the counts registered in both cameras without attenuation (assuming a parallel-hole collimator with invariant system sensitivity within the FOV). Then the geometrical mean is calculated from

$$\sqrt{P_{ant} \cdot P_{post}} = \sqrt{P_{air} \ e^{-\mu d} \cdot P_{air} \ e^{-\mu(T-d)}}$$
$$= \sqrt{P_{air}^2 \cdot e^{-\mu T}} = P_{air} \cdot e^{-\mu T/2} \quad (14.5)$$

where d is the distance from the source to the surface along the projection line toward detector A and T is the total thickness of the patient along the same projection line. The equation is valid only for point-like sources and uniform attenuation. Still, this method is used frequently in planar imaging activity quantitation.

The Chang method [9] is a postprocessing method that is applied on reconstructed SPECT images. The base for this method is the calculation on an attenuation factor averaged for all angles and determined for each voxel location within the boundary of the object. The method can be mathematically described as

$$AF_{i,j} = \frac{1}{N} \sum_{\theta} AF_{i,j,\theta} \quad \text{where} \quad AF_{i,j,\theta} = e^{\sum i,j,\theta \ \mu \Delta x}$$

$$(14.6)$$

If information about heterogeneous attenuation, expressed as a map of varying values, can be obtained by some type of transmission study (see more about this below), then this information can be included in the calculation of the attenuation factor. The Chang compensation method can be found on commercially available systems and has been successful in situations where the attenuation distribution is relatively uniform. The method may result in imperfect attenuation compensation and has inferior noise properties.

Today, the most frequently used compensation method for attenuation is as part of an iterative reconstruction method. A common feature of all iterative reconstruction methods is the calculated projection obtained by forward projecting a first-guess estimation of an activity distribution into the projection space. By comparing these calculated projections to matched measured projections using some kind of cost function, the need for an improvement (often denoted "an update") of the initial estimated activity distribution can be determined. Photon attenuation is implemented in the forward projection step before calculating the final projection bin. Information about nonuniform attenuation distribution can be included in the projection step if appropriate attenuation maps are available through transmission scans or registered CT images.

14.3.2 Measurement of Photon Attenuation

Properly correcting for attenuation in the thorax region requires a measurement of the distribution of attenuating tissue (an attenuation map) from a transmission measurement using an external radiation source mounted on the opposite side of the patient. Two measurements are required; one with the patient in site and one blank study. By calculating the quota between the two projections on a pixel-by-pixel basis, line integrals of the attenuation coefficients can be calculated from the following formula

$$\sum \mu_i = \frac{1}{\Delta x} \ln \left(\frac{P_{\text{patient}}}{P_{\text{blank}}} \right) \qquad (14.7)$$

where x is the pixel size. These -projections can then be reconstructed using either filtered backprojection or by using iterative reconstruction methods. If a radionuclide is used as a radiation source, it is generally desired to have properties so that the transmission scan can be made simultaneously to the emission scan. This implies that the radionuclide needs to be different from the main radionuclide in order to separate transmission data and have a high activity. The most commonly used radionuclide in commercial systems has been ^{153}Gd with a half-life of 242 days and two major photon energies of 97.5 keV (29.5%) and 103 keV (21.1%), respectively. The method with a radionuclide source suffers from several limitations. First, photons emitted from the main radionuclide (often ^{99m}Tc) that are scattered in the patient can be registered in the lower transmission energy window. This will lead to lower numerical values of the attenuation coefficients, because more counts are acquired than is expected and this will be treated as less attenuation. Some type of correction for the downscatter is needed. Second, the source needs to be replaced more or less on an annual basis making the method relatively expensive. Third, the spatial resolution of the camera limits the details to the major structures, such as the lungs, so the attenuation map cannot be used as an anatomical reference map. In addition to these effects and dependent on the type of SPECT system, dead time problems and related mis-positioning of events can occur mainly in the daily collection of the blank scan than may affect the values in the map.

Commercial vendors have provided several types of transmission equipments based on radionuclides. Four principles are shown in Fig. 14.8. The most common solutions have been the use of a flood source (Fig. 14.8a) (either uncollimated or collimated), a scanning line source (Fig. 14.8b) and a fixed line source imaged with either a symmetrical fan-beam

collimator (Fig. 14.8c) or an asymmetrical fan beam (Fig. 14.8d). A version of the geometry in Fig. 14.8a has been manufactured that rely on multiple replaceable line sources fixed in position such that the strongest of the line sources irradiates the thickest part of the patient where the photon attenuation dominates. The advantage is that as the line sources reduce in strength they can still be useful after reordering them. The solutions shown in Fig. 14.8c and d are found on triple-head SPECT system where one head is designated for the transmission measurement and utilizes special types of collimators. Furthermore, the dead time problems, caused by high count rates in regions of the crystal outside the patient boundary, can thereby be reduced.

The recent developments of combined SPECT/CT systems cancel most of the serious issues with radionuclide-based transmission measurements. The resolution and noise characteristics are superior and consequently, the quality of the measured attenuation coefficients is therefore high. The scaling to other photon energies is relatively accurate despite the fact that CT images are created from a broad spectrum of bremsstrahlung photon energies. The latest SPECT/CT models include diagnostic CT (spiral) with a very fast scanning time

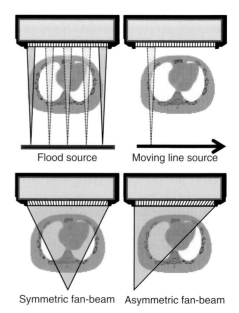

Fig. 14.8 Four common configurations for transmission measurements using a radionuclide source. The first is a fixed flood source; the second is a scanning line source. Third and fourth are fixed line sources together with a symmetrical (**c**) and an asymmetrical fan-beam collimator

and a spatial resolution that meets the requirement for a useful diagnostic modality in Radiology in contrast to the first-generation SPECT/CT system that had a spatial resolution of about 3 mm. However, care should be taken, since snaps shots from the CT does not generally represent the average attenuation caused by the breathing that is 'seen' by the SPECT camera. Artifacts can therefore be introduced in an attenuation correction. For more information on combined SPECT/CT system, see Chap. 10 in this textbook.

14.3.3 Scatter Correction Methods

Correction for scatter is most often made either in the energy domain where scatter in the photopeak energy window is modeled by collected data in additional energy windows or by using analytical methods that model the scatter on photopeak data directly. An early suggested scatter correction was the dual-energy window method (DEW), proposed by Jaszczak [10]. This method is based on an additional acquisition in a wide lower energy window. Scatter subtraction was applied by assuming that the distribution of counts in this lower energy window qualitatively equals to the distribution of scatter in the photopeak window but only differs quantitatively by a scaling factor k. A scatter-corrected projection is then calculated from

$$P(x, y)_{\text{Primary}} = P(x, y)_{\text{total}} - k \cdot P(x, y)_{\text{2nd}} \quad (14.8)$$

The main problem with this method is to obtain a proper value of k since this factor is essentially a function of the patient geometry and source distribution. Furthermore, the distribution of scatter in the lower energy window include a larger fraction of events created from multiple-scattered photons with wide angles which may then cause either over- or undercorrections in specific regions even if the k factor is accurate.

A similar approach is used in the Triple-Energy Window (TEW) method, but this method is based on two narrow adjacent-located energy windows around the photopeak window [11]. By taking the average of the acquired images pixel-by-pixel and scale by the ratio between the energy window width of the photopeak

window and the scatter windows a better scatter estimate will be obtained. Here, a scatter-corrected projection is obtained from

$$P(x, y)_{\text{Primary}} = P(x, y)_{\text{Peak}}$$
$$- \left[\frac{P(x, y)_{\text{left}}}{\Delta E_{\text{left}}} + \frac{P(x, y)_{\text{right}}}{\Delta E_{\text{right}}} \right]$$
$$\times \frac{\Delta E_{\text{Peak}}}{2} \quad (14.9)$$

This method does not rely on any scaling factor. However, the main problem here is the noise in the scatter data that is mainly a result of the narrow energy windows (Fig. 14.9) and scatter images require further processing such as low-pass filtering before subtraction. Nevertheless, this method has been successful not only for ^{99m}Tc studies but also for ^{131}I studies where the upper scatter window take into account the down scatter from the 634 keV and 723 keV photons that are emitted in the ^{131}I decay.

Figure 14.10 shows simulated point-spread functions for different point-source locations in an 11 cm radius cylindrical water phantom. The unscattered primary component has been separated and is shown as dashed lines. The shape of the scatter component in a point-spread function very much depends on the source depth. For shallow source depths, the probability for multiple scattering is low and therefore the shape of the scatter profile is quite narrow. For large source depth, the distribution becomes wider because of more events from multiple-scattered photon that results in a registered position far away from the decay location.

A variety of methods are proposed based on analytical description of scatter point-spread function as an alternative to energy window-based methods. An early paper by Axelsson et al. [12] presented a convolution-subtraction method where a scatter point-spread function (spsf) was estimated by a single exponential function obtained by a line-fitting procedure of the tails in a measured point-spread function from a point source in a cylindrical phantom.

$$P(x, y)_{\text{Primary}} = P(x, y)_{\text{Peak}} - P(x, y)_{\text{Peak}}$$
$$\otimes spsf \quad (14.10)$$

The drawback with this method is that the scatter function is stationary and dependent on an estimated

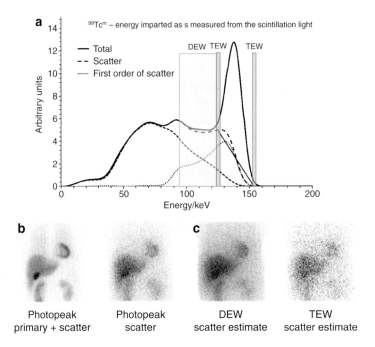

Fig. 14.9 The graph shows the location of the DEW window and the TEW windows. Image (**a**) shows the true scatter in the photon-peak energy window. Image (**b**) shows how this scatter distribution is estimated by a lower wider energy window (The DEW Method). Image (**c**) shows the scatter estimated by the TEW method where two narrow energy windows (width 4 keV) are positioned on each side of the main photon-peak window. The simulated spectrum has been divided into parts of total scatter, first order scatter, and second or more orders of scatter. It can be seen that more second or more orders of scattered event is recorded in the DEW region as compared to the photopeak region. This means that the distribution of scatter will be different in the DEW window, which will result in both over- and undercorrections when subtracting the data from the photopeak. The difference in distributions can be seen in the images. The problem of noise in the TEW windows due to the narrow energy window size is also evident

patient size and that the scatter close to the source is underestimated. A similar method based on a deconvolution process was investigated by Floyd [13]. Transmission-dependent scatter correction (TDSC) is an extension to the convolution-subtraction model in such a way that the scatter in the image is obtained by including a depth-dependent scatter function that scales the convolution kernel dependent on patient thickness. The fraction of scatter is used to scale the normalized convolving function before applying the convolution-subtraction process. The scatter fraction is determined from a generalized description of build-up functions for geometrical-mean images by Siegel et al. [14], where the buildup can be calculated as function of the depth for a given photon energy and composition

$$B(d) = a - b \cdot e^{-\mu d \beta} \quad (14.11)$$

The scatter-to-total fraction [15] can then be derived.

$$SF = 1 - \frac{1}{a - b(e^{-\mu T})^{\beta/2}} \quad (14.12)$$

and in the case of a transmission measurement

$$SF(x, y) = 1 - \frac{1}{a - b\left(\frac{P(x,y)_{\text{Patient}}}{P(x,y)_{\text{Air}}}\right)^{\beta/2}} \quad (14.13)$$

where P_{patient} and P_{air} are projections with and without a patient in site, respectively. The constants a, b and needs to be determined by experimental measurements. By including a position-dependent SF (x,y) information, Equation 14.10 will be transformed into

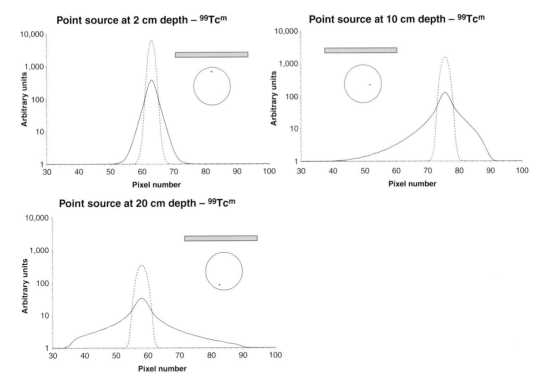

Fig. 14.10 Point-spread functions for three locations inside a cylindrical water phantom. The primary unscattered component is shown as *dashed lines*. Note the shade in distribution of the scatter as function of source depth. Also note also the nonsymmetry.

$$P(x, y)_{\text{Primary}} = P(x, y)_{\text{Peak}} - P(x, y)_{\text{Peak}}$$
$$\otimes spsf \cdot SF(x, y) \qquad (14.14)$$

An evaluation of the TDSC method using CT-based transmission data has recently been published by Willowson et al. [16]. Ljungberg and Strand [17, 18] further developed the convolution-subtraction method by use of Monte Carlo-calculated scatter line-spread functions tabulated as function of position in a cylindrical phantom. The scatter was estimated by selecting the scatter functions for each voxel that matched the voxel location as obtained from a reconstruction SPECT image.

Frey et al. [19] have developed a method called ESSE (Effective Scatter Source Estimator), in which the modeling of the scatter is incorporated in an iterative reconstruction method using precalculated scatter functions. The method has been proven to be useful and accurate for several radionuclides and also efficient when calculating the crosstalk of scatter between two energy windows [20]. However, the method has a limited accuracy in nonhomogeneous regions and in cases where activity out-of-field-of-view becomes important.

The most advanced and potentially accurate methods today are based on a real-time Monte Carlo calculation of the scatter. Floyd et al. pioneered this field already in the mid 80s, but because of limitations in computing resources the method did not reach a clinical practice [21]. However, today, it is possible to perform fast and accurate scatter modeling for an individual patient geometry and source distribution [22]. In these methods, the activity distribution at various steps in an iterative reconstruction process are linked to an external Monte Carlo-based forward projector that, based on the estimated activity distribution, calculates projection that fully include modeling of scatter in nonuniform regions. The method has been proven clinically useful mainly because of the implementation of fast variance reduction methods especially when modeling the collimator response, and studies have been made for ^{99m}Tc [23, 24] and ^{201}Tl [25]. This method can also include compensation for septum penetration in the collimator and back scatter for components behind the crystal and can therefore be useful for ^{131}I studies [26]

14.3.4 Spatial Resolution Compensation Methods

Compensation for the degradation in spatial resolution due to the collimator-response function (CRF) improves spatial resolution and provides improved quantitative accuracy for small objects. There are two classes of methods: iterative and noniterative methods. Noniterative methods include restoration filters, such as Metz and Wiener filters [27]. These filters are generally applied in the frequency domain and the usage is to filter the image data with a spatially invariant filter that described the inverse of the PSF function. They will, however, not be as effective at removing spatial varying effects as compared to iterative methods and they tend to have poor noise properties since the inverse filters generally act as a high-pass filter amplifying noise.

Some of the noniterative methods are based on the frequency distance relation (FDR) that relates the position of a source to the Fourier transform of the corresponding sinogram of the source. For a distributed source, measured activity from all sources located at the same distance from the center of rotation appears along a single line in Fourier space. One can therefore use this information in an inverse filtering method along these lines with a properly selected CRF [28,29].

In an iterative reconstruction method, the spatial resolution can be partly compensated for by including a model for distance-dependent blurring in the projector steps (forward and backward). This means that instead of forwarding the data in straight lines along the columns when calculating the projection value, the projector include the probability for a photon to pass nearby holes. This spread is often described by a distance-dependent spatially invariant Gaussian function, but images of the point-spread function can also be explicitly calculated and stored for each distance by Monte Carlo simulation for those cases where septum penetration is important (i.e., imaging with ^{131}I and ^{123}I radiopharmaceuticals). The correction method has

an effect similar to low-pass filtering, but it is not perfect in that sense that it will restore perfect resolution since some information about high spatial frequencies is permanently lost. Iterative reconstruction CRF compensation also produces different noise patterns as compared to filtered backprojection methods or iterative reconstruction without CRF correction. The correction method tends to increase the noise in the middle frequency range that may result in a blobby pattern in the reconstructed images, but noise properties can be improved by accurate modeling of CRF [30]. Some recent software programs are written to shorten acquisition time by incorporating the resolution recovery into the reconstruction process. This helps to improve the resolution properties of the image and hence signal-to-noise ratios for data acquired with less count statistics [31].

The degradation of spatial resolution is a function of the distance from the face of the collimator. Thus, a prerequisite to model CRF is the information of the distance from the center of rotation to the collimator face for every acquisition angle along with the knowledge of the collimator characteristics. For systems using circular orbits, this information is defined by the radius of rotation. For state-of-the-art SPECT system, the distance between the camera and the patient can, for each angle, be fine-tuned by sensors on the scintillation camera head. If this method is used, then a CRF correction requires the information of the varying organ-to-collimator distances for a particular projection angle. This information, however, is not always available from commercial systems or file headers.

14.3.5 Partial Volume Correction

Reconstructed SPECT images obtained by filtered backprojection or iterative reconstruction are degraded by the limited spatial resolution of the collimator system resulting in significant partial volume effects (Fig. 14.11). Because of this effect, spill-in of counts can be significant when evaluating activity in small regions located in close proximity to neighboring objects with high activity uptake. In a similar way, spill-out occurs when quantifying high activity and activity concentrations in small regions. In these cases, it might therefore be of importance to include some kind of partial volume correction (PVC).

Partial volume effects are of particular interest in clinical applications, e.g., determination of myocardial wall thickness, in quantitative brain studies where activity concentrations in small structures will be underestimated, and in dosimetry for radionuclide therapy where uptake by small tumors may be important for accurate dose assessment.

The underlying assumption for most PVC methods is that the radioactivity uptake in a specific volume is uniformly distributed and that the change in counts in this volume therefore can be used to develop a correction method. In the past, correction factors (recovery coefficients) for partial volume effects have been determined based on measurements of spheres of various sizes in physical phantoms [32–34]. The accuracy of these correction methods is, however, highly dependent on the shape of the tumor and on the background activity of the target structure. A more general approach is to minimize the resolution and penetration effects by implementing a 3D depth-dependent detector response included into the system model of an iterative reconstruction. These implementations have resulted in improved quantification accuracy for higher energy photon emitters such as ^{111}In and ^{131}I [35–37].

However, these studies show that for small targets and for targets within a high background activity, the activity recovery is not complete even when a 3D depth-dependent detector response function is included in the system model.

With the recent availability of dual modality SPECT-CT imaging with good image registration there is much incentive to use the CT-based anatomical information to correct for partial volume effects. CT-defined templates have been used for SPECT partial volume correction in myocardial studies [38] in which user-defined templates were mathematically projected to mimic the SPECT process followed by an image reconstruction to obtain a pixel-by-pixel PVC for the myocardial region. In more recent SPECT studies, the original template-based PVC was modified to implement a perturbation-based template method, which accounts for the nonlinear effects of the iterative reconstruction [37, 39, 40]. With this, PVC-improved quantitative accuracy has been demonstrated for SPECT studies with both ^{99m}Tc, ^{111}In and ^{131}I.

The method works as follows: Separate templates are generated for each target and relevant background structure by defining volume-of-interest (VIO) outlines in three dimensions on the registered anatomical

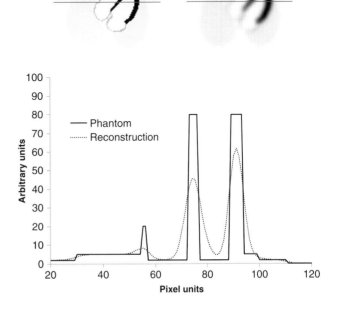

Fig. 14.11 The figure shows the effect of partial volume. The *left image* shows the real activity distribution ("phantom") and the *right figure* shows the image blurred by a Gaussian function that simulate a LEHR collimator and a clinically realistic source-to-collimator distance. The profiles through the heart show the "spill-in" into the left ventricle and "spill-out" from the myocardial region

CT image. All voxels located within the template are assigned a value of unity. Each template is then independently projected into appropriate number of angular views using an analytical (or Monte Carlo based) projector, which realistically model the SPECT imaging process. The next step is to reconstruct the reprojected template SPECT projections to transversal images of pixel-by-pixel correction factors for the VOIs in the SPECT image. Figure 14.12 shows a block diagram showing the steps for template generation, forward projection, image reconstruction and the PVC.

When reconstructing the template projections one needs to account for the nonlinearity of the iterative reconstruction algorithm. This can be done as proposed by Boening et al. [40] and Yong et al. [39], where each template is introduced as a small perturbation to the emission data set. For each of the target and background VOI defined in the image, a reconstructed template T is calculated to carry out the spill-in and spill-out correction for each of the regions defined in the image. The correction for spill-in of counts from background to target is given by

$$C_{SI}(X_j) = X_j - \sum_n T_{j,n}^{bkg} \cdot a_n \qquad (14.15)$$

where $C_{SI}(X_j)$ is the spill-in-corrected image at pixel j, X_j is the uncorrected image at pixel j, $T_{j,n}$ is the reconstructed template at pixel j for the nth background region and a_n is the average count in the uncorrected image for the nth background region. Note that nontarget regions are treated as background regions that may potentially contribute spill-in counts into the target. The PVC completes by applying the spill-out correction to the spill-in-corrected image

$$C_{SO+SI}(X_j) = \frac{C_{SI}(X_j)}{T_j^{tgt}} \qquad (14.16)$$

where $C_{SO+SI}(X_j)$ is the spill-out and spill-in-corrected image at pixel j and T^{tgt}_j is the reconstructed target template at pixel j. In patient imaging, separately defining templates for all of the background structures may not be practical since it may take a larger amount of time. A practical alternative would be to define templates for the targets and combine all of the other regions to form one background template, assuming uniform activity in this region .

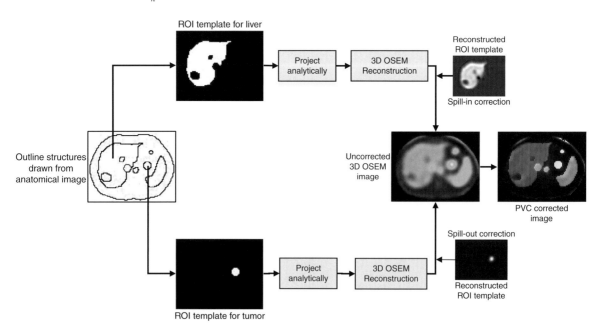

Fig. 14.12 The flowchart shows the principle steps in an image-based partial–volume correction. The user draws templates of the outline of the target (in this case a tumor) and relevant background regions from a high-resolution anatomical image. The values of each pixel in the ROIs are assigned unity. An analytical projection including simulation of distance-dependent collimator blur is then used to create projections of the templates. These projections are then reconstructed using the same reconstruction method as for the emission images. The reconstructed template images are then used to correct for the spill-in and spill-out

14.3.6 Influence of Correction Algorithms on Image Quality

Figure 14.13 shows some important factors and methods necessary to include in an quantitation procedure for SPECT. Photon attenuation is the single largest factor that degrades image quality in SPECT. Without proper compensation for attenuation, an absolute estimate of activity will often be in error by>50%. The magnitude of the effect is higher for low-energy photons and for large parts of the body with high density. Nonuniform attenuation in the head or the thorax can cause undesirable artifacts that impede both visual interpretation and activity quantitation.

Energy window-based scatter correction methods can be applied in two ways, either prior to reconstruction by simply subtracting the estimated scatter from the projection data prior to reconstruction or incorporating the scatter estimate in an iterative reconstruction method. The disadvantage of the first approach is the fact that subtracting two noise images results in an increase of the noise. This means that some kind of low-pass filtering may be necessary to apply on the data resulting in a degradation of the spatial resolution of the image. The second approach of incorporating the measured scatter estimate in the forward projection has shown to have better noise properties but may be technically more complicated to implement. Further, accurate scatter correction techniques should improve image contrast and lead to a better quantitative accuracy.

The necessity for quantitative SPECT images depends on the application. It is, however, important to understand that even if the actual number in units of MBq or MBq/mL is not used for a particular application, the quantification procedures may improve the accuracy and precision in the investigation since compensations correct for the mis-placement of counts and thus provide a better image. On the other hand, if the correction methods used are not properly setup and

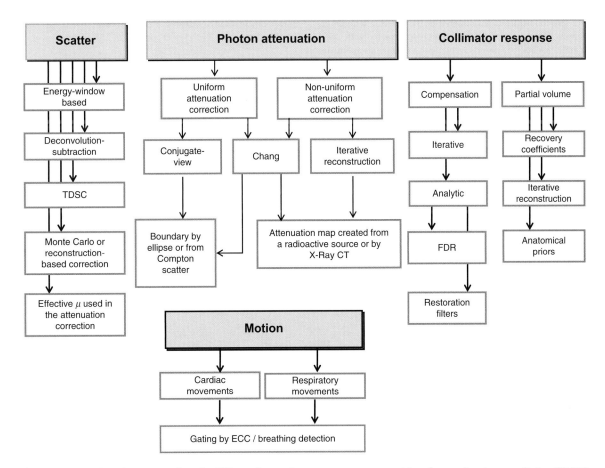

Fig. 14.13 This flowchart summarizes the different factors that are necessary to consider when performing quantitative SPECT

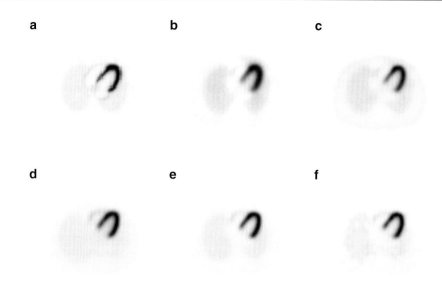

Fig. 14.14 The first image (**a**) is reconstructed data mimicking a perfect system without patient movements (the image is equal to Fig 14.7a). The second image (**b**) shows an image of the same data set reconstructed with filtered backprojection without corrections. Figure (**c**)–(**e**) shows images reconstructed with OSEM (6 iterations and 16 subsets) using nonhomogeneous attenuation correction (**c**), attenuation and scatter correction using the ESSE method (**d**), and scatter and attenuation correction together with CRF correction (**e**). (**f**) shows an image reconstructed with all correction methods but using a data set with a realistic noise level added

validated then this can lead to problems. Furthermore, in some cases, image noise can be amplified which is a degrading factor on the image quality despite the theoretical improvement due to a particular compensation.

Despite the many inherent problems with SPECT images, the recent advancement in developing correction methods for physical effects, such as photon attenuation, scatter and collimator resolution has made SPECT a quantitative tool for activity measurement. Figure 14.14 shows an example of state-of-the-art reconstruction and activity quantification method including nonuniform attenuation correction, scatter correction using the ESSE method [41] and spatial variant collimator response correction.

14.4 Applications of SPECT in Dosimetry

One of the areas in nuclear medicine applications that rely on the absolute values of the SPECT images is dosimetry in radionuclide therapy where multiple SPECT acquisitions form the base for a dose planning of the therapy. The absorbed dose is defined as the imparted energy dE within a volume of interest divided by the mass of the volume element dm or $D = dE/dm$ (1 Gy = 1 J/kg). In practice, the absorbed dose is average over a large volume than dm, which yields $D = \bar{E}/m$. Dosimetry with quantitative SPECT allows for absorbed dose estimation within an organ down to a voxel level.

14.4.1 The Basic Calculation Scheme

The basic equation for dose calculations has been given by a MIRD publication [42] and is described as

$$\int \dot{D}(t)\, dt = \tilde{A} \cdot S$$

$$= \int A(t) dt \cdot \frac{n_i E_i \varphi_i(k \leftarrow h)}{m} \qquad (14.17)$$

where n is the number of particles i per disintegration, E_i is the average energy emitted for particle i, is a geometrically related factor that describes the fraction of energy emitted from a source volume element h that is absorbed in a target volume element k. Finally, m is the mass of that target volume element. The right integral is the cumulative activity i.e., the total number of disintegrations during a time interval from time of injection to infinity (see Chap. 8 for further details).

In practice, the integral (or the area under the curve) is mostly determined by a curve-fitting procedure from a limited number of time-activity values as have been measured by a scintillation camera or SPECT. The cumulative activity then equals the area under the curve and if expressed per unit administered activity is called the residence time. Recently, He and colleagues [43] have investigated several methods to determine the residence time including both commonly used quantification planar protocols as well as quantitative SPECT and a combined hybrid method. The latter is based on defining VOIs of the major organs in a patient from a CT study and with an iterativeM-LEM method including a forward projector adjusting the activity in the VOIs to match the measured data [44]. This method has shown to be more accurate than conventional planar methods but has practical limitations in the time required for defining the VOI in 3D (mainly manual segmentation).

The estimation of risks for developing cancer due to the usage of radiation is calculated using precalculated S values that have been developed by Monte Carlo calculations for generic mathematical description of a population of interest. This is because such risk estimations are relevant only on a large population of individuals. Therefore, such mathematical descriptions represent a reference male or female i.e., an average of a large population. These S values tables have been compiled in terms of the absorbed dose (Gy) to the target volume per cumulative activity (MBqh) in the source organ. S values are embedded into useful programs, such as, the MIRDDOSE3 [45] and the newly developed OLINDA code [46]. However, the mathematical phantoms have not been developed for individual therapy planning and therefore the dose-conversion factors are not very well representative for a specific patient. To overcome this, one may need to implement the patient's own geometry and biokinetics into a dose calculation scheme. A principal flowchart showing the steps necessary to consider for 3D patient-specific SPECT (and PET) dosimetry is shown in Fig. 14.15.

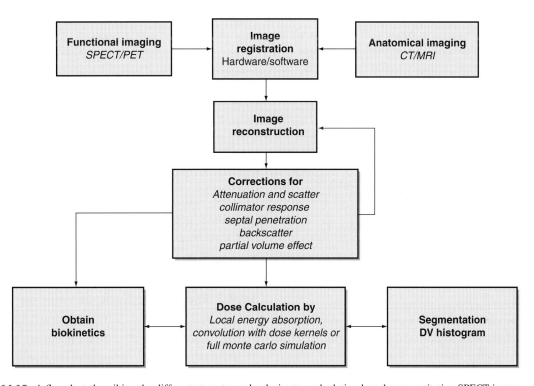

Fig. 14.15 A flowchart describing the different steps toward a dosimetry calculation based on quantitative SPECT images

14.4.2 Dose Calculation from Quantitative SPECT Imaging

Most dosimetry studies with scintillation cameras are conducted by planar scintillation camera imaging using the conjugate-view method. As described earlier, this method relies on opposite projections, and if the geometrical mean of the opposite projection is taken, the dependence on the source depth is greatly reduced. The attenuation correction then depends only on the "thickness of the patient" because the attenuation depend on the whole patient geometry and not on the source location. This is the idea behind the geometrical-mean method. First, the above statement is valid only for a point source. If extended sources are being imaged (which is always the case in clinical studies), then a correction for the source thickness needs to be made [47]. Second, if over- and underlying activities are present, this affects the quantitation, since the planar imaging is on a 2D modality and corrections needs to be made [48]. Third, scatter correction and septum penetration may not be accurately modeled and fourth, the dosimetry needs in most cases to rely on S-factors obtained from a mathematical phantom.

SPECT in combination with CT can overcome many of these drawbacks because of the inherent 3D activity determination. The methods, described below, treat each voxel as a source volume and correspondingly each voxel as a target organ. In practice, one does not store the S-factor that corresponds to each combination but the MIRD Equation 14.17 will remain valid in these cases. The results will be 3D images of absorbed dose distributions useful to obtain, for example, dose-volume histograms and other parameters related to the heterogeneity of imparted energy within the volume of interest.

14.4.3 Energy Locally Absorbed within a Voxel

In its simplest form, a dose calculation based on quantitative SPECT can assume all kinetic electron energy emitted from the radionuclide as locally absorbed within the voxel volume and disregard the energy distribution from photons. The absorbed dose is then calculated from the mass of the volume element. This assumption is not as approximate as it sounds because the spatial resolution of a SPECT image used as input is in the same order or larger compared to relevant electron ranges. Thus, the SPECT image may very well show the absorbed dose distribution from electrons. If reviewing Equation 14.17 above, this method corresponds to the case where source volume equals the target volume ($k=h$). This type of calculation may work only on pure emitting radionuclides such as ^{90}Y or when the contribution to the absorbed dose from photons can be regarded as negligible.

14.4.4 Convolution Based on Point Dose Kernels

This method use precalculated energy distribution in 3D from a point source usually stored as function of the radial distance from the point source normalized to the energy emitted per disintegration. By a mathematical convolution either in the spatial domain or in the frequency domain, the initial activity image (e.g., a SPECT image) can be converted to absorbed dose images. Berger has published point dose kernel for both photons [49] and electrons and particles [50]. Convolution of SPECT images with point-dose kernels should generally be used when the voxel size of the activity matrix is small as compared to the path length of the particles. Also note that dose kernels generally are valid for a uniform material (often water or tissue-equivalent material) and that the calculation procedure (often performed in the Fourier domain) is spatially invariant and do not take into account variations either in density or changes in energy distribution due to organ or patient boundaries. An example of a program for dosimetry that uses point dose kernels is the 3D-ID program [51].

14.4.5 Full Monte Carlo Simulation

The most accurate absorbed dose calculation, but also the most complex and computing demanding procedure, is a full radiation transport calculation using the Monte Carlo method [52]. The method in this context starts from quantitative accurate SPECT images and registered density images, usually obtained from a patient-specific CT. From this set of images, simulation of individual photon and electron interactions are performed in the 3D density volume by tracing the particles to the end by explicitly simulating all relevant interaction types. The location for a decay corresponds to the apparent voxel location in the Cartesian coordinate system and the numbers of simulated decays are proportional to the voxel values of the quantitative SPECT images. The imparted energy from each particle is then scored in a matching 3D-absorbed energy matrix as the particles are traced through the volume. When all particles are simulated, the absorbed energy in each voxel per voxel mass obtains the absorbed dose. The main advantage with full Monte Carlo simulation is that it considers the patient's geometry and that heterogeneities in density and tissue compositions can be included in the absorbed dose calculation.

There are several very competent programs in the public domain that is useful for Monte Carlo absorbed dose calculations. The EGS family of programs [53] have shown to be useful and simulation of voxel data is relatively straight forward – although the program required some programming skills. MCNP is also a program that can implement voxel information [54]. In Medical Imaging applications, the GATE Monte Carlo program [55] has gained increased interest due to its flexibility especially with complex geometries. This program is a layer of the Geant4 program from CERN and can simulate charged particles up to very high energies.

14.4.6 Considerations Related to Absorbed Dose Calculation Based on SPECT/CT Data

The new hybrid systems offer a good possibility to do accurate dosimetry both in 2D and in 3D. Today, most SPECT/CT systems are based on diagnostic CT acquisition with a spatial resolution of the order of a magnitude higher that SPECT unit. In some systems, the CT unit is useful to obtain information about the attenuation for the planar conjugate-view method by performing a full-length scan (so called scout measurement). If the scaling between pixel units and density can be determined, then this transmission image will be the

correction necessary for planar attenuation correction [56]. The high quality from diagnostic CT units makes accurate SPECT quantification possible and the known limitations with radionuclide-based transmission sources (down scatter, noise and limited spatial resolution) is eliminated by using CT.

Some issues needs consideration when doing absorbed dose calculations based on SPECT data. The most important is the fact that the SPECT images do not show the actual activity distribution. The images are affected by the particular system degradation in spatial resolution and the effect (discussed above in the partial volume section) is dependent on the source volume.

When calculating the absorbed dose, it is convenient to use the CT images if proper scaling to density can be achieved. However, in most modern system, the spatial resolution of the CT data can be in the order of a magnitude better then the SPECT information. When using high-resolution CT as mass images in the voxel-by-voxel absorbed dose calculation artifacts can be introduced where 'counts' spill out in regions of low densities. In addition, gas in the abdominal parts can result in very high absorbed doses because of low CT voxel values in combination with the blurring due to the limited spatial resolution in the SPECT images. One way to overcome this problem is to reduce the spatial resolution of the CT images by a convolution with a PSF that match the resolution of the SPECT system.

Most CT units are very fast in the image acquisition. This means that a CT image over the thorax may reflect a particular time segment of the breathing cycle more. A SPECT projection is generally acquired over a much longer time meaning that the image reflects a count distribution averaged over the whole respiration cycle. This can thus introduce artifacts in the attenuation correction and the absorbed dose calculations especially close to the lung boundaries.

Even if SPECT/CT images are accurately registered to each other in a hybrid system, there is a need for image registration when performing multiple SPECT/CT studies in order to obtain voxel-based time-activity curves. Image registration using CT-CT images are preferable here compared to SPECT-SPECT registration because of their better similarity. However, if a diagnostic CT is used, then the absorbed dose caused by multiple X-rays exposures can be significant. The problem can be reduced if the CT unit can be run in a 'low-dose' mode. The signal-to-noise ratio and spatial resolution may be reduced here, but for attenuation corrections and absorbed dose calculations, this is probably not a serious problem.

14.5 Conclusion

Today, quantitative SPECT has become a reality mainly because of the great improvement in reconstruction algorithms where the corrections for image degradation due to photon attenuation, contribution of event in the image from photons scatter in the patient, collimator and camera housing and septum penetration can be made in a consistent and natural way in the forward projector step. The limitations that existed in earlier radionuclide-based transmission measurement methods are eliminated when using high-quality attenuation maps created by CT detectors that are integrated into the SPECT gantry. Hybrid SPCT/CT systems also provide registered functional and anatomical images thus reducing the need for software registration methods, although good registration software may be required when working with multiple SPECT/CT studies. Many scatter correction methods still rely on measurements in secondary energy window, but along with the improvement in computing power, real time Monte Carlo simulation of scatter may be feasible clinically within a few years.

References

1. Ljungberg M, Strand SE (1989) A Monte Carlo program simulating scintillation camera imaging. Comput Meth Prog Bio 29:257–272
2. Ljungberg M (1998) The SIMIND Monte Carlo program. In: Ljungberg M, Strand SE, King MA (eds) Monte Carlo calculation in nuclear medicine: applications in diagnostic imaginged. IOP, Bristol/Philadelphia, pp 145–163
3. Segars WP, Lalush DS, Tsui BMW (1999) A realistic spline-based dynamic heart phantom. IEEE Trans Nucl Sci 46(3):503–506
4. Segars WP (2001) Development of a new dynamic NURBS-based cardiac-torso (NCAT) phantom. PhD Thesis, Universiy of North Carolina
5. Berger MJ, Hubbell JH (1987) XCOM: Photon Cross Sections on a Personal Computer, NBSIR 87–3597, National Bureau of Standards (former name of NIST), Gaithersburg, MD, http://physics.nist.gov/PhysRefData/Xcom/Text/version.shtml
6. Dewaraja YK, Ljungberg M, Koral KF (2000) Characterization of scatter and penetration using Monte Carlo simulation in 131-I imaging. J Nucl Med 41(1):123–130
7. Dewaraja YK, Ljungberg M, Koral KF (2000) Accuracy of 131I tumor quantification in radioimmunotherapy using SPECT imaging with an ultra-high-energy collimator: Monte Carlo study. J Nucl Med 41(10):1760–1767
8. Slomka PJ, Nishina H, Berman DS et al (2004) "Motion-frozen" display and quantification of myocardial perfusion. J Nucl Med 45(7):1128–1134
9. Chang LT (1978) A method for attenuation correction in radionuclide computed tomography. IEEE Trans Nucl Sci 25:638–643
10. Jaszczak RJ, Greer KL, Floyd CE et al (1984) Improved SPECT quantification using compensation for scattered photons. J Nucl Med 25:893–900
11. Ogawa K, Harata H, Ichihara T et al (1991) A practical method for position dependent compton-scatter correction in single photon emission CT. IEEE Trans Med Imaging 10:408–412
12. Axelsson B, Msaki P, Israelsson A (1984) Subtraction of compton-scattered photons in single-photon emission computed tomography. J Nucl Med 25:490–494
13. Floyd CE, Jaszczak RJ, Greer KL et al (1985) Deconvolution of compton scatter in SPECT. J Nucl Med 26:403–408
14. Siegel JA, Wu RK, Maurer AH (1985) The buildup factor: effect on scatter on absolute volume determination. J Nucl Med 26:390–394
15. Meikle SR, Hutton BF, Bailey DL (1994) A transmission-dependent method for scatter correction in SPECT. J Nucl Med 35:360–367
16. Willowson K, Bailey DL, Baldock C (2008) Quantitative SPECT reconstruction using CT-derived corrections. Phys Med Biol 53(12):3099–3112
17. Ljungberg M, Strand SE (1990) Scatter and attenuation correction in SPECT using density maps and Monte Carlo simulated scatter functions. J Nucl Med 31:1559–1567
18. Ljungberg M, Strand SE (1991) Attenuation and scatter correction in SPECT for sources in a nonhomogeneous object: a Monte Carlo study. J Nucl Med 32:1278–1284
19. Frey EC, Tsui BMW (1997) A new method for modeling the spatially-variant, object-dependent scatter response function in SPECT. In: Conference records of the IEEE Medical Imaging Conference, Anaheim, 1996, pp 1082–1082
20. Song X, Frey EC, Wang WT et al (2004) Validation and evaluation of model-based crosstalk compensation method in simultaneous 99mTc Stress and 201Tl rest myocardial perfusion SPECT. IEEE Trans Nucl Sci 51(1):72–79
21. Floyd CE, Jaszczak RJ, Coleman M (1985) Inverse Monte Carlo: a unified reconstruction algorithm for SPECT. IEEE Trans Nucl Sci 32:779–785
22. Beekman FJ, de Jong HW, Slijpen ET (1999) Efficient SPECT scatter calculation in non-uniform media using correlated Monte Carlo simulation. Phys Med Biol 44(8):N183–N192
23. Xiao J, de Wit TC, Staelens SG et al (2006) Evaluation of 3D Monte Carlo-based scatter correction for 99mTc cardiac perfusion SPECT. J Nucl Med 47(10):1662–1669
24. Liu S, King MA, Brill AB (2008) Accelerated SPECT Monte Carlo simulation using multiple projection sampling

and convolution-based forced detection. IEEE Trans Nucl Sci 55(1):560–568

25. Xiao J, de Wit TC, Zbijewski W et al (2007) Evaluation of 3D Monte Carlo-based scatter correction for 201Tl cardiac perfusion SPECT. J Nucl Med 48(4):637–644

26. Shaoying L, King MA, Brill AB et al (2008) Convolution-based forced detection Monte Carlo simulation incorporating septal penetration modeling. IEEE Trans Nucl Sci 55(3): 967–974

27. King MA, Schwinger RB, Doherty PW et al (1984) Two-dimensional filtering of SPECT images using the Metz and Wiener filters. J Nucl Med 25:1234–1240

28. Lewitt RM, Edholm PR, Xia W (1989) Fourier method for correction of depth dependent collimator blurring. Proc SPIE 1092:232–243

29. Xia W, Lewitt RM, Edholm PR (1995) Fourier correction for spatially variant collimator blurring in SPECT. IEEE Trans Med Imaging 14(1):100–115

30. Beekman FJ, Slijpen ET, de Jong HW et al (1999) Estimation of the depth-dependent component of the point spread function of SPECT. Med Phys 26(11):2311–2322

31. Borges-Neto S, Pagnanelli RA, Shaw LK et al (2007) Clinical results of a novel wide beam reconstruction method for shortening scan time of Tc-99m cardiac SPECT perfusion studies. J Nucl Cardiol 14(4):555–565

32. Zito F, Gilardi MC, Magnani P et al (1996) Single-photon emission tomographic quantification in spherical objects: effects of object size and background. Eur J Nucl Med Mol Imaging 23(3):263–271

33. Koral KF, Dewaraja Y (1999) I-131 SPECT activity recovery coefficients with implicit or triple-energy-window scatter correction. Nucl Instrum Methods Phys Res Sect A 422 (1–3):688–692

34. Geworski L, Knoop BO, de Cabrejas ML et al (2000) Recovery correction for quantitation in emission tomography: a feasibility study. Eur J Nucl Med Mol Imaging 27 (2):161–169

35. Dewaraja YK, Wilderman SJ, Ljungberg M et al (2005) Accurate dosimetry in 131I radionuclide therapy using patient-specific, 3-dimensional methods for SPECT reconstruction and absorbed dose calculation. J Nucl Med 46 (5):840–849

36. Ljungberg M, Sjogreen K, Liu X et al (2002) A 3-dimensional absorbed dose calculation method based on quantitative SPECT for radionuclide therapy: evaluation for 131-I using Monte Carlo simulation. J Nucl Med 43(8): 1101–1109

37. He B, Du Y, Song X et al (2005) A Monte Carlo and physical phantom evaluation of quantitative In-111 SPECT. Phys Med Biol 50(17):4169–4185

38. Da Silva AJ, Tang HR, Wong KH et al (2001) Absolute quantification of regional myocardial uptake of 99mTc-Sestamibi with SPECT: experimental validation in a Porcine model. J Nucl Med 42(5):772–779

39. Yong D, Tsui BMW, Frey EC (2005) Partial volume effect compensation for quantitative brain SPECT imaging. IEEE Trans Med Imaging 24(8):969–976

40. Boening G, Pretorius PH, King MA (2006) Study of relative quantification of Tc-99 m with partial volume effect and

spillover correction for SPECT oncology imaging. IEEE Trans Nucl Sci 53 (3-part-2):1205–1212

41. Frey EC, Tsui BMW (1993) Modeling the scatter response function in inhomogeneous scattering media. In: Conference Records of the IEEE Medical Imaging Conference, pp 1–1

42. Loevinger R, Berman M (1976) A revised schema for calculation of the absorbed dose from biologically distributed radionuclides. MIRD Phamplet No. 1, Revised. Society of Nuclear Medicine, New York

43. He B, Wahl RL, Du Y et al (2008) Comparison of residence time estimation methods for radioimmunotherapy dosimetry and treatment planning–Monte Carlo simulation studies. IEEE Trans Med Imaging 27(4):521–530

44. He B, Frey EC (2006) Comparison of conventional, model-based quantitative planar, and quantitative SPECT image processing methods for organ activity estimation using In-111 agents. Phys Med Biol 51(16):3967–3981

45. Stabin MG (1996) MIRDOSE: personal computer software for internal dose assessment in nuclear medicine. J Nucl Med 37(3):538–546

46. Stabin MG, Sparks RB, Crowe E (2005) OLINDA/EXM: the second-generation personal computer software for internal dose assessment in nuclear medicine. J Nucl Med 46 (6):1023–1027

47. Fleming JS (1979) A technique for the absolute measurement of activity using a gamma camera and computer. Phys Med Biol 24(1):178–180

48. Sjögreen K, Ljungberg M, Strand SE (2002) An activity quantification method based on registration of CT and whole-body scintillation camera images, with application to 131I. J Nucl Med 43(7):972–982

49. Berger MJ (1968) Energy deposition in water by photons from point isotropic sources: MIRD Pamphlet no. 2. J Nucl Med 9:15–25

50. Berger MJ (1971) Distribution of absorbed dose around point sources of electrons and beta particles in water and other media: MIRD Pamphlet no. 7. J Nucl Med 12:5–23

51. Kolbert KS, Sgouros G, Scott AM et al (1997) Implementation and evaluation of patient-specific three- dimensional internal dosimetry. J Nucl Med 38(2):301–308

52. Andreo P (1991) Monte Carlo techniques in medical radiation physics. Phys Med Biol 36:861–920

53. Nelson WR, Hirayama H, Rogers DWO (1985) The EGS4 Code System. Stanford Linear Accelerator Center report SLAC-265

54. Briesemeister JF (1986) MCNP-A general Monte Carlo Code for Neutron and Photon Transport Version 3A, Los Alamos National Laboratory LA-7396-M. Online document at: http://mcnp-green.lanl.gov/index.html

55. Jan S, Santin G, Strul D et al (2004) GATE: a simulation toolkit for PET and SPECT. Phys Med Biol 49(19): 4543–4561

56. Minarik D, Sjögreen K, Ljungberg M (2005) A new method to obtain transmission images for planar whole-body activity quantification. Cancer Biother Radiopharm 20(1):72–76

Quantitative Cardiac SPECT Imaging

15

Magdy M. Khalil

Contents

M.M. Khalil
Biological Imaging Centre, MRC/CSC, Imperial College London,
Hammersmith Campus, Du Cane Road, W12 0NN London, UK
e-mail: magdy.khalil@imperial.ac.uk, magdy_khalil@hotmail.com

15.1 Introduction

Nuclear cardiac imaging is a typical example that image quantitation has an important role in data interpretation and patient diagnosis. Reproducible and reliable image quantitation relies on robust techniques and well-designed computational algorithms. This in great part related to computer technology and various image-processing tools. However, the principal motivation for computer analysis is to evaluate an attribute of the image as a metric in an algorithmic manner, independent of observer bias or variability [1].

Tl-201 was one of the radionuclides that received initial attention in cardiac scintigraphy due to its analogous properties to potassium ions. It was commercially available in 1976 and utilized in patients with intermediate likelihood of coronary artery disease (CAD) and after that for risk stratification in patients with known or suspected CAD [2]. Image quantitation in myocardial perfusion imaging has passed through several steps to reach the state-of-the-art quantitation strategies seen today. Planar myocardial thallium-201 scintigraphy was the common mode of data acquisition before the advent of tomographic imaging. In that imaging procedure, a number of planar views were sequentially acquired and were known as stress and redistribution images and acquired immediately (10-min), 2–4 h, and 6–24 h poststress using mainly three planar views: anterior, anterior, 45° and 70° left anterior oblique.

Due to the planar nature of the images and absence of correction techniques for attenuation, scatter, and resolution compensation, images were interpreted with significant loss of spatial and contrast resolution. These degrading factors along with extracardiac tissue activities served to reduce the overall accuracy of the test. While the images were subjectively interpreted

M.M. Khalil (ed.), *Basic Sciences of Nuclear Medicine*, DOI: 10.1007/978-3-540-85962-8_15,
© Springer-Verlag Berlin Heidelberg 2011

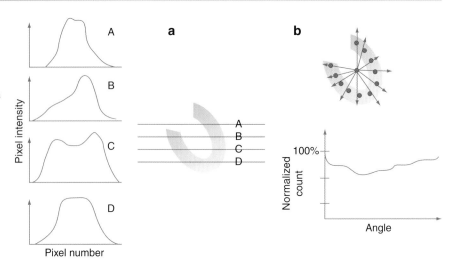

Fig. 15.1 Early methods for image quantitation in myocardial perfusion Tl-201 scintigraphy. (**a**) The quantitation is based on the peak activity determined from a series of linear horizontal profiles drawn over the myocardium while in (**b**) is based on collecting a number of circumferential radial profiles taken from a user specified centre and then constructed into a line profile

for possible myocardial ischemia, this was limited by intra- and interobserver variability, and there was early recognition for automated techniques to reproducibly assist in image quantitation. One of the initial approaches devised to quantify the myocardial planar images was based on generating linear intensity profiles of the early and late Th-201 images providing temporal and spatial representation of the tracer distribution. The method simply depended on coregistering the two data sets and reduction of the 2D images into horizontal count profiles [3]. Another approach was proposed to use a count circumferential profile to quantify the tracer uptake based on radial lines drawn from the center of the heart toward the myocardial walls at certain angular intervals [4]. Both methods are shown in Fig. 15.1.

The advent of tomographic imaging and its introduction in routine nuclear medicine has significantly improved image contrast by removing the underlying and overlying undesired structures. This has made marked improvements in image quality especially, after approval of Tc-99m-based myocardial tracers.

The introduction of Tc-99m-labeled compounds and the increase in the number of detector heads have also improved the statistical quality of the acquired images. Unlike Tl-201, with Tc-99m-labeled tracers, a longer time between injection and imaging is permitted. In addition, a relatively large dose can be administered, which is translated into a situation of high count rate and improved lesion detectability. Tc-99-based compounds also allow performing electrocardiograph (ECG)-gating myocardial perfusion

with substantial improvement to count statistics and identification of true perfusion defects from those induced by attenuation artifacts.

Further improvements to the diagnostic performance of scintigraphic myocardial perfusion images were achieved by adding x-ray computed tomography (CT) to single-photon emission computed tomography (SPECT) imaging in a new hybrid SPECT/CT or PET/CT devices (discussed in Chap. 10). Anatomically guided perfusion interpretations have opened a new gate for enhancing the diagnostic capability of SPECT imaging in providing more insights as well more information about the stenosed vessels and the affected myocardium.

SPECT and positron emission tomography (PET) are the two tomographic techniques that provide three-dimensional (3D) or four-dimensional (4D) information about heart function and perfusion/metabolism. Many factors have been associated with the development of nuclear cardiac imaging since its introduction in the field. Some of these are availability of radiopharmaceuticals, fast computer processors, and imaging devices with good characteristic performance. These developments have more progressed in the recent past because of several features, which are summarized as follows:

1. Advances in computer technology, including high-speed processors, storage media, and large-capacity memory chips have facilitated the development of various image-processing tools, providing robust data analysis, reliable data quantitation, and better

image display. Another remarkable outcome was the introduction of iterative reconstruction into the clinic, where reconstruction time was a limiting factor due to unavailability of powerful computer systems.

2. The recognition of image-degrading factors and their impact on image quality and quantitative accuracy have motivated researchers to develop and introduce new correction strategies able to enhance the diagnostic performance of cardiac protocols.

3. The practical implementation of resolution recovery in cardiac studies has been shown to influence significantly the acquisition time, the amount of the injected dose, or both.

4. New camera designs with or without semiconductor technology dedicated to cardiac imaging are relatively a new trend by which better image quality, patient convenience, and comfort as well as scanner throughouput can be realized.

5. The relatively recent introduction of SPECT/CT systems has improved the performance of attenuation correction and added a diagnostic value to myocardial perfusion imaging by providing more insights into the anatomy of coronary vessels in addition to calcium scoring and more information beyond that.

6. Molecular cardiac imaging has also become an interesting area of research and development and will exploit the potential diagnostic capabilities of radionuclide cardiac SPECT and PET tracers.

7. This last feature has encouraged a number of research groups as well as industry to manufacture multimodality small-animal imaging devices of superb spatial resolution and adequate sensitivity that could help to identify and elucidate the molecular aspects of cardiovascular disorders.

15.2 Data Acquisition

SPECT myocardial perfusion imaging has been a well-established diagnostic technique in assessment of patients with suspected or known CAD. In cardiac SPECT studies, two data sets are usually acquired: stress and rest images. The former are obtained by exercising the patient using a treadmill or by a pharmacological stress agent. The radiopharmaceutical is injected at peak exercise to be an indicator of occluded vessels when the patient undergoes tomographic scanning. The rest study is performed after injection with the patient in complete resting conditions on the same or a different day. The imaging protocol differs among institutions such that rest and stress examinations can be performed on the same day using the same radionuclide, such as Tl-201 (stress/redistribution), or Tc-99m-labeled compounds (stress/rest or rest/stress). Another protocol involves performing the stress and rest studies on two different days. The other option is to inject the patient with two different tracers (rest Tl-201/stress Tc-99m); the imaging procedure is performed the same day using an appropriate energy window setting.

Data acquisition is carried out by a rotating gamma camera equipped with one, two, or three detectors encompassing a rotational arc of at least 180°. Data reconstruction is usually performed using the analytical filtered backprojection algorithm or iterative reconstruction, with a smoothing low- pass filter applying an appropriate cutoff frequency and order.

As mentioned, the cardiac images are subjectively interpreted based on visual assessment of tracer distribution within different myocardial segments and depiction of hypoperfusion extent and severity. Although this is the gold standard approach, it remains influenced by interobserver and intraobserver variability along with the expertise of the reading staff. To reduce this variability and standardize the uptake of the tracer by the various segments, a number of software programs have been developed to aid and act as a second observer in the reading session. These methods vary in their theoretical assumptions; geometric modeling of the left ventricle (LV); 2D versus 3D approaches; thresholding and segmentation; valve definition and apical sampling, degree of automation and user intervention; whether count-based or geometric-based; or a combination of these options.

Examples of the commercially available programs are Quantitative Perfusion and Gated SPECT (QPS/QGS, Cedars-Sinai Medical Center, Los Angeles, CA); Emory Cardiac Toolbox (ECTb, Emory University, Atlanta, GA); 4D-MSPECT, which was developed at the University of Michigan Medical Center; Gated SPECT Cardiac Quantification (GSCQ, Yale, New Haven, CT) method; and others. These methods were evaluated in the literature and some found wide-spread and clinical acceptance among users in quantifying and displaying myocardial perfusion and functional parameters.

There are also some software tools developed to aid in image interpretation or to determine the quality of study interpretation. Some rely on artificial intelligence such as neural networks and case based approaches to provide increased confidence to the reading physician. Expert systems were also developed to mimic human experts and to rely on a knowledge base of heuristic rules to yield a computer-assisted patient diagnosis. In these approaches, the polar map or the reconstructed images are used as inputs for reading and quantifying the myocardial images.

15.3 Quantitative Methods

15.3.1 Quantitative Gated/Perfusion SPECT

Thie QGS/QPS method was introduced to sample, analyze, and quantify the myocardium using an ellipsoidal model [5, 6]. Data samples are extracted using equally spaced points in the longitudinal and latitudinal directions. Myocardial sampling is implemented by averaging the wall counts from the endocardial to epicardial borders rather than using the maximal pixel count along the radial profile [7]. By fitting the normal rays on the midmyocardial surface using asymmetric Gaussian functions, the endocardium and epicardium are estimated by certain percentages (i.e., 65%) of the standard deviation (SD) of the Gaussian fit. The peak of the Gaussian function is used to locate the midmyocardial point. For outlining myocardial areas of poor tracer uptake, the SDs are combined with those of each of its four spatial neighboring profiles. Further refinement is then applied by anatomical constraint of constant myocardial volume throughout the cardiac cycle [5]. This approach samples the myocardial points in a 3D ellipsoidal model through equally spaced points, regardless of the heart size; therefore, homologous points can be extracted and pooled to generate normal limit values. Due to finite sampling, the collected points are scaled to represent the curvature of the myocardium from which they are extracted [5]. This approach was developed by Cedars Sinai Medical Center in an integrated software package. An output display of the program is shown in Fig. 15.2.

15.3.2 Emory Cardiac Toolbox

The Emory Cardiac Toolbox (ECTb) method works in 3D space and uses the short-axis data set [8, 9]. The ECTb method uses Fourier analysis for wall-thickening estimation and detects a circumferential maximum count profile by applying an anatomically based model accounting for wall thickening to generate theoretical endocardial and epicardial surfaces [8, 10]. The software package integrates myocardial perfusion and function in one application. The program is automated with the possibility to change the short-axis radius and center. Data sampling is performed on the SPECT short-axis slices using a hybrid cylindrical-spherical coordinate system. Cylindrical geometry is used to sample the middle and basal part of the myocardium; the myocardial apex is sampled based on spherical modeling. The center of the coordinate system is the LV long axis, and the search space is limited by the LV radius, apex, and base. The valve plane is defined by two intersecting planes: one perpendicular to the LV long axis in the lateral half of the LV and one angled plane in the septal half of the LV. The program uses eight frames per cardiac cycle in gated myocardial perfusion SPECT studies. In case of contouring a perfusion defect, the algorithm forces the hypoperfused segment to be a smooth connection between adjacent noninfarcted portions of the wall, and because this segment is not thickening, it is pinned to its end diastolic positions [8].

15.3.3 4D-MSPECT

4D-MSPECT is a commercially available algorithm that was developed at the University of Michigan Medical Center [11, 12]. The algorithm works to process the data on the basis of a 2D gradient image from which the initial estimates of the ventricle are made. A series of 1D and 2D weighted splines are used to refine the endocardial and epicardial surface estimates. The 4D-MSPECT model also uses a cylindrical-spherical coordinate system for myocardial sampling. The former is used to sample the myocardium from the basal wall to the distal wall, and the latter is used to sample the apex. Weighted spline and data thresholding are used to refine surface estimates, and based on

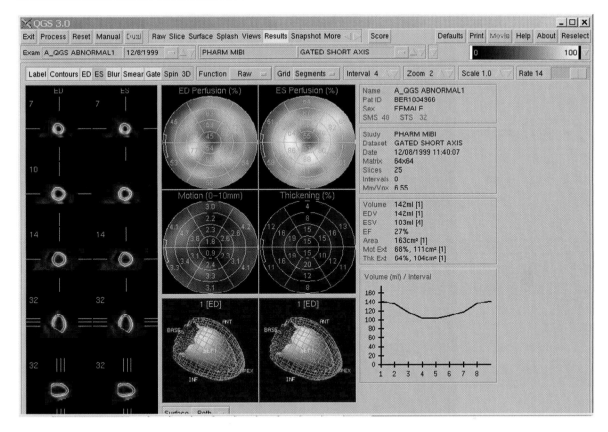

Fig. 15.2 Quantitative gated/perfusion SPECT method

Gaussian fitting, myocardial wall position and thickness are estimated. It has the capability for manual processing when the automatic module fails to accurately delineate the myocardial boundaries. 4D-MSPECT has achieved good correlations with reference techniques in evaluating the myocardial functional parameters [13]. Unlike QGS and ECTb, 4D-MSPECT differs in defining the valve plane in the sense that it permits the mitral valve plane to move as much as 20 mm inward toward the apex during systole [14]. A snapshot of 4D-MSPECT is shown in Fig. 15.3.

along all gated long-axis images. Spline curves and a threshold of 30% are used to define the LV base and the epicardial outlines to calculate the maximum circumferential profiles. The epicardial surface is defined as the outer point with 50% of peak activity, which shows a definite viable myocardial mass. Endocardial volume is estimated using a geometric technique. More refinements are performed to precisely determine the endocardial points using Fourier approximations. Finally, the ejection fraction (EF) is determined from the standard EF formula.

15.3.4 Pfast Method

pFAST stands for Perfusion and Functional Analysis for Gated SPECT (pFAST; Sapporo Medical University, Sapporo, Japan) [15, 16]. In this method, the gravity center of each short-axis image is initially determined. A long-axis central line is then identified

15.3.5 MultiDim

MultiDim (Stanford University Medical School) is a 3D method based on calculating statistical parameters of count distribution moments from the short-axis image volume [17, 18]. The method requires some

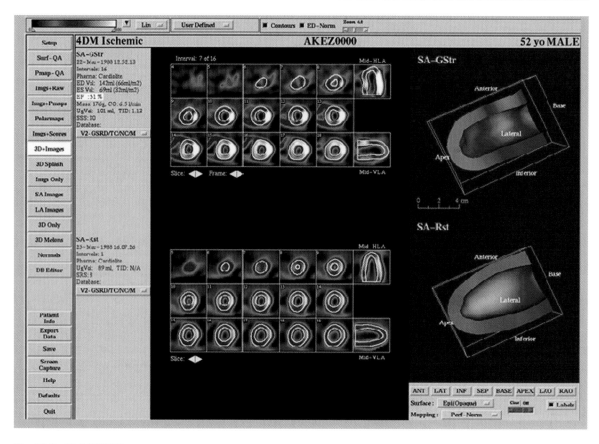

Fig. 15.3 4D-MSPECT

operator intervention for masking the LV and image thresholding. Masking is performed by manually fitting an ellipsoidal mask around the LV. Thresholding is performed by drawing a region of interest at the base of the LV cavity at end diastole and subtracting the mean value from each pixel [19]. Count sampling is carried out by radial profiles originating from the LV center using equally spaced longitudinal and latitudinal angles across the short-axis images. The endocardial wall is defined as the maxima of the first derivative of the squared activity profiles. Regional wall motion is derived from the phase and amplitude of the cyclic wave, representing the temporal variation of the first moment of the count distribution. However, the regional thickening is derived from the phase and amplitude of changes in the second moment of the density distribution multiplied by the maximum density. The volumes are calculated from the endocardial surfaces for each time segment [18].

15.3.6 Gated SPECT Cardiac Quantification

Gated SPECT Cardiac Quantification (GSCQ) is another method that is based on k-means cluster classification to separate the cardiac region from other extracardiac structures [20]. The myocardial surface boundaries are determined using hybrid count-geometric analysis for the calculation of the LV volumes and EF. The method uses thresholding and the nongated data to determine a cutoff value that serves to separate the LV volume. More refinements and constraints are carried out to remove the small remaining volumes within the image and to accurately define and obtain a clean long-axis LV binary image [21]. The long-axis images are resliced to obtain the most apical and basal slices in addition to the myocardial apex. The first apical slice is defined as the first short-axis slice containing the LV cavity, while the position of the last basal slice is defined as the last short-axis slice containing the basal limit of septum plus 10 mm toward the LV base. The algorithm models the apex as a semiellipsoid in 3D space [21].

15.3.7 Left Ventricular Global Thickening Fraction

The left ventricular global thickening fraction (LVGTF) is a count-based method that relies on fractional myocardial thickening to derive the EF, thereby avoiding the step of calculating the LV volumes [22, 23]. It depends on detection of myocardial wall thickening during systolic contraction. The method heavily depends on the partial volume effect, in which the myocardial wall thickness is less than twice the spatial resolution of the imaging system. The pixel counts in end diastolic and end systolic images are used to quantify the myocardial thickening without edge detection or geometric measurements. However, the method uses the systolic and diastolic counts in addition to geometric assumptions to derive a regional thickening fraction and hence to calculate the LV EF [22].

15.3.8 Layer of Maximum Count

Layer of Maximum Count (LMC) method is a different approach that uses the prolate-spheroid geometry to sample the myocardium; it was developed to solve the problem of small hearts [24, 25]. In patients with small hearts, most of the currently available methods tend to underestimate the LV and overestimate the EF. The midmyocardial surface is defined by the LMCs to determine the corresponding EF (i.e., EFmax). The LV EF is then calculated by performing a calibration between the EFmax and EF estimated from a reference technique, setting the intercept to zero to calculate the regression slope, which is then used to measure the EF in patients with small LVs [25–27]. The method has been evaluated in a population with small hearts versus other quantitative methods using gated blood pool and echocardiography as reference nuclear and nonnuclear techniques, respectively. In the former

situation, the LMC outperformed the other methods with moderate correlation and poor interchangeability with gated blood pool studies in patients with small LV. However, in comparison to echocardiography the same method showed a lower correlation but significant in the measurements of EF in patients with normal LV size. A drawback of the method is its dependency on other accurate techniques to derive a calibration factor required to estimate the EF for small LVs.

15.3.9 Cardiac Function Method

The cardiac function method (CAFU; Exini Diagnostics, Sweden) is a nongeometric model-based technique that uses an active shape algorithm [28]. Identification and delineation of the LV is based on a heart-shaped model, and through an iterative process the model is adjusted to optimize the fit with the image data. The algorithm uses 272 landmarks distributed in 17 layers from apex to base with 16 landmarks in each layer [29]. These landmarks are also utilized to give an estimate of myocardial wall motion and thickening. In the former, the normal distance from the landmark to the myocardial surface in both end diastolic and end systolic wall is measured, while thickening calculation is a count ratio for the landmarks in both end diastolic and end systolic frames. The LV volume is calculated using the endocardial surface and the LV valve plane with no constraint placed on basal wall motion [28, 29].

Most of the commercially available quantitative cardiac SPECT methods integrate myocardial perfusion and function in the same software package, and some have more quantitative and display features for multimodality and image fusion using SPECT, PET, and CT images. Quality assurance tools that allow the user to identify patient motion, artifacts, count density, gating problems, attenuation correction, LV segmentation and identification of myocardial boundaries, and other volumetric problems have also been embedded in these algorithms. Among those are raw data display, histogramming, valve plane fine-tuning, fusion controls, as well as measures of quality of gated SPECT studies. One of the display features of multimodality imaging is the possibility of aligning the CT vascular coronary tree on the 3D PET or SPECT functional data so that functional perfusion mapping can be visualized, with superimposition of coronary anatomy providing additional diagnostic information.

15.4 Quantification of Perfusion Abnormality

One of the earliest approaches introduced to quantify the distribution of myocardial activity in cardiac tomography was reported more than two decades ago [30]. This approach was based on quantifying the 3D activity distributions within the myocardium into a 2D polar map or "bull's-eye." The polar map is constructed through modeling the myocardium into a cylindrical and spherical coordinate system as mentioned in this chapter. Sampling the counts from the cylindrical part is implemented by drawing radial profiles from the center of the short-axis image normal to the myocardial wall (36–60 radial profiles). The maximal pixel count is recorded for each profile and plotted versus the corresponding angle to produce count circumferential curves. The apical portion of the myocardium is sampled by vertical long-axis slices to minimize the effect of partial volume. Sampling the apical portion of the myocardium is illustrated in Fig. 15.4 using different sampling approaches.

The count circumferential profiles are used to construct the polar map, which consists of concentric annuli representing the LV from the apex to the base. Furthermore, a scaling process is performed of the sampled myocardium so that the number of data points remains constant for all patients. However, the polar map distorts the heart shape, size, and geometry [31].

To determine the variability and normal limits of the tracer distribution in the myocardium, a normal database is generated based on normal patients or patients with low pretest likelihood ($<0.5\%$) of CAD. The mean value and SD are calculated from the circumferential profile of the normal data set with determination of a threshold value for segmental abnormality.

Polar maps provide quantitative measures of defect extent and severity. In QGS, myocardial sampling is not based on a circumferential profile drawn normally on the LV surface; the entire LV is modeled as a 3D structure with a standard number of equally spaced points regardless of the LV size [7]. In ECTb, the actual defect extent is calculated from the 3D activity distribution rather than from the polar map representation [9]. It is presented as a percentage of the abnormality with respect to the total myocardial volume, individual vascular territories, or actual mass of the hypoperfused myocardium.

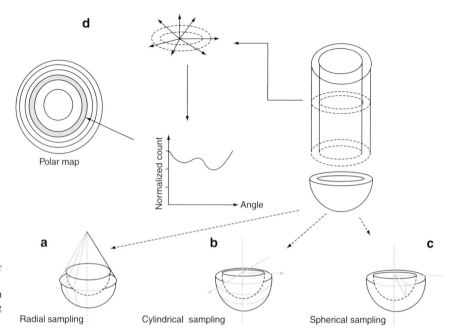

Fig. 15.4 Various methods used for sampling of myocardial apex in quantitative cardiac SPECT. (**c**) and (**d**) is one of the earlier methods used to sample the mid- and basal myocardium in addition to spherical sampling of myocardial apex

To localize the extent of the defect and to pinpoint the location, myocardial segments below a defined threshold are colored black while maintaining the color of the normal ones [32]. Defect severity is expressed in units of SD below the normal mean by a measure called defect severity or total severity score and is displayed in a polar representation referred to as a defect severity map. On this map, severity is scaled by the number of SDs below the normal to a color-coding table so that the most normal region and most abnormal region are differently colored to easily identify the abnormality. Severity score also takes into account the extent and severity of the abnormality and is measured by the number of SDs below the mean of the entire extent of the abnormality [33].

Polar maps have been a simple tool to reduce the whole LV into a 2D image that facilitates the interpretation process by looking at all segments at once. It also provides a measure of defect reversibility based on normalizing the rest images with respect to the stress images and color-coding scheme. However, volume-weighting and distance-weighting approaches serve to improve one feature over another. The former map tends to distort the defect location but offers an accurate assessment of the defect size. The latter tends to distort the defect size at the cost of improving the accuracy of the defect location. It is therefore recommended not to solely depend on a polar map without paying attention to tomographic slices [34]. Partial and significant reversibility can be determined based on certain percentages of the defect extent. Moreover, measurements of ischemic or scar fractions for a given perfusion defect can be calculated in addition to assessment of myocardial viability [35].

15.4.1 Summed Perfusion Scores

Another semiquantitative approach used to quantify tracer uptake is implemented by dividing the myocardium into 20 segments or the recommended 17 segments [36]. The perfusion of each segment is scored according to a 5-point scoring system: 0–4 (0 = normal, 1 = equivocal reduction, 2 = definite but moderate reduction, 3 = severe reduction of tracer uptake, 4 = absent uptake of radioactivity). The global measure of perfusion is then determined by summing the regional scores of all segments in stress and rest data. This scoring process results in a Summed Stress Score (SSS) and a Summed Rest Score (SRS). The difference between SSS and SRS is the Summed Difference Score (SDS), which is analogous to reversibility. High values for the SSS are an indication of large or severe defects, whereas high values of SDS provide an indication of reversibility and lower values indicate fixed or mostly fixed defects. The SRS is related to the amount of infarcted or hibernating myocardium [37]. (see Table 15.1).

These global perfusion summed scores provide a reported measure for both defect extent and severity, and they can be calculated either visually or by computer-based methods. Reproducibility and diagnostic performance have been reported in a number of studies, including those automated and conducted by human observers [38]. The SSS is employed to stratify patients into different risk groups according to the following: Individuals with SSS < 4 are considered normal or nearly normal, those with scores of 4–8 are mildly abnormal, those with scores of 9–13 are moderately abnormal, and those with SSS > 13 are severely abnormal.

Table 15.1 Summary of perfusion scores and percent abnormal myocardium in 17 and 20 segment model (Adapted from Fuster V, O'Rourke RA, Walsh RA, Poole-Wilson P. "Hurst's The Heart," 12th edn. 2007)

Perfusion index	Definition	Significance
Summed Stress Score (SSS)	Total segmental scores of stress images	Amount of infarcted, ischemic, or jeopardized myocardium
Summed Rest Score (SRS)	Total segmental scores of rest images	Amount of infarcted or hibernating myocardium
Summed Difference Score (SDS)	Difference between SSS and SRS	Amount of ischemic or jeopardized myocardium
	20 segment model	17 segment model
Percent total	SSS × 100/80	SSS × 100/68
Percent ischemic	SDS × 100/80	SDS × 100/68
Percent fixed	SRS × 100/80	SRS × 100/68

15.4.2 Percent Abnormality

Another global measure of perfusion abnormalities is calculated by normalizing the summed scores to the maximal possible score. In case of the 17-segment model and 5-point scoring system, the maximal possible score is $17 \times 4 = 68$ whereas for the 20-segment model it can be calculated as $20 \times 4 = 80$ (Table 15.1). This percentage measure is called the percentage abnormal myocardium and is applicable to other scoring systems and different myocardial segments. For example, a patient with summed scores of 17 in the 17-segment model will have a percentage abnormality of $17/68 = 40\%$, which bears diagnostic and prognostic information similar to a patient with summed scores of 20 in the 20-segment model ($20/80 = 40\%$) [39]. Expressing the amount of ischemia as percentage myocardium by this approach provides intuitive implications that are not possible with the perfusion scoring system and is applicable to other segmental models and other methods that calculate the percentage of abnormal myocardium [40]. Figure 15.5 shows a comparison between the 17- and 20-segment models.

15.4.3 Generation of Normal Limits

Different schemes were developed to generate normal databases to distinguish abnormal from normal patients in the quantification approaches mentioned. Some of these provide user-specified generation tools for normal limits that are incorporated in the software program with several options for myocardial radiotracer, patient gender, imaging protocol, processing parameters, and so on.

The Emory method is based on collecting a number of patients with a low likelihood of CAD (<0.5%) and deriving a composite pool to extract the mean and SD of the normal limits. Then, a patient study is compared to the normal database to examine and assess the perfusion defects. This approach goes through a number of steps to optimize the threshold value, which is then used to quantify perfusion abnormality in a given patient study. It has specific inherent characteristics, making it dependent on the injected radiopharmaceutical, acquisition protocol, processing parameters, and population studied. It needs a number of normal patients (20–30) or low likelihood of CAD from both genders, another group of patients with significant variation in perfusion location and severity "pilot population," and a validation group of patients to assess the performance of the algorithm in both genders with reported coronary angiography [41, 42]. Thus, approximately 150 patients are required to establish a normal database.

The group at Cedars Sinai (Los Angeles, CA) developed quantification techniques that are based on various assumptions. One requires a number of normal patients along with another group of patients with a wide range of perfusion abnormalities. The threshold of abnormality is determined by an optimization step in which the computer-generated scores are maximized with the visual scores to obtain an individual

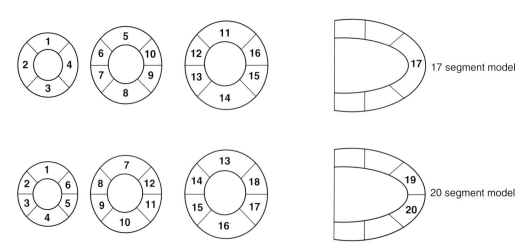

Fig. 15.5 A comparison between 17 and 20 segment models

segmental threshold. Because of the large number of patients needed to represent a large data set of segmental hypoperfusion in addition to another group of those with normal or low likelihood of the disease makes it relatively difficult to generate on-site-specific normal limits [6]. Further investigations have revealed another global assessment that combines perfusion defect extent and severity into a continuous measure referred to as the total perfusion deficit (TPD). It provides an overall assessment of hypoperfusion either by vascular territory or for the entire myocardium. In this approach, a reduction in the number of patients required for generation of normal limits is accomplished by obviating those patients with an abnormality. Furthermore, no optimization step is required to derive a segmental threshold, and the technique is based on patients with a low likelihood of the disease [43].

The methods mentioned do not permit aligning the stress with the rest images in a specific geometric orientation, and comparison of a patient study is carried out for the stress and rest separately. This perhaps limits the quantitation algorithm to precisely determine the spatial location of ischemia in stress and rest images. Furthermore, a comparison with database normal values does not account for intrapatient perfusion changes. Faber et al. have shown that by accurate image alignment, changes of 10% and 15% could be detected with false-positive rates of 15% and 10%, respectively, concluding that the mean uptake values can show a statistical significance if the difference is 10% or more in single perfusion studies of single patients [44]. On the other hand, a new measure of ischemia was developed by Slomka et al. [45] to coregister the stress and rest data. The rest images are iteratively reoriented, resized, and normalized to provide the best fit with the stress scans. They have used a new normalization technique based on 10-parameter search criteria and allows determination of the amount of ischemia in stress and rest images without a normal database.

Note from this discussion that developers vary in their representation for the defect extent and severity and differ in their definition and optimization for the threshold value on which segmental abnormality is determined [46, 47]. This has been examined by some comparative studies conducted to look at the variations that exist among the quantitative cardiac SPECT methods and to investigate their diagnostic performance versus reference techniques. These reports included evaluation for the degree of automation, summed scores (SSS, SDS, SRS), regional and total defect extent using receiver operating characteristic curves and appropriate correlation and agreement statistical tests. Some studies were also performed in comparison to coronary angiography; hence, the sensitivity, specificity, accuracy, and normalcy rates for detection of CAD were estimated for the algorithms. The absence of institutional normal limits as a cause for those variations was also investigated by some researchers if institution-specific normal databases were used. The results, however, demonstrated that significant differences among the various methods do exist in estimating the myocardial perfusion parameters [46–48].

15.5 Quantification of Myocardial Function

15.5.1 Gated Cardiac SPECT

The introduction of ECG gating to SPECT myocardial perfusion imaging has potentially improved the diagnostic and prognostic information in assessing patients with suspected or known CAD [49]. The improvement of count statistics by use of Tc-99m-based tracers, multiple detector systems, advances in computer technology and development of automated quantitative methods has allowed simultaneous acquisition of myocardial perfusion combined with ECG gated imaging in a feasible manner. As a result, assessment of patient global and regional LV function together with perfusion quantification can be carried out on a routine basis. This in turn has led to a tremendous amount of clinically relevant and valuable information for decision making in patients with CAD [50]. Figure 15.6 summarizes the steps involved in the calculation of myocardial perfusion and functional parameters.

Further diagnostic information can be obtained by coregistering data obtained from CT angiography and the metabolic/perfusion images using hybrid SPECT/CT or PET/CT systems. This allows for integrating a large amount of information that was not possible to obtain in a single imaging session. Global functional measures such as end diastolic volume (EDV), end

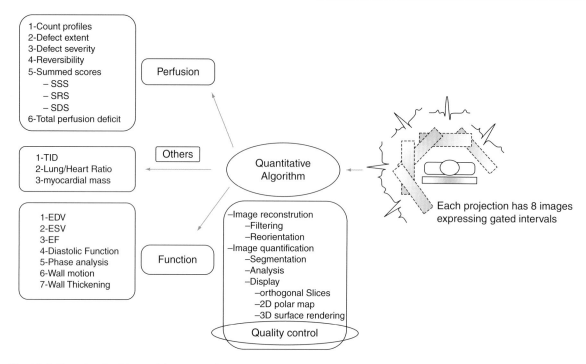

Fig. 15.6 Steps involved in acquiring, processing, and quantifying myocardial perfusion gated SPECT studies using the quantitative algorithms

systolic volume (ESV), and EF, in addition to the regional parameters such as regional wall motion and wall thickening, can be evaluated by most of the commercially available quantitative gated SPECT methods.

15.5.2 Acquisition and Processing

Myocardial perfusion gated SPECT imaging is carried out using three ECG leads placed on the patient's chest and connected to an ECG trigger device. This helps the computer system identify the beginning of the cardiac cycle (the R-R interval) and thereby it can divide the temporal changes of the heart contraction into small time intervals determined by the number of frames/cycle selected during acquisition setup. The number 8 or 16 frames per cardiac cycle is often chosen since the former provides better count statistics while the latter provides better temporal resolution. Figure 15.7 shows an acquisition for eight frames per cycle. It is also possible to use 32 frames per cardiac cycle to determine the diastolic function. However, this occurs

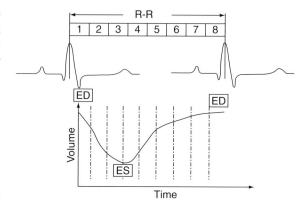

Fig. 15.7 This diagram shows the R-R interval for one heart cycle and the corresponding change in the blood volume. ECG-gating provides a mean for recording the volume change over the heart cycle. This happens by dividing the cycle into gates or frames (e.g., eight frames) or even higher 16 or 32

with significant reduction of counts collected over the cardiac frames given the same acquisition time.

The commercial methods provide several tools to process gated and ungated projection data to extract perfusion as well as functional information from gated myocardial perfusion SPECT studies. Functional information obtained from the reconstructed images are LV volumes (EDV and ESV), regional and global EF, myocardial wall motion, and wall thickening.

15.5.3 Volumes and EF Estimation

The underlying notion of ECG gating myocardial perfusion SPECT studies is to obtain several pictures of the heart during the periodic contraction. The higher the accuracy in modeling and outlining the LV in these different phases, the better is the reliability of the quantitative results. As mentioned, methods vary in their assumptions for LV geometry. Some are based on a ellipsoidal, cylindrical-spherical, or prolate-spheroidal model, and others are purely count-based techniques. One common step is the segmentation process, by which the LV should be identified and separated from other structures. Methods also vary in their segmentation for the LV as the inclusion of extracardiac tissues can confound the quantitative results [51].

Once the LV has been segmented and the valve plane defined together with determination of myocardial base and apex, outlining of myocardial boundaries can then be estimated. Different approaches have been suggested and implemented to identify endocardial and epicardial boarders as well as myocardial base and apex. Automated modes are often used to delineate the myocardial boundaries; however, in case of contouring errors, operator intervention could be helpful. This also depends on user expertise in addition to interobserver variability. Automated quality control approaches were also developed to judge the quality of the LV shape segmentation as well as valve plane definition in some software programs [52]. These quality control algorithms could provide high accuracy in identifying failure cases of LV segmentation, leading to an improvement in perfusion quantitation.

Volume-based techniques calculate the ventricular volumes by constructing a time-volume curve using either 8 or 16 frames/cycle. The maximum and minimum points on the volume curve correspond to EDV and ESV, respectively. The EF can then be calculated as a percentage:

$$EF = (EDV - ESV)/EDV*100$$

Figure 15.8 shows the output display of the ECTb for stress and rest studies together with EDV, ESV, and EF calculations.

15.5.4 Regional Function

Assessment of regional myocardial function has incremental diagnostic and prognostic information over myocardial perfusion parameters alone [53]. Myocardial wall motion and thickening are relatively not uniform as compared to myocardial perfusion. Wall motion is the excursion of the endocardium from end diastole to end systole. A 6-point scoring system is generally used to assess motion abnormality: 0 = normal, 1 = mildly hypokinetic, 2 = moderately hypokinetic, 3 = severely hypokinetic, 4 = akinetic, 5 = dyskinetic. Visual assessment of wall thickening is often based on the partial volume phenomenon, in which the intensity of the myocardial wall is proportional to the size or degree of wall thickening during cardiac contraction. A 4-point scoring system is used to assess wall thickening: 0 = normal, 1 = mildly reduced, 2 = moderately to severely reduced, 3 = no thickening.

Computer scoring for wall motion and thickening was also developed to reduce observer variability. It calculates the regional function on a segment-by-segment basis in a similar way to calculation of myocardial perfusion. In QGS, regional motion is measured as the distance (in millimeters) between a given endocardial point at end diastole and end systole perpendicular to the average midmyocardial surface between end diastole and end systole [54].

Myocardial thickening is calculated as the percentage increase in myocardial thickness and can be quantified by geometric-based, count-based, or combined methods using geometric count-based techniques [55]. The first detects the spatial position of endocardial and epicardial surfaces to calculate the myocardial thickness in both end diastole and end systole. However, count-based techniques rely on the partial volume effect.

It should be noted that normal wall motion and thickening are not always concomitant since in some pathological conditions a discordance can take place, resulting in abnormal wall motion and preserved thickening or vice versa [56].

The European guidelines stated that

Visual interpretation of myocardial wall motion and thickening remain up to the moment the conventional tool in assessing myocardial contractility in myocardial perfusion SPECT and quantitative measures provided

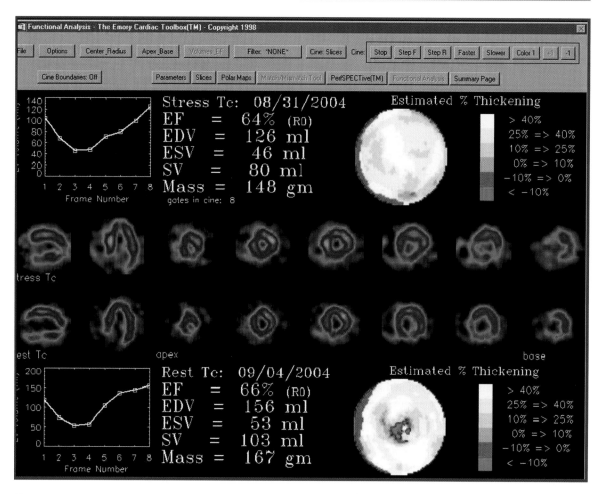

Fig. 15.8 Emory cardiac toolbox display for stress and rest studies where *left* ventricular volumes and EF in addition to wall thickening polar map are shown

by software programs shouldn't be used as the sole determinant [57].

15.5.5 Diastolic Function

In addition to the determination of the systolic function by myocardial perfusion gated SPECT, myocardial diastolic function can also be estimated which is a useful clinical indicator of LV function and precedes systolic dysfunction in many cardiac diseases. It is advisable that early diagnosis and an appropriate therapy be performed before further progression to diastolic heart failure and cardiac death [58]. Diastolic function can be evaluated by nuclear methods and

with other radiographic techniques [59]. Parameters of diastolic function are peak to filling rate (PFR), which is a clinically useful parameter describing LV filling properties; time to peak filling rate (TTFR); and the mean filling fraction (MFR/3), which is the mean filling rate over the first third of diastole.

Parameters of diastolic function require a significantly larger number of gating intervals than often are used. This higher temporal resolution is needed to accurately determine volume changes over a short period of time. The derivatives of the time-volume curve yield information about the rates of emptying and filling. Fourier fitting with three or four harmonics is often used to smooth the time-activity and derivative curves to reduce the statistical fluctuations of the acquired data.

Peak rates and average rates are usually measured in units of end diastolic volumes per second (EDV/s). Per cardiac cycle, 12, 16, or 32 frames may be employed; however, better estimation can be achieved with the highest possible framing rate. One study compared the diastolic and systolic functions using 32 frames versus 8 and 16 frames/cycle taking the gated blood pool as a reference [60]. Accurate assessment of the diastolic as well systolic function was obtained when 32 frames/cycle was applied. Furthermore, lower systematic errors for both measures were found with the highest temporal sampling. In a population of 90 patients, Akincioglu et al. derived the normal limits for PFR and TTFR as 2.62 ± 0.46 EDV/s and 164.6 ± 21.7 ms, respectively, with abnormality thresholds of PFR < 1.71 EDV/s and TTFR > 216.7 ms, respectively, applying 16 frames/cycle, and measurements were performed using the QGS software program [61].

15.5.6 Phase Analysis

Assessment of cardiac mechanical dyssynchrony is an important step for patients scheduled to undergo or who have undergone cardiac resynchronization therapy (CRT) [62]. CRT is used to improve heart function by restoring the heart rhythm contraction in patients with an irregular heartbeat, called LV dyssynchrony. Chen et al. [63] developed a tool for measuring the onset of mechanical contraction based on phase analysis of the cardiac cycle in gated myocardial SPECT imaging using Fourier transform. A phase array is extracted from the 3D count distribution in the eight bins of the gated short-axis slices. This phase array conveys information about the regional mechanical contraction in a 3D fashion, and a number of quantitative indices are derived from the phase array histogram, such as the peak of the histogram, SD of phase distribution, and phase histogram bandwidth (95% confidence interval). Phase histogram skewness and kurtosis can also be calculated, which indicate the symmetry and peakedness of the distribution, respectively. These measures correspond to specific attributes of the histogram curve and in turn should have clinical relevance in the overall assessment [9, 63] (see Fig. 12.26 in Chap. 12).

15.5.7 Tomographic ECG-Gating in Equilibrium Radionuclide Angiocardiography (ERNA)

In planar gated blood pool imaging, the anatomical geometry of the cardiac chambers limits a clear separation between right ventricle (RV) and LV. The overlapping atrial and ventricular structures obscure an accurate outlining of the RV. However, tomographic equilibrium radionuclide angiocardiography (ERNA) should be able to estimate the RV parameters more accurately than planar imaging. Adding the tomographic option to the planar gated blood pool imaging allows for better visualization of cardiac chambers and depiction of contractile motion. In this instance, SPECT data can provide better separation of the LV and RV together with information about the contractile function. ERNA can also provide an estimate of the LV and RV volumes and EF in addition to ventricular filling and emptying parameters [64]. A number of research studies were conducted to measure the normal limits for global and regional parameters of diastolic and systolic function using gated blood pool tomographic imaging [65, 66]. Figure 15.9 shows many functional parameters that can be obtained from tomographic ERNA.

A comparison between four different methods (QBS, BP-SPECT, QUBE, and 4D-MSPECT) [67–70] revealed that all methods tended to underestimate the LV volumes (EDV and ESV) with a trend of greater underestimation as the volume of the LV increased; different trends were observed among algorithms to estimate the RV volumes [71]. In LV EF estimation, most algorithms showed good correlation with the reference values with no significant trends observed across the range of EFs studied. However, all methods showed greater overestimation with an increase of the RV EF [71].

The differences observed in the study just discussed [71] are consistent with others [72], and this can be explained as caused by several reasons. The algorithmic assumptions vary among methods, which can be fixed count threshold, derivative or gradient-based edge detection, knowledge-based boundary detection, watershed voxel clustering, or neural network-based segmentation [73]. Other patient-related factors, such as definition of pulmonary outflow tract, enlarged

Fig. 15.9 Calculation of regional and global systolic and diastolic myocardial functional parameters for both RV and LV in gated blood pool SPECT using a count based method. (From [65] with permission from Springer Science+Business Media.)

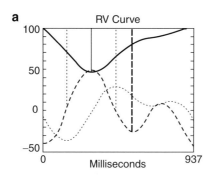

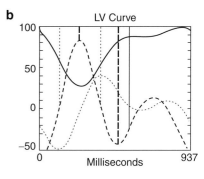

RVEF = 55%	LVEF = 63%
RVEDV = 120 ml	LVEDV = 109 ml
RVESV = 54	LVESV = 40 ml
RV avg_hr = 64 bpm	LV avg_hr = 64 bpm
RV ES_ERF = 244 msec	LV ES_ERF = 244 msec
RV peak er = −2.4 EDV/s	LV peak er = −3.2 EDV/s
RV peak fr = −1.9 EDV/s	LV peak fr = 2.8 EDV/s
RV peak fr time = 144 msec	LV peak fr time = 126 msec

ventricles, and difficulty of the RV geometry, contribute to suboptimal results of volume and EF estimation. Moreover, other technical and processing parameters are yet to be determined and practically optimized [74].

15.5.8 Transient Ischemic Dilation

Transient ischemic dilation (TID) of the LV is measured as a ratio of the LV cavity in the stress images and the LV cavity in rest images. This index has its clinical significance in multivessel stenosis and increased risk of adverse outcomes [75]. It can be calculated from both gated and ungated data sets. The normal limits are constrained by the protocol used since in some circumstances the LV chamber appears different in size, especially when different radionuclides are used (Tc-99m- vs. Tl-201-based images) or patient-detector distance varied greatly in both studies. The myocardial walls in the Tl-201 images appear thicker than in the Tc-99m images, resulting in a smaller cavity size in Tl-201 images. This should be accounted for in interpreting the results of TID. Normal limits and values of TID vary in the literature (1.012–1.40), and sources of this variability

are perhaps different radionuclides (Tc-99m, Tl-201, or both), type of stress (exercise vs. other pharmacological stressors), imaging protocol (single- or 2-day protocol), time of imaging, or other factors [76].

15.6 Factors Affecting Gated SPECT

Many variables were found to influence the performance of the quantitative gated SPECT methods in estimating the LV volumes and EF. These variables can be classified into acquisition, processing, and patient-related factors.

Selection of the matrix size, zooming factor, count density, framing rate (8 or 16 frames/cycle), and angular resolution (number of projections) and rotation arc (180° vs. 360°), collimators, radionuclide used (Tc-99m vs. Tl), and other factors were found to influence the performance of the estimation task [77–86]. Processing parameters such as reconstruction algorithm (FBP vs. iterative reconstruction), photon attenuation, scatter, resolution recovery, filtering, cutoff value, and zooming during reconstruction were also reported [87–90]. Some other factors are related to the patient and have been studied in the literature, such as irregular heart rate, gating errors (e.g. T-wave elevation), patient motion, severe perfusion defects and difficulty in outlining the myocardial boundaries, small hearts (underestimation of volumes and overestimation of EF), and high extracardiac activity [91–94]

Nevertheless, a well-defined acquisition and processing protocol could serve to optimize the results of gated studies. Moreover, quality control software tools as well as visual assessment of patient raw data are also helpful in depicting count variation and patient motion and detecting rejected heart beats.

The variations shown by the quantitative perfusion software programs were also evident in estimating the LV volumes and EF [95–97]. Relatively large agreement limits were found among methods in addition to systematic and random errors. As a result, the users should be aware of the underlying assumptions of the method used in clinical practice as well as understanding of the sources of error and technical pitfalls. Although most of the methods showed good correlations in comparison to accurate techniques in cardiac imaging achieving acceptable accuracy and reproducibility, interchangeability of values would be of limited clinical outcome, and patient monitoring must be performed in adherence to a single software program.

15.7 Conclusions

Cardiac SPECT imaging provides a tremendous amount of information about myocardial perfusion and function. Many factors are key and still contributing to the development of cardiac scintigraphy, such as radiopharmaceuticals, instrumentation, and computer technology. Software packages developed to provide such quantitative indices are helpful in patient diagnosis and have become important tools in nuclear cardiology laboratories. The quantitative parameters provided by those programs together with their automated features are unique among other cardiac imaging modalities, and to a considerable extent this has made nuclear cardiac imaging a well-established diagnostic imaging modality. Further investigations are warranted to explore the qualitative and quantitative capability of cardiac SPECT with use of hybrid imaging techniques.

A number of points should be taken into consideration when using the myocardial perfusion quantitation methods in clinical practice:

- These algorithms assist as a second observer in the reading session, and the visual assessment by an experienced reading physician must be at the forefront. Even with fully automated methods, careful inspection should be followed to check and verify the results of contour generation.
- Quantitative cardiac SPECT methods were shown to differ significantly in their performance along with the degree of automation.
- Normal limits for myocardial perfusion and function were also shown to differ among algorithms and tended to be gender specific.
- Interchangeability of these algorithms is clinically limited to use in patient monitoring or the decision-making process.
- Quantitative perfusion methods were designed to quantify the myocardial tracer uptake in a relative sense and do not provide an absolute measure of tracer distribution. Furthermore, they do not not account for image-degrading factors such as photon attenuation, scatter, and resolution effects.
- New approaches developed to evaluate perfusion defect abnormality should be extensively validated and assessed under a wide range of patient conditions with the available acquisition and processing protocols used in daily practice. Furthermore, validation studies should include not only phantom experiments but also patient data and should be compared to well-established and accurate techniques.
- For proper implementation of the quantitative methods in clinical practice and for better data interpretation, users should be aware of the basic assumptions and concepts underlying those algorithms.

References

1. Goris ML, Zhu HJ, Robinson TE (2007) A critical discussion of computer analysis in medical imaging. Proc Am Thorac Soc 4(4):347–349
2. Abidov A, Germano G, Hachamovitch R, Berman DS (2006) Gated SPECT in assessment of regional and global left ventricular function: major tool of modern nuclear imaging. J Nucl Cardiol 13(2):26–79

3. Watson DD, Campbell NP, Read EK et al (1981) Spatial and temporal quantitation of plane thallium myocardial images. J Nucl Med 22:577–584

4. Garcia E, Maddahi J, Berman D, Waxman A (1981) Space/time quantitation of thallium-201 myocardial scintigraphy. J Nucl Med 22:309–317

5. Germano G, Kavanagh PB, Waechter P, Areeda J, Van Kriekinge S, Sharir T, Lewin HC, Berman DS (2000) A new algorithm for the quantitation of myocardial perfusion SPECT. I: technical principles and reproducibility. J Nucl Med 41:712–719

6. Sharir T, Germano G, Waechter PB, Kavanagh PB, Areeda JS, Gerlach J et al (2000) A new algorithm for the quantitation of myocardial perfusion SPECT. II: validation and diagnostic yield. J Nucl Med 41:720–727

7. Germano G, Kavanagh PB, Slomka PJ, Van Kriekinge SD, Pollard G, Berman DS (2007 Jul) Quantitation in gated perfusion SPECT imaging: the Cedars-Sinai approach. J Nucl Cardiol 14(4):433–454

8. Faber TL, Cooke CD, Folks RD et al (1999) Left ventricular function and perfusion from gated perfusion images: an integrated method. J Nucl Med 40:650–659

9. Garcia EV, Faber TL, Cooke CD, Folks RD, Chen J, Santana C (2007) The increasing role of quantification in clinical nuclear cardiology: the Emory approach. J Nucl Cardiol 14(4):420–432

10. Cooke CD, Garcia EV, Cullom SJ, Faber TL, Pettigrew RI (1994) Determining the accuracy of calculating systolic wall thickening using a fast Fourier transform approximation: a simulation study based on canine and patient data. J Nucl Med 35:1185–1192

11. Ficaro EP, Quaife RA, Kritzman JN, Corbett JR (1999) Accuracy and reproducibility of 3D-MSPECT for estimating left ventricular ejection fraction in patients with severe perfusion abnormalities [abstract]. Circulation 100 (suppl):I26

12. Ficaro EP, Lee BC, Kritzman JN, Corbett JR (2007) Corridor4DM: the Michigan method for quantitative nuclear cardiology. J Nucl Cardiol 14(4):455–465

13. Schaefer WM, Lipke CS, Standke D, Kuhl HP, Nowak B, Kaiser HJ, Koch KC, Buell U (2005) Quantification of left ventricular volumes and ejection fraction from gated ^{99m}Tc-MIBI SPECT: MRI validation and comparison of the memory cardiac tool box with QGS and 4D- MSPECT. J Nucl Med 46:1256–1263

14. Ficaro EP, Kritzman JN, Corbett JR (2003) Effect of valve plane constraint on LV ejection fractions from gated perfusion SPECT [abstract]. J Nucl Cardiol 10:S23

15. Nakata T, Katagiri Y, Odawara Y, Eguchi M, Kuroda M, Tsuchihashi K, Hareyama M, Shimamoto K (2000) Two-and three-dimensional assessments of myocardial perfusion and function by using technetium-99m sestamibi gated SPECT with a combination of count- and image-based techniques. J Nucl Cardiol 7:623–632

16. Hashimoto A, Nakata T, Wakabayashi T, Kyuma M, Takahashi T (2002) Validation of quantitative gated single photon emission computed tomography and an automated scoring system for the assessment of regional left ventricular systolic function. Nucl Med Commun 23:887–898

17. Goris ML, Thompson C, Malone LJ, Franken PR (1994) Modeling the integration of myocardial regional perfusion and function. Nucl Med Commun 15:9–20

18. Everaert H, Franken PR, Flamen P et al (1996) Left ventricular ejection fraction from gated SPECT myocardial perfusion studies: a method based on the radial distribution of count rate density across the myocardial wall. Eur J Nucl Med 23:1628–1633

19. Everaert H, Bossuyt A, Franken PR (1997) Left ventricular ejection fraction and volumes from gated single photon emission tomographic myocardial perfusion images: comparison between two algorithms working in three-dimensional space. J Nucl Cardiol 4:472–476

20. Liu YH, Sinusas AJ, Khaimov D, Gebuza BI, Wackers FJ (2005) New hybrid count- and geometry-based method for quantification of left ventricular volumes and ejection fraction from ECG-gated SPECT: methodology and validation. J Nucl Cardiol 12(1):55–65

21. Liu YH (2007) Quantification of nuclear cardiac images: the Yale approach. J Nucl Cardiol 14(4):483–491

22. Smith WH, Kastner RJ, Calnon DA, Segalla D, Beller GA, Watson DD (1997) Quantitative gated SPECT imaging: a counts-based method for display and measurement of regional and global ventricular systolic function. J Nucl Cardiol 5:451–463

23. Calnon DA, Kastner RJ, Smith WH, Segalla D, Beller GA, Watson DD (1997) Validation of a new counts-based gated single photon emission computed tomography method for quantifying left ventricular systolic function: comparison with equilibrium radionuclide angiography. J Nucl Cardiol 4:464–471

24. Feng B, Sitek A, Gulberg GT (2001) The prolate spheroidal transform for gated SPECT. IEEE Trans Nucl Sci 48:872–875

25. Feng B, Sitek A, Gullberg GT (2002) Calculation of the left ventricular ejection fraction without edge detection: application to small hearts. J Nucl Med 43:786–794

26. Khalil MM, Attia A, Ali M, Ziada G, Omar A, Elgazzar A (2009) Echocardiographic validation of the layer of maximum count method in the estimation of the left ventricular EF using gated myocardial perfusion SPECT: correlation with QGS, ECTb, and LVGTF. Nucl Med Commun 30 (8):622–628

27. Khalil MM, Elgazzar A, Khalil W, Omar A, Ziada G (2005) Assessment of left ventricular ejection fraction by four different methods using ^{99m}Tc tetrofosmin gated SPECT in patients with small hearts: correlation with gated blood pool. Nucl Med Commun 26:885–893

28. Lomsky M, Richter J, Johansson L, El-Ali H, Åström K, Ljungberg M, Edenbrandt L (2005) A new automated method for analysis of gated-SPECT images based on a 3-dimensional heart shaped model. Clin Physiol Funct Imaging 25:234–240

29. Lomsky M, Richter J, Johansson L, Høilund-Carlsen PF, Edenbrandt L (2006) Validation of a new automated method for analysis of gated-SPECT images. Clin Physiol Funct Imaging 26(3):139–145

30. Garcia EV, Van Train K, Maddahi J, Prigent F, Friedman J, Areeda J et al (1985) Quantification of rotational thallium-201 myocardial tomography. J Nucl Med 26:17–26

31. Ficaro EP, Corbett JR (2004) Advances in quantitative perfusion SPECT imaging. J Nucl Cardiol 11(1):62–70

32. Klein JL, Garcia EV, DePuey EG et al (1990) Reversibility bull's eye: a new polar bull's eye map to quantify reversibility of stress-induced SPECT thallium-201 myocardial perfusion defects. J Nucl Med 31:1240–1246

33. DePuey EG, Roubin GS, DePasquale EE (1989) Sequential multivessel coronary angioplasty assessed by thallium-201 tomography. Cathet Cardiovasc Diagn 18:213–221

34. Emory Cardiac Toolbox Manual. http://www.Syntermed.com. Accessed on February 2010

35. Gibbons RJ, Miller TD, Christian T (2000) Infarct size measured by single photon emission computed tomographic imaging with 99mTc-sestamibi: a measure of the efficacy of therapy in acute myocardial infarction. Circulation 101:101–108

36. Cerqueira MD, Weissman NJ, Dilsizian V et al (2002) Standardized myocardial segmentation and nomenclature for tomographic imaging of the heart: a statement for healthcare professionals from the Cardiac Imaging Committee of the Council on Clinical Cardiology of the American Heart Association. Circulation 105:539–542

37. Hachamovitch R, Berman DS, Kiat H, Cohen I, Cabico JA, Friedman J et al (1996) Exercise myocardial perfusion SPECT in patients without known coronary artery disease: incremental prognostic value and use in risk stratification. Circulation 93:905–914

38. Hsu CC, Chen YW, Hao CL, Chong JT, Lee CI, Tan HT, Wu MS, Wu JC (2008) Comparison of automated 4D-MSPECT and visual analysis for evaluating myocardial perfusion in coronary artery disease. Kaohsiung J Med Sci 24(9):445–452

39. Germano G (2006) Quantitative analysis in myocardial SPECT imaging. In: Zaidi H (ed) Quantitative analysis in nuclear medicine imaging. Springer, New York

40. Hachamovitch R, Hayes SW, Friedman JD, Cohen I, Berman DS (2003) Comparison of the short-term survival benefit associated with revascularization compared with medical therapy in patients with no prior coronary artery disease undergoing stress myocardial perfusion single photon emission computed tomography. Circulation 107:2900–2907

41. Van Train KF, Areeda J, Garcia EV, Cooke CD, Maddahi J, Kiat H et al (1993) Quantitative same-day rest-stress technetium-99m-sestamibi SPECT: definition and validation of stress normal limits and criteria for abnormality. J Nucl Med 34:1494–1502

42. Van Train KF, Garcia EV, Maddahi J, Areeda J, Cooke CD, Kiat H et al (1994) Multicenter trial validation for quantitative analysis of same-day rest-stress technetium-99m-sestamibi myocardial tomograms. J Nucl Med 35:609–618

43. Slomka PJ, Nishina H, Berman DS et al (2005) Automated quantification of myocardial perfusion SPECT using simplified normal limits. J Nucl Cardiol 12:66–77

44. Faber TL, Modersitzki J, Folks RD, Garcia EV (2005) Detecting changes in serial myocardial perfusion SPECT: a simulation study. J Nucl Cardiol 12:302–310

45. Slomka PJ, Nishina H, Berman DS, Kang X, Friedman JD, Hayes SW, Aladl UE, Germano G (2004) Automatic quantification of myocardial erfusion stress–rest change: a new measure of ischemia. J Nucl Med 45(2):183–191

46. Wolak A, Slomka PJ, Fish MB, Lorenzo S, Acampa W, Berman DS, Germano G (2008) Quantitative myocardial-perfusion SPECT: comparison of three state-of-the-art software packages. J Nucl Cardiol 15(1):27–34, Epub 2007 Oct 29

47. Garcia EV, Santana CA, Faber TL, Cooke CD, Folks RD (2008) Comparison of the diagnostic performance for detection of coronary artery disease (CAD) of their program (QPS) with that of the Emory Cardiac Toolbox (ECTb) for automated quantification of myocardial perfusion. J Nucl Cardiol 15(3)):476

48. Knollmann D, Knebel I, Koch KC, Gebhard M, Krohn T, Buell U, Schaefer WM (2008) Comparison of SSS and SRS calculated from normal databases provided by QPS and 4D-MSPECT manufacturers and from identical institutional normals. Eur J Nucl Med Mol Imaging 35(2):311–318

49. Shaw LJ, Iskandrian AE (2004) Prognostic value of gated myocardial perfusion SPECT. J Nucl Cardiol 11(2):171–185

50. Hachamovitch R, Berman DS (2005) The use of nuclear cardiology in clinical decision making. Semin Nucl Med 35(1):62–72

51. Achtert AD, King MA, Dahlberg ST, Pretorius PH, LaCroix KJ, Tsui BM (1998) An investigation of the estimation of ejection fractions and cardiac volumes by a quantitative gated SPECT software package in simulated gated SPECT images. J Nucl Cardiol 5:144–152

52. Xu Y, Kavanagh P, Fish M, Gerlach J, Ramesh A, Lemley M, Hayes S, Berman DS, Germano G, Slomka PJ (2009) Automated quality control for segmentation of myocardial perfusion SPECT. J Nucl Med 50(9):1418–1426

53. Sharir T, Bacher-Stier C, Lewin HC et al (2000) Identification of severe and extensive coronary artery disease by post-exercise regional wall motion abnormalities in Tc-99m sestamibi gated single photon emission computed tomography. Am J Cardiol 86:1171–1175

54. Sharir T, Berman DS, Waechter PB, Areeda J, Kavanagh PB, Gerlach J, Kang X, Germano G (2001 Nov) Quantitative analysis of regional motion and thickening by gated myocardial perfusion SPECT: normal heterogeneity and criteria for abnormality. J Nucl Med 42(11):1630–1638

55. Buvat I, Bartlett ML, Kitsiou K et al (1997) A"hybrid" method for measuring myocardial wall thickening from gated PET/SPECT images. J Nucl Med 38:324–329

56. Berman DS, Germano G (eds) (1999) Clinical gated cardiac SPECT, 1st edn. Futura Publishing Company, Armonk

57. Hesse B, Lindhardt TB, Acampa W, Anagnostopoulos C, Ballinger J, Bax JJ, Edenbrandt L, Flotats A, Germano G, Stopar TG, Franken P, Kelion A, Kjaer A, Le Guludec D, Ljungberg M, Maenhout AF, Marcassa C, Marving J, McKiddie F, Schaefer WM, Stegger L, Underwood R (2008 Apr) EANM/ESC guidelines for radionuclide imaging of cardiac function. Eur J Nucl Med Mol Imaging 35(4):851–885

58. Mandinov L, Eberli FR, Seiler C, Hess OM (2000) Diastolic heart failure. Cardiovasc Res 45(4):813–825

59. Villari B, Betocchi S, Pace L, Piscione F, Russolillo E, Ciarmiello A, Salvatore M, Condorelli M, Chiariello M (1991) Assessment of left ventricular diastolic function: comparison of contrast ventriculography and equilibrium radionuclide angiography. J Nucl Med 32(10):1849–1853

60. Kumita S, Cho K, Nakajo H, Toba M, Uwamori M, Mizumura S, Kumazaki T, Sano J, Sakai S, Munakata K (2001) Assessment of left ventricular diastolic function with electrocardiography-gated myocardial perfusion SPECT: comparison with multigated equilibrium radionuclide angiography. J Nucl Cardiol 8(5):568–574

61. Akincioglu C, Berman DS, Nishina H et al (2005) Assessment of diastolic function using 16-frame ^{99m}Tc-sestamibi gated myocardial perfusion SPECT: normal values. J Nucl Med 46:1102–1108

62. Sciagrà R, Giaccardi M, Porciani MC et al (2004) Myocardial perfusion imaging using gated SPECT in heart failure patients undergoing cardiac resynchronization therapy. J Nucl Med 45:164–168

63. Chen J, Garcia EV, Folks RD, Cooke CD, Faber TL, Tauxe EL et al (2005) Onset of left ventricular mechanical contraction as determined by phase analysis of ECG-gated myocardial perfusion SPECT imaging: development of a diagnostic tool for assessment of cardiac mechanical dyssynchrony. J Nucl Cardiol 12:687–695

64. Corbett JR, Akinboboye OO, Bacharach SL, Borer JS, Botvinick EH, DePuey EG, Ficaro EP, Hansen CL, Henzlova MJ, Van Kriekinge S (2006) Quality Assurance Committee of the American Society of Nuclear Cardiology. Equilibrium radionuclide angiocardiography. J Nucl Cardiol 13(6):e56–e79

65. Nichols KJ, Van Tosh A, De Bondt P, Bergmann SR, Palestro CJ, Reichek N (2008) Normal limits of gated blood pool SPECT count-based regional cardiac function parameters. Int J Cardiovasc Imaging 24(7):717–725

66. De Bondt P, Nichols KJ, De Winter O, De Sutter J, Vanderheyden M, Akinboboye OO, Dierckx RA (2006) Comparison among tomographic radionuclide ventriculography algorithms for computing left and right ventricular normal limits. J Nucl Cardiol 13(5):675–684

67. Van Kriekinge SD, Berman DS, Germano G (1999) Automatic quantification of left ventricular ejection fraction from gated blood pool SPECT. J Nucl Cardiol 6:498–506

68. Vanhove C, Franken PR, Defrise M, Momen A, Everaert H, Bossuyt A (2001) Automatic determination of left ventricular ejection fraction from gated blood-pool tomography. J Nucl Med 42:401–407

69. Ficaro EP, Quaife RF, Kritzman JN, Corbett JR (2002) Validation of a new fully automatic algorithm for quantification of gated blood pool SPECT: correlations with planar gated blood pool and perfusion SPECT [abstract]. J Nucl Med 43(suppl):97P

70. Nichols K, Saouaf R, Ababneh AA et al (2002) Validation of SPECT equilibrium radionuclide angiographic right ventricular parameters by cardiac magnetic resonance imaging. J Nucl Cardiol 9:153–160

71. De Bondt P, Claessens T, Rys B et al (2005) Accuracy of 4 different algorithms for the analysis of tomographic radionuclide ventriculography using a physical, dynamic 4-chamber cardiac phantom. J Nucl Med 46:165–171

72. Nichols K, Humayun N, De Bondt P, Vandenberghe S, Akinboboye OO, Bergmann SR (2004) Model dependence of gated blood pool SPECT ventricular function measurements. J Nucl Cardiol 11(3):282–292

73. Port SC (2004) Tomographic equilibrium radionuclide angiography: has its time arrived? J Nucl Cardiol 11(3):242–244

74. Adachi I, Umeda T, Shimomura H, Suwa M, Komori T, Ogura Y, Utsunomiya K, Kitaura Y, Narabayashi I (2005) Comparative study of quantitative blood pool SPECT imaging with 180 degrees and 360 degrees acquisition orbits on accuracy of cardiac function. J Nucl Cardiol 12(2):186–194

75. Heston TF, Sigg DM (2005) Quantifying transient ischemic dilation using gated SPECT. J Nucl Med 46(12):1990–1996

76. McLaughlin MG, Danias PG (2002) Transient ischemic dilation: a powerful diagnostic and prognostic finding of stress myocardial perfusion imaging. J Nucl Cardiol 9(6):663–667

77. Hambye AS, Vervaet A, Dobbeleir A (2004) Variability of left ventricular ejection fraction and volumes with quantitative gated SPECT: influence of algorithm, pixel size and reconstruction parameters in small and normal-sized hearts. Eur J Nucl Med Mol Imaging 31(12):1606–1613

78. Navare SM, Wackers FJ, Liu YH (2003) Comparison of 16-frame and 8-frame gated SPET imaging for determination of left ventricular volumes and ejection fraction. Eur J Nucl Med Mol Imaging 30(10):1330–1337

79. Vallejo E, Dione DP, Bruni WL, Constable RT, Borek PP, Soares JP, Carr JG, Condos SG, Wackers FJ, Sinusas AJ (2000) Reproducibility and accuracy of gated SPECT for determination of left ventricular volumes and ejection fraction: experimental validation using MRI. J Nucl Med 41:874–882

80. Vanhove C, Franken PR, Defrise M, Bossuyt A (2003) Comparison of 180 degrees and 360 degrees data acquisition for determination of left ventricular function from gated myocardial perfusion tomography and gated blood pool tomography. Eur J Nucl Med Mol Imaging 30(11):1498–1504

81. Groch MW, Takamiya Y, Groch PJ, Erwin WD (2000 Mar) Quantitative gated myocardial SPECT: effect of collimation on left-ventricular ejection fraction. J Nucl Med Technol 28(1):36–40

82. Hyun IY M.D., Kwan J, Park KS, Lee WH (2001) Reproducibility of Tl-201 and Tc-99m sestamibi gated myocardial perfusion SPECT measurement of myocardial function. J Nucl Cardiol 8:182–187

83. Pai M, Yang YJ, Im KC, Hong IK, Yun SC, Kang DH, Song JK, Moon DH (2006) Factors affecting accuracy of ventricular volume and ejection fraction measured by gated Tl-201 myocardial perfusion single photon emission computed tomography. Int J Cardiovasc Imaging 22(5):671–681

84. Manrique A, Hitzel A, Vera P (2004) Impact of photon energy recovery on the assessment of left ventricular volume using myocardial perfusion SPECT. J Nucl Cardiol 11:312–317

85. Ficaro EP, Kritzman JN, Hamilton TW, Mitchell TA, Corbett JR (2000) Effect on attenuation corrected myocardial perfusion SPECT on left ventricular ejection fraction estimates [abstract]. J Nucl Med 41:166

86. Kumita S, Cho K, Nakajo H, Toba M, Uwamori M, Mizumura S, Kumazaki T, Sano J, Sakai S, Munakata K (2001)

Assessment of left ventricular diastolic function with electrocardiography-gated myocardial perfusion SPECT: comparison with multigated equilibrium radionuclide angiography. J Nucl Cardiol 8(5):568–574

87. Marie PY, Djaballah W, Franken PR, Vanhove C, Muller MA, Boutley H, Poussier S, Olivier P, Karcher G, Bertrand A (2005) OSEM reconstruction, associated with temporal fourier and depth-dependant resolution recovery filtering, enhances results from sestamibi and 201Tl 16-interval gated SPECT. J Nucl Med 46(11):1789–1795

88. Véra P, Manrique A, Pontvianne V et al (1999) Thallium-gated SPECT in patients with major myocardial infarction: effect of filtering and zooming in comparison with equilibrium radionuclide imaging and left ventriculography. J Nucl Med 40:513–521

89. Manrique A, Hitzel A, Gardin I, Dacher JN, Vera P (2003) Impact of Wiener filter in determining the left ventricular volume and ejection fraction using thallium-201 gated SPECT. Nucl Med Commun 24(8):907–914

90. Gremillet E, Champailler A, Soler C (2005) Fourier temporal interpolation improves electrocardiograph-gated myocardial perfusion SPECT. J Nucl Med 46: 1769–1774

91. Nichols K, Dorbala S, DePuey EG, Yao SS, Sharma A, Rozanski A (1999) Influence of arrhythmias on gated SPECT myocardial perfusion and function quantification. J Nucl Med 40:924–934

92. Kim DW, Park SA, Kim CG (2008) Gating error because of prominent T waves with ECG-gated myocardial SPECT. Clin Nucl Med 33(4):278–279

93. Kasai T, Depuey EG, Shah AA et al (2003) Impact of gating errors with electrocardiography gated myocardial perfusion SPECT. J Nucl Cardiol 10:709–711

94. Khalil MM, Elgazzar A, Khalil W et al (2005) Assessment of left ventricular ejection fraction by four different methods using 99mTc tetrofosmin gated SPECT in patients with small hearts: correlation with gated blood pool. Nucl Med Commun 26:885–893

95. Schaefer WM, Lipke CS, Standke D, Kuhl HP, Nowak B, Kaiser HJ, Koch KC, Buell U (2005) Quantification of left ventricular volumes and ejection fraction from gated ^{99m}Tc-MIBI SPECT: MRI validation and comparison of the emory cardiac tool box with QGS and 4D-MSPECT. J Nucl Med 46:1256–1263

96. Nakajima K, Higuchi T, Taki J, Kawano M, Tonami N (2001) Accuracy of ventricular volume and ejection fraction measured by gated myocardial SPECT: comparison of 4 software programs. J Nucl Med 42:1571–1578

97. Khalil MM, Elgazzar A, Khalil W (2006) Evaluation of left ventricular ejection fraction by the quantitative algorithms QGS, ECTb, LMC and LVGTF using gated myocardial perfusion SPECT: investigation of relative accuracy. Nucl Med Commun 27(4):321–332, Erratum in: Nucl Med Commun. 2006 Oct;27(10):831

Tracer Kinetic Modeling: Basics and Concepts 16

Kjell Erlandsson

Contents

K. Erlandsson
Institute of Nuclear Medicine, University College London, London, UK
e-mail: k.erlandsson@ucl.ac.uk

16.1 Introduction

In nuclear medicine all studies are dynamic. This may seem like a controversial statement as most studies performed in nuclear medicine departments consist of a single static scan. However, even in this case, the temporal dimension plays an important role in terms of the time point for the scan after administration of the tracer as well as its length.

In general, in nuclear medicine studies, a radio-tracer is administered by intravenous injection and clinical information is obtained from the uptake of the tracer in different organs or tissues. The uptake is determined by the delivery, retention, and clearance of the tracer [1]. The delivery and clearance rates are dependent on the blood flow while the retention is determined by the extraction of the tracer from blood to tissue as well as the metabolism of the tracer in tissue or binding of tracer molecules to specific or unspecific binding sites. All these processes are dynamic, which, together with the physical decay of the radionuclide, lead to a tracer distribution that changes over time. Therefore, in order to determine quantitative parameters related to physiological or biochemical processes, it is necessary to obtain information about the time course of the tracer in different organs or tissues. This can be done with a dynamic data acquisition protocol, consisting of a series of scans performed over a period of time after administration of a radio-tracer. When sufficient knowledge has been obtained regarding the general behavior of a tracer, it may be possible to develop simplified study protocols based on single scan techniques, which can

---

This chapter is dedicated to the memory of Prof. Lyn S Pilowsky.

M.M. Khalil (ed.), *Basic Sciences of Nuclear Medicine*, DOI: 10.1007/978-3-540-85962-8_16,
© Springer-Verlag Berlin Heidelberg 2011

provide relevant information related to the biological function of interest [2].

With dynamic data acquisition, quantitative values for physiological or biochemical parameters can be determined by applying mathematical tools to the dynamic data sets. This procedure is known as "kinetic analysis".

Dynamic data acquisition involves repeated PET or SPECT scans over a period of time, and result in time-activity curves (TACs) representing the time course of activity concentration in different parts of the image. TACs can be generated for various volumes of interest (VOIs) or alternatively for individual voxels if parametric images are required. Absolute quantification of radioactivity is needed and therefore correction for physical effects such as attenuation and scatter are essential. Correction for partial volume effects (PVE) may also be needed. PVE correspond to contribution of information between adjacent image regions due to the limited spatial resolution usually associated with PET or SPECT data.

Kinetic analysis is done using a mathematical model of tracer behavior [3], usually a compartmental model consisting of a series of compartments, representing tracer concentration in various regions or states, and first order rate constants that govern the transfer of tracer between compartments. In order to determine the parameters of the model, it is necessary to have information about the tracer delivery in the form of an input function, ideally representing the time-course of tracer concentration in arterial blood or plasma.

Kinetic analysis can be useful within different clinical areas, such as cardiology, oncology, and neurology, where tracers such as ^{15}O-H$_2$O, ^{18}F-FDG, and ^{123}I-IBZM can be used to quantify values of blood flow, metabolic rate of glucose, and neuroreceptor binding, respectively. In this chapter, we shall describe the basic mathematical tools and concepts used in tracer kinetic modeling. Practical applications are discussed in the next chapter.

16.2 Compartmental Modeling

16.2.1 Definitions and Assumptions

In kinetic modeling theory, the term "steady state" is used for the situation when the concentration of a compound in a compartment does not change with time. The term "equilibrium" is used for the situation when all compartments in the model are in steady-state.

A series of assumptions are needed to proceed with tracer kinetic modeling. The most important of these are [4]:

1. The physiological processes that affect the measurements (e.g., blood flow) are in a steady state condition throughout the experiment.
2. The radio-ligands used are administered in tracer concentrations, and therefore do not affect the physiological or biochemical processes being studied.
3. The tracer concentration within a compartment is homogeneous – i.e., instant mixing is assumed.

16.2.2 Compartmental Models

Physiological or biochemical systems are often described using compartmental models, in which a tracer is assumed to be transferred between a number of different compartments, which can represent separate regions in space (e.g., vascular, interstitial, or intracellular space), or alternatively different chemical states (e.g., parent compound, metabolic products or receptor bound tracer molecules). The rate of transfer from one compartment to another is proportional to the concentration in the compartment of origin and to a first order rate constant. In general, a compartmental model is described by a system of differential equations, where each equation corresponds to the sum of all transfer rates to and from a specific compartment, i:

$$\frac{\mathrm{d}}{\mathrm{d}t}C_i(t) = \sum_{\substack{j=1,..N \\ j \neq i}} \left(k_{ij}C_j(t) - k_{ji}C_i(t) \right); \qquad (16.1)$$

$$i = 1,..N$$

where $C_i(\cdot)$ is the tracer concentration in compartment i, N is the number of compartments in the model, and k_{ij} is the rate constant for transfer to compartment i from compartment j.

Compartmental models can be either reversible or irreversible. The irreversible models are those which contain at least one compartment that does not have an outflow.

In nuclear medicine, a single-index nomenclature is normally used to denote the rate constants. The rate constants for transfer from blood to tissue and from tissue to blood are called K_1 and k_2, respectively, and additional rate constants in the model are called k_3, k_4, etc. These symbols are sometimes qualified with asterisks or primes when necessary. Traditionally, a capital K is used in K_1, while lower case k:s are used for the other rate constants. This is to reflect that K_1 corresponds to a clearance term, which leads to a distinction in terms of units. While k_i, $i \geq 2$, are expressed in units of (min^{-1}), K_1 is expressed in same units as blood flow: (mL/min/mL) or (mL/min/g) (mL of blood/plasma per minute per mL or g of tissue).

16.2.3 Solving Compartmental Models – The Laplace Transform

The Laplace transform is a useful tool when it comes to solving systems of linear first order differential equation, such as Equation 16.1. The Laplace transform is defined as:

$$F(s) = \int_0^\infty e^{-st} f(t) dt \qquad (16.2)$$

where s is a complex Laplace-space variable.

Using the properties listed in Table 16.1, it is possible to obtain solutions for complex compartmental systems. In particular, the property relating the transform of the derivative of a function to that of the original function is the key to the solution. After taking the Laplace transform of both sides in each equation, the terms are

Table 16.1 Laplace transform pairs

Time domain	Laplace domain
$f(t)$	$F(s)$
k	k/s
e^{kt}	$1/(s-k)$
$ag(t)+bh(t)$	$aG(s) + bH(s)$
$g'(t)$	$sG(s) - g(0)$
$g(t) \otimes h(t)$	$G(s)H(s)$

k, a and b are constants, t and s are variables, $g(\cdot)$, $G(\cdot)$, $h(\cdot)$ and $H(\cdot)$ are functions, represents derivation and "ox" convolution. (NB: "ox" above represents a symbol consisting of a circle and a cross)

rearranged into the transform of a simple function, such as a sum of constants and exponential functions, and the inverse Laplace transform can then be found.

In the case of biological systems, the solution can often be expressed as:

$$C_T(t) = H_N(t) \otimes C_a(t) \qquad (16.3)$$

where $C_a(\cdot)$ and $C_T(\cdot)$ are the input and output functions, respectively, $\otimes$ represents the convolution operation, and $H_N(\cdot)$ is the impulse response function of the model, which has the following general form [5]:

$$H_N(t) = \sum_{i=1}^N \phi_i e^{-\theta_i t} \qquad (16.4)$$

where ϕ_i and θ_i are functions of the individual rate constants of the model (K_1, k_2...), and N is the number of compartments. Irreversible compartments correspond to terms in $H_N(\cdot)$ with $\theta_i = 0$, i.e., a constant. The number of terms (constants or exponential terms) in the impulse response function is equal to the number of tissue compartments in the model.

Appendix A contains examples of Laplace transform-derived solutions for a number of different compartmental models. Sometimes, it may be necessary to use the technique of partial fractions expansion [6] to find the individual terms of the impulse response function. Once the impulse response function has been determined, the individual parameters (K_1, k_2...) can be estimated. This is an inverse problem, where an equation of type 16.3 represents the forward model, and which can be solved using an iterative procedure. For nonlinear systems, it may not be possible to find an analytic solution for the impulse response function, in which case, the forward step can be calculated based on the original differential equations using a numerical technique, such as the Runge–Kutta method [7].

16.2.4 The 1-Tissue Compartment Model – Blood Flow

From a physiological point of view, the term "blood flow" refers to the volume of blood delivered to an organ per unit of time, often expressed in (mL/min), while "perfusion" refers to the volume of blood delivered per unit of time and per unit of tissue-mass (mL/min/g) or per unit of tissue-volume (mL/min/ mL). In the context of tracer kinetic modeling, the two terms are used interchangeably with the latter definition. It has recently been recommended that this quantity be expressed in the units (mL/min/cm^3) in order to accentuate the distinction between volume of blood (mL) and volume of tissue (cm^3) [8].

A model for quantifying blood flow was developed 6 decades ago [9]. It was based on the Fick principle, which states that the rate of change of the tracer concentration in tissue is proportional to blood flow and to the difference in the arterial and venous concentrations:

$$\frac{d}{dt}C_T(t) = F(C_a(t) - C_v(t)) \qquad (16.5)$$

where $C_T(\cdot)$, $C_a(\cdot)$, and $C_v(\cdot)$ are the tracer concentrations in tissue and in arterial and venous blood, respectively, F is blood flow, and t is time.

Assuming that the tracer concentration in tissue is at equilibrium with that in venous blood at all times $\{C_T(t)/C_v(t)=V_T \ \forall \ t\}$, Equation 16.5 can be rewritten as follows [10]:

$$\frac{d}{dt}C_T(t) = FC_a(t) - \frac{F}{V_T}C_T(t) \qquad (16.6)$$

The constant V_T is known as "volume of distribution" (see below).

The Kety-Schmidt model is valid only for tracers that are fully extracted from blood to tissue. This is true for many of the tracers used for measuring blood flow, such as ^{15}O-H$_2$O, ^{13}N-NH$_4$, and ^{133}Xe. On the other hand, if the tracer is not fully extracted (as is the case for e.g., ^{82}Rb), this may be taken into account using the extraction fraction, E, defined as the amount of tracer trapped in the first pass to the amount delivered. The extraction fraction can be calculated using the Renkin-Crone formula [11, 12]:

$$E = 1 - e^{-PS/F} \qquad (16.7)$$

where PS is the permeability surface area product, expressed in (mL/min/mL) or (mL/min/g).

Replacing F by FE in Equation 16.6 and including the constants $K_1 = FE$ and $k_2 = K_1/V_T$ leads to:

$$\frac{d}{dt}C_T(t) = K_1C_a(t) - k_2C_T(t) \qquad (16.8)$$

Equation 16.8 can be interpreted as the operational equation for the simple compartmental system shown in Fig. 16.1, and has the solution (see Appendix A):

$$C_T(t) = K_1e^{-k_2t} \otimes C_a(t) \qquad (16.9)$$

The model in Fig. 16.1 is sometimes referred to as a two-compartment model and represented with the k_2-arrow directed from the tissue compartment back to blood. This may seem intuitively logical; however, it does not correspond to the actual mathematical relationship between the input and output functions. In practice, the arterial blood TAC is just used as an input function and blood is not actually treated as a compartment in a mathematical sense. A better choice of nomenclature is therefore to name the model depending on the number of tissue compartments it contains. Hereby, the model in Fig. 16.1 would be called a 1-tissue compartment (1-TC) model.

16.2.5 Multitissue Compartment Models – Neuroreceptor Mapping

Neuroreceptor mapping deals with studies of the systems that control the chemical transmission of neuronal signals across the synapse between two neurons. When an electrical impulse reaches the end of the presynaptic nerve cell, a series of events are initiated: Neurotransmitter substance is released from vesicles within the presynaptic cell into the synaptic cleft. The neurotransmitter diffuses across to the postsynaptic cell and binds to specific receptors, triggering a new electrical impulse. The neurotransmitter substance in the synapse is reabsorbed into the presynaptic cell via channels known as transporters, in order to make way for a new neuronal signal. The neurotransmitter can also bind to receptors on the presynaptic cell, which

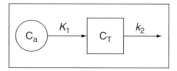

Fig. 16.1 The blood flow model (1-TC). C_a and C_T are the tracer concentrations in arterial blood and in tissue, respectively, and K_1 and k_2 are rate constants

would lead to modulation of the signal transmission across the synapse. In psychiatric studies, it is of interest to measure the concentration of different receptors or transporters in different brain regions. This can be achieved using radiotracers that bind specifically to the receptors or transporters of interest.

16.2.5.1 *In Vitro* Quantification

For historical reasons, the theory for quantification of neuroreceptor binding *in vivo* is based on the theory for *in vitro* binding assays, involving incubation of a receptor-enriched preparation with a radioligand. This theory is based on the law of mass action, which states that the ligand binds to receptors (association) at a rate proportional to the concentration of ligand and to the concentration of receptors, and that the resultant ligand-receptor complex breaks down (dissociation) at a rate proportional to the concentration of the complex [13], which is described in the following equation:

$$\frac{\mathrm{d}}{\mathrm{d}t}[RL] = k_{\mathrm{on}}[R][L] - k_{\mathrm{off}}[RL] \qquad (16.10)$$

where $[R]$, $[L]$, and $[RL]$ are the concentrations of receptors, ligand, and receptor-ligand complex, respectively, and k_{on} and k_{off} are the rate constants for association and dissociation, respectively. Equation 16.10 can be represented as a simple two-compartment model with the rate constants $k_{\mathrm{on}}[R]$ and k_{off} (Fig. 16.2). In practice, $k_{\mathrm{on}}[R]$ can be assumed to be constant only if $[R] >> [L]$ (tracer conditions).

In *in vitro* experiments, a state of equilibrium will be reached after some time, in which, the rate of association is equal to the rate of dissociation, and the following relation is obtained:

$$k_{\mathrm{on}}[R][L] = k_{\mathrm{off}}[RL]$$

$$\Leftrightarrow$$

$$\frac{[R][L]}{[RL]} = \frac{k_{\mathrm{off}}}{k_{\mathrm{on}}} \equiv K_D \qquad (16.11)$$

The constant K_D is known as the equilibrium dissociation constant. Its reciprocal value is defined as the affinity of the ligand for the receptor. Thus, a low K_D value corresponds to high affinity.

For *in vivo* experiments, a different set of symbols are used: Free ligand, $F = [L]$, bound ligand, $B = [RL]$, and total receptor-concentration, $B_{\mathrm{max}} = [R]+[RL]$. With these symbols, we can rewrite Equation 16.11 as follows:

$$B = \frac{B_{\mathrm{max}}F}{K_D + F} \qquad (16.12)$$

This is the Michaelis-Menten equation, and describes the relation between bound and free ligand equilibrium concentrations [14]. If B is plotted as a function of F, this equation corresponds to a saturation curve, which initially rises linearly ($B/F \approx B_{\mathrm{max}}/K_D$, $F << K_D$) and then gradually plateaus, asymptotically approaching a constant level ($B \approx B_{\mathrm{max}}, F >> K_D$). By measuring a series of corresponding B and F values, it is possible to estimate the parameters B_{max} and K_D. A simple solution is obtained after rewriting Equation 16.12 as follows:

$$\frac{B}{F} = \frac{B_{\mathrm{max}}}{K_D} - \frac{1}{K_D}B \qquad (16.13)$$

If (B/F) is plotted as a function of B, this equation describes a straight line with a slope of $(-1/K_D)$ and an intercept of (B_{max}/K_D). This is the Scatchard method [15] (see Fig. 16.3).

The analysis above is valid for any values of B and F. Under tracer conditions, defined by $B << B_{\mathrm{max}}$ (or $F << K_D$), Equation 16.13 reduces to:

$$\frac{B}{F} \approx \frac{B_{\mathrm{max}}}{K_D} \equiv BP \qquad (16.14)$$

where BP is the binding potential [16], which is the most important parameter in *in vivo* neuroreceptor studies. As most human *in vivo* studies are performed under tracer conditions, in order to avoid

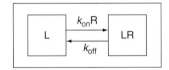

Fig. 16.2 The *in vitro* model. L, R, and LR represent concentration of ligand, receptors, and ligand-receptor complex, respectively, and k_{on} and k_{off} are constants

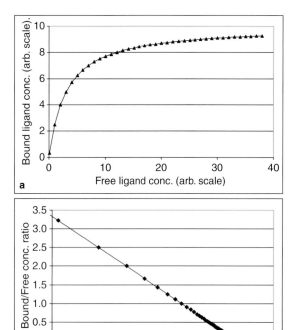

a

b

Fig. 16.3 The relationship between free and bound ligand concentration as expressed in the Michaelis-Menten equation. (**a**) Bound vs. free concentration with $B_{max} = 10$ and $K_d = 3$ in arbitrary units. (**b**) Same data displayed with bound over free vs. bound concentration. All points are on a straight line with a slope of $-1/K_d$, a y-intercept of B_{max}/K_d, and an x-intercept of B_{max}

pharmacological effects of the ligand, it is not possible to estimate the values of B_{max} and K_D separately – only their ratio, BP, can be estimated.

16.2.5.2 *In Vivo* Quantification

The *in vivo* neuroreceptor model can be seen as a combination of the Fick principle (blood flow) and the law of mass-action (receptor binding). Apart from binding to specific receptors, most neuroreceptor tracers will also bind to so-called nonspecific binding sites, consisting mainly of macromolecules such as proteins. As opposed to specific binding, nonspecific binding is not saturable and not displaceable. The most general neuroreceptor model therefore consists of

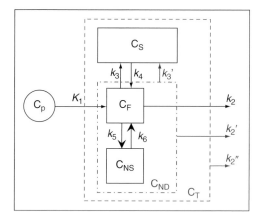

Fig. 16.4 Combined illustration of the 3-TC, 2-TC, and 1-TC models for neuroreceptor quantification. C_p is the concentration of unmetabolized tracer in plasma, C_F, C_{NS}, and C_S are the concentrations of free, nonspecifically bound, and specifically bound tracer in tissue, respectively, C_{ND} is the concentration of nondisplaceable tracer in tissue ($C_{ND} = C_F + C_{NS}$), and C_T is the total concentration of tracer in tissue. The sets of rate constants used in the different models are: $\{K_1, k_2–k_6\}$ (3-TC), $\{K_1, k_2', k_3', k_4\}$ (2-TC), and $\{K_1, k_2''\}$ (1-TC model)

three tissue compartments (see Fig. 16.4), and can be described as follows:

$$\begin{cases} \dfrac{d}{dt}C_F(t) = K_1 C_p(t) - (k_2 + k_3 + k_5)C_F(t) \\ \qquad\qquad + k_4 C_S(t) + k_6 C_{NS}(t) \\ \dfrac{d}{dt}C_S(t) = k_3 C_F(t) - k_4 C_S(t) \\ \dfrac{d}{dt}C_{NS}(t) = k_5 C_F(t) - k_6 C_{NS}(t) \end{cases}$$

$$(16.15)$$

where $C_p(\cdot)$, $C_F(\cdot)$, $C_S(\cdot)$, and $C_{NS}(\cdot)$ are the tracer concentrations in plasma and in the compartments for free, specifically bound, and nonspecifically bound tracer, respectively, and K_1, $k_2–k_6$ are rate constants.

With six free parameters (K_1, $k_2–k_6$), the 3-TC model is normally too complex to be practically useful. All the parameters may not be identifiable,[1] given the limited amount of information available, namely one input function and one TAC representing the

---

[1] Parameter identifiability means that a change in the parameter values should always lead to a change in the output function [17].

sum of all tissue compartments. Therefore, it is often necessary to reduce the complexity of the model by reducing the number of compartments. The 3-TC model would thereby be converted to a 2-TC or even a 1-TC model. This can be done when the data are equally well described by the simpler model, which is consistent with rapid exchange between two or more compartment and allows for them to be considered in equilibrium at all time.

It is important to note that when the compartmental structure of the model changes, the meaning of the rate constants also changes, and it may be appropriate to use different symbols in the different models. Therefore, in the 2-TC model, k_2 and k_3 become k_2' and k_3', and in the 1-TC model, k_2 becomes k_2'' [18]. Many authors do not make this distinction, however, which makes it necessary to clarify which model the parameters refer to in each case.

The 2-TC model (Fig. 16.4) is obtained by merging the compartments for free and nonspecifically bound tracer into one compartment, known as the nondisplaceable (ND) compartment. The 2-TC model can be described as follows:

$$\begin{cases} \dfrac{\mathrm{d}}{\mathrm{d}t}C_{ND}(t) = K_1 C_p(t) - (k_2' + k_3')C_{ND}(t) + k_4 C_S(t) \\ \dfrac{\mathrm{d}}{\mathrm{d}t}C_S(t) = k_3' C_{ND}(t) - k_4 C_S(t) \end{cases}$$

$$(16.16)$$

where $C_{ND}(\cdot)$ is the tracer concentration in the nondisplaceable compartment (free and nonspecifically bound tracer), and k_2' and k_3' are rate constants specific to this model.

This simplification implicitly involves the assumption that equilibrium is rapidly established between the F- and NS-compartments, and that the free fraction in tissue, f_{ND}, is constant during the experiment. f_{ND} is defined as:

$$f_{ND} = \left[\frac{C_F}{C_F + C_{NS}}\right]_{eq} = \left[\frac{C_F}{C_{ND}}\right]_{eq} = \frac{k_6}{k_5 + k_6} \quad (16.17)$$

The last equality is obtained from the last differential equation in (16.15) together with the equilibrium condition $\mathrm{d}C_{NS}(t)/\mathrm{d}t = 0$. The constant f_{ND} to improve readability cannot be directly measured. The relationships between the rate constants in the 2-TC and 3-TC

models can be derived by equating the transport rates between compartments in the two models:

$$k_2'C_{ND} = k_2 C_F = k_2 f_{ND}C_{ND} \; \Leftrightarrow \; k_2' = f_{ND}k_2$$
$$k_3'C_{ND} = k_3 C_F = k_3 f_{ND}C_{ND} \; \Leftrightarrow \; k_3' = f_{ND}k_3$$

$$(16.18)$$

In the 1-TC model (Fig. 16.4), one single compartment represents nondisplaceable and specifically bound tracer in tissue. It can be described as follows:

$$\frac{\mathrm{d}}{\mathrm{d}t}C_T(t) = K_1 C_p(t) - k_2''C_T(t) \qquad (16.19)$$

where $C_T(\cdot)$ is the total concentration of nondisplaceable and specifically bound tracer in tissue, and k_2'' is a rate constant specific to this model. This simplification implicitly involves the assumption of rapid equilibration between the ND- and S-compartments, and as above we obtain:

$$k_2''C_T = k_2'C_{ND} \Leftrightarrow k_2'' = k_2'\left(1 + \frac{k_3'}{k_4}\right)^{-1} \quad (16.20)$$

The 1-TC model for neuroreceptor quantification is mathematically equivalent to the one used for blood flow above (Fig. 16.1). The difference is that, while the main parameter of interest in the case of blood flow measurements is the uptake rate constant, K_1, which reflects blood flow ($K_1=FE$), in the case of neuroreceptor studies, the main parameter of interest is the washout rate constant, k_2'', reflecting the amount of tracer retention in the target tissue due to receptor binding ($BP_{ND} = k_3'/k_4$ [see below]).

Figure 16.5 shows an example of TACs corresponding to a SPECT study using the NMDA receptor tracer [^{123}I]CNS 1261 [19]. The tissue curves were generated with the 2-TC model using rate constants averaged over the values estimated in a number of subjects (see Table 16.2).

16.3 Input Function Issues

A factor that complicates the quantification procedure is the presence of radioactive metabolites. Such metabolites can be produced in peripheral organs (liver, kidneys, lungs, etc.), and released back into the

Fig. 16.5 Time-activity
curves corresponding to the
NMDA receptor SPECT
tracer ^{123}I-CNS 1261 with
bolus injection; (**a**) arterial
plasma input function
(NB: log-scale), (**b**) tissue
curves for various brain
regions: Frontal cortex (FC),
striatum (Str), temporal cortex
(TC), thalamus (Tha), and
white matter (WM)

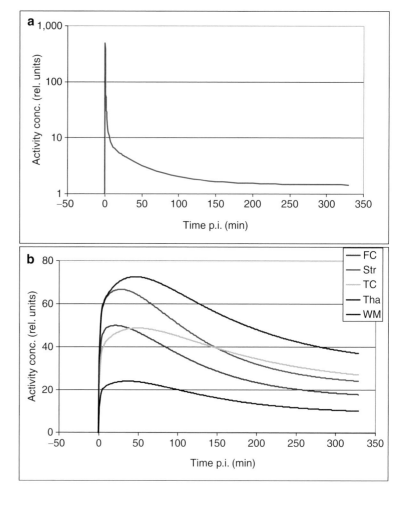

Table 16.2 Average rate constants for the 2-TC model for the SPECT tracer [^{123}I]CNS 1261

	K_1 (mL/min/mL)	k_2' (min^{-1})	k_3' (min^{-1})	k_4 (min^{-1})
FC	0.172	0.023	0.018	0.036
Str	0.215	0.018	0.016	0.058
TC	0.145	0.019	0.039	0.037
Tha	0.227	0.033	0.106	0.049
WM	0.076	0.025	0.078	0.075

FC frontal cortex, *Str* striatum, *TC* temporal cortex, *Tha* thalamus, *WM* white matter

blood stream. If the metabolites can cross the blood–brain barrier (BBB), it will be necessary to use a more complex model with more parameters, resulting in increased variability, which often makes the tracer intractable as a quantitative imaging tool. This problem can be avoided by appropriate tracer selection.

However, radioactive metabolites in the blood stream can, in general, not be avoided, and metabolite-correction of the arterial input function is therefore needed. For this purpose, high-pressure liquid chromatography (HPLC) can be used to determine the fraction of radioactivity in arterial plasma corresponding to metabolites.

The measured input function is also affected by nonspecific binding in plasma. Tracer bound to protein molecules is not available for transportation across the BBB. Usually, it is assumed that equilibrium is reached quickly between free and protein-bound tracer in plasma, and the free fraction in plasma, f_p, is thereby assumed to be constant during the experiment. f_p is defined as:

$$f_p = \left[\frac{C_{p,F}}{C_{p,F} + C_{p,NS}} \right]_{eq} = \left[\frac{C_{p,F}}{C_p} \right]_{eq} \qquad (16.21)$$

where C_p, $C_{p,F}$, and $C_{p,NS}$ are the total concentration and the concentrations of free and of protein-bound unmetabolized tracer in plasma, respectively. In principle, it is possible to measure f_p (e.g., by ultrafiltration), but these measurements often have high variability. The input function is discussed further in the next chapter.

$$V_T \equiv \left[\frac{C_T(t)}{C_p(t)} \right]_{eq} = \frac{K_1}{k_2} \left(1 + \frac{k_3}{k_4} + \frac{k_5}{k_6} \right)$$
$$= \frac{K_1}{k_2'} \left(1 + \frac{k_3'}{k_4} \right) = \frac{K_1}{k_2''} \qquad (16.22)$$

This equation shows that V_T is independent of blood flow: Both K_1 and k_2 depend on blood flow, but their ratio does not, and neither do the rate constants k_3-k_6.

16.4 Outcome Measures

The basic parameters in a compartmental model are the rate constants (K_1, k_2...). These so-called microparameters can usually not be determined with a high degree of precision, due to noise present in the data (mainly related to limited counting statistics in the photon detection process). Therefore various macroparameters are usually used instead as outcome measures. The macroparameters, typically formed from functions of the individual rate constants, are more robust and can be easily interpreted in terms of the impulse response function itself [5]. For reversible tracers, the macroparameters of interest are the volume of distribution and the binding potential.

16.4.1 Volume of Distribution

One of the most robust outcome measure is the "total volume of distribution," V_T, defined as the ratio between tracer concentration in tissue and in plasma at equilibrium. V_T is expressed in units of (mL/mL) or (mL/g), i.e., mL of blood/plasma per mL or g of tissue. V_T is useful in neuroreceptor studies, since it is dependent on the receptor concentration in the target tissue but independent of blood flow (see below). It is numerically equal to a quantity known as the partition coefficient. In theory, V_T can be obtained as the integral of the impulse response function $\left(V_T = \int_0^\infty H(t) dt \right)$ [5].

When using compartmental modeling, V_T can be calculated from the rate constants with expressions derived by equilibrium analysis of the differential equations that describe each model. Thus we obtain the following expressions for the 3-TC, 2-TC, and 1-TC models (see Appendix B, Equations 16.31a–c):

16.4.2 Binding Potential

The principal outcome measure in neuroreceptor studies is binding potential, BP. However, in *in vivo* studies, it can be difficult to accurately estimate BP according to Equation 16.14 independent of some nonspecific components. In the past, several alternative definitions of the term binding potential were used, which would sometimes lead to confusion. Therefore, recently, a consensus was reached among researches in the field, and three different types of *in vivo* binding potentials were defined: BP_F, BP_p, and BP_{ND} [8]. All three are defined in terms of concentration ratios at equilibrium – concentration of specifically bound tracer vs. a reference concentration. The difference between the three lies in which concentration is used as a reference. For BP_F, the reference concentration is that of free tracer in plasma, which at equilibrium is equal to the free concentration in tissue ($C_{p,F} \equiv f_p C_p = C_F \equiv f_{ND} C_{ND}$); for BP_p it is the total concentration of parent compound in plasma ($C_p \equiv C_{p,F} + C_{p,NS}$); and for BP_{ND}, the concentration of nondisplaceable tracer in tissue ($C_{ND} \equiv C_F + C_{NS}$):

$$BP_F \equiv \left[\frac{C_S}{C_{p,F}} \right]_{eq}; \quad BP_p \equiv \left[\frac{C_S}{C_p} \right]_{eq};$$
$$BP_{ND} \equiv \left[\frac{C_S}{C_{ND}} \right]_{eq} \qquad (16.23)$$

Another difference with *in vitro* studies is that *in vivo* measurements do not reflect the total receptor concentration, B_{max}. Some fraction of the receptors may be occupied by the endogenous transmitter substance (dopamine, serotonin...), by some drug administered to the patient, or by the tracer itself.

In vivo studies reflect the concentration of available receptors, B_{avail}.

As for V_T, the various *BP*-values can be derived from the model parameters. Also, if a brain region exists that is known not to have any specific binding, this can be used as a reference region to derive *BP*-values from V_T values. This approach usually yields more robust results as compared to estimating the *BP*-values directly from the rate constants. The relations between *BP*, V_T, and model parameters is summarized in Table 16.3. The derivation of the formulas for BP_F is given in Appendix B (Equation 16.32).

Of the three *in vivo* *BP*-measures, BP_F is the one that comes closest to the *in vitro* definition in Equation 16.14, but it can be difficult to determine in practice. The use of BP_p requires the assumption that f_p is constant between scans or across groups of subjects. BP_{ND} requires the same assumption regarding f_{ND}, but has the advantage that it can be estimated using the reference tissue model (see below), which does not require arterial sampling.

It is generally assumed that any factor that affects the BP values, apart from B_{avail}, such as K_D, f_p, or f_{ND}, is constant across different brain regions, subjects, and/or clinical conditions. Thereby, any change in *BP* would reflect a change in B_{avail}. For example, the fraction of receptors occupied by a drug (occupancy, *O*) can be estimated by measuring *BP* of a tracer that binds to the same kind of receptors before (BP_{base}) and after giving the drug (BP_{drug}) [8, 13]:

$$O \equiv 1 - \frac{B_{avail,drug}}{B_{avail,base}} = 1 - \frac{BP_{drug}}{BP_{base}} \quad (16.24)$$

where *BP* in BP_{base} and BP_{drug} represents either BP_F, BP_p, or BP_{ND}.

Table 16.3 Calculation of binding potential *in vivo*

Name	Definition	3-TC model	2-TC model	Volume of distribution
BP_F	$\frac{B_{avail}}{K_D}$	$\frac{k_3}{k_4}$	$\frac{1}{f_p}\frac{K_1 k_3'}{k_2' k_4}$	$\frac{1}{f_p}(V_T - V_{ND})$
BP_p	$f_p \frac{B_{avail}}{K_D}$	$f_p \frac{k_3}{k_4}$	$\frac{K_1 k_3'}{k_2' k_4}$	$V_T - V_{ND}$
BP_{ND}	$f_{ND}\frac{B_{avail}}{K_D}$	$\frac{k_3}{k_4}\left(\frac{k_6}{k_5+k_6}\right)$	$\frac{k_3'}{k_4}$	$\frac{V_T - V_{ND}}{V_{ND}}$

V_{ND} is the volume of distribution for non-displaceable tracer, as obtained from a reference region

16.5 Parameter Estimation Methods

16.5.1 Reference Tissue Models

The modeling approaches discussed so far were all based on the availability of an arterial input function. Traditionally, this would be obtained by repeated arterial sampling throughout the experiment, but that is an invasive and labor-intensive procedure, and it would be a clear advantage if it could be avoided. In some cases, the input function can be obtained directly from the images, if an appropriate blood pool can be identified. This approach is useful in cardiac studies, where the left ventricle or the aorta can be used.

As an alternative, the input function can be built into the model itself, utilizing the fact that different tissue regions are exposed to the same input function. An advantage with this method over the direct image-derived input function method is that no metabolite correction is needed. One such approach, which is often used in brain studies, is the reference tissue or reference region model. If a brain region can be identified, which is devoid of specific binding, the TAC for this "reference region" can be used as an indirect input function for the target region. Two alternative models that have been proposed are: The full reference tissue model (FRTM) [20, 21], based on the 2TC-model, and the simplified reference tissue model (SRTM) [22], based on the 1-TC model (see Fig. 16.6). The impulse response functions for the two models are given by Equations 16.33 and 16.35, respectively.

In principle, FRTM is dependent on the six rate constants: $K_1, k_2', k_3', k_4, {}^R K_1,$ and ${}^R k_2'$, where the first four belong to the target region and the latter two to the reference region. However, K_1 and ${}^R K_1$ enter the model only as a ratio: $R_1 = K_1/{}^R K_1$. Furthermore, it can be assumed that the volume of distribution of the nondisplaceable compartment (V_{ND}) is the same for both regions: $K_1/k_2' = {}^R K_1/{}^R k_2' \Leftrightarrow k_2' = R_1 {}^R k_2'$, and thereby, the number of parameters for this model can be reduced to 4. SRTM has, in principle, the following three parameters: $R_1, k_2'',$ and ${}^R k_2'$. However, with the same assumption as above regarding V_{ND}, we can write: $k_2'' = R_1 {}^R k_2'/(1 + BP_{ND})$, and thereby, we can obtain BP_{ND} directly as one of three model parameters. A fast, linearized version of SRTM, appropriate for voxel-based analysis, has been proposed [23].

As an illustration, Fig. 16.7 shows simulated data corresponding to the SPECT tracer ^{123}I-ADAM, which binds to serotonin transporters (presynaptic reuptake channels; 5-HTT), and can be used for measuring occupancy of antidepressant drugs. The data were generated based on average parameters from a number of subjects determined using SRTM [24]. Time-activity curves are shown for the midbrain, which is the region with highest 5-HTT concentration, and for cerebellum, which was used as a reference

region. The parameters used were: $R_1 = 0.85$, $k_2' = 0.030$ min^{-1}, and $BP_{ND} = 1.14$.

16.5.2 Spectral Analysis

By combining Equations 16.3 and 16.4 we get:

$$C_T(t) = C_a(t) \otimes \sum_{i=1}^{N} \phi_i e^{-\theta_i t} = \sum_{i=1}^{N} \phi_i \left(C_a(t) \otimes e^{-\theta_i t} \right)$$

$$= \sum_{i=1}^{N} \phi_i \Psi_i(t)$$

In the method of spectral analysis [25], a library of basis functions, $\Psi_i(t)$, is first generated for a suitable range of θ_i values. The problem is then solved using nonnegative least squares fitting, resulting in a limited number of components, with nonzero coefficients, ϕ_i. The number of nonzero components corresponds to the number of model-compartments, which therefore does not need to be determined beforehand. (Two adjacent nonzero coefficients, ϕ_i and ϕ_{i+1} should in this context be regarded as one single component, with a θ value somewhere between θ_i and θ_{i+1}.)

The spectral analysis method is not strictly valid for reference tissue models, where negative components in theory can occur. Therefore, a more general method was later developed using the basis pursuit denoising

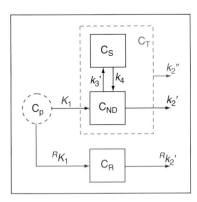

Fig. 16.6 Combined illustration of the full and the simplified reference region models. C_p is the (unknown) concentrations of nonmetabolized tracer in plasma, C_{ND} and C_S are the concentrations of nondisplaceable and specifically bound tracer in the target tissue, respectively, C_T is the total concentration of tracer in tissue, and C_R is the tracer concentration in the reference region. The sets of rate constants corresponding to the full and simplified models are: $\{K_1, k_2', k_3', k_4, {}^R K_1, {}^R k_2'\}$ and $\{K_1, k_2'', {}^R K_1, {}^R k_2'\}$, respectively

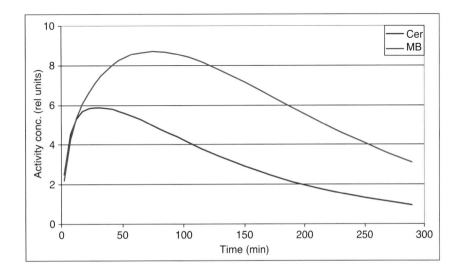

Fig. 16.7 Time-activity curves for the 5-HTT SPECT tracer ^{123}I-ADAM. The two curves represent midbrain (MB) and cerebellum (Cer), which were used as reference regions

technique [26]. Spectral analysis is discussed further in the next chapter.

16.5.3 Graphical Analysis

An alternative approach to solving the differential equations describing the kinetic models is to integrate them. This can yield equations which lend themselves to graphical analysis. The basic idea is that, after an appropriate transformation, the data can be plotted in a graph and a straight line be fitted to the points. The slope and intercept of the fitted line will reflect certain characteristics of the tracer uptake or binding. The Logan method [27] was developed specifically for reversible tracers, and is obtained by plotting $y(t) = \int_0^t C_T(\tau)\mathrm{d}\tau / C_T(t)$ vs. $x(t) = \int_0^t C_p(\tau)\mathrm{d}\tau / C_T(t)$. After a certain amount of time, a straight line is obtained with a slope equal to V_T. This result is independent of the assumed compartmental structure of the model, as shown in Appendix D (Equations 16.36 and 16.37).

This approach is also known as linearization, since it converts a nonlinear parameter estimation problem into a linear one. For this reason, it is also relatively fast, and thereby useful in voxel-based analysis. A limitation of the approach is that it may result in bias with noisy data due to correlation in the noise structure between the dependent and independent variables [28]. A more robust approach has been proposed [29]. A reference region version of the Logan method

has also been developed [30]. There is a corresponding method for irreversible tracers, known as the Patlak plot, which is covered in the next chapter.

16.5.4 The Constant Infusion Approach

In conventional studies, the tracer is administered with a single injection over a short time period – a so called "bolus injection." An alternative approach is to use a constant infusion protocol, where tracer is being continuously administered slowly throughout the experiment. The aim is to establish a true equilibrium situation, which allows for direct estimation of V_T as the ratio of tissue and plasma activity concentration, in accordance with the definition (Equation 16.22) [31]. Equilibrium can be reached more rapidly by using a combination of constant infusion and an initial bolus injection (a "bolus/infusion," B/I, protocol) [32]. This approach is particularly useful in "challenge studies," in which the radiotracer is displaced by a cold competitor. It is also useful in situations when a linear model is not applicable, such as in the case of "multiple ligand concentration receptor assays" [33, 34]. In these studies, low concentrations of the radioligand are used in order to estimate B_{max} and K_D separately. B/I paradigms have also been used in order to avoid arterial sampling by replacing it with venous sampling at equilibrium [35].

Figure 16.8 shows an example of TACs corresponding to a B/I study using the SPECT tracer

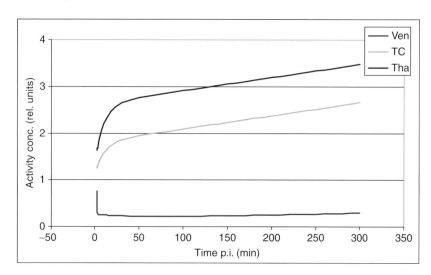

Fig. 16.8 Time-activity curves for the NMDA receptor SPECT tracer ^{123}I-CNS 1261 with bolus-infusion administration. The different curves correspond to venous plasma (Ven), temporal cortex (TC), and thalamus (Tha)

[^{123}I]CNS 1261 [35] (cf. Fig. 16.5). The graph shows curves fitted to data averaged over a number of subjects. For this tracer, a true equilibrium was not reached, since the curves are straight but not horizontal. Therefore a "slope-correction" was needed in the computation of V_T. Model comparison

16.6 Model Comparison

Choosing a quantification method involves a trade-off between bias, variance, and practicality. A model with more parameters will always give a better fit to the data (as judged by the residual sum of squares), but this may be because it is fitting the noise in the data rather than the actual signal. A model with less parameters will lead to less variability in the results, but can also lead to bias, if the model does not properly describe the underlying physiological or biochemical processes. There are various statistical methods for determining the best model to use, based on the residuals of the fit and on the number of parameters [36–38]. The use of various different models and comparison of the estimated outcome measures is an approach that has been recommended in order to avoid systematic errors related to one particular model. In terms of practicality, it may be appropriate to also consider methods based on simplified data acquisition protocols, such as reference tissue methods, constant infusion methods, or even methods based on single scan protocols. However, these methods should always first be validated versus more complex and accurate ones (see e.g., [39]). The next chapter includes further discussions on model selection.

16.7 Applications – Schizophrenia

PET and SPECT studies have been used for many years in psychiatric research. A wide range of tracers have been developed for imaging different neurotransmitter (especially dopamine and serotonin) systems. These tracers have allowed for studies which aid in the drug development process by providing information on drug delivery, mechanism of action, and occupancy levels at targets of interest. Below, we present some illustrative examples, based on work from the research career of Prof. Lyn S Pilowsky, who sadly passed away in 2007.

Antipsychotic drugs are used for treatment of schizophrenic patients, and their therapeutic effect is believed to be related to blockade of postsynaptic dopamine D_2-receptors. They can be classified into two groups: Typical and atypical (or first and second generation) drugs. The atypical antipsychotics are advantageous in that they produce less Parkinsonian side effects than the typical ones, while preserving high clinical efficacy. Pilowsky et al. [40] used the SPECT tracer ^{123}I-IBZM to compare the atypical drug Clozapine with the typical drug Haloperidol. They showed that Clozapine produced a lower level of D_2/D_3 receptor blockade in the striatum (a central brain structure), which would explain the lower level of Parkinsonian side effects.

Different theories emerged regarding the mechanism of action of atypical drugs, involving either different receptor types or different brain regions. To investigate the importance of blocking serotonin-(5-HT) 2A receptors, Travis et al. [41] used the SPECT tracer ^{123}I-R91150, and found no correlation between clinical efficacy of atypical antipsychotics and 5-HT$_{2A}$ receptor blockade. In order to investigate the extrastriatal D_2 receptor blockade, Pilowsky et al. [42] used ^{123}I-epidepride, a D_2/D_3 receptor tracer with higher affinity than ^{123}I-IBZM. The higher affinity was needed due to the much lower concentration of D_2 receptors outside the striatum. They found that, while typical antipsychotics produces high D_2 receptor occupancy in both striatal and extrastriatal regions (temporal cortex), Clozapine produced high occupancy only in extrastriatal regions. This could explain the clinical efficacy of atypical drugs with low Parkinsonian side effects. However, this finding remained controversial for some time due to methodological issues, which were eventually solved [43]. The finding was also supported by the results of a recent meta-analysis, which pools data from several published PET and SPECT studies [44].

16.8 Conclusions

In this chapter, we have described the basic mathematical tools and concepts used in tracer kinetic modeling for quantification of physiological or biochemical parameters *in vivo* with PET or SPECT. Summaries of the basic theory discussed here can be found in [45, 46]. The next chapter describes various methods used in practice for parameter estimation and discuss some examples of practical applications. Finally, as a word of caution, I would just like to remind the reader that: "All models are wrong, but some are useful."[2]

Acknowledgments The author would like to thank Prof. Brian F Hutton (University College London, UK) and Prof. Roger N Gunn (Glaxo Smith Kline, London, UK and University of Oxford, UK) for valuable comments and suggestions.

Appendix A – Compartmental Models

Expressions for the impulse response functions for the 1-TC and 2-TC models are derived below. $L\{\cdot\}$ represents the Laplace transform, Laplace-domain functions are identified with a tilde, and s is a complex Laplace domain variable.

The 1-TC Model

$$\frac{\mathrm{d}}{\mathrm{d}t}C_T(t) = K_1 C_p(t) - k_2'' C_T(t)$$

$$\Leftrightarrow$$

$$L\left\{\frac{\mathrm{d}}{\mathrm{d}t}C_T(t)\right\} = L\{K_1 C_p(t) - k_2'' C_T(t)\}$$

$$\Leftrightarrow$$

$$s\hat{C}_T(s) - C_T(0) = K_1 \hat{C}_p(s) - k_2'' \hat{C}_T(s)$$

$$\Rightarrow$$

With initial condition, $C_T(0){=}0$:

$$\hat{C}_T(s) = \frac{K_1}{s + k_2''}\hat{C}_p(s) \tag{16.25}$$

$$\Leftrightarrow$$

$$C_T(t) = K_1 \mathrm{e}^{-k_2'' t} \otimes C_p(t)$$

$$\Leftrightarrow$$

Impulse response function:

$$H_1(t) = K_1 \mathrm{e}^{-k_2'' t} \tag{16.26}$$

The 2-TC Model

$$\begin{cases} \dfrac{\mathrm{d}}{\mathrm{d}t}C_{ND}(t) = K_1 C_p(t) - (k_2' + k_3')C_{ND}(t) + k_4 C_S(t) \\ \dfrac{\mathrm{d}}{\mathrm{d}t}C_S(t) = k_3' C_{ND}(t) - k_4 C_S(t) \end{cases}$$

$$\Leftrightarrow$$

$$\begin{cases} s\hat{C}_{ND}(s) - C_{ND}(0) = K_1 \hat{C}_p(s) - (k_2' + k_3')\hat{C}_{ND}(s) + k_4 \hat{C}_S(s) \\ s\hat{C}_S(s) - C_S(0) = k_3' \hat{C}_{ND}(s) - k_4 \hat{C}_S(s) \end{cases}$$

With initial conditions, $C_{ND}(0) = C_S(0) = 0$:

$$\Rightarrow$$

$$\begin{cases} (s + k_2' + k_3')\hat{C}_{ND}(s) = K_1 \hat{C}_p(s) + k_4 \hat{C}_S(s) \\ (s + k_4)\hat{C}_S(s) = k_3' \hat{C}_{ND}(s) \end{cases}$$

$$\Leftrightarrow$$

$$\begin{cases} \hat{C}_{ND}(s) = \left(s + k_2' + k_3' - \dfrac{k_3' k_4}{s + k_4}\right)^{-1} K_1 \hat{C}_p(s) \\ \hat{C}_S(s) = \dfrac{k_3'}{s + k_4}\hat{C}_{ND}(s) \end{cases}$$

$$\Rightarrow$$

$$\hat{C}_T(s) \equiv \hat{C}_{ND}(s) + \hat{C}_S(s) = \left(1 + \frac{k_3'}{s + k_4}\right)\hat{C}_{ND}(s)$$

$$= \left(\frac{s + k_3' + k_4}{s + k_4}\right)\left(\frac{s + k_4}{(s + k_2' + k_3')(s + k_4) - k_3' k_4}\right)K_1 \hat{C}_p(s)$$

$$= \left(\frac{s + k_3' + k_4}{s^2 + (k_2' + k_3' + k_4)s + k_2' k_4}\right)K_1 \hat{C}_p(s) \tag{16.27}$$

Find poles:

$$s^2 + (k_2' + k_3' + k_4)s + k_2' k_4 = 0$$

$$\Leftrightarrow$$

$$s = -\frac{1}{2}\left(k_2' + k_3' + k_4 \mp \sqrt{(k_2' + k_3' + k_4)^2 - 4k_2' k_4}\right) \equiv -\theta_{1,2}$$

$$\sim \sim \sim$$

---

[2] Quote usually attributed to George Box.

Partial fraction expansion:

$$\frac{\phi_1}{s+\theta_1} + \frac{\phi_2}{s+\theta_2} = K_1 \frac{s + k_3' + k_4}{s^2 + (k_2' + k_3' + k_4)s + k_2'k_4}$$
$$(16.28)$$

$$\Leftrightarrow$$

$$\begin{cases} \phi_1 = K_1 \dfrac{k_3' + k_4 - \theta_1}{\theta_2 - \theta_1} \\[2mm] \phi_2 = -K_1 \dfrac{k_3' + k_4 - \theta_2}{\theta_2 - \theta_1} \end{cases}$$

$$\sim \sim \sim$$

$$(16.27) + (16.28)$$

$$\Rightarrow$$

$$\hat{C}_T(s) = \left(\frac{\phi_1}{s+\theta_1} + \frac{\phi_2}{s+\theta_2} \right) \hat{C}_p(s) \qquad (16.29)$$

$$\Leftrightarrow$$

$$C_T(t) = \left(\phi_1 e^{-\theta_1 t} + \phi_2 e^{-\theta_2 t} \right) \otimes C_p(t)$$

$$\Leftrightarrow$$

Impulse response function:

$$H_2(t) = \phi_1 e^{-\theta_1 t} + \phi_2 e^{-\theta_2 t} \qquad (16.30)$$

Appendix B – Outcome Measures

Volume of Distribution

For the 1-TC model we obtain:

$$\frac{\mathrm{d}}{\mathrm{d}t} C_T(t) = K_1 C_p(t) - k_2'' C_T(t) = 0$$

$$\Rightarrow \qquad\qquad (16.31a)$$

$$V_T \equiv \left[\frac{C_T(t)}{C_p(t)} \right]_{eq} = \frac{K_1}{k_2''}$$

for the 2-TC model:

$$\begin{cases} \dfrac{\mathrm{d}}{\mathrm{d}t} C_{ND}(t) = K_1 C_p(t) - (k_2' + k_3')C_{ND}(t) + k_4 C_S(t) = 0 \\[2mm] \dfrac{\mathrm{d}}{\mathrm{d}t} C_S(t) = k_3' C_{ND}(t) - k_4 C_S(t) = 0 \end{cases}$$

$$\Rightarrow$$

$$\begin{cases} \left[\dfrac{C_{ND}(t)}{C_p(t)} \right]_{eq} = \dfrac{K_1}{k_2'} \\[3mm] \left[\dfrac{C_S(t)}{C_{ND}(t)} \right]_{eq} = \dfrac{k_3'}{k_4} \end{cases} \qquad (16.31b)$$

$$\Rightarrow$$

$$V_T \equiv \left[\frac{C_{ND}(t) + C_S(t)}{C_p(t)} \right]_{eq} = \left[\frac{C_{ND}(t)(1 + k_3'/k_4)}{C_p(t)} \right]_{eq}$$
$$= \frac{K_1}{k_2'} \left(1 + \frac{k_3'}{k_4} \right)$$

and similarly for the 3-TC model:

$$V_T \equiv \left[\frac{C_F(t) + C_{NS}(t) + C_S(t)}{C_p(t)} \right]_{eq}$$
$$= \frac{K_1}{k_2} \left(1 + \frac{k_3}{k_4} + \frac{k_5}{k_6} \right) \qquad (16.31c)$$

Binding Potential

Expressions for calculating BP_F from different model parameters can be derived as shown below, using the identities $k_3 = k_{on}B_{avail}$, $k_4 = k_{off}$, $k_3' = f_{ND}k_3$, $k_2' = f_{ND}k_2$, and $K_1/k_2 = f_p$ (from $f_p[C_p]_{eq} = [C_F]_{eq}$ and $K_1[C_p]_{eq} = k_2[C_F]_{eq}$):

$$BP \equiv \frac{B_{max}}{K_D} \geq BP_F \equiv \frac{B_{avail}}{K_D} = \frac{B_{avail}k_{on}}{k_{off}} = \frac{k_3}{k_4}$$
$$= (1/f_{ND})(k_3'/k_4) = \frac{1}{f_p}\frac{K_1 k_3'}{k_2' k_4}$$
$$(16.32)$$

Appendix C – Reference Tissue Models

The Simplified Reference Tissue Model

$$\begin{cases} \dfrac{\mathrm{d}}{\mathrm{d}t} C_T(t) = K_1 C_p(t) - k_2'' C_T(t) \\[2mm] \dfrac{\mathrm{d}}{\mathrm{d}t} C_R(t) = {}^R K_1 C_p(t) - {}^R k_2' C_R(t) \end{cases}$$

$$\Leftrightarrow$$

From (16.25):

$$\begin{cases} \hat{C}_T(s) = \dfrac{K_1}{s + k_2''} \hat{C}_p(s) \\[2mm] \hat{C}_R(s) = \dfrac{{}^R K_1}{s + {}^R k_2'} \hat{C}_p(s) \end{cases}$$

$$\Rightarrow$$

$$\left(\text{with } R_1 = \dfrac{K_1}{{}^R K_1} \right):$$

$$\hat{C}_T(s) = R_1 \dfrac{s + {}^R k_2'}{s + k_2''} \hat{C}_R(s)$$

$$= R_1 \hat{C}_R(s) + R_1 \dfrac{{}^R k_2' - k_2''}{s + k_2''} \hat{C}_R(s)$$

$$\Rightarrow$$

$$C_T(t) = R_1 C_R(t) + R_1 \left({}^R k_2' - k_2'' \right) e^{-k_2'' t} \otimes C_R(t)$$

$$\Leftrightarrow$$

Impulse response function:

$$H_{1R}(t) = R_1 \delta(t) + R_1 \left({}^R k_2' - k_2'' \right) e^{-k_2'' t} \qquad (16.33)$$

where $\delta(t)$ is the Dirac delta-function.

The Full Reference Tissue Model

$$\begin{cases} \dfrac{d}{dt} C_{ND}(t) = K_1 C_p(t) - (k_2' + k_3') C_{ND}(t) + k_4 C_S(t) \\[2mm] \dfrac{d}{dt} C_S(t) = k_3' C_{ND}(t) - k_4 C_S(t) \\[2mm] \dfrac{d}{dt} C_R(t) = {}^R K_1 C_p(t) - {}^R k_2' C_R(t) \end{cases}$$

From (16.25) and (16.29):

$$\begin{cases} \hat{C}_T(s) = \left(\dfrac{\phi_1}{s + \theta_1} + \dfrac{\phi_2}{s + \theta_2} \right) \hat{C}_p(s) \\[2mm] \hat{C}_R(s) = \dfrac{{}^R K_1}{s + {}^R k_2'} \hat{C}_p(s) \end{cases}$$

$$\Rightarrow$$

$$\hat{C}_T(s) = \left(\dfrac{\phi_1}{s + \theta_1} + \dfrac{\phi_2}{s + \theta_2} \right) \dfrac{s + {}^R k_2'}{{}^R K_1} \hat{C}_R(s)$$

$$\Leftrightarrow$$

$$\left(\text{with } R_1 = \dfrac{K_1}{{}^R K_1} \right):$$

$$\hat{C}_T(s) = \dfrac{R_1}{\theta_2 - \theta_1} \left(\dfrac{k_3' + k_4 - \theta_1}{s + \theta_1} - \dfrac{k_3' + k_4 - \theta_2}{s + \theta_2} \right)$$

$$\times \left(s + {}^R k_2' \right) \hat{C}_R(s)$$

$$= \dfrac{R_1}{\theta_2 - \theta_1} \left((k_3' + k_4 - \theta_1) \left(1 + \dfrac{{}^R k_2' - \theta_1}{s + \theta_1} \right) \right.$$

$$\left. - (k_3' + k_4 - \theta_2) \left(1 + \dfrac{{}^R k_2' - \theta_2}{s + \theta_2} \right) \right) \hat{C}_R(s)$$

$$= R_1 \hat{C}_R(s) + \dfrac{R_1}{\theta_2 - \theta_1} \left(\dfrac{(k_3' + k_4 - \theta_1)({}^R k_2' - \theta_1)}{s + \theta_1} \right.$$

$$\left. - \dfrac{(k_3' + k_4 - \theta_2)({}^R k_2' - \theta_2)}{s + \theta_2} \right) \hat{C}_R(s)$$

$$\Leftrightarrow$$

$$\hat{C}_T(s) = R_1 \hat{C}_R(s)$$

$$+ \left(\dfrac{\rho_1}{s + \theta_1} + \dfrac{\rho_2}{s + \theta_2} \right) \hat{C}_R(s) \qquad (16.34)$$

where

$$\begin{cases} \rho_1 = R_1 \dfrac{(k_3' + k_4 - \theta_1)({}^R k_2' - \theta_1)}{\theta_2 - \theta_1} \\[3mm] \rho_2 = -R_1 \dfrac{(k_3' + k_4 - \theta_2)({}^R k_2' - \theta_2)}{\theta_2 - \theta_1} \end{cases}$$

$$\sim \sim \sim$$

$$(16.34)$$

$$\Rightarrow$$

$$C_T(t) = R_1 C_R(t) + \left(\rho_1 e^{-\theta_1 t} + \rho_2 e^{-\theta_2 t} \right) \otimes C_R(t)$$

$$\Leftrightarrow$$

Impulse response function:

$$H_{2R}(t) = R_1 \delta(t) + \rho_1 e^{-\theta_1 t} + \rho_2 e^{-\theta_2 t} \qquad (16.35)$$

Appendix D – Logan Graphical Analysis

1-TC Model

$$\frac{\mathrm{d}}{\mathrm{d}t}C_T(t) = K_1 C_p(t) - k_2'' C_T(t)$$

$$\Leftrightarrow$$

$$C_T(t) - C_T(0) = K_1 \int_0^t C_p(\tau)\mathrm{d}\tau - k_2'' \int_0^t C_T(\tau)\mathrm{d}\tau$$

with $C_T(0)=0$:

$$\Leftrightarrow$$

$$\frac{\int_0^t C_T(\tau)\mathrm{d}\tau}{C_T(t)} = \frac{K_1}{k_2''}\frac{\int_0^t C_p(\tau)\mathrm{d}\tau}{C_T(t)} - \frac{1}{k_2''}$$

$$\Rightarrow$$

$$\frac{\int_0^t C_T(\tau)\mathrm{d}\tau}{C_T(t)} = V_T \frac{\int_0^t C_p(\tau)\mathrm{d}\tau}{C_T(t)} + const. \qquad (16.36)$$

2-TC Model

$$\begin{cases} \frac{\mathrm{d}}{\mathrm{d}t}C_{ND}(t) = K_1 C_p(t) - (k_2' + k_3')C_{ND}(t) + k_4 C_S(t) \\ \frac{\mathrm{d}}{\mathrm{d}t}C_S(t) = k_3' C_{ND}(t) - k_4 C_S(t) \end{cases}$$

$$\Leftrightarrow$$

$$\begin{cases} C_{ND}(t) - C_{ND}(0) = K_1 \int_0^t C_p(\tau)\mathrm{d}\tau - (k_2' + k_3') \\ \qquad\qquad \times \int_0^t C_{ND}(\tau)\mathrm{d}\tau + k_4 \int_0^t C_S(\tau)\mathrm{d}\tau \\ C_S(t) - C_S(0) = k_3' \int_0^t C_{ND}(\tau)\mathrm{d}\tau - k_4 \int_0^t C_S(\tau)\mathrm{d}\tau \end{cases}$$

with $C_{ND}(0)=C_S(0)=0$:

$$\Leftrightarrow$$

$$\begin{cases} C_T(t) = K_1 \int_0^t C_p(\tau)\mathrm{d}\tau - k_2' \int_0^t C_{ND}(\tau)\mathrm{d}\tau \\ C_S(t) = k_3' \int_0^t C_{ND}(\tau)\mathrm{d}\tau - k_4 \int_0^t C_S(\tau)\mathrm{d}\tau \end{cases}$$

$$\Leftrightarrow$$

$$\begin{cases} \dfrac{\int_0^t C_{ND}(\tau)\mathrm{d}\tau}{C_T(t)} = \dfrac{K_1}{k_2'}\dfrac{\int_0^t C_p(\tau)\mathrm{d}\tau}{C_T(t)} - \dfrac{1}{k_2'} \\ \dfrac{\int_0^t C_S(\tau)\mathrm{d}\tau}{C_T(t)} = \dfrac{k_3'}{k_4}\dfrac{\int_0^t C_{ND}(\tau)\mathrm{d}\tau}{C_T(t)} - \dfrac{1}{k_4}\dfrac{C_S(t)}{C_T(t)} \end{cases}$$

$$\Rightarrow$$

$$\frac{\int_0^t C_T(\tau)\mathrm{d}\tau}{C_T(t)} \equiv \frac{\int_0^t C_{ND}(\tau) + C_S(\tau)\mathrm{d}\tau}{C_T(t)} = \frac{K_1}{k_2'}\frac{\int_0^t C_p(\tau)\mathrm{d}\tau}{C_T(t)}$$

$$-\frac{1}{k_2'} + \frac{k_3'}{k_4}\left(\frac{K_1}{k_2'}\frac{\int_0^t C_p(\tau)\mathrm{d}\tau}{C_T(t)} - \frac{1}{k_2'}\right)$$

$$-\frac{1}{k_4}\frac{C_S(t)}{C_T(t)}$$

$$= \frac{K_1}{k_2'}\left(1 + \frac{k_3'}{k_4}\right)\frac{\int_0^t C_p(\tau)\mathrm{d}\tau}{C_T(t)} - \frac{1}{k_2'}\left(1 + \frac{k_3'}{k_4}\right)$$

$$-\frac{1}{k_4}\frac{C_S(t)}{C_T(t)}$$

$$\Leftrightarrow$$

$$\frac{\int_0^t C_T(\tau)\mathrm{d}\tau}{C_T(t)} = V_T \frac{\int_0^t C_p(\tau)\mathrm{d}\tau}{C_T(t)} - \frac{1}{k_2''} - \frac{1}{k_4}\frac{C_S(t)}{C_T(t)}$$

$$\Rightarrow$$

with $C_S(t)/C_T(t)$=constant (pseudoequilibrium):

$$\frac{\int_0^t C_T(\tau)\mathrm{d}\tau}{C_T(t)} = V_T \frac{\int_0^t C_p(\tau)\mathrm{d}\tau}{C_T(t)} + const. \qquad (16.37)$$

References

1. Cunningham VJ, Gunn RN, Matthews JC (2004) Quantification in positron emission tomography for research in pharmacology and drug development. Nucl Med Commun 25:643–646

2. Laruelle M (2000) The role of model-based methods in the development of single scan techniques. Nucl Med Biol 27:637–642

3. Carson RE (1991) The development and application of mathematical models in nuclear medicine. J Nucl Med 32:2206–2208

4. Leenders KL (2003) In: PET pharmacokinetic course manual. Maguire RP, Leenders KL (eds) Chap. 1, University of Groningen, Groningen, The Netherlands and McGill University, Canada

5. Gunn RN, Gunn SR, Cunningham VJ (2001) Positron emission tomography compartmental models. J Cereb Blood Flow Metab 21:635–652

6. Arfken G (1985) Mathematical methods for physicists. Academic, San Diego

7. Press WH, Teukolsky SA, Vetterling WT, Flannery BP (1992) Numerical recipes in C: the art of scientific computing. Cambridge University Press, Cambridge

8. Innis RB, Cunningham VJ, Delforge J, Fujita M, Gjedde A, Gunn RN, Holden J, Houle S, Huang SC, Ichise M, Iida H, Ito H, Kimura Y, Koeppe RA, Knudsen GM, Knuuti J, Lammertsma AA, Laruelle M, Logan J, Maguire RP, Mintun MA, Morris ED, Parsey R, Price JC, Slifstein M, Sossi V, Suhara T, Votaw JR, Wong DF, Carson RE (2007) Consensus nomenclature for in vivo imaging of reversibly binding radioligands. J Cereb Blood Flow Metab 27:1533–1539

9. Kety SS, Schmidt CF (1948) The nitrous oxide method for the quantitative determination of cerebral blood flow in man: theory, procedure and normal values. J Clin Investig 27:476–483

10. Kety SS (1951) The theory and applications of the exchange of inert gas at the lungs and tissues. Pharmacol Rev 3:1–41

11. Renkin EM (1959) Transport of potassium-42 from blood to tissue in isolated mammalian skeletal muscles. Am J Physiol 197:1205–1210

12. Crone C (1963) The permeability of capillaries in various organs as determined by use of the "indicator diffusion" method. Acta Physiol Scand 58:292–305

13. Kerwin RW, Pilowsky LS (1995) Traditional receptor theory and its application to neuroreceptor measurements in functional imaging. Eur J Nucl Med 22:699–710

14. Michaelis L, Menten ML (1913) Die kinetik der invertinwirkung. Biochem Z 49:1333

15. Scatchard G (1949) The attractions of proteins for small molecules and ions. Ann NY Acad Sci 51:660–665

16. Mintun MA, Raichle ME, Kilbourn MR, Wooten GF, Welch MJ (1984) A quantitative model for the in vivo assessment of drug binding sites with positron emission tomography. Ann Neurol 15:217–227

17. Scheibe PO (2003) Identifiability analysis of second-order systems. Nucl Med Biol 30:827–832

18. Koeppe RA, Holthoff VA, Frey KA, Kilbourn MR, Kuhl DE (1991) Compartmental analysis of [^{11}C]flumazenil kinetics for the estimation of ligand transport rate and receptor distribution using positron emission tomography. J Cereb Blood Flow Metab 11:735–744

19. Erlandsson K, Bressan RA, Mulligan RS, Gunn RN, Cunningham VJ, Owens J, Wyper D, Ell PJ, Pilowsky LS (2003) Kinetic modelling of [^{123}I]-CNS 1261 – a novel SPET tracer for the NMDA receptor. Nucl Med Biol 30:441–454

20. Cunningham VJ, Hume SP, Price GR, Ahier RG, Cremer JE, Jones AK (1991) Compartmental analysis of diprenorphine binding to opiate receptors in the rat in vivo and its comparison with equilibrium data in vitro. J Cereb Blood Flow Metab 11:1–9

21. Lammertsma AA, Bench CJ, Hume SP, Osman S, Gunn K, Brooks DJ, Frackowiak RS (1996) Comparison of methods for analysis of clinical [^{11}C]raclopride studies. J Cereb Blood Flow Metab 16:42–52

22. Lammertsma AA, Hume SP (1996) Simplified reference tissue model for PET receptor studies. Neuroimage 4:153–158

23. Gunn RN, Lammertsma AA, Hume SP, Cunningham VJ (1997) Parametric imaging of ligand-receptor binding in PET using a simplified reference region model. Neuroimage 6:279–287

24. Erlandsson K, Sivananthan T, Lui D, Spezzi A, Townsend CE, Mu S, Lucas R, Warrington S, Ell PJ (2005) Measuring SSRI occupancy of SERT using the novel tracer [^{123}I] ADAM: a SPECT validation study. Eur J Nucl Med Mol Imaging 32:329–336

25. Cunningham VJ, Jones T (1993) Spectral analysis of dynamic PET studies. J Cereb Blood Flow Metab 13:15–23

26. Gunn RN, Gunn SR, Turkheimer FE, Aston JAD, Cunningham VJ (2002) Positron emission tomography compartmental models: A basis pursuit strategy for kinetic modelling. J Cereb Blood Flow Metab 22:1425–1439

27. Logan J, Fowler JS, Volkow ND, Wolf AP, Dewey SL, Schlyer DJ, MacGregor RR, Hitzemann R, Bendriem B, Gatley SJ et al (1990) Graphical analysis of reversible radioligand binding from time-activity measurements applied to [N-^{11}C-methyl]-(–)-cocaine PET studies in human subjects. J Cereb Blood Flow Metab 10:740–747

28. Slifstein M, Laruelle M (2000) Effects of statistical noise on graphic analysis of PET neuroreceptor studies. J Nucl Med 41:2083–2088

29. Ogden RT (2003) Estimation of kinetic parameters in graphical analysis of PET imaging data. Stat Med 22:3557–3568

30. Logan J, Fowler JS, Volkow ND, Wang GJ, Ding YS, Alexoff DL (1996) Distribution volume ratios without blood sampling from graphical analysis of PET data. J Cereb Blood Flow Metab 16:834–840

31. Carson RE (2000) PET physiological measurements using constant infusion. Nucl Med Biol 27:657–660

32. Carson RE, Channing MA, Blasberg RG, Dunn BB, Cohen RM, Rice KC, Herscovitch P (1993) Comparison of bolus and infusion methods for receptor quantitation: application to [^{18}F]cyclofoxy and positron emission tomography. J Cereb Blood Flow Metab 13:24–42

33. Kawai R, Carson RE, Dunn B, Newman AH, Rice KC, Blasberg RG (1991) Regional brain measurement of Bmax and KD with the opiate antagonist cyclofoxy: equilibrium studies in the conscious rat. J Cereb Blood Flow Metab 11:529–544

34. Holden JE, Jivan S, Ruth TJ, Doudet DJ (2002) *In vivo* receptor assay with multiple ligand concentrations: an equilibrium approach. J Cereb Blood Flow Metab 22:1132–1141

35. Bressan RA, Erlandsson K, Mulligan RS, Gunn RN, Cunningham VJ, Owens J, Cullum ID, Ell PJ, Pilowsky LS (2004) A bolus/infusion paradigm for the novel NMDA receptor SPET tracer $[^{123}$I]CNS 1261. Nucl Med Biol 31:155–164

36. Akaike H (1974) A new look at the statistical model identification. IEEE Trans Automat Contr 19:716–723

37. Cunningham VJ (1985) Non-linear regression techniques in data analysis. Med Inform (Lond) 10:137–142

38. Schwarz G (1978) Estimating the dimension of a model. Ann Statist 6:461–464

39. Ogden RT, Ojha A, Erlandsson K, Oquendo MA, Mann JJ, Parsey RV (2007) *In vivo* quantification of serotonin transporters using $[^{11}$C]DASB and positron emission tomography in humans: modeling considerations. J Cereb Blood Flow Metab 27:205–217

40. Pilowsky LS, Costa DC, Ell PJ, Murray RM, Verhoeff NP, Kerwin RW (1992) Clozapine, single photon emission tomography, and the D2 dopamine receptor blockade hypothesis of schizophrenia. Lancet 340:199–202

41. Travis MJ, Busatto GF, Pilowsky LS, Mulligan R, Acton PD, Gacinovic S, Mertens J, Terriere D, Costa DC, Ell PJ, Kerwin RW (1998) 5-HT2A receptor blockade in patients with schizophrenia treated with risperidone or clozapine. A SPET study using the novel 5-HT2A ligand ^{123}I-5-I-R-91150. Br J Psychiatry 173:236–241

42. Pilowsky LS, Mulligan RS, Acton PD, Ell PJ, Costa DC, Kerwin RW (1997) Limbic selectivity of clozapine. Lancet 350:490–491

43. Erlandsson K, Bressan RA, Mulligan RS, Ell PJ, Cunningham VJ, Pilowsky LS (2003) Analysis of D2 dopamine receptor occupancy with quantitative SPET using the high-affinity ligand $[^{123}$I]epidepride: resolving conflicting findings. Neuroimage 19:1205–1214

44. Stone JM, Davis JM, Leucht S, Pilowsky LS (2009) Cortical dopamine D2/D3 receptors are a common site of action for antipsychotic drugs – an original patient data meta-analysis of the SPECT and PET in vivo receptor imaging literature. Schizophrenia Bulletin 35:789–797

45. Ichise M, Meyer JH, Yonekura Y (2001) An introduction to PET and SPECT neuroreceptor quantification models. J Nucl Med 42:755–763

46. Slifstein M, Laruelle M (2001) Models and methods for derivation of in vivo neuroreceptor parameters with PET and SPECT reversible radiotracers. Nucl Med Biol 28:595–608

Tracer Kinetic Modeling: Methodology and Applications

17

M'hamed Bentourkia

Contents

17.1 Introduction

Positron emission tomography (PET) is a medical imaging technique based on the simultaneous detection of pairs of 511-keV gamma radiations emitted by the annihilation of positrons within the subject following administration of a radiotracer. The radiotracer could be any pharmacological molecule or a natural molecule, such as water ($H_2{}^{15}O$) or carbon monoxide (^{11}CO, $C^{15}O$), where an atom or a group of atoms are replaced with a positron emitting isotope. These two particularities (i.e., radiation emission and radiotracer labeling) provide the functionality and the versatility of PET. In addition, the use of PET to measure noninvasively biochemical and physiological reactions in a tissue as a function of time greatly contributes to a new avenue in medicine. PET has a picomolar sensitivity and can acquire images in frames of 10 s in humans and almost 3 s in small animals, providing dynamic insights in living tissues. Moreover, and since a tissue can be imaged by an appropriate radiotracer, both diseased and healthy tissues can be measured by PET. Among such applications are cancer and cognitive studies. These advantageous particularities of PET are exploited, however, at a substantially high cost, which can mainly be because of the necessity to include a cyclotron as part of the imaging center and to involve radiochemists or radiopharmacists and physicists to work within the same team in addition to clinicians.

If the technology of PET allows the calculation of physiological parameters and provides parametric images, these calculated parameters are subject to some hindrances, among them the low spatial resolution, the partial volume effect (PVE), the scattered radiation, the parallax error, and others. Because the dose of radiotracer administered to the patient is limited, the imaging apparatus is based on larger crystals (detectors) to possibly count enough of the emitted photons to produce an acceptable image for visual observations or for quantification The result of this constraint is the limitation of the spatial resolution, which translates to a non- or partial detection of small-size objects, such as small tumors or blood vessels [1–4]. By the same process, if a small-size object is detected, the intensity of this object in the image appears underestimated due to the PVE [5–11]. The PVE not only reduces the intensity of the signal but also expands it to its surrounding.

M. Bentourkia
Department of Nuclear Medicine and Radiobiology, Université de Sherbrooke, Canada
e-mail: Mhamed.Bentourkia@USherbrooke.ca

M.M. Khalil (ed.), *Basic Sciences of Nuclear Medicine*, DOI: 10.1007/978-3-540-85962-8_17,
© Springer-Verlag Berlin Heidelberg 2011

In PET imaging, the most important factors affecting the images are the attenuation and scatter. The emitted photons at a site in the subject do not all reach the detectors. Most of the photons in whole-body scanners are subject to deflections by Compton interactions at certain angles and with decreased energies. The energy window settings for photon detection, for which the lower bound is generally set around 400 keV, could reduce the number of detected scattered photons, mainly those at large angles (i.e., at low energies). Accordingly, because of the energy resolution of the detection system, the energy discrimination unfortunately accepts the scattered photons at high energy and reduces the number of the nonscattered photons. Meanwhile, the scatter correction procedures appreciably correct for scatter [12]. The attenuated photons can be compensated by measuring the subject densities, and this is accomplished by transmission measurements with rotating sources or using x-ray images obtained with a computed tomographic (CT) scanner. The rotating sources generate noisy transmission images and necessitate a longer scanning time, while the CT scanner, even faster, provides high-resolution images but at energies of 30–120 keV in comparison to the 511 keV in PET emission. A conversion is thus necessary, which could produce a bias [13–18].

The image reconstruction, either statistical or analytical, generates errors at two levels. First, there is a trade-off between the preservation of the spatial resolution and the noise in the images. A cutoff in the frequency for the analytical image reconstruction procedures, mainly filtered backprojection (FBP), is equivalent to lowering the number of iterations in iterative procedures (maximum likelihood-expectation maximization, MLEM; ordered subsets expectation maximization, OSEM, etc.), and both produce smooth images [19–26]. Second, a uniform image reconstruction procedure applied to data dynamically acquired in time frames of different durations and of different statistics depending on the dose and duration of the radiotracer injection, on the tissue uptake and accumulation of the radiotracer, and on the metabolites could not be appropriate.

At the beginning of medical imaging, there was image reconstruction to visually observe tissue behavior or pathologies. Until now, in clinical imaging, image reconstruction is mandatory on the whole for diagnoses. Visual observations are subjective, and some clinicians are attempted to apply quantitative alternatives such as contrast rates and standard uptake values (SUVs). In research, however, the operators rely on kinetic modeling to extract physiological parameters that could be compared to other subject values or to values extracted from the same subject data in different conditions or at different times. The kinetic modeling procedure allows representation of the dynamically acquired images of a specific tissue in terms of subprocesses. These subprocesses reflect the molecular interactions of the radiotracer in tissue. The biochemical transformations of the radiotracer are governed by rate constants. Only the labeled molecules are measured. The formed molecules, after the dissociation of the radiotracer, can be recombined to form the previous molecule. Rather than looking at an intensity image as a whole where the radiotracer can be in the blood vessels, in the interstitial space, or in any form within the cells, the kinetic modeling allows extraction of an image of a single state of the radiotracer or of a single rate constant. If a process is fast, it can be ignored, and this depends on the framing time resolution. In practice, each biochemical process is represented by a compartment, and the compartments are linked by rate constants. The kinetic modeling can be applied to a homogeneous region of interest (ROI) or to voxels considered individually. The kinetic model satisfactorily adjusts an ROI since the time course of this ROI is made of an average over several voxels. Meanwhile, the individual voxels having noisy time-activity curves (TACs) are difficult to adjust. However, if the noise in the voxels is acceptable, this procedure produces parametric images more useful than ROI fitting.

In PET imaging, an image voxel is a measure of the radioactivity emerging from several tissue cells, from the extravascular and extracellular space, and from the capillaries perfusing the tissue. When applying kinetic modeling, the compartments of the concentration of the radiotracer in blood and in tissue in any form are included. The cells represented by a single voxel could not be homogeneous; thus, the kinetic model generates averaged parameter values for the voxel. If we compare a voxel in the image to a coincidence in the projection space, they would be comparable as in both cases the intensities include contributions from different cells and from different components, except that in the projection the intensity is summed in a tube over several emitting sites in the subject, which produces more statistics in the projection TAC, thus facilitating its adjustment with the model and providing more accurate kinetic parameters. The accuracy in kinetic modeling at the projection level is more appreciated when we think that there are no more inaccuracies introduced by the reconstruction procedures as described here, and that a single parametric image can be optimally reconstructed. Meanwhile, image voxels or voxels grouped in an ROI could be considered representing a homogeneous tissue, thus providing more precise kinetic parameters than from projections that provide global parameters. A few authors explored the possibility of calculating parametric images from the projections, and this technique is not yet popular [27–36].

The factors affecting the calculated parameter values as discussed can be considered as physical factors inherent in PET imaging. Other factors, such as the definition of the imaging protocol, the choice of the appropriate kinetic model, and the determination of the input function, can be considered methodological factors.

A kinetic model aims at calculating specific physiological parameters. The biochemical transformations of the radiotracer in the tissue should be known; alternatively, when established with PET, the processes should be validated by other quantitative techniques. The calculated parameters should also be confirmed by a gold standard technique that includes the units of the parameter of interest. The PET imaging should contribute more emphasis than the other techniques due to its functionality, versatility in using quasi-unlimited labeled radiotracers, specificity, and sensitivity.

In the present chapter, we focus on the kinetic modeling from the images. We discuss the effects of the physical and methodological factors on the accuracy of the kinetic parameters.

17.2 Input Function

PET imaging provides the distribution of the radiotracer concentration as a function of time in the subject body. This radiotracer could selectively target specific tissues, but at any time, it is observed in the vascular system. In fact, the detected photons could be emitted by the native radiotracer as administered, or they might originate from molecules produced by radiotracer transformations, which are still labeled by the

positron-emitting isotope, and that is what happens in most cases. The labeled molecules, as administered (free radiotracer), after transformation and accumulation within the cells (metabolism), after transformation in the cells or in the blood and rejected in the blood (metabolites), or excreted from the cells, which can be filtered out by the kidneys or can enter the cells again (recirculation), all contribute to the measured signal with PET. All radiotracers are transported in the blood and delivered to the cells. As an example, ^{18}F-fluorodeoxyglucose (^{18}F-FDG) enters brain cells and accumulates as ^{18}F-FDG-6-PO$_4$ after phosphorylation (metabolism), and it can recombine to ^{18}F-FDG and be sent back in blood (recirculation). ^{11}C-acetate produces carbon dioxide (^{11}C-CO$_2$), which is transported in blood and cannot enter the cells (metabolites).

The data measured with PET in tissue in a certain interval of time depend on several factors, among them the dose of the administered radiotracer (administered means injected or inhaled); the duration of tracer administration; the behavior of the radiotracer in tissue; and the time of data collection. In any case, and to quantify the data, the knowledge of the radiotracer delivered to tissue must be known as a function of time. Physically speaking, the radiotracer delivered to tissue represents the input or excitation. The data measured with PET represents the output or the response of tissue to the excitation. Suppose a system, represented as a black box, receives an excitation and naturally generates a response to this excitation as depicted in Fig. 17.1.

The goal of the analysis is to describe what was achieved within the black box. It is generally hard to guess the work done within the black box if the input and response were only punctual in time. Therefore, it is hoped that the problem can be solved by repeating the measurements at several time points. Because we use mathematics to solve this problem, we thus need an equal number or more of equations than variables. In PET imaging, the input function (function of time) is defined by the concentration of the radiotracer in

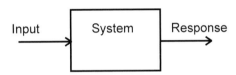

Fig. 17.1 Diagram of a black box system receiving an excitation and generating a response

blood, such as ^{15}O-O$_2$ bound to red blood cells. Also, the radiotracer such as ^{18}F-FDG can be transported by the plasma. For these reasons, the input function can also be called the blood curve or plasma curve, where the word *curve* replaces the word *function*.

To emphasize how to determine what happens within the system in Fig. 17.1, we use the example of the most popular radiotracer in PET, which is ^{18}F-FDG. ^{18}F-FDG was studied in mice; its retention, phosphorylation, and excretion were reported in several organs [37]. Also, ^{18}F-FDG can be found either as injected or after being phosphorylated. Other workers reported complementary findings with either fluorine or carbon isotopes [38–42]. The ^{18}F-FDG compartmental model was finally stated as three compartments describing the spaces the radiotracer occupies and the biochemical processes or states under which the isotope appears, as shown in Fig. 17.2.

In this model in which the number of compartments was defined by biochemical analyses, the dashed rectangle represents what the PET scanner measures in tissue. There is the vascular compartment around the tissue where the radiotracer is transported in plasma. The radiotracer passes from the blood vessels to the interstitial compartment with a rate constant K_1 without any transformation; it can exit from the extracellular space to the vascular space with a rate constant k_2; it can enter the cell and be phosphorylated (metabolized) and then kept there for about 1.5 h [42], or it can recombine back to ^{18}F-FDG and exit from the cells with the rate constant k_4. By analogy to Fig. 17.1, C$_{PET}$ in Fig. 17.2 represents the black box. By measuring the input function and the system response, it is possible to understand what happens in the system.

The input function is mandatory for all types of quantification in PET imaging. Prior to any PET quantitative study, a protocol of measurements and analyses needs to be stated. The protocol depends mainly on the radiotracer used, the injection dose, the tissue of interest, the acquisition duration, and so on. Generally, the measured data are reconstructed in time frames in which the images are positioned at the midscan of time intervals. The first frames should be narrow to observe the uptake of the radiotracer, especially for bolus injections. The sampling of the input function should be as narrow as possible at the beginning of tracer injection to accurately describe the peak of the function. An erroneous input function in shape would not allow a good fit of the tissue data, while an erroneous function of its amplitude would generate biased rate constant values, especially the perfusion K_1. With the usual statistics in PET imaging either for human measurements or in small animals, 5-s scans during the first minute are possible to obtain, and these have enough statistics to allow accurate data fitting. Correspondingly, the input function has to be defined at similar times or to be interpolated at these time points.

In kinetic modeling from the images, the input function can be determined by several techniques:

- Manual sampling
- Automatic sampling
- Image-based input function
- Population-based input function

Manual sampling: The manual withdrawal of blood samples from an arm vein for humans and from a tail vein for small animals is usually employed. The procedure is the most accurate and precise; at the same time, it is the most cumbersome. Because arterial sampling is technically difficult, catheters are placed in a vein of a warmed hand or in the tail vein of a small animal heated on a pad. The heating allows arterialization of the venous blood [43, 44]. The effect of heating the arm is to increase the blood supply in response to heating; consequently, the concentration of the radiotracer in the arterial blood remains almost unchanged in the venous blood as the tissue at that place does not uptake the radiotracer or uptakes little of it. The approach of heating the hand was well suited for measuring radioactive tracer amounts of glucose and other substrates in arterialized venous blood in

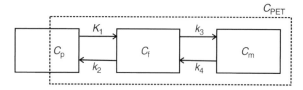

Fig. 17.2 Diagram of the three-compartment ^{18}F-FDG (fluorodeoxyglucose) model. C_p, C_f, and C_m are the compartments for plasma and free and metabolized tracer, respectively. C$_{PET}$ represents what the scanner measures in a voxel or in a region of interest (ROI). The transfer of the radiotracer between the compartments is regulated by the rate constants K_1–k_4. Note that K_1 is the perfusion and has units in milliliters/gram/minute, while k_2–k_4 have units in 1/minute. The partially measured plasma compartment by positron emission tomography (PET) translates in the inclusion of a fraction of the input function in the kinetic model equation

comparison to arterial blood samples [45–47]. The venous blood samples should be withdrawn as frequently (about every 5 s) as possible, at least in the first minute after the start of the bolus injection of the radiotracer, to accurately define the time course of the radiotracer in blood. The subsequent few samples should be made at 30 s intervals, and the last samples could be spaced by 5 or 10 min or more; a final sample is necessary some 5–30 s after the end of the PET scan. The blood sampling time must be longer than the PET acquisition time to allow interpolations at the midscan times of the imaging frames.

The blood samples need further analyses. In most cases, as with ^{18}F-FDG, the whole blood is measured for radioactivity in defined volumes, the samples are centrifuged to separate the plasma, then volumes of plasma are measured for radioactivity in well counters; finally, the well counter is calibrated to the PET scanner by measuring the same concentration of radiotracer. Some of the blood measurements can serve also for the assessment of metabolites, blood glucose, blood gases, and so on.

Automatic sampling: Automatic blood sampling was introduced to simplify the operators' task; after placing the catheter, the radioactivity in the blood is automatically measured. The blood flows in the tube by continuous and automatic pumping. The blood then passes in a gap where a detector counts the radioactivity emitted by a defined volume of blood [48–51]. The main problems with this procedure are the contamination of blood radioactivity from previous samples, even if the tubes are well heparinized, and this effect causes a dispersion of the input function that does not reflect the reality of the blood supply to a tissue. Even though the tubing between the subject and the detector is short (50 cm in rat and mice [51]), there is a delay because the radioactivity measured in the blood samples does not match the exact time of the arrival of blood at the tissue of interest. Generally, these techniques allow measurement of the radioactivity in the whole blood, while for ^{18}F-FDG, for example, the plasma radioactivity is needed. In this case, one or a few samples are separately analyzed after centrifugation to calculate the ratio of plasma to whole blood radioactivity and to use this factor to scale the measured blood radioactivity in the counter, hypothesizing that no metabolites are created in the time course of the measurement. Another limitation regarding blood sampling (whether manual or automatic) is

the limited amount of blood in small animals such as mice, especially in repeated measurements in the same session or in separate sessions, such as the study of the effect of medication or an activation. Some techniques process blood sampling by automatically reinjecting the withdrawn blood in the animal after counting the radioactivity.

Image-based input function: Due to these difficult and risky procedures, methods to extract the input function from the images have been processed. The idea was tempting as there is no need for blood sampling, measuring, calibrating, and other difficult tasks. Mathematically, there is no or a little delay and dispersion in the input function. Meanwhile, the limitation of the spatial resolution of PET drastically affects the quantification of the input function using this technique. This effect can be seen in two ways: PVE and spillover. PVE is the result of underestimation of the emitted radioactivity from a small-size structure. Spillover is the contamination in the images of neighboring structures by the emitted radioactivity from a tissue.

In cardiac studies, the left ventricle (LV) and the atrium were used to provide the input function by means of ROIs generally corrected for spillover and partial volume [52–54]. In the case of imaging tumors or organs other than the heart, the input curve was directly derived from PET images of arteries or with the recourse to CT or magnetic resonance images (MRIs) [55–59]. Here also, when plasma radioactivity or metabolites are needed, some normalization has to be made to the image-derived input function. The most promising approach is based on the separation of blood from tissue components in dynamic PET imaging. The calculations, generally based on principle component analysis, allow obtaining blood images from which the input function is determined with reduced influence of spillover. However, this procedure does not correct for PVE. Mainly, two algorithms have been used in these objectives: factor analysis of dynamic structures (FADS) [60–65] and independent component analysis (ICA) [66–69].

Population-based input function: Another approach to circumvent blood sampling is the population-based input function, which requires previously collected data from blood sampling; these data are normalized with one or a few blood samples to obtain the input function of a specific measurement [70–72]. In this case, the subjects and the PET measurements have to be in similar conditions and environments.

Other reported works used different approaches to estimate the input curve or to quantify the PET data without the use of a predefined input function [63, 73–76].

The blood supply to a tissue in PET imaging could be made through a bolus or an infusion of the radiotracer through the duration of the scan. The bolus injection is usually processed to assess the state of a tissue such as in diagnostic imaging or to estimate its response to an external effect such as activation. The response could be punctual or as a function of time. The infusion is preferentially used to observe in real time the behavior of a tissue while directly acting on some factors influencing the tissue [77, 78].

As for the tissue time-activity curve for which the unit is expressed in counts/voxel/seconds or in becquerels/voxel, the input function is thus calculated in these same units. If the tissue TAC and the input function are both extracted from the images, there is no need to calibration in becquerels or other units as the factor of calibration in tissue TAC and in input function is the same, and it cancels out.

Meanwhile, the same input function cannot serve in kinetic modeling for several organs or tissues in the same subject and within the same scan if a specific tissue is subjected to a local task or treatment. This can particularly be illustrated in the following example: This example is extracted from a work reporting the real-time monitoring of cancer treatment with photodynamic therapy (PDT). In summary, two mammary tumors were grown on the back of rats. The rats were injected with photosensitizers 24 h prior to the PET scan and treatment. The treatment consisted of illuminating one tumor with a red light ($\lambda = 670$ nm), and the other tumor served as a control [79, 80]. The heart was simultaneously imaged with the tumor to extract the input curve from the images of the LV.

The injection consisted of an infusion of ^{18}F-FDG for 2 h. The PET scan started and ended with the radiotracer infusion. Thirty minutes after the start of the scan, a tumor was illuminated for 30 min, and the control tumor was masked. Figure 17.3a shows the fit of the model to the data from myocardial septum, and Fig. 17.3b displays a modified ^{18}F-FDG compartmental model fitting the treated tumor [80]. As can be seen in Fig. 17.3b, the blood supply to the tumor did not behave in similar manner as in the heart.

17.3 Model and Data-Based Methods and Parameter Estimation

Actually, in the clinic, patients are generally imaged for disease diagnoses. Therefore, the measured data of these patients are individually analyzed and archived. There is no need (or almost no need) to quantify these

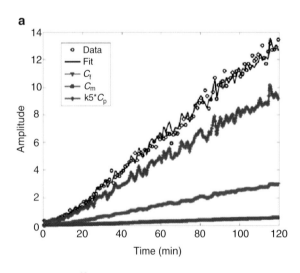

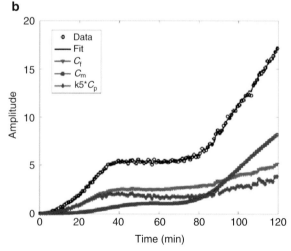

Fig. 17.3 (a) ^{18}F-FDG (fluorodeoxyglucose) kinetic fit to septum time-activity curve (TAC) in normal rat heart with continuous infusion of ^{18}F-FDG for 120 min. C_f, C_m, and $k_5 * C_p$ are free ^{18}F-FDG, metabolized ^{18}F-FDG, and blood compartments, respectively. (b) ^{18}F-FDG kinetic fit to treated tumor

data as the quantification needs specific protocols with several measurements to be statistically significant; appropriate tools for data analyses; more time for the PET scanning; and persons with specialized skills for the measurements and analyses. Usually, the patients are injected with the radiotracer, isolated in a room for the time of radiotracer uptake, and then scanned for a minimal time but sufficient for the diagnosis. These types of measurements are reconstructed in volume images, and the clinicians provide their observations by visually reading intensity images; sometimes, they use such basic tools as zooming, averaging ROI voxels, fusing images, plotting profiles, and so on.

The mostly used radiotracer in the clinic is ^{18}F-FDG, especially for its uptake and accumulation in most tissues without generating metabolites; for its property in glucose metabolism assessment; and for its long half-life (109 min), which permits acquisition of images with good statistics. ^{18}F-FDG is recognized for its use in a valuable technique for studying glucose metabolism in tumors, with glucose utilization in malignant tissues higher than that in normal tissue, and has shown great success in tumor detection and cancer staging. The accurate staging is crucial in choosing the appropriate therapy. The potential of ^{18}F-FDG PET in cancer staging is now well recognized [81–83]. Usually, patient follow-up is evaluated with morphological changes measured by anatomical imaging modalities such as CT and MRI, which are less adequate [84, 85].

The quantification of PET data is mostly performed in research; the planned study requires a group of subjects in the same conditions, measured with the same protocol, and the data analyzed with the same tools. The results are statistically analyzed, and clear conclusions are reported with parameter values produced as tables and graphs. The results of such studies can serve as a basis or support for other studies. The quantification is deduced from mathematical models reflecting functional changes in tissues. In fact, the data collected by PET have their origin from various signals. As stated, the measured photons are issued from blood or tissue. By further insights, the photons emitted from blood could originate from the plasma or from the hemoglobin as a form of the native radiotracer or as metabolites that cannot enter the cells. In the extravascular space, the photons can be issued by any form of the biochemical transformations of the radiotracer as long as the daughter molecules have enough mean life to contribute to the measured signal

during the time of the measurement. Each of these components participating to the whole signal could be isolated. One can proceed with kinetic modeling by extracting the individual components, which are mostly formed by exponential functions. The parameters of these exponentials (i.e., coefficients, exponents, and other extrapolated values) have to be linked to physiological parameters.

The model-based kinetic modeling techniques are the most popular as the proposed models have been validated with standard approaches such as biochemical analyses, biopsies, autoradiography, and in vitro experiments. The compartment models are used most often. Once the biochemical transformations of a radiotracer can be represented by compartments, mathematical equations can then be set. The sequence of images must be dynamic (i.e., PET scans starting with the radiotracer injection). The time framing should be optimal to collect enough photons during an interval of time. It should be optimal also to be able to measure the physiological changes during the PET measurements. These restrictions, and others, effectively contribute to the precision of the calculated data. An example is the kinetic modeling of the ^{15}O-H$_2$O (or ^{15}O$_2$, ^{15}O-CO) which has a half-life of 2 min. The framing should be short to allow measuring a few frames. However, the photon collection is low not only due to the short half-life but also because ^{15}O-H$_2$O is freely diffusible and cannot produce images contrasting the tissue. The kinetic modeling is thus difficult to apply on a voxel basis as the TACs are noisy. In the case of ^{15}O-H$_2$O and for several other compartment models, these can be simplified or approximated to generate more accurate results, even on the voxel basis [86].

The data-based parameter estimation approaches rely on the calculation of global parameters with a reduced number of these parameters and with less confinement on their values. Since these parameters are directly extracted from the data, such as slopes and intercepts of functions, their units are not appropriately determined. They have to be rearranged to correspond to parameters determined by standard techniques. The spectral analysis and the graphical analysis discussed further in this chapter are among this category. The force of these approaches is their ease of use. Their weakness is their sensitivity to noise. Also, in their general form, the data-driven techniques do not allow the reconstruction of isolated components of the signal as the model-based techniques do, for which there are specific functions describing specific components.

When calculating parametric imaging and applying the kinetic model to each dynamic image voxel individually, at first sight, this approach is inappropriate because not all image voxels obey the radiotracer behavior as prescribed in the kinetic model. Some voxels contain no radioactivity at all, or they contain noise, scatter, or a mixture of intensities from heterogeneous tissues and blood. The procedure of modeling has to start with discriminating the area where the kinetic model has to be applied either by thresholding on image intensity or by ROI drawing. The area selected has to be done on an appropriate image frame where the contrast is optimal. Finally, we mention that the kinetic modeling aims are to determine the response of a tissue in a specific state depending on the input function, which can be done as a bolus or as a continuous infusion during the PET scan.

17.3.1 Dynamic Three-Compartment Model of ^{18}F-FDG

The model of ^{18}F-FDG as depicted in Fig. 17.2 can be translated to mathematical equations to calculate the four rate constants and to reproduce each of the two compartments C_f and C_m individually. These parameters allow learning about the biology and the physiology of the cells. The behavior of each compartment as a function of time is expressed as [42]:

$$\frac{dC_f(t)}{dt} = K_1 C_p(t) - (k_2 + k_3)C_f(t) + k_4 C_m(t)$$
$$\frac{dC_m(t)}{dt} = k_3 C_f(t) - k_4 C_m(t) \qquad (17.1)$$

The solutions to these equations are given by where the symbol $\otimes$ represents the convolution operator. The constants α_1 and α_2 represent combinations of the rate constants:

$$\alpha_1 = \left[k_2 + k_3 + k_4 - \sqrt{(k_2 + k_3 + k_4)^2 - 4k_2 k_4} \right]/2$$

$$\alpha_2 = \left[k_2 + k_3 + k_4 + \sqrt{(k_2 + k_3 + k_4)^2 - 4k_2 k_4} \right]/2$$

$$(17.3)$$

To reproduce the measured data with PET as described in the model of Fig. 17.2, we have to add a fraction of $C_p(t)$ to the sum of $C_f(t)$ and $C_m(t)$ as

$$C_{PET}(t) = C_f(t) + C_m(t) + k_5 C_p(t) \qquad (17.4)$$

which, by means of Eq. 17.3, becomes

$$C_{PET}(t) = \frac{K_1}{\alpha_2 - \alpha_1} \left[(k_3 + k_4 - \alpha_1)e^{-\alpha_1 t} \right.$$
$$\left. + (\alpha_2 - k_3 - k_4)e^{-\alpha_2 t} \right] \otimes C_p(t) + k_5 C_p(t)$$

$$(17.5)$$

where k_5 is called the tissue blood volume or tissue vascular fraction. This is why only a portion of the C_p compartment is seen by PET (Fig. 17.2). Obviously, the tissue blood volume measured by PET in an ROI or in a voxel represents the signal emerging from the whole blood in that region, while in Eq. 17.5, a fraction of C_p is counted in the model instead of a fraction of the whole blood. In fact, Eq. 17.5 should contain $k_5 C_b(t)$ instead of $k_5 C_p(t)$ as the scanner measures whole blood not plasma concentration of radiotracer. Phelps et al. demonstrated that the signal measured in the red blood cells at time of injection accounts for 80% of that measured in plasma, and this ratio increases with time to reach about 87% after 60 min with a slope of 0.0012/min [42]. The counts measured in the red blood cells were attributed to the inclusion of ^{18}F-FDG-6-PO$_4$. The concentration of the radiotracer in the whole blood C_{wb} can be calculated in the brain as [42]

$$C_{wb} = \frac{C_p[RBC]/[Plasma]0.85HCT}{1 - 0.85HCT} + C_p \qquad (17.6)$$

$$C_f(t) = \frac{K_1}{\alpha_2 - \alpha_1}[(k_4 - \alpha_1)e^{-\alpha_1 t} + (\alpha_2 - k_4)e^{-\alpha_2 t}] \otimes C_p(t)$$
$$C_m(t) = \frac{K_1 k_3}{\alpha_2 - \alpha_1}[e^{-\alpha_1 t} - e^{-\alpha_2 t}] \otimes C_p(t) \qquad (17.2)$$

where [RBC]/[Plasma] is the ratio of red blood cells to plasma ^{18}F-FDG concentration. HCT is the hematocrit, which accounts for the proportion of blood volume that is occupied by red blood cells and was assigned 0.39 for brain. The cerebral hematocrit correction factor is 0.85. Other works reported different ways to calculate C_{wb} [87, 88].

Knowing $C_{PET}(t)$ and $C_p(t)$ at several time points, the parameters K_1 to k_5 are calculated by least squares fitting or by other means by adjusting the right member of Eq. 17.5 to $C_{PET}(t)$. Finally, the metabolic rate for glucose (MRGlc) is calculated as

$$MRGlc(\mu moles/100g/\min)$$

$$= \frac{gl(\text{mg of glucose}/100\,\text{ml of plasma})}{LC\,0.182(\text{mg}/\mu moles)}$$

$$\times \frac{K_1(\text{ml}/g/\min)k_3(1/\min)}{k_2(1/\min) + k_3(1/\min)} \quad (17.7)$$

Here, gl is the concentration of glucose in plasma, and LC is the lumped constant. LC is taken in the human brain as 0.42 [42] and 0.52 [89]. However, more than one report has increased this value to more than 0.8 [90, 91]. The MRGlc is in micromoles of glucose/100 g of tissue/min. Sometimes, MRGlc can be expressed in milliliters of tissue instead of grams of tissue. The factor 0.182 in the denominator accounts for the molecular mass of glucose, which is 182 g/mole.

By using the Levenberg–Marquardt algorithm [92] to adjust the model (right member of Eq. 17.5) to the measured data $C_{PET}(t)$ (left member of Eq. 17.5), the rate constants K_1–k_4 and the tissue blood volume k_5 are calculated (Fig. 17.4). At the beginning of the fitting procedure, the initial values of the five parameters to fit and globally taken from the literature are supplied. These are continuously and iteratively modified during the calculations until the model adjusts the data. In Fig. 17.4, we see how C_f increases rapidly as a function of the bolus injection of ^{18}F-FDG, then it decreases, while C_m continuously increases during the 1-h measurement. The decrease of C_f means that the radiotracer is either flowing through k_3 into the cells or returning back through k_2 to the vascular space. The increase of C_m means that ^{18}F-FDG is transformed to ^{18}F-FDG-6-PO$_4$ in the cells, where it is retained as it cannot be further transformed for use by the cells.

Equation 17.2 expresses the two compartments individually, and these are shown in Fig. 17.4c.

$C_f(t)$ and $C_m(t)$ are the response of the tissue to the input function, and they depend on the input function as it is translated by the convolution operation in Eq. 17.2. The intrinsic response of the tissue can be considered without the convolution operation with $C_p(t)$. In other words, if we repeat the measurements in the same conditions and in the same patient but with different input functions, we shall get the same rate constants. This is what is actually processed when a group of subjects is measured and the radiotracer delivered to the tissue of interest varies in the subjects. Examples of C_{if} and C_{im} (i.e., intrinsic compartments) are reconstructed by means of Eq. 17.2 from the calculated rate constants and are displayed in Fig. 17.4d.

17.3.2 Autoradiographic Model of ^{18}F-FDG

The autoradiographic approach not only simplifies the calculation of the parameters and is suited for parametric imaging in the brain but also simplifies the PET data acquisition as it consists of a single scan some time after the bolus injection of the radiotracer. The approach is also encouraging since the subject does not occupy the scanner for longer time as for the dynamic studies. In fact the measurement is compared to analytical data generated from parameters (rate constants) in a sample of population. The simulated radiotracer compartments $C'_f(t)$ and $C'_m(t)$ by means of the measured input function and population-based rate constants are compared to the measured TAC of the tissue, and MRGlc is calculated as [93]

$$MRGlc = \frac{gl}{LC} \frac{K'_1 K'_3}{k'_2 + k'_3} \left[\frac{C_{PET}(T)}{C'_f(T) + C'_m(T)} \right] \quad (17.8)$$

17.3.3 Graphical Analysis of ^{18}F-FDG

The graphical analysis was first described by Patlak et al. [94, 95], and it is often called the Patlak plot. It was originally applied to ^{18}F-FDG, but it can be used with other radiotracers, such as with ^{13}N-ammonia [96]. The method assumes that $k_4 = 0$ in the ^{18}F-FDG

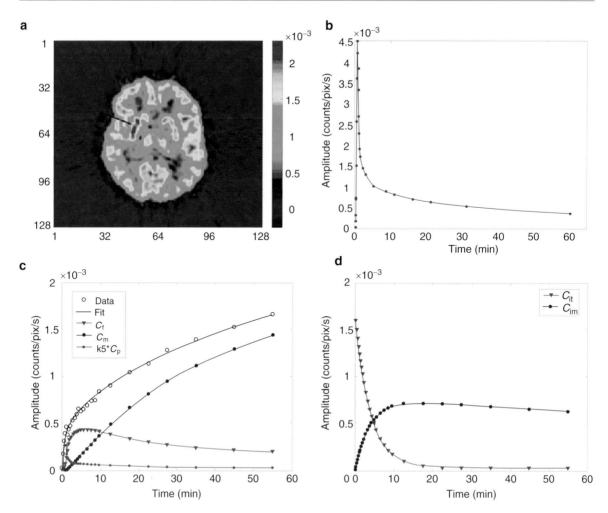

Fig. 17.4 (**a**) Image slice of a brain measured with positron emission tomography (PET) in a healthy young volunteer. The *arrow* indicates the region of the putamen, which is fitted with the kinetic model of ^{18}F-FDG (fluorodeoxyglucose) as shown in (**c**). (**b**) The input function used in the kinetic modeling. (**c**) The

data from the putamen were accurately fitted, and the compartments C_f, C_m, and k_5*C_p are also displayed. (**d**) Reproduction of the intrinsic tissue response for the free and metabolized radiotracer compartments (Eq. 17.2 without convolution)

model (Eqs. 17.3 and 17.5), and the values for α_1 and α_2 (Eq. 17.3) become

$$\begin{aligned} \alpha_1 &= 0 \\ \alpha_2 &= k_2 + k_3 \end{aligned} \qquad (17.9)$$

and if we omit the blood compartment, and replacing k_4, α_1, and α_2 by their new values, Eq. 17.5 becomes

$$C_{\mathrm{PET}}(t) = \frac{K_1}{k_2 + k_3}\left[k_3 + k_2 e^{-(k_2 + k_3)t}\right] \otimes C_p(t) \quad (17.10)$$

By assuming $C_p(t)$ is a constant relative to the exponential,

$$C_{\mathrm{PET}}(t) = \frac{K_1}{k_2 + k_3}\left[k_3 \int_0^t C_p(u)du + \frac{k_2}{k_2 + k_3}C_p(t)\right]$$

$$(17.11)$$

and dividing both sides by $C_p(t)$, we obtain

$$C_{\mathrm{PET}}(t)/C_p(t) = \frac{K_1 k_3}{k_2 + k_3}\int_0^t C_p(u)du/C_p(t) + \frac{K_1 k_2}{(k_2 + k_3)}$$

$$(17.12)$$

This equation is of the form $y = ax + b$, where the slope $\frac{K_1 k_3}{k_2 + k_3}$ can be calculated from the last data points of the TACs, where the ^{18}F-FDG is metabolized and accumulates in tissue. MRGlc is then calculated as expressed in Eq. 17.7. Figure 17.5a–c shows the input function and a tissue TAC with adjustment of the last frames as described in Eq. 17.12. Figure 17.5d depicts the bias in MRGlc values obtained with the graphical method in comparison to the dynamic method by which the TACs were adjusted according to Eq. 17.5.

17.3.4 Spectral Analysis

An example of the exponential-based data analysis approach is spectral analysis [32–34, 73, 97]. Suppose a volume of tissue (either a voxel or an ROI) produces a dynamic signal $C_{PET}(t)$. Within this volume, there is a blood component that emits photons from either the original radiotracer C_p or from metabolites. The mathematical representation of the collected signal with PET can be written as

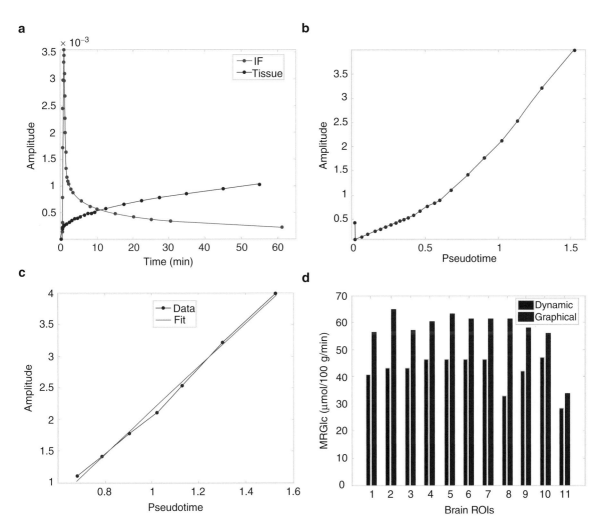

Fig. 17.5 Graphical analysis of ^{18}F-FDG-PET (fluorodeoxy-glucose-positron emission tomographic) brain data from a normal young volunteer. (**a**) Manually sampled input function and left hemicortex tissue time-activity curves (TACs). (**b**) Modified tissue TAC according to Eq. 17.12; (**c**) Last data frames adjusted with a regression line (Eq. 17.12). (**d**) Comparison of metabolic rate for glucose (MRGlc) values calculated in 11 brain regions with dynamic and graphical analyses

$$C_{\text{PET}}(t) = \sum_{i=1}^{N} A_i \exp(-B_i t) \otimes C_p(t)$$
$$+ BV.C_b(t) \qquad (17.13)$$

This general expression is equivalent to that of ^{18}F-FDG (Fig. 17.2, Eq. 17.5). The rate constants considered as the microparameters or rate constants in Eq. 17.5 are replaced here by macroparameters A and B. Also, the C_{PET} data include the radioactivity emitted from the whole blood ($C_b(t)$) as represented by BV.$C_b(t)$, that is, a fraction of total radioactivity in blood TAC and BV stands for tissue blood volume. Equation 17.13 can be decomposed to match a pharmacokinetic model such as for ^{18}F-FDG (Eq. 17.5), or it can be used to decompose a PET signal in its compartments, helping to design a pharmacokinetic model.

When the number of compartments is not known, it is possible to generate several compartments identified with the exponential functions $\exp(-B_i t)$ in Eq. 17.13. This is accomplished by generating N values for B within an interval [Bmin Bmax] corresponding to possible physiological parameters. The accuracy of the values of B depends on the sampling in the interval [Bmin Bmax] and thus on the number N of the starting values. This is the procedure of spectral analysis. $C_b(t)$ can be replaced with the plasma function $C_p(t)$ when these are equivalent, or it can be replaced by a functional ratio as seen for ^{18}F-FDG (Eq. 17.6) [42] or as in the case of ^{11}C-acetate [98]:

$$C_p(t) = [1 - a_0(1 - \exp(-t\log(2)/m))]C_p(t) \quad (17.14)$$

where a_0 and m are parameters accounting for metabolites.

Let us design N exponential functions E_{ij} at M time values t ($i = 1{:}N$, $j = 1{:}M$) corresponding to the M PET frames. These exponential values have to be multiplied by the amplitudes A_i, $i = 1{:}N$ as in Eq. 17.13. Finally we insert $C_b(t)$, still evaluated at the M frame times, at the last line of the matrix of exponentials and call it $E_{N+1,1}$, $E_{N+1,2}$, ... $E_{N+1,M}$. Correspondingly, we insert BV at the last position of the amplitudes A_i and call it A_{N+1}. Note that $C_b(t)$ and BV could be equally inserted at the beginning of E_{ij} and A_i, respectively. Equation 17.13 written in a matrix form becomes

$$C_{\text{PET}}(t_1 t_2, \ldots, t_m) = [A_0\, A_1\, A_2 \ldots A_{N+1}]$$

$$\times \begin{bmatrix} E_{01} & E_{02} & E_{03} & \ldots & E_{0M} \\ E_{11} & E_{12} & E_{13} & \ldots & E_{1M} \\ E_{21} & E_{22} & E_{23} & \ldots & E_{2M} \\ & & \cdot & & \\ & & \cdot & & \\ & & \cdot & & \\ E_{N+1,1} & E_{N+1,2} & E_{N+1,3} & \ldots & E_{N+1,M} \end{bmatrix}$$
$$(17.15)$$

Note that Eq. 17.15 could be written in the usual way as $C_{\text{PET}}{}^T = E^T.A^T$, where T is the matrix transpose. Equation 17.15 is of the form $y = A.x$ and can be solved with the linear least squares with nonnegativity constraints algorithm [99], which returns $N + 1$ values of the amplitudes A_i having either positive or null values. The indices of the nonnull values of A_i allow selection of the corresponding exponentials E_i and hence the corresponding values of B_i. Of course, BV = A_{N+1} and $C_b(t) = E_{N+1}$. The matrix (Eq. 17.15) can be solved for an ROI or for a voxel. If the equation is solved at the voxel basis, parametric images can be produced for amplitudes (A_i), exponents (B_i), or for any compartment intensity. It is evident that from the parameters A_i and B_i one can retrieve the microparameters as the K_i for ^{18}F-FDG from which the metabolism of glucose can be calculated (Eq. 17.7) [33, 34].

Alternatively, without recourse to the model, parameters can be accessed directly or graphically from the solutions to Eq. 17.15 [32, 73, 97, 100]. This approach is termed the data-driven modeling technique, in comparison to the model-driven technique [100].

As an example of spectral analysis, we applied the technique to PET data measured in normal rats with ^{13}N-ammonia through the heart (Fig. 17.6a) [33]. The measured data were reconstructed in 24 frames: 12×5 s; 8×30 s, 4×150 s. We used the TAC from an ROI manually drawn on the image blood pool within the LV as the input function. We set $N = 100$ for B_i values (Eq. 17.15), equally distributed and constrained between 10^{-5} and 0. The solutions gave the coefficients A_i as plotted in Fig. 17.6c. Among the B_i initial values, we extracted those corresponding to indices of A_i, and these are plotted in Fig. 17.6d. Note that BV is reported at $B = 0$ in Fig. 17.6d.

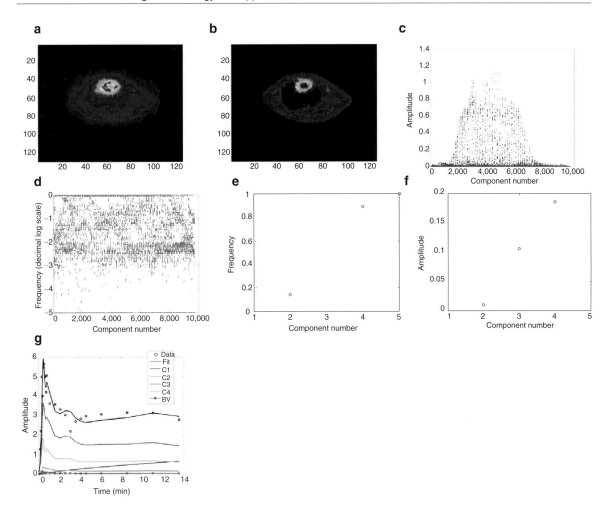

Fig. 17.6 Example of application of spectral analysis to images obtained with ^{13}N-ammonia through the midventricle of a rat heart. The voxels from the whole rat were individually decomposed with spectral analysis. (**a**) Image slice of the rat through the heart. (**b**) Reconstructed image from the parameters obtained with spectral analysis for the interval of $\log 10(B_i)$ between -5 and -0.5 (see Eq. 17.15). (**c**) Plot of all A_i values. (**d**) Plot of all $\log 10(B_i)$ values. (**e**) Plot of the B_i values of a single voxel. (**f**) Plot of the A_i values of a single voxel (same voxel as in **e**) . (**g**) Plot of the reconstructed individual time-activity curves (TACs) with their total (Fit) accurately adjusting the data, based on Eq. 17.15 and parameters in Fig. 17.6e and 17.6f. Here BV represents BV.$C_b(t)$

Figure 17.6e, f presents the frequencies B_i and the coefficients A_i for a single image voxel. By means of Eq. 17.15 and the values of A_i and B_i in Fig. 17.6e, f, the TACs of each component were built, and the result is reported in Fig. 17.6g with the total of the TACs as the fit to the measured TAC. The sequence of images was reconstructed from the sum of the individual TACs in each voxel calculated for $-5 < \log 10(B_i) < -0.5$ and the corresponding A_i, and the last image frame is displayed in Fig. 17.6b. In this application, the spectral analysis calculations returned a maximum

of four components excluding the blood volume, while the compartment model usually has two compartments [101]. There might be a split of components due to noise or to the inaccurate sampling of the $N\,B_i$ values. If a true B value does not appear in the sampled B_i values, the model generally compensates for this component by generating one or two B_i values with different amplitudes around the true B value. In previous work, the blood component was found to split into arterial and venous blood [33]. The inaccuracies could also be caused by noise and by inaccuracy of the input function, which undoubtedly contained spill-over from tissue.

17.3.5 Standard Uptake Value

Among the fast and simple quantitative methods is the standard uptake value (SUV). When we say quantitative, this means the data analyses produce parameter values not only in percentages but also in absolute values with proper units. The image itself is quantitative since it contains values of the radioactivity concentration. Values such as the mean, the median, the variance, and the contrast can help quantify regions versus other regions. In common language, quantification of PET data means extraction by calculations of physiological, biological, and pharmacological parameter absolute values in precise units that can be compared with other techniques. The SUV is termed semiquantitative. It has no units. It is calculated as [102–104]

$$SUV = \frac{C_{PET}}{(Dose/w)} = \frac{C_{PET}w}{Dose} \qquad (17.16)$$

where C_{PET} (becquerels/kilogram) is the mean intensity in an ROI and is measured in a given interval of time in a steady state with minimal variation, Dose (becquerels) is the injected dose of the radiotracer, and w (kilograms) is the body weight of the subject. The SUV is not robust, and it is a function of several factors:

1. The radiotracer is not equally distributed in the body in tissue as in fat.
2. The PVE and spillover affect the C_{PET} value.
3. C_{PET} is a measure of the whole radiotracer without distinction of blood and tissue compartments.
4. The nonsteady state of the radiotracer in tissue during the time of C_{PET} measurement produces uncertainties.

More than 1 h postinjection, the tissue, specifically the tumors, continues to uptake the radiotracer. At first sight according to Eq. 17.16, SUV values in the same patient and with the same injected dose only reflect the intensity of the ROIs as Dose/w is a common value for all patient tissues. More comments on SUV can be found in [105, 106].

17.4 Sources of Errors in Kinetic Modeling

The sources of errors in quantitative nuclear imaging should be regarded at several levels:

1. Design of the acquisition protocols: dose of injected radiotracer, duration of injection, duration of the measurements, time framing of the scans versus input function and interpolation, blood sampling, and patient preparation
2. Data corrections for physical aspects: dead time, normalization, randoms, positron range, noncollinearity of annihilation photons, image uniformity through the field of view (FOV), attenuation, scatter, and PVE
3. Data analyses: image reconstruction, calibration, patient motion, organ motion, choice of appropriate kinetic model, delineation of tissue of interest, and determination of input functions

We discuss next most of these factors with reference to some applications.

17.4.1 Design of the Acquisition Protocols

The radiotracer used in imaging affects the images depending on its half-life, its injection amount, its injection duration, and its behavior in the body. For example, measurement with ^{15}O-water, a freely diffusible radiotracer with a half-life of 2 min, will not produce images with contrasted brain tissues even with a dose of 35 mCi, in comparison to 10 mCi with ^{18}F-FDG (Fig. 17.7). If the injection of ^{15}O-water is extended for more than 1 min, the statistics in the images would be poorer since only a fraction of the injected radiotracer is measured at a given time.

Injected dose: The measured signal in tissue is generally proportional to the amount of the injected radiotracer in some limits. A greater dose will not be translated in an intense signal as there is saturation of receptor sites, transporters, diffusion, or at least limitation of the demand. Above all, the dose of radioactivity is limited by the possible risk of harm to the subject or by the effect on the measurement itself at the cell levels and in producing detection dead time.

a

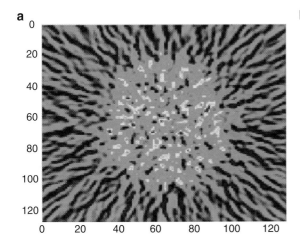

b

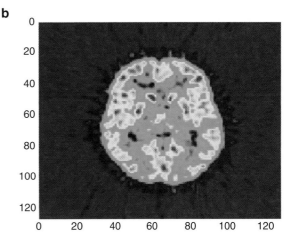

Fig. 17.7 Examples of ^{15}O-water and ^{18}F-FDG (fluorodeoxy-glucose) images in a normal brain showing the difference in structure appearance. The two measurements were carried out in the same patient during the same positron emission tomographic (PET) session. The two images reconstructed with filtered back-projection were obtained through the same brain slice

Meanwhile, the injection could be made as a bolus or as an infusion as long as the scan duration. In fact, in kinetic modeling, the response of the tissue to an excitation is represented by exponentials governed by rate constants, and the whole is convolved with the input function. Thus, the response of the tissue is unique with either a bolus or an infused injection [107].

Time framing: On the other hand, the collection of the PET data should be made optimal in terms of time framing. To describe the uptake of the radiotracer that translates in the determination of the tissue perfusion (K_1 rate constant), the first frames should be short enough. The later frames generally represent less variation in signal intensity as a function of time in addition to the low emission rate due to the physical radioactive decay of the radiotracer and to its biological extraction and elimination from the tissue. They are thus collected over longer time intervals.

These considerations are valid as far as there is no external perturbation of the tissue behavior such as by activation or by pharmacological stress. With some radiotracers, like ^{13}N-ammonia in the myocardium and ^{18}F-FDG in tumors or in brain, their accumulation in tissue produces well-contrasted images in the last frames, and these frame images are commonly used for tissue delimitation and ROI drawing. The length of the overall measurement in dynamic studies has a direct impact on the calculated parameters. The physiological parameters extracted from the same TAC of different time lengths could vary considerably. Thus, an optimal duration of the scan has to be considered.

In the next example, a young normal individual was measured for a brain study with ^{18}F-FDG, and a frontal region produced the data in Fig. 17.8a. When modeling only the first 20 min (Fig. 17.8b) and reproducing the data for the entire 60 min, although the 20-min TAC was accurately fitted, extending the plot to 60 min appears to diverge from the measured data. Similar examples are shown in Fig. 17.8c, d, respectively, for 120 and 160 min, reproducing the fit using rate constants and tissue blood volume calculated for 60 min. Quantitatively, the MRGlc calculated from the same TAC measured in 60 min but considering initial intervals of 20, 30, 40, 50, and 60 min, respectively, produced MRGlc values of 58.21, 44.74, 49.60, 46.48, and 43.33 μmol/100 g/min. The errors with respect to the MRGlc value at 60 min were 1.34, 1.03, 1.14, 1.07, and 1.00, respectively. Why is there so much discrepancy between these values? If the measured TAC is accurate (obeys the model) and precise (no statistical variations in the frame data), then it can be reproduced by the model from any part of it, and the returned parameters are equivalent.

To verify this hypothesis, we made an analytical TAC (simulated TACsim) using the rate constants from the fit to the measured 60-min TAC. We used the same time framing, the same input function, and the same algorithm, and the value of MRGlc was the same when fitting TACsim for 20, 30, 40, 50, and 60 min. If we again reproduce the plots in Fig. 17.8b by extrapolation of the fit obtained from the parameter model to the early 20 min of TACsim, the extrapolated

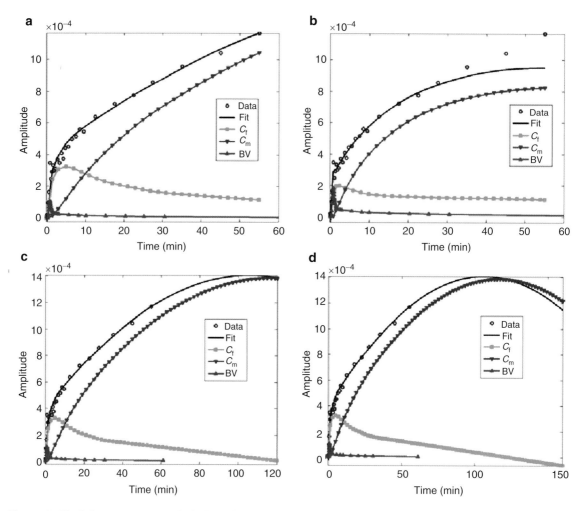

Fig. 17.8 The fitting parameters to a brain tissue time-activity curve (TAC; here a brain frontal region) do not reproduce nonmeasured tissue at extended times: (**a**) accurate fit to TAC measured in 60 min; (**b**) same data as in (**a**) fitted for 20 min and

fit reproduced for 60 min; (**c**) and (**d**) parameters extracted from fit to TAC in (**a**) and reproducing the model at extended times of 120 and 160 min, respectively

function perfectly matches the TACsim at 60 min. The simulation is manifestly different from the actual measured data not only for the noise, which influences the rate constant determination, but also for the value of the rate constants, especially the k_4, which seems to be a function of the measurement time length. The extrapolation of data at further times has its importance when comparing tissue behavior in an activation or treatment to its baseline in the same scan session using a single or a double injection, with a bolus or an infusion. An example of this application is the activation in a brain study or a tumor treatment (Fig. 17.3).

In the case of brain activation, brain images are acquired after a bolus injection of ^{18}F-FDG, for example, while the brain is at rest. Then, starting with a second injection, brain activation is initiated. The goal of the study is to calculate the MRGlc in both rest and activated states. The problem is that the collected data in the activated state unfortunately include tissue response to the first injection. In myocardial measurement of perfusion with ^{13}N-ammonia, one could consider the remaining radioactivity from the first injection as constant with time when measuring tissue response with the second injection. This approximation is acceptable since the intensity of the signal at the baseline appears low and varies slowly at times far from the bolus injection.

Patient preparation: Subject preparation has an important role in the success of data acquisition. Unfortunately, the dimensions of the PET scanners currently do not accept all patient sizes. The subjects with claustrophobia, those who cannot lie on the scanner bed for the duration of the scan, or those for whom it is difficult to withdraw blood samples have to be particularly prepared or excluded from quantitative studies. The subjects to be scanned should fast for some 4–10 h prior to the study. The subjects should be comfortably installed on the scanner bed and warned not to move until the end of the scan. The scanner room should be quiet, dimly lit, and warm enough to accommodate the patient. Some supports at the neck and at the legs could be installed to add some comfort to the patient. It is known that the movements of the subject during the scanning automatically corrupt the data, while the data could also be corrupted when the subject feels some pain or is uncomfortably installed even if the subject does not move, especially in brain imaging. Prior to the scan, the subject should use the restroom and empty the bladder. The subject should be secured and be well informed of the procedures of the study.

17.4.2 Data Corrections for Physical Aspects

In this section, we do not intend to review the physical principles of the factors affecting the quality of the images. Instead, we summarize the impact of these factors on the accuracy of the data. Usually, the optimal doses of different radiotracers and for diverse organ imaging are predefined. These should be acceptable for the patient and not provoke dead time in photon detections. Lower doses also should consider the effective detection and signal formation in successive short intervals of time in the case of quantitative dynamic studies or in cardiac gated studies as the dose is split on several frame or gate images. In noisy images acquired with low doses of radiotracers or when the radiotracer uptake in a tissue is low, the analyses become difficult either in tissue delimitation or in assessing the physiological parameters by model fitting. In some cases of data analyses, such as the modeling of dynamic

^{18}F-FDG data, as far as the model converges in fitting the data points, the results are acceptable. However, these same noisy data analyzed with the graphical analysis method would generate approximate results as this model is sensitive to noise.

The scan corrections for detection normalization and randoms, and at a certain extent for attenuation and scatter, are technically accepted based on manufacturer guides [108, 109]. Meanwhile, daily quality control should be done before proceeding with any scan [110]. The attenuation and scatter corrections are both dependent on the accuracy of the transmission measurement. When based on the rotating transmission sources, and to reduce the time of the study and the dose to thesubject, the transmission scans are made shortly. Consequently, the transmission image is noisy, and the structures are not well delimited; this uncertainty impinges on the attenuation coefficients used to restore the attenuated counts in the emission image, which directly amplifies the emission image noise. When the attenuation correction is processed based on CT images, a slight uncertainty is introduced when converting (or segmenting) CT images from high-resolution and low-energy x-ray images to low-resolution and high-energy PET images. The scatter undoubtedly causes significant change in TAC shapes and provokes smoothing in neighboring voxels. Consequently, the kinetic parameters are affected by the contribution of scatter at the site of interest [111–114].

The positron range (1 mm or less) and the noncollinearity emission of annihilation photons (diverging from 180° by a fraction of a degree on average) affect the accuracy of the positioning of the emission sites. These factors are included in the spatial resolution of the scanner and are not corrected in current PET studies. The scatter in the detectors (crystals), especially in small-animal scanners based on individual crystals, and the PVE are other factors that are usually counted as part of the spatial resolution of the system. These factors affect the signal at the boundaries of the measured structures and of course reduce the signal amplitude within the structure. Except for PVE in small structures, these effects introduce marginal uncertainties. Image uniformity (parallax effect) can be assessed by measuring a cylinder phantom filled with a uniform concentration of radioactivity in a solution. The phantom should cover at least half of the FOV diameter. Once the data are corrected for all effects, including radioactive decay, the image should appear uniform in intensity. By taking a profile through the image, the amplitude should appear constant. The same measurement could be used to check the axial uniformity. For more accurate measurements of these and other topics, refer to the recommendations of the National Electrical Manufacturers Association (NEMA) [1, 3, 115, 116]. The effect of image nonuniformity on parameter estimates is minor if the structure of interest has limited extent in the FOV. This effect is more apparent when comparing two or more structures located at different positions in the image.

17.4.3 Data Analyses

Apart from the different corrections, the PET data have to be reconstructed to match the measured object and to qualitatively or quantitatively assess the distribution of the radiotracer concentration in the subject. Before the reconstruction, many projections or sinograms have to be grouped depending on coincident detector rings and angular views. This necessary operation to reduce the data size reduces the spatial resolution. At this level of grouping the projections, there is a compromise between the noise and the spatial resolution since the individual projections (before grouping) have fewer counts. During the reconstruction procedure by any method, there is also a compromise between the high-resolution and noisy images on one hand and the smooth and less-noisy images on the other hand. Most of reconstructed images are made smooth by reducing the high-frequency data values. In iterative reconstruction techniques, the noise is reduced by lowering the number of iterations.

Reconstruction algorithm: The impact on the smoothing in kinetic modeling allows a better fit of the data, resulting in less variation in the parameter values, while this operation blurs the contours of the structures. In cardiac studies in small-animal imaging, the difference is significant since the heart is so small, and the blurring can expand to several voxels. Figure 17.9 shows two images obtained with ^{18}F-FDG in the rat through the heart and reconstructed with the MLEM algorithm [117] for 10 and 20 iterations. The patterns in the two images are apparent in smoothness, granularity, and spatial resolution where the myocardium appears thinner in Fig. 17.9b and in

the intensity of the voxels as represented by the color bar beside each image.

When defining the ROIs around the blood pool and tissue, the amplitudes of the corresponding TACs appear clearly affected, as can be seen in Fig. 17.9c, d. The algorithm tends to elevate the voxels with higher intensity and lower those with low intensities within the image. Since the 24 frame images were reconstructed separately, the shapes of the TAC do not suffer a bias, but they appear with different shapes. Quantitatively, by summing the intensity of the whole TAC, the values at 20 iterations with respect to those at 10 iterations for blood and tissue were respectively found: 93% and 106%, respectively. The effect of this variance directly affects the value of the perfusion (K_1), which is inversely proportional to the input function integral and proportional to the signal rise in tissue TAC. In ^{18}F-FDG-PET studies, the error in K_1 is directly transferred to the MRGlc values.

Calibration errors: The calibration in curies or in becquerels of the PET images is not necessary in kinetic modeling except if they have to match the units of input function. If the input function is extracted from the images, there would be no need to convert to other units since in the equation of the kinetic model the conversion factor will cancel as it appears in the PET and input function data. The most significant errors, although difficult to quantify, originate from the determination of input function. Any of the operations of blood withdrawal from subjects, centrifugation, extraction of volumes, measurements in the well counter, and cross calibration with the scanner undoubtedly introduces errors. The measurements with a blood counter need to be calibrated. When extracting the input function from the images or by means of a blood counter, there would be a normalization to assess the ratio of the plasma radioactivity to that of the whole blood. The input function determined from a blood counter should be taken with care due to contamination of blood radioactivity from previous samples (Fig. 17.10).

Motion: Patient motion and organ motion highly contribute to uncertainties in parameter estimates. The motion of tissues during imaging results in a superposition of counts in the same voxels emerging from these tissues, thus forming heterogeneous voxels. This effect is mostly encountered in lung and abdominal imaging in general due to respiration.

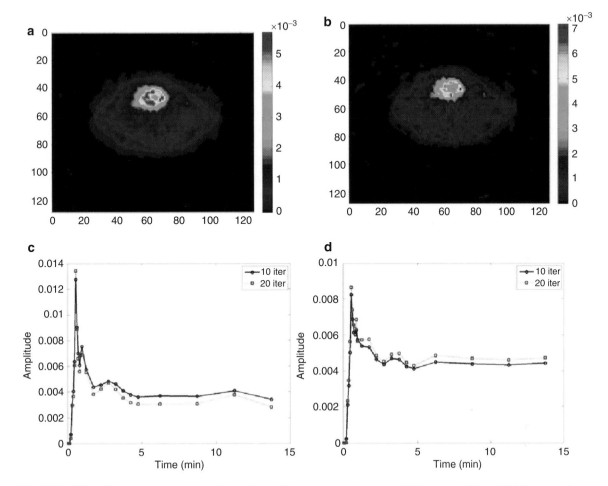

Fig. 17.9 Effect of image reconstruction with maximum likelihood expectation maximization (MLEM) on time-activity curves (TACs) of blood and tissue defined by regions of interest (ROIs) respectively set around the left ventricle blood pool and on anterior myocardial segment. (**a**) and (**b**) Images of a rat through the heart obtained with 10 and 20 iterations, respectively. (**c**) and (**d**) Comparison of 10- and 20-iteration TACs of blood and tissue, respectively

Cardiac imaging suffers from movement of both the lungs and the heart. For lung cancer, it is hard to locate a small tumor with precision. In cardiac studies, a high signal from blood is always added to the signal emerging from tissue. Note that PVE, scatter, and filtering during image reconstruction are all additional contributors to tissue movement. The sum of these contributions is generally called the spillover effect. One can observe the spillover effect in Fig. 17.4c, where the blood component appears low in brain tissue and high in myocardium at the early frames corresponding to the peak of the bolus injection (Fig. 17.9d).

Quantitatively, when the kinetic model is applied to a TAC, it is supposed that the TAC is obtained from a homogeneous tissue. If the source of the contamination is known as the spillover from blood to myocardial tissue or from tissue to blood, and since both TACs are known, weight factors are generally introduced in the kinetic model equation to account for the fraction of the contaminating component. However, this approach adds more parameters to be adjusted by the model.

Model selection: The main tasks for kinetic modeling in the images is to select (or to design) the kinetic model with appropriate and independent parameters to accurately fit the data. The data corrections should be done to include the decay correction prior to kinetic modeling. The tissue to be modeled has to be well delimited on the images. The input function should be corrected for spillover, metabolites, time delay,

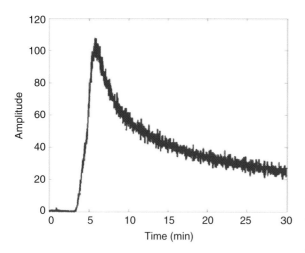

Fig. 17.10 Example of input function determined with a blood counter. The slow decay of this function resulted from the high contamination from previous sample radioactivity; even the 50-cm tube from the rat to the counter contained heparin

and dispersion. If the plasma input function is needed in kinetic modeling, it cannot be replaced by a blood function. The tissue TAC contains a fraction of radioactivity emitted by blood, and this fraction is accounted as tissue blood volume. In some approaches, an ROI is considered made of tissue and blood, and the kinetic modeling expresses the blood contribution as a fraction of the input function. Unless plasma and blood functions are similar, an error is introduced in using the same function for tissue blood volume and input function. The measured PET signal in an ROI can be represented as the sum of the concentration of the radioactivity in tissue and blood. Supposing the blood function is known and expressing the kinetic model as the convolution of exponentials with blood function, the model can be expressed as

$$C_{\text{PET}}(t) = \left(A_1 e^{-B_1 t} + A_2 e^{-B_2 t}\right) \otimes C_b(t) + BV.C_b(t) \tag{17.17}$$

where $C_b(t)$ and BV are the blood function and tissue blood volume, respectively. This equation is similar to that in Eq. 17.5. However, in other works [101], the expression is slightly different:

$$C_{\text{PET}}(t) = (1 - BV)\left(A_1 e^{-B_1 t} + A_2 e^{-B_2 t}\right) \otimes C_b(t) + BV.C_b(t) \tag{17.18}$$

This form of equation translates the quantity measured in a voxel or an ROI in a fraction coming from blood (BV) and the rest coming from tissue $(1 - BV)$, thus their sum makes 100%. Equation 17.17, however, stipulates that the measured signal is made of tissue, as represented by the convolution of the exponentials with C_b, plus the contribution from blood. The difference between Eqs. 17.17 and 17.18 is the underestimation of the amplitudes A_1 and A_2 in Eq. 17.18 by the factor $1 - BV$.

Input function: The kinetic modeling depends on the sampling in both the input function and the PET data. The convolution of input function with the TACs supposes the two functions are expressed in terms of the same time points. Except when the input function and TACs are extracted from images, the two functions do not have the same times, and interpolations to common time points are mandatory. Fundamentally, one could not interpolate data at intermediate time points if the function representing these data is not known, and this is the case for the input function and TACs. Generally, a linear interpolation is performed between the nearest data values.

ROI definition: Among the most important and frequent errors in PET imaging is the ROI determination. These errors are implicit in PET data in which the voxel is already a mixture of several aggregates of cells that could not fully obey the kinetic model. At the boundary of a normally homogeneous tissue, the voxels are contaminated by neighboring tissues due to PVE or organ movement. In the case of small-size structures, the region could hardly be delimited as it contains a few voxels. In larger structures, one can draw the ROI within the structure image. However, in both small- and large-size structures, the ROIs manually drawn are subjective. The intensity is not uniform in a tissue structure even when ignoring the noise. Consequently, the mean value in an ROI depends a lot on the ROI drawing itself, and this effect is more delicate because the ROI drawing is rarely reproducible. However, there are several algorithms based on anatomy (e.g., in dual modality imaging), on discrimination in image intensities, or on the time course of voxel intensities. The automatic ROI drawing is reproducible; meanwhile, it necessitates the intervention of the operator to select the structure of interest and to decide some initial parameter values in either two-dimensional (2D) or three-dimensional (3D) imaging.

17.5 Conclusions

The potential of PET imaging could be considered unlimited in the sense of the unlimited radiotracers that can be used for medical or pharmacological studies. By its versatility, PET is becoming a link between several disciplines. Meanwhile, the absolute parameter values provided by PET still present uncertainties that can be enhanced at several levels: in the instrument itself mainly by improving the detection efficiency, the spatial resolution, and the energy resolution; in the data corrections for the physical aspects and to take advantage of the whole injected dose of the radiotracer; in optimized protocols of measurements; and finally in utilizing appropriate and automatic data analysis procedures.

References

1. Karp JS, Daube-Witherspoon ME, Hoffman EJ, Lewellen TK, Links JM, Wong WH, Hichwa RD, Casey ME, Colsher JG, Hitchens RE, Muehllehner G, Stoub EW (1991) Performance standards in positron emission tomography. J Nucl Med 32:2342–2350
2. Hasegawa T, Wada Y, Murayama H, Nakajima T (1999) Basic performance of PET scanner, EXACT HR+, with adjustable data-acquisition parameters. IEEE Trans Nucl Sci 40(3):652–658
3. Adam LE, Karp JS, Daube-Witherspoon ME, Smith RJ (2001) Performance of a whole-body PET scanner using curve-plate NaI(Tl) detectors. J Nucl Med 42:1821–1830
4. Suk JY, Thompson CJ, Labuda A, Goertzen AL (2008) Improvement of the spatial resolution of the MicroPET R4 scanner by wobbling the bed. Med Phys 35(4):1223–1231
5. Hoffman EJ, Huang SC, Phelps ME (1979) Quantitation in positron emission computed tomography: 1. Effects of object size. J Comput Assist Tomogr 3:299–308
6. Meltzer CC, Leal JP, Mayberg HS, Wagner HJ, Frost JJ (1990) Correction of PET data for partial volume effects in human cerebral cortex by MR imaging. J Comput Assist Tomogr 14:561–570
7. Rousset OG, Ma Y, Evans AC (1998) Correction for partial volume effects in PET: principle and validation. J Nucl Med 39:904–911
8. Meltzer C, Kinahan P, Greer P, Nichols TE, Comtat C, Cantwell MN, Lin MP, Price JC (1999) Comparative evaluation of MR-based partial volume correction schemes for PET. J Nucl Med 40:2053–2065
9. Aston JAD, Cunningham VJ, Asselin MC, Hammers A, Evans AC, Gunn RN (2002) Positron emission tomography partial volume correction: estimation and algorithms. J Cereb Blood Flow Metab 22:1019–1034
10. Boussion N, Hatt M, Lamare F, Bizais Y, Turzo A, Cheze-Le Rest C, Visvikis D (2006) A multiresolution image based approach for correction of partial volume effects in emission tomography. Phys Med Biol 51:1857–1876
11. Soret M, Bacharach SL, Buvat I (2007) Partial volume effect in PET tumor imaging. J Nucl Med 48:932–945
12. Watson CC (2000) New, faster, image-based scatter correction for 3D PET. IEEE Trans Nucl Sci 47:1587–1594
13. Kinahan PE, Townsend DW, Beyer T et al (1998) Attenuation correction for a combined 3D PET/CT scanner. Med Phys 25:2046–2053
14. Burger C, Goerres G, Schoenes S et al (2002) PET attenuation coefficients from CT images: experimental evaluation of the transformation of CT into PET 511-keV attenuation coefficients. Eur J Nucl Med Mol Imaging 29:922–927
15. Kinahan PE, Hasegawa BH, Beyer T (2003) X-ray-based attenuation correction for positron emission tomography/computed tomography scanners. Semin Nucl Med 33: 166–179
16. Watson CC, Rappoport V, Faul D et al (2006) A method for calibrating the CT-based attenuation correction of PET in human tissue. IEEE Trans Nucl Sci 53:102–107
17. Carney JP, Townsend DW, Rappoport V et al (2006) Method for transforming CT images for attenuation correction in PET/CT imaging. Med Phys 33:976–983
18. Townsend WD (2008) Positron emission tomography/computed tomography. Semin Nucl Med 38:152–166
19. Shepp LA, Vardi Y (1982) Maximum likelihood reconstruction for emission tomography. IEEE Trans Med Imaging MI-1:113–122
20. Kak AC, Slaney M (1998) Principles of computerized tomographic imaging. IEEE Press, New York
21. Hudson H, Larkin R (1994) Accelerated image reconstruction using ordered subsets of projection data. IEEE Trans Med Imaging 13:601–609
22. Defrise M, Kinahan PE, Townsend DW, Michel C, Sibomana M, Newport DF (1997) Exact and approximate rebinning algorithms for 3-D PET data. IEEE Trans Med Imaging 16:145–158
23. Alenius S, Ruotsalainen U (1997) Bayesian image reconstruction for emission tomography based on median root prior. Eur J Nucl Med 24:258–265
24. Kinahan PE, Rodgers JG (1989) Analytic 3D image reconstruction using all detected events. IEEE Trans Nucl Sci 36:964–968
25. Liu X, Comtat C, Michel C et al (2001) Comparison of 3-D reconstruction with 3D-OSEM and with FORE-OSEM for PET. IEEE Trans Med Imaging 20:804–814
26. Popescu LM, Matej S, Lewitt RM (2004) Iterative image reconstruction using geometrically ordered subsets with list-mode data. Nucl Sci Symp Conf Rec 6:3536–3540
27. Huesman RH (1984) A new fast algorithm for evaluation of regions of interest and statistical uncertainty in computed tomography. Phys Med Biol 29:543–552
28. Carson RE, Lange K (1985) The EM parametric image reconstruction algorithm. J Am Stat Assoc 80:20–22
29. Maguire RP, Calonder C, Leenders KL (1997) An investigation of multiple time/graphical analysis applied to projection data: theory and validation. J Comput Assist Tomogr 21:327–331

30. Huesman RH, Reutter BW, Zeng GL, Gullberg TL (1998) Kinetic parameter estimation from SPECT cone-beam projection measurements. Phys Med Biol 43:973–982

31. Matthews J, Bailey D, Price P, Cunningham V (1997) The direct calculation of parametric images from dynamic PET data using maximum-likelihood iterative reconstruction. Phys Med Biol 42:1155–1173

32. Meikle SR, Matthews JC, Cunningham V, Bailey DL, Livieratos L, Jones T, Price P (1998) Parametric image reconstruction using spectral analysis of PET projection data. Phys Med Biol 43:651–666

33. Bentourkia M (2003) PET kinetic modeling of ^{13}N-ammonia from sinograms in rats. IEEE Trans Nucl Sci 50(1):32–36

34. Bentourkia M (2003) PET kinetic modeling of ^{11}C-acetate from projections. Comput Med Imaging Graph 27: 373–379

35. Arhjoul L, Bentourkia M (2007) Assessment of glucose metabolism from the projections using the wavelet technique in small animal PET imaging. Comp Med Imaging Graph 31:157–165

36. Kamasak ME, Bouman CA, Morris ED, Sauer K (2005) Direct reconstruction of kinetic parameter images from dynamic PET data. IEEE Trans Med Imaging 24(5): 636–650

37. Gallagher MB, Fowler JS, Gutterson NI, MacGregor RR, Wan CN, Wolf AP (1978) Metabolic trapping as a principle of radiopharmaceutical design: some factors responsible for the biodistribution of [^{18}F] 2-deoxy-2-fluoro-D-glucose. J Nucl Med 19(10):1154–1161

38. Raichle ME, Larson KB, Phelps ME et al (1975) In vivo measurement of brain glucose transport and metabolism employing glucose-11C. Am J Physiol 228:1936–1948

39. Kuhl DE, Phelps ME, Hoffman EJ et al (1977) Initial clinical experience with 18F-2-deoxy-D-glucose for determination of local cerebral glucose utilization by emission computed tomography. Acta Neurol Scand 56(64): 192–193

40. Reivich M, Kuhl D, Wolf A et al (1977) Measurement of local cerebral glucose metabolism in man with 18F-2-fluoro-2-deoxy-D-glucose. Acta Neurol Scand 56(64): 192–193

41. Sokoloff L, Reivich M, Kennedy C et al (1977) The [14C] deoxyglucose method for the measurement of local cerebral glucose utilization: theory, procedure and normal values in the conscious and anesthetized albino rat. J Neurochem 28(5):897–916

42. Phelps ME, Huang SC, Hoffman EJ, Selin C, Sokoloff L, Kuhl DE (1979) Tomographic measurement of local cerebral glucose metabolic rate in humans with (F-18)2-fluoro-2-deoxy-D-glucose: validation of method. Ann Neurol 6:371–388

43. Nauck MA, Lie H, Siegel EG, Niedmann PD, Creutzfeldt W (1992) Critical evaluation of the "heated-hand-technique" for obtaining "arterialized" venous blood: incomplete arterialization and alterations in glucagon responses. Clin Physiol 12:537–552

44. MacDonald IA (1999) Arterio-venous differences to study macronutrient metabolism: introduction and overview. Proc Nutr Soc 58:871–875

45. McGuire EAH, Helderman JH, Tobin JD, Andres R, Berman M (1976) Effects of arterial versus venous sampling on analysis of glucose kinetics in man. J Appl Physiol 41:565–573

46. Abumrad NN, Rabin D, Diamond MP, Lacy WW (1981) Use of heated superficial hand vein as an alternative site for the measurement of amino acid concentrations and for the study of glucose and alanine kinetics in man. Metabolism 30:936–940

47. Sonnenberg E, Keller U (1982) Sampling of arterialized heated-hand venous blood as a non-invasive technique for the study of ketone body kinetics in man. Metabolism 31:1–5

48. Boellaard R, van Lingen A, van Balen SC, Hoving BG, Lammertsma AA (2001) Characteristics of a new fully programmable blood sampling device for monitoring blood radioactivity during PET. Eur J Nucl Med 28(1):81–89

49. Yamamoto S, Tarutani K, Suga M, Minato K, Watabe H, Iida H (2001) Development of a phoswich detector for a continuous blood-sampling system. IEEE Trans Nucl Sci 48:1408–1411

50. Pain F, Laniece P, Mastrippolito R, Gervais P, Hantraye P, Besret L (2004) Arterial input function measurement without blood sampling using a β-microprobe in rats. J Nucl Med 45:1577–1582

51. Convert L, Morin-Brassard G, Cadorette J, Archambault M, Bentourkia M, Lecomte R (2007) A new tool for molecular imaging: the microvolumetric β blood counter. J Nucl Med 48:1197–1206

52. Gambhir SS, Schwaiger M, Huang SC, Krivokapich J, Schelbert HR, Nienaber CA, Phelps ME (1989) Simple noninvasive quantification method for measuring myocardial glucose utilization in humans employing positron emission tomography and fluorine-18 deoxyglucose. J Nucl Med 30(3):359–366

53. Iida H, Rhodes CG, de Silva R, Araujo LI, Bloomfield PM, Lammertsma AA, Jones T (1992) Use of the left ventricular time-activity curve as a noninvasive input function in dynamic oxygen-15-water positron emission tomography. J Nucl Med 33(9):1669–1677

54. Lin KP, Huang SC, Choi Y, Brunken RC, Schelbert HR, Phelps ME (1995) Correction of spillover radioactivities for estimation of the blood time-activity curve from the imaged LV chamber in cardiac dynamic FDG PET studies. Phys Med Biol 40(4):629–642

55. Ohtake T, Kosaka N, Watanabe T, Yokoyama I, Moritan T, Masuo M, Iizuka M, Kozeni K, Momose T, Oku S et al (1991) Noninvasive method to obtain input function for measuring tissue glucose utilization of thoracic and abdominal organs. J Nucl Med 32(7):1432–1438

56. Germano G, Chen BC, Huang SC, Gambhir SS, Hoffman EJ, Phelps ME (1992) Use of the abdominal aorta for arterial input function determination in hepatic and renal PET studies. J Nucl Med 33(4):620–622

57. Litton JE (1997) Input function in PET brain studies using MR-defined arteries. J Comput Assist Tomogr 21(6): 907–909

58. Hoekstra CJ, Hoekstra OS, Lammertsma AA (1999) On the use of image-derived input functions in oncological fluorine-18 fluorodeoxyglucose positron emission tomography studies. Eur J Nucl Med 26(11):1489–1492

59. Watabe H, Channing MA, Riddell C, Jousse F, Libutti SK, Carrasquillo JA, Bacharach SL, Carson RE (2001) Noninvasive estimation of the aorta input function for measurement of tumor blood flow with. IEEE Trans Med Imaging 20(3):164–174

60. Barber DC (1980) The use of principal components in the quantitative analysis of gamma camera dynamic studies. Phys Med Biol 25(2):283–292

61. Di Paola R, Bazin JP, Aubry F, Aurengo A, Cavailloles F, Herry JY et al (1982) Handling of dynamic sequences in nuclear medicine. IEEE Trans Nucl Sci 29:1310–1321

62. Wu HM, Hoh CK, Choi Y, Schelbert HR, Hawkins RA, Phelps ME et al (1995) Factor analysis for extraction of blood time-activity curves in dynamic FDG-PET studies. J Nucl Med 36(9):1714–1722

63. Bentourkia M (2005) Kinetic modeling of PET data without blood sampling. IEEE Trans Nucl Sci 52(3):697–702

64. Kim J, Herrero P, Sharp T, Laforest R, Rowland DJ, Tai YC et al (2006) Minimally invasive method of determining blood input function from PET images in rodents. J Nucl Med 47(2):330–336

65. Shoghi KI, Rowland DJ, Laforest R, Welch MJ (2006). Characterization of spillover and recovery coefficients in the gated mouse heart for noninvasive extraction of input function in microPET studies: feasibility and sensitivity analysis. IEEE Nucl Sci Symp 4:2134–2136

66. Lee JS, Lee DS, Ahn JY, Cheon GJ, Kim SK, Yeo JS, Seo K, Park KS, Chung JK, Lee MC (2001) Blind separation of cardiac components and extraction of input function from H(2)(15)O dynamic myocardial PET using independent component analysis. J Nucl Med 42(6):938–943

67. Magadan-Mendez M, Kivimaki A, Ruotsalainen U (2004). ICA separation of functional components from dynamic cardiac PET data. NSS & MIC Conference

68. Naganawa M, Kimura Y, Ishii K, Oda K, Ishiwata K, Matani A (2005) Extraction of a plasma time-activity curve from dynamic brain PET images based on independent component analysis. IEEE Trans Biomed Eng 52 (2):201–210

69. Chen K, Chen X, Renaut R, Alexander GE, Bandy D, Guo H, Reiman EM (2007) Characterization of the image-derived carotid artery input function using independent component analysis for the quantitation of [18F] fluorodeoxyglucose positron emission tomography images. Phys Med Biol 52(23):7055–7071

70. Takikawa S, Dhawan V, Spetsieris P, Robeson W, Chaly T, Dahl R, Margouleff D, Eidelberg D (1993) Noninvasive quantitative fluorodeoxyglucose PET studies with an estimated input function derived from a population-based arterial blood curve. Radiology 188(1):131–136

71. Eberl S, Anayat AR, Fulton RR, Hooper PK, Fulham MJ (1997) Evaluation of two population-based input functions for quantitative neurological FDG PET studies. Eur J Nucl Med 24(3):299–304

72. Wakita K, Imahori Y, Ido T, Fujii R, Horii H, Shimizu M, Nakajima S, Mineura K, Nakamura T, Kanatsuna T (2000) Simplification for measuring input function of FDG PET: investigation of 1-point blood sampling method. J Nucl Med 41(9):1484–1490

73. Cunningham VJ, Jones T (1993) Spectral analysis of dynamic PET studies. J Cereb Blood Flow Metab 13:15–23

74. Lammertsma AA, Hume SP (1996) Simplified reference tissue model for PET receptor studies. Neuroimage 4: 153–158

75. Feng D, Wong KP, Wu CM, Siu WC (1997) A technique for extracting physiological parameters and the required input function simultaneously from PET image measurements: theory and simulation study. IEEE Trans Inf Technol Biomed 1(4):243–254

76. Bentourkia M (2006) Kinetic modeling of PET-FDG in the brain without blood sampling. Comput Med Imaging Graph 30:447–451

77. Carson RE, Breier A, de Bartolomeis A, Saunders RC, Su TP, Schmall B, Der MG, Pickar D, Eckelman WC (1997) Quantification of amphetamine-induced changes in [11C] raclopride binding with continuous infusion. J Cereb Blood Flow Metab 17:437–447

78. Ito H, Hietala J, Blomqvist G, Halldin C, Farde L (1998) Comparison of the transient equilibrium and continuous infusion method for quantitative PET analysis of [11C] raclopride binding. J Cereb Blood Flow Metab 18:941–950

79. Bérard V, Rousseau J, Cadorette J, Hubert L, Bentourkia M, van Lier JE, Lecomte R (2006) Dynamic imaging of transient metabolic processes by small animal positron emission tomography for the evaluation of photosensitizers in photodynamic therapy of cancer. J Nucl Med 47:1119–1126

80. Bentourkia M, Boubacar P, Bérard V, van Lier JE, Lecomte R (2007) Kinetic modeling of PET data and FDG continuous infusion in rat tumors simultaneously treated with PDT. IEEE Nuclear Science Symposium and Medical Imaging Conference, October 28 – November 3, 2007

81. Delbeke D (1999) Oncological applications of FDG PET imaging: brain tumors, colorectal cancer, lymphoma and melanoma. J Nucl Med 40:591–603

82. Lucas JD, O'Doherty MJ, Cronin BF et al (1999) Prospective evaluation of soft tissue masses and sarcomas using fluorodeoxyglucose positron emission tomography. Br J Surg 86:550–556

83. Sugawara Y, Zasadny KR, Grossman HB, Francis IR, Clarke MF, Wahl RL (1999) Germ cell tumor: differentiation of viable tumor, mature teratoma, and necrotic tissue with FDG PET and kinetic modeling. Radiology 211: 249–256

84. Kubota K, Yamada S, Ishiwata K, Ito M, Ido T (1992) Positron emission tomography for treatment evaluation and recurrence detection compared with CT in long-term follow-up cases of lung cancer. Clin Nucl Med 17: 877–881

85. Hunter GJ, Hamberg LM, Choi N, Jain RK, McCloud T, Fischman AJ (1988) Dynamic T1-weighted magnetic resonance imaging and positron emission tomography in patients with lung cancer: correlating vascular physiology with glucose metabolism. Clin Cancer Res 4:949–955

86. Bol A, Melin JA, Vanoverschelde JL, Baudhuin T, Vogelaers D, De Pauw M, Michel C, Luxen A, Labar D,

Cogneau M, Robert A, Heyndrickx GR, Wijns W (1993) Direct comparison of (nitrogen-13) ammonia and (oxygen-15)water estimates of perfusion with quantification of regional myocardial blood flow by microspheres. Circulation 87(2):512–525

87. Wahl ML, Ce Asselin M, Nahmias C (1999) Regions of interest in the venous sinuses as input functions for quantitative PET. J Nucl Med 40:1666–1675

88. Lee JS, Su KH, Lin JC et al (2008) A novel blood-cell-two-compartment model for transferring a whole blood time activity curve to plasma in rodents. Comput Meth Programs Biomed 92(3):299–304

89. Reivich M, Alavi A, Wolf A, Fowler J, Russell J, Arnett C, MacGregor RR, Shiue CY, Atkins H, Anand A (1985) Glucose metabolic rate kinetic model parameter determination in humans: the lumped constants and rate constants for [18F]fluorodeoxyglucose and [11C]deoxyglucose. J Cereb Blood Flow Metab 5(2):179–192

90. Graham MM, Muzi M, Spence AM, O'Sullivan F, Lewellen TK, Links JM, Krohn KA (2002) The FDG lumped constant in normal human brain. J Nucl Med 43:1157–1166

91. Hasselbalch SG, Madsen PL, Knudsen GM, Holm S, Paulson OB (1998) Calculation of the FDG lumped constant by simultaneous measurements of global glucose and FDG metabolism in humans. J Cereb Blood Flow Metab 18:154–160

92. PressWH TSA, Vetterling WT, Flannery BP (1988) Numerical recipes in C: the art of scientific computing. Cambridge University Press, New York

93. Hutchins G, Holden J, Koeppe R, Halama J, Gatley S, Nickles R (1984) Alternative approach to single-scan estimation of cerebral glucose metabolic rate using glucose analogs, with particular application to ischemia. J Cereb Blood Flow Metab 4:35–40

94. Patlak CS, Blasberg RG, Fenstermacher JD (1983) Graphical evaluation of blood-to-brain transfer constants from multiple-time uptake data. J Cereb Blood Flow Metab 3:1–7

95. Gjedde A, Wienhard K, Heiss W et al (1985) Comparative regional analysis of 2-fluorodeoxyglucose and methylglucose uptake in brain of four stroke patients. With special reference to the regional estimation of the lumped constant. J Cereb Blood Flow Metab 5:163–178

96. Kitsukawa S, Yoshida K, Mullani N et al (1998) Simple and Patlak models for myocardial blood flow measurements with nitrogen-13-ammonia and PET in humans. J Nucl Med 39:1123–1128

97. Turkheimer F, Sokoloff L, Bertoldo A, Lucignani G, Reivich M, Jaggi JL, Schmidt K (1998) Estimation of component and parameter distributions in spectral analysis. J Cereb Blood Flow Metab 18(11):1211–1222

98. Buck AH, Wolpers HG, Hutchins GD, Savas V, Mangner TJ, Nguyen N, Schwaiger M (1991) Effect of carbon-11-acetate recirculation on estimates of myocardial oxygen consumption by PET. J Nucl Med 32(10):1950–1957

99. Lawson CL, Hanson RJ (1974) Solving least squares problems. Prentice-Hall, Englewood Cliffs, p 161, Chapter 23

100. Gunn RN, Gunn SR, Cunningham VJ (2001) Positron emission tomography compartmental models. J Cereb Blood Flow Metab 21:635–652

101. Muzik O, Beanlands RSB, Hutchins GD, Mangner TJ, Nguyen N, Schwaiger M (1993) Validation of nitrogen-13-ammonia tracer kinetic model for quantification of myocardial blood flow using PET. J Nucl Med 34:83–91

102. Huang SC (2000) Anatomy of SUV. Nucl Med Biol 27:643–646

103. Lucignani G, Paganelli G, Bombardieri E (2004) The use of standardized uptake values for assessing FDG uptake with PET in oncology: a clinical perspective. Nucl Med Commun 25:651–656

104. Thie JA (2004) Understanding the standardized uptake value, its methods, and implications for usage. J Nucl Med 45:1431–1434

105. Zasadny KR, Wahl RL (1993) Standardized uptake values of normal tissues at PET with 2-[fluorine-18]-fluoro-2-deoxy-D-glucose: variations with body weight and a method for correction. Radiology 189:847–850

106. Keyes JWJ (1995) SUV: standard uptake or silly useless value? J Nucl Med 36:1836–1839

107. Gunn RN, Gunn SR, Turkheimer FE, Aston JAD, Cunningham VJ (2002) Positron emission tomography compartmental models: a basis pursuit strategy for kinetic modelling. J Cereb Blood Flow Metab 22(12):1425–1439

108. Defrise M, Townsend DW, Bailey D, Geissbuhler A, Michel C, Jones T (1991) A normalization technique for 3D PET data. Phys Med Biol 36(7):939–952

109. Bailey DL, Jones T (1997) A method for calibrating three-dimensional positron emission tomography without scatter correction. Eur J Nucl Med 24:660–664

110. Thomas MDR, Bailey DL, Livieratos L (2005) A dual modality approach to quantitative quality control in emission tomography. Phys Med Biol 50:N187–N194

111. Cherry SR, Huang SC (1995) Effects of scatter on model parameter estimates in 3D PET studies of the human brain. IEEE Trans Nucl Sci 42(4):1174–1179

112. Iida H, Narita Y, Kado H et al (1998) Effect of scatter and attenuation correction on quantitative assessment of regional cerebral blood flow with SPECT. J Nucl Med 39:181–189

113. Kim KM, Watabe H, Shidahara M, Onishi Y, Yonekura Y, Iida H (2001) Impact of scatter correction in the kinetic analysis of a D2 receptor ligand SPECT study. IEEE Nuclear Science Symposium Conference Record

114. Chow PL, Rannou FR, Chatziioannou AF (2005) Attenuation correction for small animal PET tomographs. Phys Med Biol 50(8):1837–1850

115. National Electrical Manufacturers Association (2001) NEMA standards publication NU 2-2001. National Electrical Manufacturers Association, Rosslyn

116. International Electrotechnical Commission (1998) IEC Standard 61675-1: Radionuclide imaging devices – characteristics and test conditions. Part 1. Positron emission tomographs. International Electrotechnical Commission, Geneva

117. Selivanov V, Lapointe D, Bentourkia M, Lecomte R (2001) Cross-validation stopping rule for ML-EM reconstruction of dynamic PET series: effect on image quality and quantitative accuracy. IEEE Trans Nucl Sci 48:883–889

Contents

A. Douraghy (✉)
Department of Molecular and Medical Pharmacology, Crump Institute for Molecular Imaging, David Geffen School of Medicine at UCLA, 570 Westwood Plaza, CNSI-4345, Building 114, Mail Code 177010, Los Angeles, CA 90095-1770, USA
e-mail: adouraghy@gmail.com

A.F. Chatziioannou
Department of Molecular and Medical Pharmacology, Crump Institute for Molecular Imaging, David Geffen School of Medicine at UCLA, 570 Westwood Plaza, CNSI-4345, Building 114, Mail Code 177010, Los Angeles, CA 90095-1770, USA
e-mail: archatziioann@mednet.ucla.edu

18.1 Introduction

This chapter provides the reader with an introductory look into the significance of preclinical imaging relative to human medicine. The concept of translating preclinical research to the clinical realm is presented with a focus on the primary human disease model, the mouse. Here, the term Small Animal Imaging (SAI) is used to describe preclinical imaging of mice. The fundamental operating principles of the various SAI technologies and primary differences with their clinical counterparts are described. First generation and state-of-the-art instruments are reviewed as well as the utility of combining these technologies into multimodality instruments. Considerations in small animal use, such as anesthesia and radiation dose are followed by a brief look at SAI center design. The application of SAI in the areas of cardiology, neurology, and oncology are reviewed and finally, a perspective on the future of SAI is given. This is not meant to be a comprehensive review, but rather a primer for the biomedical student or researcher to become familiarized with the overall field of preclinical imaging. For further information the reader is referred to external sources of literature.

18.2 What Is Small Animal Imaging?

18.2.1 Translational Medicine

Currently, clinical understanding and treatment of human disease is largely applied on the macro scale of tissue and organ manifestations of disease, as well as in traditional pathology reports. Recent advances in biomedical research have identified large numbers of molecules and signaling pathways that potentially promote or limit disease [1] suggesting that the future of disease diagnosis and treatment will be based on an understanding of the molecular considerations involved. *Molecular* or *Personalized Medicine* can be defined as the study of the underlying molecular mechanisms of disease and the development of targeted treatments which act at the molecular level. The overall understanding of how these molecular components interact with each other, in the cell, organ, and organism is termed the *Systems Biology* approach [2]. The shift toward this new paradigm for understanding and treating disease is critically dependent on the development of the necessary tools, and their effective use in exploring its fundamental molecular basis. Molecular medicine is just beginning and much needs to be done in order to bridge the gap between laboratory science and treating patients in the clinic. Our developing understanding of the molecular basis necessitates the two-way transfer of information between basic sciences and clinical practice. *Translational Medicine* is the process by which this exchange takes place [3–9]. Systems Biology and Translational Medicine are integrated approaches which encompass several scientific disciplines such as genomics, proteomics, transgenic animal models, structural biology, biochemistry, and imaging technologies among several others [9]. At the center of this exchange are small animal models of disease, which, provide a view of disease in vivo through direct observation of the molecular scenario via SAI technologies.

18.2.2 The Mouse

Some of the more common animal models for studying mammalian disease biology include nonhuman primates, cats, dogs, pigs, and rodents. This introduction focuses almost exclusively on the mouse (murine) model as it is widely used and makes up more than 90% of all mammalian animal studies of disease [10]. The mouse is the established model of choice for several reasons which include a high genetic homology with man, well-developed methodology for genetic manipulation, quick reproduction cycle, relatively low cost of maintenance, and its small size allowing for rapid screening at the system and organ level [11]. By targeting specific regions of the genome

using DNA swapping methods such as homologous recombination, mouse genes can be "knocked-in," "knocked-out", or overexpressed [12–14]. These and other manipulation techniques allow study of the genotypic basis and the expression of phenotypes of normal and diseased states of biological processes [15]. The ability to disable or alter specific genes in the mouse genome has prompted a revolution in our understanding of mammalian disease. This is attested by the 2007 Nobel Prize in Physiology or Medicine as well as the undertaking of long-term global commitments to creating libraries containing knockout mouse models for every gene [16, 17]. Recent milestones in the biological sciences such as the mapping and sequencing of the human and mouse genomes, while in themselves significant, have only underscored our limited understanding of the role of mammalian genes within the system of organs, tissues, and the organism.

18.2.3 Small Animal Imaging

Clinical imaging, while extremely useful in diagnosing and treating disease, is still largely nonspecific and operates on the macro scale of viewing tissues and organs. As such, clinical imaging techniques are not yet optimized for identifying the underlying molecular mechanisms involved in disease. SAI on the other hand promises to image more specific molecular scenarios involving the genes, proteins, and cells of human disease. There is a multitude of known, and still unknown, information about genes, proteins, cellular interactions, and their molecular pathways in diseased states. Biological researchers are constantly discovering genes and proteins that are involved in disease. Most often, these are part of multilevel and complex interactions involving several molecular players. Researchers may want to know where specific proteins of a gene are expressed, their level of expression, and how their distribution and level changes over time [18]. SAI facilitates the functional study of these multicomponent interactions and can give insight to their kinetic rates, intracellular signaling mechanisms, and so forth [18]. SAI provides us with a very powerful set of tools to formulate and answer these types of questions.

SAI provides a means of directly observing in vivo the biological and physiological processes over time in

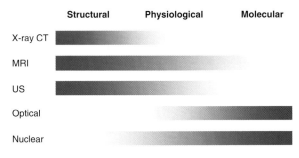

Fig. 18.1 The useful range of the primary imaging modalities relative to one another for imaging structure and function

the same animals, while providing an anatomical reference of the structures in which these processes take place. The effective use of SAI technologies must consider the imaging requirements needed to answer the biological questions at hand. Each imaging modality has strengths and weaknesses and is characterized by its different spatial and temporal resolution and sensitivity for function and structure [19]. The reason that several different modalities exist is because each operates in a defined parameter space that renders it well suited for some applications and unsuitable for others [19]. Figure 18.1 illustrates the useful range of the primary imaging modalities relative to one another for imaging structure and function. Often, combining imaging modalities in studies can complement their strengths and weaknesses to improve the overall performance and the quality of the information gathered. As the field advances, SAI technologies will offer increasing sensitivity and resolution to quantify specific biological targets in vivo [18]. Animal models and the means by which to study them undoubtedly play a central and critical role in the continuing investigation of fundamental biological processes and our ability to develop treatment therapies to more accurately target disease.

18.3 Principles and Technologies

18.3.1 Overview

Several clinical imaging technologies such as Magnetic Resonance Imaging (MRI), x-ray Computed Tomography (CT), Ultrasound (US), Single Photon Emission Computed Tomography (SPECT), and Positron Emission Tomography (PET) have been adapted for the imaging of small animals. These small animal counterparts are commonly referred to as the "micro" modalities, given their enhanced spatial resolution capabilities. These modalities, including the more animal-specific ones of Autoradiography (AR) and Optical Imaging (OI), are reviewed in this section.

In each modality, radiation is utilized to collect information from the tissue under investigation through X-rays (CT), Radio-waves (MRI), High-frequency sound waves (US), Charged particles (AR), Visible and Infrared light (OI), and Gamma-rays (SPECT/PET) [19]. As such, the possible imaging scenarios arising from the different physics principles employed in each provide unique information. These possibilities must be considered against the biological questions at hand, as each major modality measures fundamentally different information [19]. The modalities are roughly grouped into two categories based on their capability to image *structure* and/or *function*. The modalities of microCT, microMRI, and ultrasound mostly image anatomical structures. Yet, each one has the ability to relay some functional information, particularly MRI. The other modalities, optical and radionuclide imaging, offer little anatomical information and are most often used to image physiological and molecular information. Table 18.1 details some of the general performance parameters and applications for the different SAI modalities. Parameters of interest include the basis of information gathering, spatial resolution (and whether or not the information is depth dependent), time scale, sensitivity, ability to quantify information, and the type of information arrived at. These parameters are discussed in more detail for each modality.

The ability to image animal models noninvasively and in vivo provides biomedical researchers with an extremely powerful set of tools with which to investigate human disease. Noninvasive in vivo imaging provides, by definition, several advantages. One advantage is the ability to study the same animal over time. In other words, the entire time course of a radiolabeled probe biodistribution, disease progression, or therapeutic response can be determined in a single animal. The result is a substantial reduction in the number of animals used since the need to sacrifice animals at various time points is virtually eliminated. This also improves the speed of obtaining results and can remove interanimal differences which

Table 18.1 Physical basis of information, general performance parameters, and applications for the different small animal imaging modalities

Modality	Basis	Spatial resolution	Depth dependent	Time scale	Sensitivity (mol/l)	Quantitative	Information
CT	X-rays	~20 μm	No	min	–	+	Structural
							Physiological
MRI	Radio-waves	~20 μm	No	min-h	10^{-3}–10^{-5}	++	Structural
							Physiological
							Molecular
Ultrasound	High-frequency sound waves	~50 μm	Yes	s-min	–	+	Structural
							Physiological
Autoradiography	Charged particles	~5 μm	Yes	h-weeks	10^{-11}–10^{-12}	+++	Structural
							Physiological
							Molecular
SPECT	γ-ray photons	<1 mm	No	min-h	10^{-10}–10^{-11}	+++	Physiological
							Molecular
PET	Annihilation photons	~1 mm	No	min-h	10^{-11}–10^{-12}	+++	Physiological
							Molecular
Fluorescence	Visible-NIR	Several mm	Yes	s-min	10^{-9}–10^{-12}	No	Physiological
							Molecular
Bioluminescence	Visible-NIR	Several mm	Yes	s-min	10^{-15}–10^{-17}	No	Molecular

are introduced when multiple animals are required. The reduction in animals can also reduce the financial expense of studies, although this is not always the case as some of the imaging instruments and their operational costs are still high. With the increased dissemination and awareness of SAI and the development of newer technologies, the costs associated with imaging can surely be reduced, further facilitating its widespread use.

18.3.2 Structural Imaging

18.3.2.1 Micro X-Ray Computed Tomography

Micro x-ray Computed Tomography (microCT) provides the ability to noninvasively scan small animals and to produce high-resolution tomographic images detailing anatomy such as bone and cartilage [20,21]. In microCT, an x-ray source is used to transmit a polychromatic beam of x-rays through the subject at hundreds of equally spaced angular projections.

A detector is used on the opposite side to measure the x-ray flux. The x-ray flux is proportional to the level of attenuation of the x-rays by the tissues and represents the tissue density. The projections are reconstructed using mathematical algorithms to determine the x-ray attenuation in each voxel (volume element) of the image volume. Uses of microCT range from the need to overlay anatomical information for the localization of radioisotope tracer distributions from SPECT and PET studies to the ability to image tumor nodules in the mouse lungs and other tissues. A more detailed description of microCT and its applications is available elsewhere [20, 21].

The spatial resolution of microCT can be as high as a few tens of microns. The spatial resolution is primarily determined by the x-ray focal spot size, the geometry of the mouse relative to the source and detector, and the detector element size [20]. The most common microCT system geometry consists of a stationary subject and an x-ray source-detector pair that rotates around the subject, similar to most clinical CT systems.

Fig. 18.2 The main differences between microCT and clinical CT are in the energies of the x-ray beams used and in the spatial resolution. The x-ray tube in microCT is typically operated at a voltage of 40–80 kVp as opposed to 80–140 kVp for clinical systems producing x-ray beams with different energy spectra (Figure courtesy of Dr. Richard Taschereau, University of California, Los Angeles)

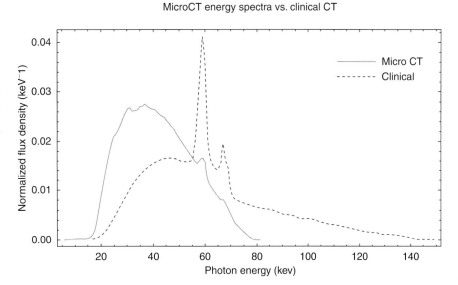

The main differences between microCT and clinical CT are in the energies of the x-ray beams used and in the spatial resolution. The x-ray tube in microCT is typically operated at a voltage of 40–80 kVp as opposed to 80–120 kVp for clinical systems. This produces x-ray beams with different energy spectra (clinical data from reference [22]), as shown in Fig. 18.2. Thus, the beam *effective energy*, which describes its penetration power, is also different [23]. Given the nonlinear x-ray attenuation of materials (in this case tissue) as a function of energy, different effective energies will lead to different ratios between the attenuation coefficients of the materials under observation.

The attenuation of x-rays depends on the atomic number (Z), the density of the material composition, and the energy of the x-rays. Figure 18.3 shows the mass attenuation coefficient for water and cortical bone as a function of energy. The shaded area denotes the useful range of preclinical x-rays. Attenuation of a given x-ray beam is given as:

$$I_t = I_0 \cdot e^{-\int_0^t \mu(E)\,dt}$$

where, I_t represents the intensity of the attenuated beam after it passes through the subject with an initial intensity of I_0, $\mu(E)$ is the energy-dependent linear attenuation coefficient (cm^{-1}), and t is the thickness of the material that the beam traverses.

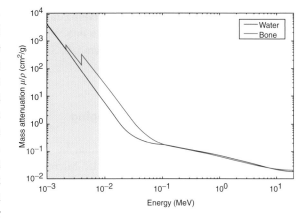

Fig. 18.3 Mass attenuation coefficient for water and cortical bone as a function of x-ray energy. The shaded area represents the useful energy range of x-rays for preclinical imaging. Note the log scale on both axes (Data taken from National Institute of Standards and Technology [NIST] website)

The projections are used in the image reconstruction process to solve for the μ values, which yield the CT numbers at each location. The CT numbers represent attenuation of the tissue normalized to the attenuation of water:

$$CT\# = \frac{(\mu_{\text{tissue}} - \mu_{\text{water}})}{\mu_{\text{water}}} \cdot 1{,}000$$

Since the x-ray beam is polychromatic by nature, lower energy x-rays are preferentially absorbed as the beam traverses the material, changing the effective beam energy and thus, the measured attenuation coefficients. This effect is referred to as *beam hardening* and results in image artifacts during reconstruction [24]. One method to alleviate beam hardening is to filter the x-ray beam between the source and the subject using materials such as Aluminum or Molybdenum. These materials preferentially absorb some of the lower energy x-rays, which only contribute to radiation dose at the surface and not to the image formation. Several methods have been suggested for reducing beam hardening using software and hardware techniques [25–27].

Detection of x-rays can be done using direct or indirect detection methods. Pixilated flat-panel amorphous selenium detectors can be used to convert x-rays directly to an electric charge which represents the x-ray flux [28, 29]. In indirect detection, scintillating screens such as Gadolinium Oxysulfide (GOS) or Cesium Iodide CsI(Tl) are used to convert x-ray energies to visible light. These screens are optically coupled to solid-state visible light detectors [30, 31].

18.3.2.2 Magnetic Resonance Imaging

Small animal Magnetic Resonance Imaging (MRI), also referred to as microMRI and MR Microscopy, utilizes magnetic fields and Radio-frequency (RF) signals to collect information about the nuclei of endogenous hydrogen atoms. The nuclei of the hydrogen atoms are positively charged protons that induce a magnetic moment along the proton axis. When an external magnetic field is applied by the MR magnet, a fraction of the protons orient their spin with the external field. The application of a RF perturbs the nuclei to higher energy states as they absorb the RF energy, termed *excitation*. Upon switching the external magnetic field, the protons undergo *relaxation* and will emit energy in the form of a unique RF that is characteristic of their density and tissue relaxation properties. Since hydrogen is present in all tissues as water (H_2O), a great deal of information regarding differences in soft tissue densities can be extracted using MRI. The RF information regarding the tissue characteristics is used to form a tomographic image. Similar imaging techniques can be used to extract information from the nuclei of other atoms such as ^{31}P, ^{13}C, and ^{3}He [32].

Small animal MRI typically uses magnetic fields with strengths between 4.7 and 9.4 Tesla and small bore sizes of 20–40 cm in diameter [18]. The sensitivity of MRI is determined by its signal-to-noise ratio (SNR). The signal is proportional to the number of nuclei detected in the voxel of resolution. Therefore, there is a trade-off between increased resolution (smaller voxels) and the SNR. To overcome this limitation, higher field strengths and specialized RF coils are often used to maximize the SNR [33]. In vivo images of anatomy with a resolution of less than a hundred microns can be achieved with MRI. An excellent review of MRI techniques for imaging small animals has been published [34].

The potential of MRI is, however, not only in anatomical imaging. Contrast agents can be used to provide enhanced information in MRI studies [35]. Paramagnetic or ferromagnetic compounds which localize in regions of interest can be introduced to the tissue. These materials are not detected directly but rather are used to alter the RF signal of the surrounding protons. MRI can also measure physiological function such as water diffusion and blood oxygen levels which are used in functional MRI of the brain. MR can also be used in spectroscopy applications, termed MR spectroscopy. In this technique, applying selective RF pulses can reveal accurate information about the molecular composition of materials in vitro as well as in vivo. Resonance frequencies from the nuclei present in the sample are plotted on a frequency spectrum and the peaks are used to identify and quantify the tissue constituents [36]. MRI has been shown to be capable of imaging several subjects simultaneously and can be used in high-throughput applications [37].

18.3.2.3 Ultrasound

Ultrasound (US) uses sound waves at high frequencies in the 2–20 MHz range to produce images of tissue structure. At very high frequencies, typically in the 20–60 MHz range, this type of imaging is commonly referred to as small animal US or US microscopy. US can also be used to measure blood velocities when used in Doppler mode. The basic components of an US system are the transducer and a processing computer with software for image reconstruction and visualization. The transducer uses a piezoelectric crystal element to transmit sound waves and to record their reflections through the tissue. The size and frequency of the transducer will determine the field-of-view (FOV) and the spatial and temporal resolutions achievable. Sound waves travel at velocities relative to the *acoustic impedance* of the medium they are traveling in. The acoustic impedance is the product of the transmission velocity of sound and the density of the medium. Therefore, the acoustic impedance depends mostly on the tissue density. In soft tissues this value is typically 1,540 m/s [38]. An acoustic impedance mismatch at the boundary of adjacent tissues of different compositions causes incident sound waves to be reflected back toward the transducer. Larger mismatches in the tissue densities result in more reflected waves, resulting in higher signal intensities. Air-filled cavities such as lungs, or hard structures such as bones are not well suited for US imaging and can cause image artifacts since the majority of sound waves will be reflected at these surfaces. Another effect of these materials is to cause an overall attenuation of the sound wave which also decreases the depth of beam penetration in tissue.

The spatial resolution in US is comprised of the axial and lateral resolution components. The axial resolution is in the direction parallel to the beam and depends on the wave pulse length and frequency. In the axial component, the pulse length must be shorter than the distance separating two structures for them to be resolved. The lateral resolution is in the direction perpendicular to the axis of the beam. It depends on the beam width and frequency. Figure 18.4 shows the

axial and lateral resolution components relative to the transducer and sound beam profile. The axial and lateral resolutions both improve with increasing beam frequency. To be able to visualize structures in small animals with high spatial resolution, high frequency transducers are desirable. Ultrasonic biomicroscopy (UBM) uses very high frequencies of sound to generate resolutions in the several tens of microns [39]. The drawback is that increasing the frequency also results in a decrease in the depth of penetration by the beam. This however does not produce as much of a problem in small animals as in humans since a depth of penetration more than 2 cm is typically not needed for mice.

B-mode imaging is the most common imaging format in US. It is a real-time, gray-scaled, two-dimensional cross section of the FOV covered by the beam width. Three-dimensional imaging is also possible with US systems. These systems mechanically scan the area being imaged and use pixel correlation methods to align image slices together [40].

US has the ability to provide real-time temporal information from the structures being imaged. The temporal resolution is an important consideration in applications such as small animal cardiac imaging (echocardiography) since mice have heart rates in excess of 500 beats/min. The temporal resolution in US is determined by the imaging frame rate. For cardiac imaging, there must be enough frames covering the full cardiac cycle. The temporal resolution is however not critical when imaging static structures. For high frame rates, hardware capable of fast image processing is needed to be able to visualize the acquired data in real time. In general, the highest frequency available should be used for SAI as it produces the highest spatial and temporal resolutions.

Doppler imaging refers to the use of sound wave frequency shifts to determine the velocity of blood flow through a vessel. Objects such as red blood cells moving away or toward the transducer will cause reflected sound waves to have lower and higher frequencies, respectively, than the original waves. This is known as Doppler Shift. The measured velocities can be color coded (red – moving toward, blue – moving away) and superimposed onto the gray-scaled images [41, 42].

Contrast-enhanced US imaging is also possible with the use of microbubbles of inert gas. The bubbles act as highly reflecting media and increase the signal

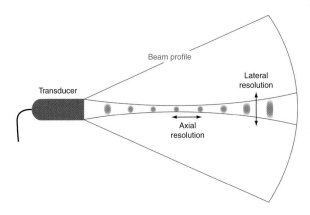

Fig. 18.4 Axial and lateral resolution components relative to the ultrasound transducer and sound beam profile. The lateral component changes along the beam profile, while the axial component depends only on the wave pulse length and frequency

level detected by the transducer. Microbubble contrast agents can also be used to target specific regions of disease as the inherent chemical of electrostatic properties of the microbubble shell can target receptors that bind to the shell [43]. For a review of the molecular imaging applications of US the reader is referred to other sources [43].

US provides a portable, cost-effective, and simple means of imaging small animals noninvasively and in real time without the use of ionizing radiation. US acquires dynamic images which can be quantified to produce useful structural and functional information. One limitation of US is that its performance (resolution, accuracy, image quality, etc.) is dependent on the skill and experience of the user [38]. For this reason, image acquisition and interpretation should be performed by the same individual whenever possible to improve repeatability and to minimize between-study variations.

18.3.3 Functional Imaging

18.3.3.1 Optical Imaging

Optical Imaging (OI) is largely limited to small animals as there are few clinical opportunities for its use other than intravital, or breast and brain imaging given the poor tissue penetration of light [44–49]. OI techniques can be used to study gene expression, cell trafficking, and drug efficacy among several other applications. Of the techniques that utilize visible light for imaging, this summary focuses on Fluorescence Imaging (FI) and Bioluminescence Imaging (BI). FI and BI provide a high-throughput and cost-effective means for researchers to investigate a wide variety of biological and physiological functions in the whole-body mouse [50]. Advantages of OI include its high sensitivity, probe stability (as there is no radioactive decay over time), and its nonionizing nature. There is also potential for using techniques of spectral differentiation to follow multiple light emitting targets in the same study [51]. Here, we briefly describe the concept of FI and BI technology as well as the interaction of light with tissues. For a more thorough review of in vivo optical imaging the reader is referred to additional sources [52–54].

Fluorescence Imaging

In Fluorescence imaging, an excitation light source at a defined wavelength is used to excite a molecule called a *fluorophore*. The fluorophore in turn reemits light at a longer wavelength (lower energy) during a period known as its fluorescence lifetime [59]. Each fluorophore has unique optical properties in terms of its signal intensity and excitation and emission wavelengths. The gene for Green Fluorescent Protein (GFP) from jellyfish is the most common fluorophore used and has been cloned and used to assay reporter genes [52, 55, 60]. Many fluorescent reporter probes have NIR emissions and are thus more capable of overcoming absorption in tissue for the reasons described earlier. In FI, the signal intensities are higher than in BI, but there is also a background *autoflourescence* [61]. Autofluorescence is the natural fluorescence of tissues which is due to endogenous fluorophores such as keratin, NAD(P)H, collagen, and ellastin. Autofluorescence results in a reduction in the SNR and contrast of the signal. For fluorophores located deeper within tissues, both excitation and emission become more difficult as the depth of penetration of the source and signal become poorer, respectively.

Bioluminescence Imaging

In Bioluminescence imaging, light is collected without the use of excitation sources. Instead, enzymes are used to catalyze reactions where the product is visible light. Firefly Luciferase and Renilla Luciferase are the most commonly used bioluminescence enzymes for imaging reporter gene expression in small animals [54, 62, 63]. Luciferase, in the presence of oxygen and ATP, converts substrates into light. The in vitro and in vivo emission spectra of luciferase covers the range above 600 nm where transmission through tissues is higher. Red-shifted luciferase, which has emissions at higher wavelengths, has also been developed and offers superior tissue penetration [64]. Luciferase-encoding genes have been extensively used as reporter genes for protein expression [55]. In BI, there is no inherent autofluorescence background as in FI, allowing for high SNR and image contrast as well as the ability to detect very low-level signals. Figure 18.5 shows three mice with tumors expressing luciferase imaged using bioluminescence and fluorescence techniques.

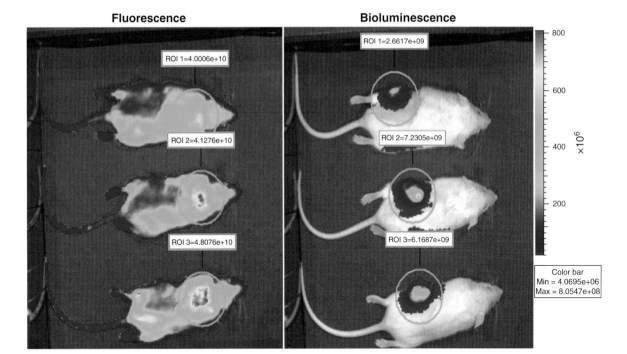

Fig. 18.5 The images above show three mice with tumors expressing Luciferase. The bioluminescence images on the *right* show the low background and specific signal to the tumor, whereas the fluorescence images on the *left* (acquired 2 min later) show the heterogeneous background associated with endogenous fluorophores that include blood, fur, and skin (Images courtesy of Dr. David Stout, University of California, Los Angeles)

Detectors

Optical imaging systems are among the most cost-effective and easy to operate within the array of SAI technologies. These systems require a light detector, light-proof enclosure, excitation source with emission and excitation filters, and a lens. Inexpensive silicon Charged Coupled Devices (CCDs) coupled to a lens are used to measure light emitted from the surface of the animal subject. Temperature-cooled CCDs are very sensitive devices where the charge collected in each pixel corresponds to the signal intensity (i.e., photon flux). These are the same type of solid-state sensors found in digital cameras. Optical signal intensity images are usually superimposed on photographs to provide anatomical localization of signal sources at the surface. Important specifications when choosing an optical imaging system include the CCD's quantum efficiency, image uniformity, dynamic range, resolution, SNR, noise (dark current and read noise), and cooling requirements [55].

Interaction of Light with Tissue

In x-ray and radionuclide imaging, *scatter* and *attenuation* occur when x-rays and γ-ray photons interact with tissue constituents. These interactions are analogous to the *scatter* and *absorption* of visible light in tissues. However, the exact mechanisms of light interaction in tissues are different from those of higher-energy photons. The useful wavelengths of light for OI range from ultra violet (UV) (~400 nm) to the near infrared (NIR) (~800 nm) regions. Light is made up of electromagnetic waves whose wavelength (λ) is given by:

$$\lambda = c_0/v$$

where c_0 is the speed of light in vacuum (3.0×10^8 m/s) and v is the frequency. The energy of the light wave is given by the product of the frequency and the Planck constant ($h = 6.626 \times 10^{-34}$ Js) and is typically on the order of ~1–3 electron Volts (eV).

Light scatter is the redirection of light photons – or, the reflection, refraction, and diffraction of light caused by cells, lipids, and other tissue components which change the linear path of light propagation due to the changing indices of refraction [55]. Significant scatter of light within tissues leads to diffusion of light signals at small distances from the source. Since the amount of scatter is a function of the distance traversed, signals originating deeper in tissues will have a broader distribution at the surface. This is easily confirmed by holding a laser-pointer to one's index finger and observing the spread of the exiting light. Rayleigh scatter (elastic scatter with no energy loss) is dominant in tissues, although Raman scatter (inelastic scatter with energy transfer) can also occur [56].

Absorption is the transfer of the light photon energy to a molecule, resulting in a loss of the incident photon. The energy transferred can be lost in the molecular environment (nonradiative decay) or result in the reemission of a light photon (radiative decay). The time scale of radiative decay can be *fluorescent* (1–10 ns) or *phosphorescent* (10^{-3}–10 s) [56]. Absorption causes attenuation of optical photons and thus, a reduction in the signal intensity. Absorption is strongly nonlinear as a function of depth and leads to increasingly obscure signal quantification at the tissue surface [51]. Absorption may be as much as ten-fold per cm of tissue, at near infrared wavelengths and much higher at shorter wavelengths [1]. Several molecules in tissues contribute to the absorption of light. The most significant absorbers in the visible and NIR regions are oxyhemoglobin and deoxyhemoglobin, whereas water is dominant at wavelengths greater than 900 nm. Figure 18.6 shows the absorption of hemoglobin and water as a function of wavelength. For this reason, reporter probes with spectral emissions of greater than 600 nm are preferred due to the relatively low absorption in tissue at these wavelengths [57]. The scattering and absorption coefficients, which can be determined experimentally, are used to describe the level of scattering and absorption for a medium [58].

Optical Tomography

Due to the large amount of scattering and depth dependence of their signals, neither fluorescence imaging nor bioluminescence imaging are quantitative in terms of

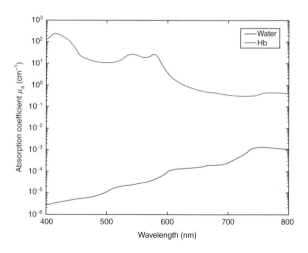

Fig. 18.6 Absorption coefficient (μa) of water and arterial blood hemoglobin (Hb) as a function of wavelength for the visible light spectrum. Note the log scale on the vertical axis (Data courtesy of Dr. George Alexandrakis, University of Texas at Arlington)

their measured signal intensities. Virtually, no information arrives unscattered to the surface and as a result, there is limited localization of the signals. The need for quantifying optical signals within tissues has prompted significant interest in the area of optical tomography (OT) [65–74]. In OT, multiple views from around the subject are used to determine depth information, which is analogous to CT and radionuclide tomographic reconstruction. This determination enhances the spatial resolution and improves source localization. However, OT is significantly more difficult to realize than radionuclide or x-ray tomographic reconstruction techniques. This is mostly due to the fact that optical photons undergo several scattering interactions in tissue prior to exiting, and that these interactions are highly dependent on the path of the light given the different tissues and organs traversed. Different photon propagation models can be used to take into account the various scattering and absorption properties of the tissue. This is called the forward problem. Image reconstruction algorithms are then used to solve the signal concentrations in the image volume distribution, called the inverse problem.

18.3.3.2 Radionuclide

Radionuclide imaging includes the modalities of Autoradiography (AR), Single Photon Emission

Computed Tomography (SPECT), and Positron Emission Tomography (PET). These techniques all involve the injection of a radiolabeled tracer and the visualization of its biodistribution in tissues and organs, usually across the entire body of small animals in a single study. A large number of radiolabeled tracers have been developed for clinical and preclinical use [75]. Radionuclide imaging techniques provide highly sensitive and quantitative measurements of tracer concentrations from deep inside tissues. Disadvantages of radionuclide techniques include the use of ionizing radiation, which contributes a radioactive dose to the animal, as well as the radioactive decay of radionuclides, which cannot be controlled and contribute background signals that must be cleared biologically to achieve strong SNRs.

18.3.3.3 Autoradiography

Autoradiography (AR) is a technique in which the distribution of a tracer is imaged onto a film emulsion showing the position and signal intensity of its uptake. The animal subject is injected with the tracer, which is allowed to distribute within the tissues. Following biodistribution, the animal is sacrificed, imbedded in a cellulose gel, and then rapidly frozen using freezing liquid. Sagittal sections of the frozen block are made one at a time using a microtome blade which cuts slices in the range of 5–200 μm thick [76]. The sections are freeze-dried and pressed against a photographic film emulsion which is then placed inside a light-tight environment for up to several weeks. The radiation exposes the film's silver halide grains and after adequate exposure, the film is developed to make two-dimensional autoradiograms, which show the localization and signal level of the tracer biodistribution at a specific time point [77]. Factors which influence the exposure are the energy and half-life of the radionuclide, the dose to the animal, the section thickness, and the film sensitivity [78].

Common radionuclides for tagging molecules for use in autoradiography include electron emitters such as carbon-14 (^{14}C) and tritium (^{3}H). The spatial resolution is inversely related to the energy of the electron emissions, as lower energies will have shorter ranges in the photographic emulsion. ^{3}H (18.6 keV) and ^{14}C (156 keV) provide a higher spatial resolution relative to other electron emitters. On x-ray film, the resolution

of ^{14}C is about 25 μm at the Full-Width at Half-Maximum (FWHM) [78]. Thicker slices also contribute to a loss of spatial resolution.

For quantification, a radioactive scale can be placed on the film for reference (densitometry). Regions-of-Interest (ROIs) from the section (i.e., tissues and organs) can also be excised and counted in a radiation counting instrument for more accurate quantification. Computer-assisted autoradiography approaches have been developed and it is also possible to reconstruct data from autoradiograms to form tomographic data sets, but this requires software algorithms and can be tedious [79, 80].

One drawback of AR is that each animal provides only a snapshot in time of the process being studied. To obtain information regarding the radiotracer timescale, several animals are required. Thus, longitudinal studies in the same animal are not possible and interanimal variability is introduced when using multiple subjects. Small animal PET (discussed later) can overcome this limitation since it allows for in vivo repeatable imaging of animals. PET however, is often not suitable for imaging structures in the brain and other applications where the high spatial resolution afforded by autoradiography is desirable. The spatial resolution achievable with autoradiography is less than a few hundred microns which is approximately one order of magnitude better than PET. Comparisons of AR and PET have been used to validate the quantification of PET and also suggest that there may be benefits to using AR for making preliminary assessments regarding the PET spatial resolution for specific studies [78, 81]. For further reading on the principles and applications of autoradiography the reader is referred to additional sources [82].

18.3.3.4 Single Photon Emission Computed Tomography

Using radiolabeled tracers, small animal Single Photon Emission Computed Tomography (SPECT) can be used to measure slow kinetic processes due to the relatively long half-lives of the available single photon emitting tracers. This makes SPECT well suited for tracking labeled molecules with slow blood clearance and requiring longer localization times, such as peptides, antibodies, and hormones [83]. The most commonly used SPECT radionuclides are Technetium-99

(^{99m}Tc) and Iodine-123 (^{123}I), with half-lives of 6.02 h and 13.2 h, respectively. Applications of SPECT in small animals include brain imaging, gene expression, cardiac studies, and the imaging of tumors. There is also potential for imaging two radiolabed tracers of different energies simultaneously using SPECT. This can be advantageous since many molecular pathways have multiple components, or interact with other pathways. To achieve this, the SPECT detectors must have an energy resolution good enough to distinguish between the different energies being used [84].

The main components of a SPECT system are the image-forming element (collimator) and the detector. There are two main categories of small animal SPECT systems. The first is clinical SPECT systems which have been modified with pinhole collimators. These designs use detectors comprised of continuous scintillator crystals, typically Sodium Iodide (NaI), coupled to an array of photomultiplier tubes. The second category is the dedicated small animal SPECT system. These systems use either parallel-hole or pinhole collimators with detectors of pixilated arrays of small (1–2 mm) scintillator elements coupled to Position-Sensitive Photomultiplier Tubes (PSPMTs), or solid-state semiconductor devices. Collimators can be made of lead, tungsten, copper, or even gold.

In terms of spatial resolution, SPECT has the advantage when compared to PET because it does not face the same resolution limitations caused by the physics of positron range and noncollinearity [85]. The spatial resolution in small animal SPECT is a combination of the collimator and detector intrinsic resolutions. For parallel-hole collimators, the resolution is limited by the geometry of the collimator being used (i.e., aperture and septal thickness). Pinhole collimators, which

are more common in small animal SPECT imaging, can provide very high resolutions through magnification of the object compared to parallel-hole collimators, as shown in Fig. 18.7 [86–89].

For pinhole collimators, septal penetration at the edges of the pinholes can lead to spatial resolution loss. Additional degradation in the spatial resolution is due to gamma-ray interactions at oblique angles, which cause position miscalculation due to depth of interaction effects within the detector [90]. The spatial resolution depends on the pinhole diameter, the magnification, and the intrinsic spatial resolution of the detector. The magnification factor (M) is a function of the object-to-pinhole distance (s_1) and the pinhole-to-detector distance (s_2):

$$M = \frac{s_2}{s_1}$$

The pinhole diameter (d) and s_1 determine the pinhole collection efficiency (E):

$$E = \left(\frac{d}{s_1}\right)^2$$

One major limitation in SPECT systems is their low geometric efficiency due to the small apertures of the pinhole collimator or the high-resolution parallel-hole collimators. The efficiency can be improved by increasing the pinhole diameter or collimator element size, at the expense of spatial resolution.

Another method for increasing the SNR is to increase the dose of the injected tracer. SPECT tracers usually have a higher specific activity than PET tracers, which allows for the dose to the animal to be of a higher concentration while remaining within the limits

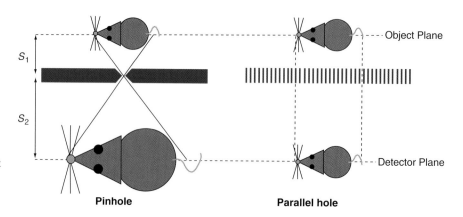

Fig. 18.7 Pinhole collimators provide high resolution through magnification of the object compared to parallel-hole collimators, which do not magnify the object. Note that the actual subject image will be inverted on the pinhole detector plane

of the injection volume (discussed in the section on Animal Usage).

Multiple-pinhole and coded-aperture designs have also been developed to increase the sensitivity of small animal SPECT systems [91–93]. In these designs, multiple pinholes are used to increase the detection efficiency (i.e., n pinholes $= n \times$ detection efficiency of one pinhole). This requires special reconstruction algorithms to reconstruct the multiple projection data.

Small animals such as mice have a greatly reduced thickness for photons to travel through (~2 cm) compared with humans (~20 cm), which greatly reduces the scatter and attenuation of gamma-rays. This allows the use of lower energy isotopes and for small animal SPECT to be more quantitative compared to clinical SPECT [90]. For a thorough review of small animal SPECT the reader is referred to further reading [83, 90, 94].

18.3.3.5 Positron Emission Tomography

PET can noninvasively quantify the temporal and spatial biodistribution of a molecule tagged with a positron-emitting radioactive probe [85,95–97]. Small animal PET provides the ability to study processes dynamically in real time, as well as longitudinally in the same animal model. Biological and physiological processes that can be studied quantitatively using small animal PET include perfusion, metabolism, protein expression, and enzyme activity among several others [98]. Information obtained using PET can facilitate the direct comparison of studies performed in animal models with those in the clinical setting. In pharmacological research, PET can be used to perform rapid in vivo screening of pharmacokinetics for drug candidates by visualizing and quantifying their biodistrubution, occupancy at specific biological targets, and efficacy [99].

Small animal PET technology is similar in many ways to clinical PET. Clinical PET scanners typically have a spatial resolution on the order of 1 ml. An important consideration in small animal systems is that the spatial resolution should be able to resolve tracer distributions in the organs and structures of the mouse. Given the volumetric ratio of humans to the average mouse (2,000:1), an improvement of the same order would ideally need to be realized for the resolution of small animal PET. The resolution of the typical small animal PET system is however on the order of

1 µl, which provides a volumetric resolution improvement of ~100 over their clinical counterparts [98]. Small animal PET detectors can have detector elements less than 2 mm across. Noncollinearity plays a small role in resolution loss due to the small ring diameters of these scanners. Thus, the current spatial resolution achievable in small animal PET approaches the limit determined by the positron range of the radioisotope [100].

The absolute system sensitivity is an important consideration since the SNR of the reconstructed images is determined by the number of counts in each element of the image volume [101]. The main parameters which determine the sensitivity are the solid angle coverage and the intrinsic efficiency of the detectors for 511 keV annihilation events. The solid angle can be increased by placing the detectors closer to the subject [102]. In addition to these factors, the SNR is also affected by the injected dose and the total acquisition time. Increasing the injection activity can improve counting statistics and thus, the SNR. The limiting factor in this case is the count rate capability of the system due to the close proximity of the animal to the detectors. High-activity injections can also cause random coincidence rates to increase substantially, leading to a reduction in the SNR. The injection volumes must also be kept within a limit that does not perturb the biological processes under consideration (discussed in the section on Animal Usage). Injection activities for mice typically range from 50 to 200 µCi and do not result in significant dead times for most small animal PET scanners [11].

The attenuation of annihilation photons in humans can be upwards of 90% in the abdominal area [101]. In mice, attenuation is typically on the order of 20–40% and can be compensated for by using attenuation correction methods which assume a homogenous attenuation coefficient (usually equal to water) over the volume of the mouse. Alternatively, transmission scanning using an external 511 keV source can also be used.

Currently, the most common tracer used in both clinical and small animal studies is [18F]-2-fluoro-2-deoxy-D-glucose (FDG). One of the most common uses of FDG in mice is in oncology. FDG is retained in tumor cells at the same rate as glucose uptake and phosphorylation and is therefore reflective of regional glucose metabolism, which can be used to identify hypermetabolic cell populations.

Another application of PET is in imaging reporter gene expression. A PET reporter gene expresses a protein that can trap or bind a PET reporter probe. The reporter gene is driven by the same promoter as the gene of interest and the promoter can be used to "switch" expression of the gene *on* or *off*. The gene product leads to an enzyme or receptor that is capable of trapping the reporter probe, the level of which is proportional to the level of reporter gene expression. In this way, the location, magnitude of expression, and time course of expression levels of any gene that is introduced in a mouse can be monitored in vivo [101]. Applications of reporter genes include monitoring of cell trafficking, metastases, and cell-cell interactions among other scenarios. Measuring gene expression in small animals provides an experimental platform from which to develop methods of measuring gene expression in humans. For a more complete review of reporter gene imaging techniques the reader is referred to [103–106].

PET tracers can also be used to label antibody fragments which can target receptors on the cell surface [107,108]. These antibody fragments have a high affinity for tumors and are rapidly cleared from the blood, providing researchers with a new type of PET imaging agent. Figure 18.8 shows the tumor uptake of three different antibody fragments in mice at 20 h postinjection.

18.3.4 First Generation and State-of-the-Art Instruments

18.3.4.1 CT

The first microscale CT systems for research were developed with the goal of rapidly providing high-

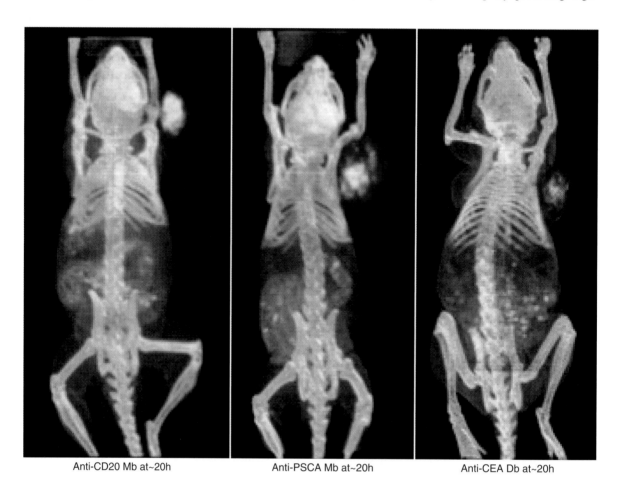

Anti-CD20 Mb at~20h   Anti-PSCA Mb at~20h   Anti-CEA Db at~20h

Fig. 18.8 PET images (with CT overlay) of tumor uptake using three different antibody fragments in mice at 20 h postinjection (Figure courtesy of Dr. Anna Wu and Dr. Tove Olafsen, University of California, Los Angeles)

resolution structural images of laboratory specimens [109,110] and small animals [111, 112]. Succeeding generations of commercially developed preclinical CT systems are still geared toward cost-effective and high-throughput scanning of small animals, while offering several other versatile functions. The CT module of the Inveon system from Siemens Preclinical Solutions (Knoxville, TN, USA) allows the operator to adjust the FOV and scan resolution, down to 15 μm, while also providing a real-time image reconstruction tool. The CT Subsystem from Gamma Medica-Ideas, Inc. (Northridge, CA, USA) contains a variable focal spot x-ray, which allows the user to select between 15 μm high-resolution or rapid low-dose scanning modes. The eXplore CT 120 from GE Healthcare (London, United Kingdom) combines high resolution with fast scanning speed so that dynamic perfusion imaging can be performed in small animals.

18.3.4.2 MRI

The developers of the first clinical MRI systems immediately realized that the technology could be adapted to imaging of laboratory animals. Small animal MRI provides higher spatial resolution than clinical MRI, where the resolution is usually limited to ~1 mm. Initial efforts in the 1980s were focused on overcoming the largest challenge in microMRI, namely the limited SNR [113, 114]. This has primarily been addressed by using more sensitive RF coils, higher magnetic fields, and specially designed pulse sequences [115]. MRI techniques such as diffusion imaging [116] and fMRI [117] have further improved the information that can be obtained in small animals. Over the past several years, many studies have been performed which demonstrate the usefulness of MRI for observing anatomy and physiological function in small animals [35, 118, 119]. Bruker Biospin Corporation (Billerica, MA, USA) offers several preclinical MRI systems with a range of magnetic field strengths, bore sizes, and image analysis software packages.

18.3.4.3 Ultrasound

The field of small animal US has advanced with the advent of instruments which are capable of achieving submillimeter spatial resolution using high frequencies (20-60 MHz). Instrumentation operating in this frequency range has proven capable of imaging various structures in mice [39, 120, 121]. Recent developments in US microscopy include the use of high-frequency continuous-wave [122] and pulsed-wave [123] transducers as well as color Doppler techniques [124] for imaging of the microcirculation. The VS40 system from Visualsonics (Toronto, Ontario, Canada) is capable of selecting frequencies in the range of 19–55 MHz, corresponding to a lateral resolution of 100 and 60 μm, respectively, and has been used to image mouse embryos and adult animals [125].

18.3.4.4 Optical

The IVIS product line from Caliper Life Sciences (Hopkinton, MA, USA) has in vivo optical imaging systems which can image bioluminescence as well as three-dimensional fluorescence [126]. The Maestro imaging system from Cambridge Research and Instrumentation, Inc. (Woburn, MA, USA) offers multispectral fluorescence in vivo imaging. This system uses a liquid crystal tunable filter to select a 10–20 nm bandpass of light to reach the detector [127]. This allows for spectral differentiation of the autofluorescence signal and higher SNRs. The Kodak Image Station In-Vivo FX product line from Kodak Molecular Imaging Systems (New Haven, CT, USA) is a multimodality imaging system that provides coregistered planar fluorescence, radioisotope, and x-ray imaging on a single platform [128].

18.3.4.5 SPECT

Several academic research centers and commercial vendors have developed high-resolution high-sensitivity SPECT scanners in recent years. The U-SPECT-I system (University Medical Center Utrecht, Netherlands) uses 75 gold micropinholes which are focused on ROIs of the small animal to maximize detection yield of gamma-ray photons. This method, called the Scanning Focus Method (SFM), has been shown to reduce noise, streak artifacts, and background activity while achieving a spatial resolution of 0.35 mm using 0.3 mm pinholes [129, 130]. A proposed U-SPECT-III system configuration using 135 gold pinholes is expected to eliminate depth-of-interaction effects encountered by the pinhole design and achieve intrinsic spatial resolution of better than 150 µm [131].

FastSPECT II (University of Arizona, AZ, USA) uses a modular scintillation camera design. Each camera is comprised of a 5 mm thick NaI scintillator crystal coupled to PMTs using a quartz light guide. FastSPECT II has an exchangeable aperture and adjustable camera position which allow the user to select the magnification, and FOV – parameters which change the system sensitivity and resolution to match the chosen imaging task [132]. Another small animal SPECT system, SemiSPECT (University of Arizona, AZ, USA) uses eight compact detectors based on pinhole apertures and solid-state cadmium zinc telluride (CZT) detectors (intrinsic efficiency of 40% for 140 keV) to achieve a spatial resolution of 1.4 mm [133].

NanoSPECT (Bioscan Inc., USA) is a commercial scanner which uses a design of multiplexed multiple tungsten pinholes [134]. This system has been used with 2 mm pinholes, which allow a spatial resolution of 1.6 mm, to obtain high-resolution images of rat kidneys [135].

The LumaGEM gamma camera from Gamma Medica-Ideas uses an array of NaI crystals coupled to an array of PSPMTs. Changeable pinhole apertures can be used and this scanner has demonstrated a 1.3 mm spatial resolution using 1.0 mm pinholes [136]. The Flex Triumph (Gamma Medica-Ideas Inc., USA) multimodality scanner has achieved the first dual-isotope mouse SPECT imaging capability by using high-resolution CZT detectors with an energy resolution of 4.5% at 140 keV [84].

18.3.4.6 PET

The first dedicated small animal PET systems were introduced in the 1990s. Several systems used similar scintillator-PMT based designs to achieve high spatial resolutions in animal models. Hammersmith Hospital (London, UK), in collaboration with CTI PET Systems, Inc. (Knoxville, TN, USA) developed the initial rodent scanner which used BGO block detectors [137]. Several other dedicated animal scanners were introduced shortly thereafter, including the Sherbrooke APD-PET, MicroPET, YAP-PET, HIDAC-PET, and TierPET [138–142]. Several of these scanners have

led to subsequent generations of animal PET scanners which are now offered as commercial systems.

The PET module of the Inveon from Siemens Preclinical Solutions incorporates PET, SPECT, and CT imaging onto a single platform. The Inveon PET detectors use LSO crystals and PSPMTs to achieve a 1.4 mm spatial resolution with a detection sensitivity greater than 10% (100 keV lower energy window) [143, 144]. The GE eXplore vista PET/CT system (London, United Kingdom) uses a lutetium-yttrium-oxyorthosilicate (LYSO) – gadolinium orthosilicate (GSO) phoswich detector to retrieve depth-of-interaction information. It has a 1.6 mm spatial resolution and 4% sensitivity (250 keV lower energy window) [145, 146]. The Philips Mosaic small animal PET system from Philips Medical Systems (Andover, MA, USA) uses GSO with single channel PMTs to achieve a spatial resolution of 2.7 mm and sensitivity of 1.3% (400 keV threshold) [147, 148]. The LabPET system of the Gamma Medica-Ideas, Inc. uses a phoswich-APD detector design and can achieve a mean axial spatial resolution of 1.38 mm and sensitivity of 2.1% (450 keV threshold) [149, 150]. For a more thorough review of small animal PET systems the reader is referred to other sources [151, 152].

The RatCAP PET system developed at Brookhaven National Laboratory consists of a miniaturized ring of LSO crystals that can be mounted to the head of a conscious rat [153, 154]. Signals from the crystals are read out via optical fibers which send light signals to APDs. The RatCAP allows for animal studies without the use of anesthesia, which can have profound effects on the study outcome.

18.3.5 Multimodality Imaging

Multimodality imaging refers to the combination of two or more SAI modalities in studies of the same subject. No single SAI modality discussed in this chapter can provide information on all aspects of structure and function in the animal subject. The combination of complementary or contrasting modalities can greatly enhance the information provided in the study. As described earlier, the imaging modalities can be divided roughly into two groups: those that image structure (CT, MRI, Ultrasound) and those that image function or molecular information (SPECT, PET, Optical). One method of combining modalities is to image the subject on multiple image platforms and to overlay the data using software image registration techniques. A second method is to build multiple capabilities into the scanner hardware, in which case, the image registration is inherent to the system geometry. These multimodality instruments can be further subdivided into those that image different signals of interest using the same detector and those that use side-by-side placement of different detector technologies. In each case, there are always factors to consider in order to minimize interference between the different signals that are present.

An easy to use tool for viewing, analyzing, and registering multiple volumetric image data sets known as AMIDE (A Medical Imaging Data Examiner) is available to researchers [155].

An example of combining similar imaging modalities is in PET-SPECT or Optical-PET applications. A researcher may want to simultaneously image more than one molecular target to determine their association with one another. In an example of contrasting modalities, structural information from CT or MRI can provide anatomic localization for physiological or molecular data from SPECT or PET, something which is often highly desirable. The benefits of structural and functional information are not only in localization, but can also lead to more accurate corrections for attenuation and scatter of radionuclide techniques, therefore improving quantification of tracer activities [156].

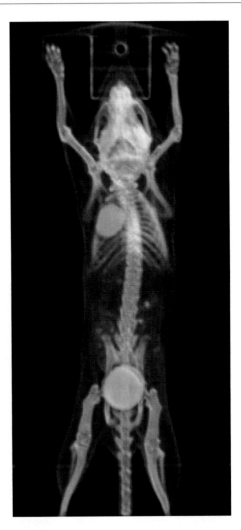

Fig. 18.9 Overlay of PET and CT datasets taken from a single subject (Figure courtesy of Dr. David Stout, University of California, Los Angeles)

18.3.5.1 Radionuclide-CT

The greatest use of combining radioisotope and CT data is in providing anatomic localization of tracer distributions, as shown in the PET-CT image in Fig. 18.9. Without anatomical information, localization and identification of nonspecific, and even specific, tracers in molecular imaging studies can be difficult [157]. This is especially important in animal studies since the small stature of mice places organs and structures of interest in close proximity to one another.

In clinical CT systems, the x-ray beam energy (80–120 kVp) can overlap with the energies of single photon emitting radionuclides, making signal discrimination virtually impossible given current detector technologies. In small animal CT, differences between the x-ray beam energy (40–80 kVp) and most single photon emitting radionuclides are slightly larger, allowing them

to be more easily discernable from one another [19]. In PET, this is usually not a problem since 511 keV annihilation gamma-rays have a much larger energy than the x-rays and shielding of the PET detectors from the x-rays can easily be achieved [19].

Several SPECT-CT systems have been developed for imaging small animals using either the same detector module [158–160], or side-by-side placement of SPECT and x-ray detectors [158, 161]. PET-CT systems can incorporate simultaneous imaging capability in a single detector [162], in coplanar configurations [157], or side-by-side as in the case of most small animal PET-CT systems [163–165]. Alternatively, multimodality PET-CT can also be achieved using separate PET and CT systems and software image registration [166, 167]. Recently, systems incorporating tri-modalities of PET-SPECT and CT have also been developed [144, 168].

18.3.5.2 PET-MRI

The ability of MRI to resolve soft tissues using non-ionizing radiation while achieving high contrast and high spatial resolution make it particularly useful and indeed more attractive for anatomic localization compared to x-ray CT, especially when soft tissues are of interest. Figure 18.10 shows a fused image from a mouse in a dual-modality PET-MRI study. The enhanced soft tissue contrast can provide enhanced ROI definition, leading to more accurate PET tracer quantification [32]. Given the very high sensitivity of PET for molecular probes, the combination of PET and MRI makes for a particularly powerful multimodality tool. An added advantage to PET-MRI imaging is the potential reduction of the resolution-limiting positron range by the MR magnetic field [169–171].

There are several challenges of physics which hinder the combination of these two modalities. PET

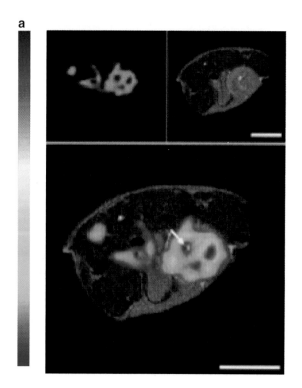
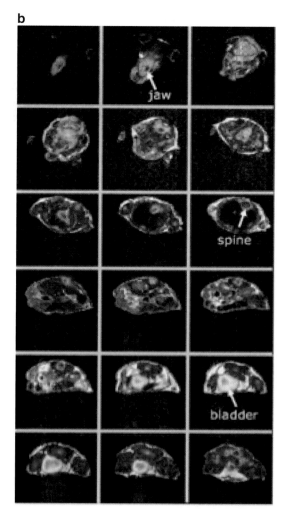

Fig. 18.10 Simultaneous in vivo PET and MR imaging. (**a**) Mouse FDG tumor imaging. (*upper left*) PET image (*upper right*) MR image, and (*lower*) fused PET and MR image. One transaxial image slice is shown. (**b**) Fused PET and MR images of a mouse. Transaxial sections from top of the head to the bladder are shown. (Scale bars = 5 mm) The same false-color look-up table is used in both (**a**) and (**b**) (Images courtesy of Dr. Ciprian Catana, Siemens Preclinical Solutions, Knoxville, Tennessee)

detector PMTs and front-end electronics, and indeed any ferromagnetic materials, can interfere with the MR magnetic field homogeneity and gradient field linearity and introduce RF noise as a result [32]. PMTs on the other hand are highly sensitive to the magnetic fields of MR. For these reasons, standard PET detectors cannot be placed directly within the MR bore [19].

Several PET-MRI solutions have been proposed and are currently under development. One possibility is to use PET inserts in which light from scintillator elements inside the bore is channeled to PMTs outside the FOV via optical fibers [172–174]. Another opportunity for PET-MR imaging has been made possible with the relatively recent introduction of silicon-based Avalanche Photodiode (APD) light detectors for use with PET [138, 175, 176]. APDs can potentially replace PMTs and be placed directly in the MR magnet as they are immune to magnetic fields. APD-based PET inserts have shown to have a strong potential for successful PET-MRI imaging [177–180]. Figure 18.11 shows a schematic diagram of an APD-based MRI-compatible PET insert placed inside a preclinical MRI system.

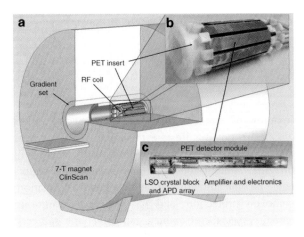

Fig. 18.11 (**a**) Drawing of PET-MRI combination showing the PET insert placed inside the MRI scanner, matching the centers of both fields of view. (**b**) Photograph of the MRI-compatible PET insert consisting of ten radially arranged detector modules. (**c**) Single PET detector module showing the LSO scintillator block, APD array, and preamplifier built into a MRI-compatible copper shielding (Reprinted with permission from Judenhofer MS et al. (2008) Nature Medicine. Macmillan, 14(4):459–65), copyright

18.3.5.3 Optical-Radionuclide

Both optical techniques (Fluorescence and Bioluminescence) and PET imaging have extremely high sensitivity. PET has the advantage of being quantitative for signals originating in any location, while the depth-dependent attenuation of light in tissues makes quantification of optical techniques difficult. The difference in the measured signal between optical and PET imaging can be thought of as qualitative vs. quantitative information gathering. The choice of which modality to use is often arrived at based on the study scope and requirements, as is addressed in the next sections. There are several advantages to imaging both PET and optical probes, either across instruments, or more preferably, on the same imaging platform.

Simultaneous reporter gene imaging using optical and PET probes is highly desirable since it allows for the correlation of the two signals. In this scenario, injecting small animals with a tracer containing both a radionuclide and optical imaging substrate would allow the tracking of its movement and pharmacokinetics in conjunction with the light signal it produces when it comes in to contact with its enzyme. One of the potentials of this is in the use of the PET signal to provide additional information regarding the optical probe. Optical-PET fusion reporter genes which contain both a PET and an optical reporter gene have also been created. Such reporter probes have been successfully used to image herpes simplex virus type-1 thymidine kinase (HSV1-tk) [167, 181–183] and melanoma gene expression [184]. These double- and triple- fusion reporter probes can be used in several ways to increase the range of measurable processes. One method is to allow for the PET signal to be used for quantification of optical signal sensitivity and specificity as a function of depth [60, 183].

Monomolecular Multimodality Imaging Agents (MOMIAs) have also been developed [185]. MOMIAs are single molecules that can emit both PET and optical signals and can allow for the normalization of detection sensitivities between the two modalities.

With PET, a single longitudinal study is often not feasible due to the relatively short half-lives of the radionuclides used. On the other hand, optical imaging allows for the controlled release of enzyme substrates that can prolong the light emission. Thus, PET can potentially provide early quantitative data, while optical techniques can be used to monitor longer-term changes in the subject [186]. The opposite can also be true, where optical techniques can provide preliminary signal information which can then be quantified using PET.

While it is possible to use image registration for combining information from independently obtained optical and PET images [167], it is certainly more desirable to acquire the two signals using the same instrument. The development of dual-modality optical-radionuclide instrumentation is of high interest since it will provide biological researchers with a powerful and novel tool for conducting the types of studies described earlier. In addition, most systems being developed aim to acquire optical projections from around the subject, which will be used for tomographic reconstruction of fluorescence and bioluminescence sources as described in the section on Optical Tomography.

A current design for simultaneously imaging optical and PET signals involves the use of a solid-state Complementary Metal-Oxide-Semiconductor (CMOS) detector. In this design, a microarray of lenses is used to focus light onto detectors placed around the subject. Initial results have shown that it is feasible to use this device as an insert in a clinical PET scanner to image photons from fluorescence without degrading the PET signal [187]. A different approach uses a Cadmium Teluride (CdTe) high-resolution gamma camera and CCD to image gamma-rays and photons from fluorescence [188], respectively. A third system has demonstrated use of the same PMT-based detector module to image both annihilation photons and bioluminescence photons [189–191].

18.3.6 Qualitative vs. Quantitative Imaging

The concept of using molecular imaging to provide signal quantification at the source has multiple levels of answers. These range from a simple qualitative decision about a signal being increased or decreased, *up* or *down*, to a more conventional in biology log order quantification, to the absolute quantification of the number of enzymatic reactions taking place in each second at the target site. Even though many researchers are striving for the latter definition in tight confidence intervals in an attempt to provide

a truly quantitative explanation of the underlying biology [85,192], the fact is that biological research has made significant progress by using simpler quantification schemes that lend themselves to easier data interpretation and higher-throughput methodologies. A prime example of this approach is traditional bioluminescence imaging, which tends to serve at an earlier stage of the discovery process and feeds into more quantitative, but lower throughput and higher cost, imaging modalities [52]. The information gathered using optical imaging can be further quantified using more quantitative techniques, such as PET and SPECT.

Molecular imaging (Optical, PET, SPECT) quantification can be further improved by using information from anatomical imaging (CT, MRI) for better delineation of regions-of-interest (ROIs). In this case, accurate coregistration of images is important. As a stand-alone modality, CT can be used to define the 3-Dimensional margins of tumors and to evaluate their growth or response to treatment. Contrast agents containing iodine can provide high-resolution detail of vasculature, but quantification is limited. Accurate quantification of tissue attenuation using CT numbers is confounded by beam hardening (described earlier). Certain types of MR imaging (Paramagnetic compounds, diffusion, spectroscopy) can be of high value when quantitative information is required, as described in the section on Magnetic Resonance Imaging.

18.4 Animal Usage

Imaging of small animals presents several issues which are not manifest in the clinical environment and must be taken into consideration for successful imaging. Animal considerations of particular importance include animal sedation, temperature regulation, pathogen protection, and physiological monitoring among other factors which can affect the subjects. One factor common to the clinic and to small animals is the radiation dose the subject receives during the imaging procedure. If not monitored properly, these effects can confound the experimental outcomes and even lead to premature mortality. Considerations for these and other issues in the context of the overall imaging center design can produce better, more accurate, and highly repeatable studies in small animals. In general, increased familiarity with the species being used can only help to improve the quality of the experimental results and more importantly, can minimize the discomfort and stress the animals endure in our care. There are several resources available to researchers for educating themselves regarding animal handling issues [193–196].

18.4.1 Anesthesia and Physiological Considerations

Anesthesia is necessary to sedate animals during virtually all imaging procedures. It is used as a means of minimizing image motion artifacts which affect the results and lead to poor data quantification. There will, however, always be some inherent blurring due to breathing and cardiac motion during in vivo imaging, but these effects can also be reduced substantially using gating techniques (described in the Cardiology section in Applications). In mice, anesthetic agents can be administered via intraperitoneal or tail vein injection (ketamine, xylazine), or through inhalation (isoflurane, halothane). Inhalation is usually preferred since it allows control of the depth, duration, and rate of anesthesia. For more detailed information on small animal anesthesia the reader is referred to [197–199].

Due to rapid heat loss given their high surface area to mass ratio, mice must be maintained at a temperature range of 21–25°C to maintain their normal body temperature of 37.4°C [90]. Under anesthesia, mice can reach hypothermic states within minutes if they are not properly warmed [200]. Warming animals is also important as it has shown to affect the uptake of radiolabled tracers in nuclear imaging studies [201]. To mitigate the effects of environmental factors and general stress on animal physiology, mice should be maintained in a constant environment for several days prior to performing imaging studies. Dietary conditions, temperature, and the type of anesthesia used can all affect tumor uptake of tracers. The effects of these conditions have been studied and standard imaging protocols for optimizing visualization of tumor xenografts using FDG have been developed [201].

Many studies use transgenic mice with compromised immune systems so that tumor and disease investigations are not complicated by the immune system response. Severe Combined Immunodeficient (SCID) mice are unable to produce lymphocytes and are highly susceptible to environmental pathogens. These mice must be protected using a physical barrier. The self-contained mouse imaging chamber shown in Fig. 18.12 can serve several of the requirements of animal handling in addition to protection from pathogens [202]. A chamber can provide a repeatable and

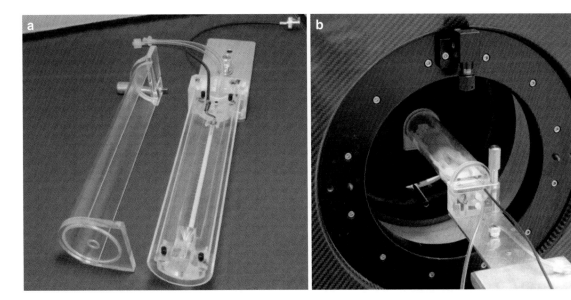

Fig. 18.12 (a) Self-contained mouse imaging chamber with top removed and (b) chamber containing a mouse placed inside a microPET Focus 220 scanner from Siemens Preclinical Solutions

reliable method for anesthesia delivery and warming while ensuring repeatable animal positioning in the same imaging system or between instruments.

Other physiological conditions of interest include the respiratory rate, heart rate, circadian rhythm, and blood oxygen content [199]. Animal respiration can be monitored using a video camera that visualizes, but is not contained within the FOV. Heart rates can be measured with electric leads from an Electrocardio-gram (ECG) device that monitors electrical activity on the animal surface. Both respiration and heart rate monitoring are important for the animal status and can also be used in gating methods. Gating techniques use breathing and cardiac motion to trigger the acquisition of image data and can significantly reduce motion artifacts.

Another important consideration when imaging mice is the injection volume of radiolabeled tracers or contrast agents. The injection volume must ensure that there are no adverse effects on the animal physi-ology which can compromise the experimental out-come. Mice can be injected safely with about 10% of their total blood volume (25 ml), which corresponds to approximately 2.5 ml [101, 203].

18.4.2 Radiation Dose

In x-ray microCT, the dose delivered to the subject is a function of the x-ray tube current (milliamperes per second [mAs]), beam hardness (i.e., filtration), and the desired image quality (i.e., photon flux). For high SNR ratios, large x-ray photon fluxes are required, resulting in significant radiation doses to mice. The doses may be high enough to induce changes in the physiology of the animals, affecting the experimental outcome. Tables for whole-body radiation dose estimates in mice imaged with typical microCT scan parameters have been calcu-lated and published [204]. These tables can guide inves-tigators in estimating the average whole-body dose to animals and to ensure that dose levels remain well below the LD50/30 of ~7 Gy for mice, which is the 50% – 30 day mortality rate for a single dose received. More detailed simulations have estimated dose distributions in mouse organs and structures [205] and have shown that bony structures receive the highest dose while soft tissues receive lower and more homogenous dose dis-tributions [206].

In nuclear studies, the dose is a function of the administered activity, the radioactive and biological half-lives of the radiopharmaceutical, and the dose dis-tribution. Whole-body dose estimates for small animal PET and SPECT for a variety of radiolabeled tracers have been simulated for localized and distributed sources in ellipsoid mouse phantoms [207]. Estimates of doses from 18-Fluorine compounds for specific organs in mice have also been made (Table 18.2) using a voxelized mouse phantom, as shown in Fig. 18.13 [208].

For better quality, high-resolution imaging, and good SNRs, more signal counts are desirable. We cannot however, simply raise the x-ray flux or increase injection activities due to dose and physiological con-siderations. This is especially true in multimodality

Table 18.2 Radiation dose estimates for F-18 compounds in a voxelized mouse phantom (in mGy) from 18-Fluorine com-pounds for specific organs and for a typical injection of 7.4 MBq (Data courtesy of Dr. Richard Taschereau, University of California, Los Angeles)

	FDG	FLT	F-ion
Bladder	4,000	3,100	2,500
Whole body	105	100	80
Heart	425	95	60
Kidneys	195	105	115
Liver	40	95	60
Brain	100	90	95
Bone marrow	75	70	300
Spine	35	30	560

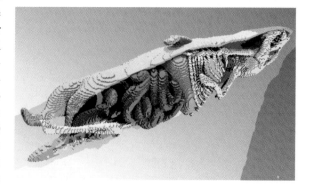

Fig. 18.13 Voxelized mouse phantom used in simulation stud-ies (Image courtesy of Dr. Richard Taschereau, University of California, Los Angeles)

imaging where the subject receives multiple radiation doses. Therefore, improvements in imaging system sensitivities are needed, which will remain a significant area of small animal imaging instrumentation research in the near future.

18.5 Small Animal Imaging Center Design

With the increasing recognition of small animal imaging as a requirement for biomedical research into human disease, dedicated SAI facilities are quickly becoming permanent establishments in academic, pharmaceutical, and other research settings. These facilities can be developed as shared resource centers in order to offset the high start-up costs, and can also help promote scientific collaborations. Defining the role of a SAI center early on is the single most important consideration as it will determine the design objectives and planning requirements. When designing a SAI facility, a comprehensive design allowing for an optimized workflow is important. The most common animal imaging studies, instrumentation needs, and an estimation of the subject throughput should be determined. Other considerations include technical staffing requirements and the financial support needed to maintain services while allowing for the incorporation of technology which would advance future imaging capabilities.

Animal housing and maintenance should be on-site and adjacent to the imaging instrumentation allowing for a high-throughput smooth-functioning queue. In a facility performing multimodality imaging on separate instruments, complimentary modality scanners should be placed in close proximity to one another. Scanners requiring minimal technical assistance, such as optical and ultrasound imaging, should be placed in locations where researchers can conduct their own imaging studies and not interfere with other ongoing activities in the center. The responsibilities of the technical staff should be focused on nuclear, CT, and MRI instrumentation due to their special training requirements.

A dedicated computing network infrastructure is necessary for reconstructing tomographic images as the computational requirements are substantial. Reconstructions should be performed immediately after imaging studies are concluded, providing end

users quick and easy access to their study results and to ensure that the study was performed correctly. Computational components such as reconstruction, data tracking, archiving, retrieval, and transfer should be communicated via a network backbone and dedicated computational resources. A database can be used to record the details and study parameters and to track the history of each subject.

All scans should follow standard operating procedures (SOPs) to ensure repeatability between imaging studies. Additional SOPs include those required for hazardous material handling and storage, radiation handling and safety, radioactive and immuno-compromised animal handling, anesthesia usage, data storage and retrieval, and the scheduling of experiments. For a more thorough review of SAI facility design considerations the reader is referred to [200, 209].

18.6 Applications

18.6.1 Cardiology

The development of high-resolution SAI has opened the door for investigations into models using transgenic mice which exhibit phenotypes of human cardiovascular disease. Cardiac imaging in small animals includes observations of overall heart function as well as imaging of molecular events. One consideration regarding cardiac activity in mice is the effect of anesthetics on cardiac function [210]. Inhaled anesthetics are much easier to control and provide more stable and physiologically relevant heat rates. Inhaled isoflurane is preferred in cardiac studies as it produces minimal cardiac depression [211]. Another challenge in obtaining accurate structural information in the mouse heart is its small size (~0.5 cm diameter). By using anatomical measurements of the heart, several cardiac parameters of interest can be determined. These include the [210]:

- *Fractional Shortening* – Relative difference in the left ventricle (LV) dimensions from end-diastole to end-systole.
- *Ejection Fraction* – End-diastolic volume that is ejected per beat, which measures heart contractility.
- *Stroke Volume* – Difference between the end-diastolic and end-systolic volumes.

• *Cardiac Output* – Amount of blood pumped by the LV into the aorta each minute, product of stroke volume, and heart rate.

MicroCT, ultrasound, and MRI can all be used to measure these parameters. Echocardiogram imaging using ultrasound is usually the preferred method given its ease of use and the ability to image cardiac function in real time. The requirement of real-time cardiac imaging, given the average mouse heart rate of ~500 beats/min, is a frame rate high enough to capture the cardiac cycle. Typically, frame rates of 800 images/s are sufficient to capture the full cardiac cycle [212]. B-mode ultrasound imaging can provide a 2D image of the heart, while imaging in M-mode uses a single beam through the heart to image the beam path, which is plotted as a function of time. This is useful for making accurate measurements of parameters such as wall thickness, LV dimensions, and cardiac mass. Doppler imaging can be used for measuring the blood flow of the aorta. Recent advances in ultrasound such as digital acquisition and data storage for off-line processing have improved the usefulness of this technology for assessing cardiac function. Ultrasound has also been used to study the heart of mice in the embryonic stage [213].

Imaging of heart function using microCT is also possible. Often with CT, gating methods are used to produce a dynamic 4D image of the heart (3D over time) [214, 215]. Gating refers to the use of ECG information from the cardiac cycle to trigger the acquisition during the imaging scan, or to perform postacquisition segmentation of the data based on the cycle information. MicroCT [214–216], MRI [217], and PET [218] can be used in conjunction with gating techniques to remove motion artifacts during cardiac studies. MRI has also demonstrated usefulness for accurate measurements of cardiac parameters [219, 220]. Another use of MRI has been in imaging atherosclerotic plaques in the mouse aorta [221, 222]. SPECT has been used for myocardial perfusion studies in mice [223]. Figure 18.14a shows a series of micro-PET images where the passage of an FDG tracer bolus through the RV cavity, lungs, and LV chamber of a mouse over time is captured while Fig. 18.14b shows a series of Time Activity Curves (TAC) for volumes-of-interest in the mouse RV and LV chamber and over the whole body. Nuclear medicine allows for imaging of molecular markers and pathways involved in cardiac disease. These types of studies can provide insight into

opportunities for clinical intervention. These studies include radionuclide imaging of heart failure, angiogenesis, apoptosis, and atherosclerosis in small animal models. Optical and microPET imaging have been used to provide insight into cardiac cell transplantation biology [224]. Reporter gene expression in cardiac cells has also been performed in living animals using microPET, which may eventually be applied to human gene therapy studies [225]. Stem cell therapy, which is emerging as an approach to treating heart disease, has shown that stem cell transplantation can promote function and prevent remodeling of the heart muscle. Stem cell techniques have been combined with several small animal imaging modalities such as MRI, SPECT, and PET to investigate their role in cardiac therapy [226].

Angiogenesis is the formation of new microvasculature and is a critical component of organ repair, but also of tumor development [227]. It is a complex process which involves interactions between many molecules and cell types. Several factors involved in the process of mediating cellular events in angiogenesis have been identified. Some of the more important angiogenic factors include Vascular Endothelial Growth Factor (VEGF) (endothelial cell adhesion), the integrin $\alpha v\beta 3$ (ligand recognition), and Matrix Metalloproteinases (MMPs) (vascular remodeling). Radionuclide labeled molecules such as VEGF ligands, $\alpha v\beta 3$ antagonists, and MMP inhibitors have been used to target each of these angiogenic factors in vivo [228–231]. Angiogenesis can also be visualized using MRI perfusion [232, 233], ultrasound for blood flow to tumors [234], and microCT for vascularization using contrast agents [235]. These techniques can lead to the development and evaluation of methods for inhibiting angiogenesis.

Apoptosis, or programmed cell death, is associated with many cardiovascular diseases [228]. Phosphatidyl Serine (PS), a plasma membrane phospholipid, is expressed on the surfaces of cells undergoing apoptosis and provides a target for imaging. Annexin-V is a protein that has a high affinity for PS and has been labeled with ^{99m}Tc for imaging of apoptosis [231, 236].

18.6.2 Neurology

In vivo imaging provides less invasive methods of exploring brain function in small animals. The brain (including the central nervous system) is important

a

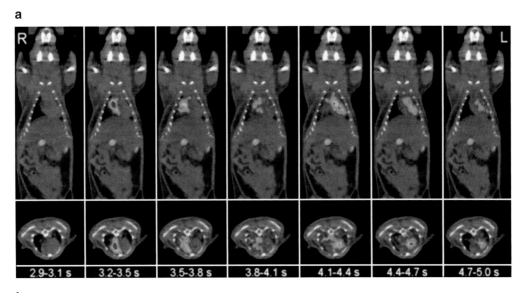

b

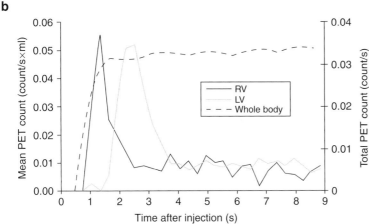

Fig. 18.14 (**a**) Consecutive 0.3-s frames show passage of a FDG tracer bolus through RV cavity, lungs, and LV chamber of a mouse on coronal and transverse slices. Times are those after start of image acquisition. For better anatomic orientation, PET scan is overlaid with coregistered CT scan.

(**b**) Time–activity curves derived for volumes of interest placed in RV and LV chamber and over whole body (total count on secondary y-axis) (From Kreissl MC et al. (2006) J Nucl Med 47(6):974–980 with permission from Society of Nuclear Medicine)

since it is the coordinator and central processing unit of many physiological processes. In many ways, relatively little is known about mammalian brain function. Most animal brain studies are conducted on nonhuman primates and rats. There are several advantages to using rats, including their role as the neurological model of choice historically and their larger brain size relative to the mouse (×5). The development of high spatial resolution instruments, however, has also brought mice into the foray of neurological imaging models as well, and detailed maps of the mouse brain are available [237, 238]. Small animal brain imaging is almost

completely dominated by various MRI techniques. SPECT and PET are also used to some extent, while optical and ultrasound imaging have minimal usefulness in the brain given the barrier presented by the skull. Ultrasound can be useful for brain studies during embryonic development [120]. A few of these techniques and applications offered by the SAI modalities are described here, with a focus on MRI.

MRI is a powerful tool for brain imaging because it offers both high sensitivity and high spatial resolution. There are several mechanisms in MRI which can be used to provide optimal contrast and to produce images with dramatic differences between tissue types of interest. These techniques can be used to detect blood oxygenation, regional blood volume, blood flow, diffusion of water, neuronal connections, brain damage, and plasticity after stroke [56]. Excellent reviews of the uses of MRI for neurological imaging have been written elsewhere [35, 239].

Ischemic stroke, which is a decrease in the blood supply to the brain, most often results in some level of morbidity (loss of function) and is a leading cause of disability in the elderly. The brain is capable of reorganizing its connections following a stroke to restore some level of function. This restoration of function is associated with plastic changes in the neurons of the brain [240]. Functional MRI (fMRI) has been used to study plasticity in the rat brain at different time points in response to external stimuli [241]. This method uses blood flow and blood oxygenation (hemodynamics) in the brain to detect the oxygen utilization level of neurons. The fMRI techniques of Blood Oxygenation Level-Dependent (BOLD), Cerebral Blood Flow (CBF)-weighted, and Cerebral Blood Volume (CBV)-weighted techniques can all be used in functional imaging of neuronal activity [241]. Diffusion tensor imaging (DTI) or manganese-enhanced MRI (MEMRI) fMRI techniques can also detect changes in neuronal connectivity. DTI allows the detection of water diffusion and can be used to infer white-matter connectivity, which shows the parts of the brain that are connected to each other. MEMRI is based on the introduction of Mn^{2+} ions to brain tissues, which are thought to play a role in synaptic transmission [242]. MEMRI has been used to detect changes in neuronal connectivity after stroke in a rat model [243]. Understanding the mechanisms of spontaneous functional recovery can assist researchers in the design of effective neuro-rehabilitative strategies.

In the brain, PET and SPECT can also be used to measure regional blood volume and flow, oxygenation and glucose consumption as well as to quantify receptors in drug uptake. The saturation of dopamine transporter probes in rats and dopamine receptor occupancy of cerebral binding sites in mice has been studied using SPECT and PET, respectively [132, 244, 245]. Endogenous dopamine release in mice has also been visualized using SPECT [246]. The study of these receptor-ligand interactions in the brain can be useful in determining the functional efficacy of novel drugs. PET has also been used to study neurotransmitter activity [247, 248].

18.6.3 Oncology

The use of SAI in oncology research has been well established and is still rapidly expanding. In this section, only a select number of applications using SAI techniques in the study of cancer are mentioned.

Prior to SAI, tumors from transgenic cancer animal models could be visualized only on autopsy and tissue histology [249]. With the advent of SAI, subjects can be screened at the macrolevel of whole-body anatomy and physiology prior to and during cancer therapy. New methods of study such as tracking the spread of metastatic disease and following treatment response have become available to the researcher. While all of the SAI modalities are useful in oncology studies, MRI, optical, and radionuclide imaging are particularly powerful as they provide the most information related to the physiological and molecular changes that occur in tissue, often before anatomical changes are apparent. A powerful potential of optical and radionuclide techniques in this respect is the extremely high sensitivity they provide, which aids in the differentiation between healthy and diseased tissue as is the goal in early cancer detection.

The study of xenograft tumors in small animals using radiolabeled compounds is relatively simple since they can be implanted away from major organs [101]. Fluorine-18-based compounds such as FDG and [18F]-3-fluoro-3-deoxy-L-thymidine (FLT), which are commonly used in clinical PET imaging [85, 250], are also used for imaging glucose metabolism and DNA replication in small animals, respectively [99, 251]. One of the most powerful uses of PET is in its ability to monitor cancer therapy treatments by looking at cellular uptake of FDG and FLT [252]. These and other PET molecular probes can be used to specifically target molecular-level scenarios involving signal transduction, metabolites, tumor-specific antigens, or the expression of a particular gene among others [249]. A recently developed radiolabeled cytosine probe, 1-(2-deoxy-2-[18F]fluoroarabinofuranosyl)-cytosine (FAC), specifically targets immune activity in response to tumors [253]. Deoxycytidine kinase (DCK) enzyme activity varies significantly among subjects and across different tumor types and is a critical determinant of tumor responses to certain nucleoside analog drugs. Figure 18.15 shows how FAC is preferentially taken up in (DCK) positive tumors. Tumor response following

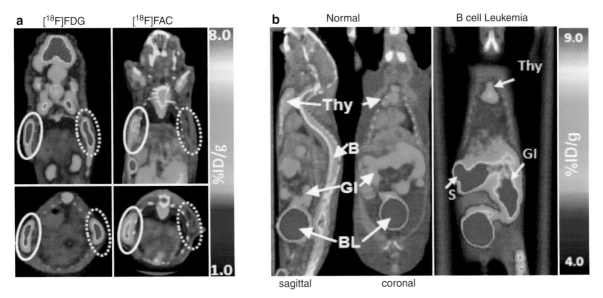

Fig. 18.15 Deoxycytidine kinase (DCK) enzyme activity varies significantly among subjects and across different tumor types and is a critical determinant of tumor responses to certain nucleoside analog drugs. (**a**) FAC is preferentially taken up in (DCK) positive tumors. FDG and FAC imaging of DCK positive (*left*) and DCK negative (*right*) tumors. (**b**) In the B cell leukemia model, there is a striking increase in the spleen FAC signals compared to those detected in healthy mice. These signals reflect the accumulation of DCK-expressing leukemic cells in the spleen. Thy – thymus; BL – bladder; L – liver; S – spleen; GI – gastrointestinal tract; LN – lymph nodes; B – bone/bone-marrow (Figure courtesy of Rachel Laing, University of California, Los Angeles)

photodynamic therapy can also be visualized using PET [254]. Another class of imaging agent, radiolabeled antibody fragments, have been used to image anitigen-positive xenografts in mice [108, 255]. For all the examples mentioned, the challenge in using PET remains in developing probes with high target specificity and low background levels.

MRI has proved to be a useful tool for developing and validating small animal cancer models in the brain [256], kidney [257], prostate [258], and other organs [249]. Using MRI, tumor growth in these organs and other tissues can be measured over time. During cancer therapy, treatment efficacy can be monitored as well [249, 259]. Angiogenesis, which is known to play a role in tumor vasculature formation, has been studied using MRI, CT and Ultrasound [260], and PET [252] and the efficacy of antiangiogenic agents can be determined [261, 262]. Detailed characterizations of tumor composition can be made, often through imaging of the tumor vasculature and oxygenation. In both MRI and CT, this can be done by using contrast agents in conjunction with various techniques to study dynamic processes such as diffusion, perfusion, and flow to [249, 263–265]. CT is a useful tool for tumor imaging given its ability to rapidly image animals with a high spatial resolution and it has been used to study lung nodules in mice [266, 267].

Optical imaging has shown usefulness in studies dealing with tumor cell proliferation [268], treatment response [269], high-throughput assessment of tumor development and metastatic spread [50], reporter gene imaging for measurements of neoplastic disease [270], NIR fluorescent probe imaging of tumors [271], and receptor-targeted optical imaging using NIR [272], among several other uses.

18.7 Future Directions

The field of preclinical imaging has rapidly evolved during the last decade or so to include new detector technologies in addition to the constant improvements in existing modalities. There are many rapidly evolving technologies on the horizon that will continue to bring preclinical imaging technologies, often in combination with other complementary technologies, into the forefront of biomedical research of human disease.

One relevant area of complementary technology is that of microfluidics. Microfluidic chip technologies allow for the manipulation of fluids in channels with dimensions on the order of tens of micrometers [273]. Microfluidics allows for a wide variety of experimental and practical applications to be performed rapidly on the micro scale. This includes cell cultures and radiolabeled probe synthesis [274] among many other biological analyses and chemical syntheses applications. Microfluidic technology has also been combined with scintillation detectors or solid state detectors such as APDs to provide novel methods of imaging beta particles emitted from radioisotopes [275, 276]. This class of preclinical imaging devices allows for repeatable quantification of metabolic activity in cells.

Novel techniques for combining PET and MRI imaging technologies have shown that this tool will soon become commercially available. Among the several advantages of obtaining anatomical information using MRI rather than CT are the excellent soft tissue contrast and nonionizing nature of MRI. There are currently many groups actively working toward the development of this technology [32, 180, 277, 278].

Optoacoustic imaging is a technology based on the photoacoustic effect, in which sound or pressure waves result from localized heating of tissue using light, such as a laser. Optoacoustic imaging can be used to obtain images of structures in turbid environments. This technique has been used to image cerebral oxygen levels noninvasively [279] as well as in combination with gold nanoparticles which can target cancer cells in vivo [280]. Similarly, thermoacoustic imaging can be used to image small animals noninvasively and without the effects of ionizing radiation [281]. Hyperspectral imaging uses spectral information collected over the visible and infrared regions of the electromagnetic spectrum to enhance tomographic reconstruction techniques [282, 283].

References

1. Luker GD, Luker KE (2008) Optical imaging: current applications and future directions. J Nucl Med 49:1–4
2. Kitano H (2002) Systems biology: a brief overview. Science 295:1662–1664
3. Marincola F (2003) Translational medicine: a two-way road. J Transl Med 1:1
4. Sartor RB (2003) Translational research: bridging the widening gap between basic and clinical research. Gastroenterology 124:1178
5. Humes HD (2005) Translational medicine and the National Institutes of Health road map: steep grades and tortuous curves. J Lab Clin Med 146:51–54
6. Sonntag K-C (2005) Implementations of translational medicine. J Transl Med 3:33
7. O'Connell D, Roblin D (2006) Translational research in the pharmaceutical industry: from bench to bedside. Drug Discov Today 11:833–837
8. Littman BH, Di mario L, Plebani M, Marincola FM (2007) What's next in translational medicine? Clin Sci 112:217–227
9. Zerhouni EA (2005) Translational and clinical science – time for a new vision. N Engl J Med 353:1621–1623
10. Malakoff D (2000) SUPPLIERS: the rise of the mouse. Biomedicine's model mammal. Science 288:248–253
11. Cherry SR, Gambhir SS (2001) Use of positron emission tomography in animal research. Inst Lab Animal Res J 42:219–232
12. Hanahan D (1989) Transgenic mice as probes into complex systems. Science 246:1265–1275
13. Misra R, Duncan S (2002) Gene targeting in the mouse. Endocr 19:229–238
14. Ryan MJ, Sigmund CD (2002) Use of transgenic and knockout strategies in mice. Semin Nephrol 22:154–160
15. Nolan PM et al (2000) A systematic, genome-wide, phenotype-driven mutagenesis programme for gene function studies in the mouse. Nat Genet 25:440–443
16. Vogel G (2007) Nobel prizes: a knockout award in medicine. Science 318:178–179
17. Grimm D (2006) Mouse genetics: a mouse for every gene. Science 312:1862–1866
18. Cherry SR (2004) In vivo molecular and genomic imaging: new challenges for imaging physics. Phy Med Biol 49:R13
19. Cherry SR (2006) Multimodality in vivo imaging systems: twice the power or double the trouble? Ann Rev Biomed Eng 8:35–62
20. Paulus MJ, Gleason SS, Kennel SJ, Hunsicker PR, Johnson DK (2000) High resolution x-ray computed tomography: an emerging tool for small animal cancer research. Neoplasia 2:62–70
21. Ritman EL (2004) Micro-computed, tomography – current status and developments. Annu Rev Biomed Eng 6:185–208
22. Matscheko G, Carlsson GA (1989) Measurement of absolute energy spectra from a clinical CT machine under working conditions using a compton spectrometer. Phys Med Biol 34:209–222
23. Bushberg JT, Seibert JA, Leidholdt EM Jr, Boone JM (2002) The Essential physics of medical imaging, 2nd edn. Williams & Wilkins, Lippincott
24. Brooks RA, Chiro GD (1976) Beam hardening in X-ray reconstructive tomography. Phy Med Biol 21:390
25. Hsieh J, Molthen RC, Dawson CA, Johnson RH (2000) An iterative approach to the beam hardening correction in cone beam CT. Med Phys 27:23–29
26. Chow PL, Rannou FR, Chatziioannou AF (2004) Towards a beam hardening correction for a microCT scanner. Mol Imaging Biol 6:77–78

27. Yan CH, Whalen RT, Beaupre GS, Yen SY, Napel S (2000) Reconstruction algorithm for polychromatic CT imaging: application to beam hardening correction. IEEE Trans Med Imaging 19:1–11

28. Zhao W, Rowlands JA (1995) X-ray imaging using amorphous selenium: feasibility of a flat panel self-scanned detector for digital radiology. Med Phys 22:1595–1604

29. Zhao W et al (1997) Digital radiology using active matrix readout of amorphous selenium: construction and evaluation of a prototype real-time detector. Med Phys 24:1834–1843

30. Nagarkar VV et al (1998) Structured CsI(Tl) scintillators for X-ray imaging applications. IEEE Trans Nucl Sci 45:492–496

31. Shepherd JA, Gruner SM, Tate MW, Tecotzky M (1994) In: X-ray and ultraviolet sensors and applications. Hoover RB, Williams MB (eds) 24–30 (SPIE) http://spie.org/x648.html?product_id=211910

32. Pichler BJ, Wehrl HF, Judenhofer MS (2008) Latest advances in molecular imaging instrumentation. J Nucl Med 49:5S–23S

33. Doty FD, Entzminger G, Kulkarni J, Pamarthy K, Staab JP (2007) Radio frequency coil technology for small-animal MRI. NMR Biomed 20:304–325

34. Driehuys B et al (2008) Small animal imaging with magnetic resonance microscopy. ILAR J 49:35–53

35. Benveniste H, Blackband S (2002) MR microscopy and high resolution small animal MRI: applications in neuroscience research. Prog Neurobiol 67:393–420

36. Bollard ME, Stanley EG, Lindon JC, Nicholson JK, Holmes E (2005) NMR-based metabonomic approaches for evaluating physiological influences on biofluid composition. NMR Biomed 18:143–162

37. McConville P, Moody JB, Moffat BA (2005) High-throughput magnetic resonance imaging in mice for phenotyping and therapeutic evaluation. Curr Opin Chem Biol 9:413–420

38. Coatney RW (2001) Ultrasound imaging: principles and applications in rodent research. ILAR J 42:233–247

39. Foster SF, Pavlin CJ, Harasiewicz KA, Christopher DA, Turnbull DH (2000) Advances in ultrasound biomicroscopy. Ultrasound Med Biol 26:1–27

40. Wirtzfeld LA et al (2005) A new three-dimensional ultrasound microimaging technology for preclinical studies using a transgenic prostate cancer mouse model. Cancer Res 65:6337–6345

41. Krix M et al (2003) Comparison of intermittent-bolus contrast imaging with conventional power Doppler sonography: quantification of tumour perfusion in small animals. Ultrasound Med Biol 29:1093–1103

42. Ferrara K, DeAngelis G (1997) Color flow mapping. Ultrasound Med Biol 23:321–345

43. Liang H-D, Blomley MJK (2003) The role of ultrasound in molecular imaging. Br J Radiol 76:S140–S150

44. Villringer A, Chance B (1997) Non-invasive optical spectroscopy and imaging of human brain function. Trends Neurosci 20:435–442

45. Ntziachristos V, Yodh AG, Schnall M, Chance B (2000) Concurrent MRI and diffuse optical tomography of breast after indocyanine green enhancement. Proc Natl Acad Sci USA 97:2767–2772

46. Intes X et al (2003) In vivo continuous-wave optical breast imaging enhanced with indocyanine green. Med Phys 30:1039–1047

47. Obrig H, Villringer A (2003) Beyond the visible-imaging the human brain with light. J Cereb Blood Flow Metab 23:1–18

48. Li A et al (2003) Tomographic optical breast imaging guided by three-dimensional mammography. Appl Opt 42:5181–5190

49. Zhang Q et al (2005) Coregistered tomographic x-ray and optical breast imaging: initial results. J Biomed Opt 10:024033

50. Paroo Z et al (2004) Validating bioluminescence imaging as a high-throughput, quantitative modality for assessing tumor burden. Mol Imaging 3:117–124

51. Ntziachristos V, Ripoll J, Wang LV, Weissleder R (2005) Looking and listening to light: the evolution of whole-body photonic imaging. Nat Biotechnol 23:313–320

52. Massoud TF, Gambhir SS (2003) Molecular imaging in living subjects: seeing fundamental biological processes in a new light. Genes Dev 17:545–580

53. Weissleder R, Ntziachristos V (2003) Shedding light onto live molecular targets. 9:123–128

54. Contag CH, Bachmann MH (2002) Advances in in vivo bioluminescence imaging of gene expression. Annu Rev Biomed Eng 4:235–260

55. Choy G, Choyke P, Libutti SK (2003) Current advances in molecular imaging: noninvasive in vivo bioluminescent and fluorescent optical imaging in cancer research. Mol Imaging 2:303–312

56. Ntziachristos V, Leroy-Willig A, Tavitian B (2007) Textbook of in vivo imaging in vertebrates. Wiley, New York

57. Rice BW, Cable MD, Nelson MB (2001) In vivo imaging of light-emitting probes. J Biomed Opt 6:432–440

58. Pham TH et al (2000) Quantifying the absorption and reduced scattering coefficients of tissuelike turbid media over a broad spectral range with noncontact Fourier-transform hyperspectral imaging. Appl Opt 39:6487–6497

59. Weissleder R, Pittet MJ (2008) Imaging in the era of molecular oncology. 452:580–589

60. Park JM, Gambhir SS (2005) Multimodality radionuclide, fluorescence, and bioluminescence small-animal imaging. Proc IEEE 93:771–783

61. Troy T, Jekic-McMullen D, Sambucetti L, Rice B (2004) Quantitative comparison of the sensitivity of detection of fluorescent and bioluminescent reporters in animal models. Mol Imaging 3:9–23

62. Bhaumik S, Gambhir SS (2002) Optical imaging of Renilla luciferase reporter gene expression in living mice. Proc Natl Acad Sci USA 99:377–382

63. Greer LF III, Szalay AA (2002) Imaging of light emission from the expression of luciferases in living cells and organisms: a review. Luminescence 17:43–74

64. Loening AM, Wu AM, Gambhir SS (2007) Red-shifted Renilla reniformis luciferase variants for imaging in living subjects. Nat Meth 4:641–643

65. Ntziachristos V, Bremer C, Weissleder R (2003) Fluorescence imaging with near-infrared light: new technological advances that enable in vivo molecular imaging. Eur Radiol 13:195–208

66. Bremer C, Ntziachristos V, Weissleder R (2003) Optical-based molecular imaging: contrast agents and potential medical applications. Eur Radiol 13:231–243

67. Bluestone AY, Stewart M, Lasker J, Abdoulaev GS, Hielscher AH (2004) Three-dimensional optical tomographic brain imaging in small animals, part 1: hypercapnia. J Biomed Opt 9:1046–1062

68. Hielscher AH (2005) Optical tomographic imaging of small animals. Curr Opin Biotechnol 16:79–88

69. Zacharakis G, Ripoll J, Weissleder R, Ntziachristos V (2005) Fluorescent protein tomography scanner for small animal imaging. IEEE Trans Medl Imaging 24:878–885

70. Alexandrakis G, Rannou FR, Chatziioannou AF (2005) Tomographic bioluminescence imaging by use of a combined optical-PET (OPET) system: a computer simulation feasibility study. Phys Med Biol 50:4225–4241

71. Chaudhari AJ et al (2005) Hyperspectral and multispectral bioluminescence optical tomography for small animal imaging. Phys Med Biol 50:5421–5441

72. Alexandrakis G, Rannou FR, Chatziioannou AF (2006) Effect of optical property estimation accuracy on tomographic bioluminescence imaging: simulation of a combined optical-PET (OPET) system. Phys Med Biol 51 (8):2045–2053

73. Wang G, Shen H, Durairaj K, Qian X, Cong W (2006) The first bioluminescence tomography system for simultaneous acquisition of multiview and multispectral data. Int J Biomed Imaging 1–8, www.ncbi.nlm.nih.gov/pmc/articles/PMC2324039/pdf/IJBI2006-58601.pdf

74. Lv Y et al (2007) Spectrally resolved bioluminescence tomography with adaptive finite element analysis: methodology and simulation. Phys Med Biol 52:4497–4513

75. Welch MJ, Redvanly CS (2001) Handbook of radiopharmaceuticals. Wiley, New York

76. Ullberg S, Larsson B (1981) Whole-body autoradiography. Meth Enzymol 77:64–80

77. Hall MD, Davenport AP, Clark CR (1986) Quantitative receptor autoradiography. Nature 324:493–494

78. Schmidt KC, Smith CB (2005) Resolution, sensitivity and precision with autoradiography and small animal positron emission tomography: implications for functional brain imaging in animal research. Nucl Med Biol 32:719–725

79. Kuhar MJ, Lloyd DG, Appel N, Loats HL (1991) Imaging receptors by autoradiography: computer-assisted approaches. J Chem Neuroanat 4:319–327

80. Zhao W, Ginsberg MD, Smith DW (1995) Three-dimensional quantitative autoradiography by disparity analysis: theory and applications to image averaging of local cerebral glucose utilization. J Cereb Blood Flow Metab 15:552–565

81. Toyama H et al (2004) Absolute quantification of regional cerebral glucose utilization in mice by 18F-FDG small animal PET scanning and 2-14C-DG autoradiography. J Nucl Med 45:1398–1405

82. Phelps ME, Mazziotta JC, Schelbert HR (1986) Positron emission tomography and autoradiography – principles and applications for the brain and heart. Raven, New York

83. Meikle SR, Kench P, Kassiou M, Banati RB (2005) Small animal SPECT and its place in the matrix of molecular imaging technologies. Phys Med Biol 50:R45

84. Wagenaar DJ et al (2006) In vivo dual-isotope SPECT imaging with improved energy resolution. IEEE Nuclear Science Symposium Conference Record **6**, 3821–3826

85. Phelps ME (2004) PET: molecular imaging and its biological applications. Springer, Berlin

86. Strand S-E et al (1994) Small animal imaging with pinhole single-photon emission computed tomography. Cancer 73:981–984

87. Weber DA et al (1994) Pinhole SPECT: an approach to in vivo high resolution SPECT imaging in small laboratory animals. J Nucl Med 35:342–348

88. Jaszczak RJ, Li J, Wang H, Zalutsky MR, Coleman RE (1994) Pinhole collimation for ultra-high-resolution, small-field-of-view SPECT. Phys Med Biol 39(3):425

89. Beekman F, van der Have F (2007) The pinhole: gateway to ultra-high-resolution three-dimensional radionuclide imaging. Eur J Nucl Med Mol Imaging 34:151–161

90. Kupinski MA, Barrett HH (2005) Small-animal SPECT imaging. Springer, New York

91. Meikle SR et al (2001) An investigation of coded aperture imaging for small animal SPECT. IEEE Trans Nucl Sci 48:816–821

92. Meikle SR et al (2002) A prototype coded aperture detector for small animal SPECT. IEEE Trans Nucl Sci 49:2167–2171

93. Schramm NU et al (2003) High-resolution SPECT using multipinhole collimation. IEEE Trans Nucl Sci 50:315–320

94. Madsen MT (2007) Recent advances in SPECT imaging. J Nucl Med 48:661–673

95. Phelps ME, Hoffman EJ, Mullani NA, Ter-Pogossian MM (1975) Application of annihilation coincidence detection to transaxial reconstruction tomography. J Nucl Med 16:210–224

96. Phelps ME (1999) Positron emission tomography provides molecular imaging of biological processes. Proc Natl Acad Sci USA 97:9226–9233

97. Phelps ME (2000) PET: the merging of biology and imaging into molecular imaging. J Nucl Med 41:661–681

98. Hutchins GD, Miller MA, Soon VC, Receveur T (2008) Small animal PET imaging. ILAR J 49:54–65

99. Myers R (2001) The biological application of small animal PET imaging. Nucl Med Biol 28:585–593

100. Levin CS, Hoffman EJ (1999) Calculation of positron range and its effect on the fundamental limit of positron emission tomography system spatial resolution. Phys Med Biol 44:781

101. Chatziioannou AF (2002) Molecular imaging of small animals with dedicated PET tomographs. Eur J Nucl Med 29:98–114

102. Cherry SR (2006) The 2006 Henry N. Wagner lecture: of mice and men (and positrons) – advances in PET imaging technology. J Nucl Med 47:1735–1745

103. Gambhir SS et al (1999) Imaging adenoviral-directed reporter gene expression in living animals with positron emission tomography. Proc Natl Acad Sci USA 96:2333–2338

104. Herschman HR et al (2000) Seeing is believing: non-invasive, quantitative and repetitive imaging of reporter gene expression in living animals, using positron emission tomography. J Neurosci Res 59:699–705

105. Gambhir SS, Barrio JR, Herschman HR, Phelps ME (1999) Assays for noninvasive imaging of reporter gene expression. Nucl Med Biol 26:481–490

106. Gambhir SS et al (2000) Imaging transgene expression with radionuclide imaging technologies. Neoplasia 2:118–138

107. Hu S-Z et al (1996) Minibody: a novel engineered anti-carcinoembryonic antigen antibody fragment (single-chain Fv-CH3) which exhibits rapid, high-level targeting of xenografts. Cancer Res 56:3055–3061

108. Wu AM et al (2000) High-resolution microPET imaging of carcinoembryonic antigen-positive xenografts by using a copper-64-labeled engineered antibody fragment. Proc Natl Acad Sci USA 97:8495–8500

109. Boone J, Alexander G, Seibert J (1993) A fluoroscopy-based computed tomography scanner for small specimen research. Investig Radiol 28:539–544

110. Holdsworth DW, Drangova M, Schulenburg KS, Fenster A (1990) A table-top CT system for high-resolution volume imaging. Proc Soc Photo Instrum Eng 1231:239–245

111. Paulus MJ et al (1999) A new X-ray computed tomography system for laboratory mouse imaging. IEEE Trans Nucl Sci 46:558–564

112. Seguin FH, Burstein P, Bjorkholm PJ, Homburger F, Adams RA (1985) X-ray computed tomography with 50-μm resolution. Appl Opt 24:4117–4123

113. Eccles CD, Callaghan PT (1986) High resolution imaging – the NMR microscope. J Magn Reson 68:393–398

114. Johnson GA, Thompson MB, Gewalt SL, Hayes CE (1986) Nuclear magnetic resonance imaging at microscopic resolution. J Magn Reson 68

115. Johnson GA, Benveniste H, Engelhardt RT, Qiu H, Hedlund LW (1997) Magnetic resonance microscopy in basic studies of brain structure and function. Ann NY Acad Sci 820:139–148

116. Zhang J et al (2003) Three-dimensional anatomical characterization of the developing mouse brain by diffusion tensor microimaging. Neuroimage 20:1639–1648

117. Tenney JR, Duong TQ, King JA, Ferris CF (2004) fMRI of brain activation in a genetic rat model of absence seizures. Epilepsia 45:576–582

118. Benveniste H, Kim K, Zhang L, Johnson GA (2000) Magnetic resonance microscopy of the C57BL mouse brain. Neuroimage 11:601–611

119. Maronpot RR, Sills RC, Johnson GA (2004) Applications of magnetic resonancy microscopy. Toxicol Pathol 32

120. Turnbull DH, Bloomfield TS, Baldwin HS, Foster FS, Joyner AL (1995) Ultrasound backscatter microscope analysis of early mouse embryonic brain development. Proc Natl Acad Sci USA 92:2239–2243

121. Aristizábal O, Christopher DA, Foster FS, Turnbull DH (1998) 40-MHz echocardiography scanner for cardiovascular assessment of mouse embryos. Ultrasound Med Biol 24:1407–1417

122. Christopher DA, Burns PN, Foster FS (1996) High frequency continuous wave Doppler ultrasound system for the detection of blood Flow in the microcirculation. Ultrasound Med Biol 22:1196–1203

123. Christopher DA, Starkoski BG, Burns PN, Foster FS (1997) High frequency pulsed doppler ultrasound system for detecting and mapping blood flow in the microcirculation. Ultrasound Med Biol 23:997–1015

124. Kruse DE, Silverman RH, Fornaris RJ, Coleman DJ, Ferrara KW (1998) A swept-scanning mode for estimation of blood velocity in the microvasculature. IEEE Trans Ultrason Ferroelectr Freq Control 45:1437–1440

125. Foster FS et al (2002) A new ultrasound instrument for in vivo microimaging of mice. Ultrasound Med Biol 28:1165–1172

126. Caliper Life Sciences: IVIS Optical imaging systems. http://www.caliperls.com/.

127. Cambridge research instruments: maestro optical imaging system. http://www.cri-inc.com/.

128. Kodak: in-vivo image station. http://www.carestream-health.com/in-vivo-multispectral-system-fx.html.

129. Vastenhouw B, Beekman F (2007) Submillimeter total-body murine imaging with U-SPECT-I. J Nucl Med 48:487–493

130. Beekman FJ et al (2005) U-SPECT-I: a novel system for submillimeter-resolution tomography with radiolabeled molecules in mice. J Nucl Med 46:1194–1200

131. Beekman FJ, Vastenhouw B (2004) Design and simulation of a high-resolution stationary SPECT system for small animals. Phys Med Biol 49:4579

132. Acton PD, Choi S-R, Plossl K, Kung HF (2002) Quantification of dopamine transporters in the mouse brain using ultra-high resolution single-photon emission tomography. Eur J Nucl Med Mol Imaging 29:691–698

133. Kim H et al (2006) SemiSPECT: a small-animal single-photon emission computed tomography (SPECT) imager based on eight cadmium zinc telluride (CZT) detector arrays. Med Phys 33:465–474

134. Lackas C et al (2005) T-SPECT: a novel imaging technique for small animal research. IEEE Trans Nucl Sci 52:181–187

135. Forrer F et al (2006) In vivo radionuclide uptake quantification using a multi-pinhole SPECT system to predict renal function in small animals. Eur J Nucl Med Mol Imaging 33:1214–1217

136. MacDonald LR et al (2001) Pinhole SPECT of mice using the LumaGEM gamma camera. IEEE Trans Nucl Sci 48:830–836

137. Bloomfield PM et al (1995) The design and physical characteristics of a small animal positron emission tomograph. Phys Med Biol 40:1105

138. Lecomte R, Cadorette J, Richard P, Rodrigue S, Rouleau D (1994) Design and engineering aspects of a high resolution positron emission tomography for small animal imaging. IEEE Trans Nucl Sci 41:1446–1452

139. Cherry SR et al (1997) MicroPET: a high resolution pet scanner for imaging small animals. IEEE Trans Nucl Sci 44:1161–1166

140. Del Guerra A, Di Domenico G, Scandola M, Zavattini G (1998) YAP-PET: first results of a small animal positron emission tomograph based on YAP:Ce finger crystals. IEEE Trans Nucl Sci 45:3105–3108

141. Jeavons AP, Chandler RA, Dettmar CAR (1999) A 3D HIDAC-PET camera with sub-millimetre resolution for imaging small animals. IEEE Trans Nucl Sci 46:468–473

142. Weber S et al (1999) Evaluation of TierPET system. IEEE Trans Nucl Sci 46:1177–1183

143. Siemens Preclinical Solutions: Inveon

144. Gleason SS et al (2006) A new highly versatile multimodality small animal imaging platform. IEEE Nucl Sci Symp Conf Rec 4:2447–2449

145. Wang Y, Seidel J, Tsui BMW, Vaquero JJ, Pomper MG (2006) Performance evaluation of the GE healthcare eXplore VISTA dual-ring small-animal PET scanner. J Nucl Med 47:1891–1900

146. GE Healthcare: eXplore Vista PET/CT

147. Huisman M, Reder S, Weber A, Ziegler S, Schwaiger M (2007) Performance evaluation of the Philips MOSAIC small animal PET scanner. Eur J Nucl Med Mol Imaging 34:532–540

148. Philips Medical Systems: Mosaic HP. http://www. medical.philips.com/main/products/preclinical/products/ mosaic_hp/

149. Gamma Medica-Ideas: LabPET. http://www.gm-ideas. com/index.php?option = com_content&task = view&id = 107&Itemid = 36

150. Bergeron M et al (2007) Performance evaluation of the LabPET APD-based digital PET scanner. Nucl Sci Symp Conf Rec 2007(6):4185–4191

151. Larobina M, Brunetti A, Salvatore M (2006) Small animal PET: a review of commercially available imaging systems. Curr Med Imaging Rev 2:187–192

152. Levin CS, Zaidi H (2007) Current trends in preclinical PET system design. PET Clinic 2:125–160

153. Shokouhi S et al (2005) System performance simulations of the RatCAP awake rat brain scanner. IEEE Trans Nucl Sci 52:1305–1310

154. Woody C et al (2004) RatCAP: a small, head-mounted PET tomograph for imaging the brain of an awake RAT. Nucl Inst Methods Phys Res A 527:166–170

155. Loening AM, Gambhir SS (2003) AMIDE: a free software tool for multimodality medical image analysis. Mol Imaging 2:131–137

156. Hasegawa BH et al (2002) In Medical imaging 2002: physiology and function from multidimensional images. 1–15 (SPIE) http://spie.org/x648.html?product_id=463620

157. Goertzen AL, Meadors AK, Silverman RW, Cherry SR (2002) Simultaneous molecular and anatomical imaging of the mouse in vivo. Phys Med Biol 47(24):4315

158. Iwata K, Wu MC, Hasegawa BH (2000) Design of combined X-ray CT and SPECT system for small animals. IEEE Nucl Sci Symp Conf Rec 3:1608–1612

159. Weisenberger AG et al (2003) SPECT-CT system for small animal imaging. IEEE Trans Nucl Sci 50:74–79

160. Zingerman Y, Golan H, Gersten A, Moalem AA (2008) Compact CT/SPECT system for small-object imaging. Nucl Inst Methods Phy Res A 548:135–148

161. Kastis GA et al (2004) Compact CT/SPECT small-animal imaging system. IEEE Trans Nucl Sci 51:63–67

162. Fontaine R et al (2005) Architecture of a dual-modality, high-resolution, fully digital positron emission tomography/computed tomography (PET/CT) scanner for small animal imaging. IEEE Trans Nucl Sci 52:691–696

163. Seidel J et al (2002) Features of the NIH ATLAS small animal PET scanner and its use with a coaxial small animal volume CT scanner. IEEE Proc Biomed Eng Symp 4:545–548

164. Khodaverdi M, Pauly F, Weber S, Schroder G, Ziemons K, Sievering R, Halling H (2001) Preliminary studies of a micro-CT for a combined small animal PET/CT scanner, Conference Record of the 2001 IEEE Nuclear Science Symposium and Medical Imaging Conference, San Diego, CA, USA, 3:1605–1606

165. Liang H et al (2007) A microPET/CT system for in vivo small animal imaging. Phys Med Biol 52:3881

166. Chow PL, Stout DB, Komisopoulou E, Chatziioannou AF (2006) A method of image registration for small animal, multi-modality imaging. Phys Med Biol 51:379

167. Deroose CM et al (2007) Multimodality imaging of tumor xenografts and metastases in mice with combined small-animal PET, small-animal CT, and bioluminescence imaging. J Nucl Med 48:295–303

168. Siemens Preclinical Solutions: Inveon. http://www.medical. siemens.com/siemens/en_US/gg_nm_FBAs/files/brochures/ preclinical/Inveon.pdf

169. Raylman RR, Hammer BE, Christensen NL (1996) Combined MRI-PET scanner: a Monte Carlo evaluation of the improvements in PET resolution due to the effects of a static homogeneous magnetic field. IEEE Trans Nucl Sci 43:2406–2412

170. Wirrwar A et al (1997) 4.5 tesla magnetic field reduces range of high-energy positrons – potential implications for positron emission tomography. IEEE Trans Nucl Sci 44:184–189

171. Hammer BE, Christensen NL, Heil BG (1994) Use of a magnetic field to increase the spatial resolution of positron emission tomography. Med Phys 21:1917–1920

172. Shao Y et al (1997) Development of a PET detector system compatible with MRI/NMR systems. IEEE Trans Nucl Sci 44:1167–1171

173. Shao Y et al (1997) Simultaneous PET and MR imaging. Phys Med Biol 42:1965

174. Slates RB et al (1990) A study of artefacts in simultaneous PET and MR imaging using a prototype MR compatible PET scanner. Phys Med Biol 44:2015

175. Lecomte R et al (1996) Initial results from the sherbrooke avalanche photodiode positron tomograph. IEEE Trans Nucl Sci 43:1952–1957

176. Levin CS, Foudray AMK, Olcott PD, Habte F (2003) Investigation of position sensitive avalanche photodiodes for a new high resolution PET detector design. Nucl Sci Symp Conf Rec 4:2262–2266

177. Marsden PK, Strul D, Keevil SF, Williams SCR, Cash D (2002) Simultaneous PET and NMR. Br J Radiol 75:S53–S59

178. Pichler BJ et al (2006) Performance Test of an LSO-APD Detector in a 7-T MRI scanner for simultaneous PET/MRI. J Nucl Med 47:639–647

179. Raylman RR et al (2006) Simultaneous MRI and PET imaging of a rat brain. Phys Med Biol 51:6371

180. Catana C et al (2006) Simultaneous acquisition of multi-slice PET and MR images: initial results with a MR-compatible PET scanner. J Nucl Med 47:1968–1976

181. Jacobs A et al (1999) Functional coexpression of HSV-1 thymidine kinase and green fluorescent protein: implications for noninvasive imaging of transgene expression. Neoplasia 1:154–161

182. Ray P, Wu AM, Gambhir SS (2003) Optical bioluminescence and positron emission tomography imaging of a novel fusion reporter gene in tumor xenografts of living mice. Cancer Res 63:1160–1165

183. Ray P, De A, Min J-J, Tsien RY, Gambhir SS (2004) Imaging tri-fusion multimodality reporter gene expression in living subjects. Cancer Res 64:1323–1330

184. Li C et al (2006) Dual optical and nuclear imaging in human melanoma xenografts using a single targeted imaging probe. Nucl Med Biol 33:349–358

185. Zhang Z, Liang K, Bloch S, Berezin M, Achilefu S (2005) Monomolecular multimodal fluorescence-radioisotope imaging agents. Bioconjug Chem 16:1232–1239

186. Culver J, Akers W, Achilefu S (2008) Multimodality molecular imaging with combined optical and SPECT/PET modalities. J Nucl Med 49:169–172

187. Peter J, Unholtz D, Schulz RB, Doll J, Semmler W (2007) Development and initial results of a tomographic dual-modality positron/optical small animal imager. IEEE Trans Nucl Sci 54:1553–1560

188. Celentano L et al (2003) Preliminary tests of a prototype system for optical and radionuclide imaging in small animals. IEEE Trans Nucl Sci 50:1693–1701

189. Prout DL, Silverman RW, Chatziioannou AF (2004) Detector concept for OPET – a combined PET and optical imaging system. IEEE Trans Nucl Sci 51:752–756

190. Prout DL, Silverman RW, Chatziioannou AF (2005) Read-out of the optical PET (OPET) detector. IEEE Trans Nucl Sci 52:28–32

191. Douraghy A, Rannou FR, Silverman RW, Chatziioannou AF (2008) FPGA electronics for OPET: a dual-modality optical and positron emission tomograph. IEEE Trans Nucl Sci 55:2541–2545

192. Kim S-J et al (2006) Quantitative micro positron emission tomography (PET) imaging for the in vivo determination of pancreatic islet graft survival. Nat Med 12:1423–1428

193. Fox JG, Cohen BJ, Loew FM (1984) Laboratory animal medicine. Academic, Orlando

194. Hendrich H (2004) The laboratory mouse. Academic, Amsterdam

195. Suckow MA, Danneman P, Brayton C (2001) The laboratory mouse. CRC Press, Boca Raton

196. National Research Council (1996) Guide for the care and use of laboratory animals. National Academy, Washington

197. Flecknell PA (1993) Anaesthesia of animals for biomedical research. Br J Anaesth 71:885–894

198. Szczesny G, Veihelmann A, Massberg S, Nolte D, Messmer K (2004) Long-term anaesthesia using inhalatory isoflurane in different strains of mice–the haemodynamic effects. Lab Anim 38:64–69

199. Hildebrandt I, Su H, Weber WA (2008) Anesthesia and other considerations for in vivo imaging of small animals. ILAR J 49:17–26

200. Stout D et al (2005) Small animal imaging center design: the facility at the UCLA crump institute for molecular imaging. Mol Imaging Biol 7:393–402

201. Fueger BJ et al (2006) Impact of animal handling on the results of 18F-FDG PET studies in mice. J Nucl Med 47:999–1006

202. Suckow C et al (2008) Multimodality rodent imaging chambers for use under barrier conditions with gas anesthesia. Mol Imaging Biol 11(2):100–106

203. Wernick MN, Aarsvold JN (2004) Emission tomography: the fundamentals of PET and SPECT. Elsevier Academic, San Diego

204. Boone JM, Velazquez O, Cherry SR (2004) Small-animal X-ray dose from micro-CT. Mol Imaging 3:149–158

205. Segars WP, Tsui BMW, Frey EC, Johnson GA, Berr SS (2004) Development of a 4-D digital mouse phantom for molecular imaging research. Mol Imaging Biol 6:149–159

206. Taschereau R, Chow PL, Chatziioannou AF (2006) Monte Carlo simulations of dose from microCT imaging procedures in a realistic mouse phantom. Med Phys 33:216–224

207. Funk T, Sun M, Hasegawa BH (2004) Radiation dose estimate in small animal SPECT and PET. Med Phys 31:2680–2686

208. Taschereau R, Chatziioannou AF (2007) Monte Carlo simulations of absorbed dose in a mouse phantom from 18-fluorine compounds. Med Phys 34:1026–1036

209. Klaunberg BA, Davis JA (2008) Considerations for laboratory animal imaging center design and setup. ILAR J 49:4–16

210. Johnson K (2008) Introduction to rodent cardiac imaging. ILAR J 49:27–34

211. Roth DM, Swaney JS, Dalton ND, Gilpin EA, Ross J Jr (2002) Impact of anesthesia on cardiac function during echocardiography in mice. Am J Physiol Heart Circ Physiol 282:H2134–H2140

212. Strotmann J, Wiesmann F, Frantz S (2004) Cardiac imaging in a small animal model. Vis J 6:46–49

213. Jouannot E et al (2006) High-frequency ultrasound detection and follow-up of Wilms' tumor in the mouse. Ultrasound Med Biol 32:183–190

214. Badea CT, Fubara B, Hedlund LW, Johnson GA (2005) 4-D Micro-CT of the mouse heart. Mol Imaging 4:110–116

215. Drangova M, Ford NL, Detombe SA, Wheatley AW, Holdsworth DW (2007) Fast retrospectively gated quantitative four-dimensional (4D) cardiac micro computed tomography imaging of free-breathing mice. Investig Radiol 42:85–94

216. Badea C, Hedlund LW, Johnson GA (2004) Micro-CT with respiratory and cardiac gating. Med Phys 31:3324–3329

217. Cassidy PJ et al (2004) Assessment of motion gating strategies for mouse magnetic resonance at high magnetic fields. J Magn Reson Imaging 19:229–237

218. Yang Y, Rendig S, Siegel S, Newport DF, Cherry SR (2005) Cardiac PET imaging in mice with simultaneous cardiac and respiratory gating. Phys Med Biol 50:2979–2989

219. Weiss RG (2001) Imaging the murine cardiovascular system with magnetic resonance. Circ Res 88:550–551

220. Nahrendorf M et al (2003) Cardiac magnetic resonance imaging in small animal models of human heart failure. Med Image Anal 7:369–375

221. Hockings PD et al (2002) Repeated three-dimensional magnetic resonance imaging of atherosclerosis development in innominate arteries of low-density lipoprotein receptor-knockout mice. Circulation 106:1716–1721

222. Fayad ZA et al (1998) Noninvasive in vivo high-resolution magnetic resonance imaging of atherosclerotic lesions in genetically engineered mice. Circulation 98:1541–1547

223. Wu MC et al (2003) Pinhole single-photon emission computed tomography for myocardial perfusion imaging of mice. J Am Coll Cardiol 42:576–582

224. Wu JC et al (2003) Molecular imaging of cardiac cell transplantation in living animals using optical

bioluminescence and positron emission tomography. Circulation 108:1302–1305

225. Wu JC, Inubushi M, Sundaresan G, Schelbert HR, Gambhir SS (2002) Positron emission tomography imaging of cardiac reporter gene expression in living rats. Circulation 106:180–183

226. Chang GY, Xie X, Wu JC (2006) Overview of stem cells and imaging modalities for cardiovascular diseases. J Nucl Cardiol, Abstracts of Original Contributions 11th Annual Scientific Session 13:554–569

227. Carmeliet P (2005) Angiogenesis in life, disease and medicine. Nature 438:932–936

228. Dobrucki LW, Sinusas AJ (2005) Cardiovascular molecular imaging. Semin Nucl Med 35:73–81

229. Sinusas AJ (2004) Imaging of angiogenesis. J Nucl Cardiol 11:617–633

230. Haubner R et al (1999) Radiolabeled alpha-v-beta-3 integrin antagonists: a new class of tracers for tumor targeting. J Nucl Med 40:1061–1071

231. Haubner R et al (2001) Noninvasive imaging of alpha-v-beta-3 integrin expression using 18F-labeled RGD-containing glycopeptide and positron emission tomography. Cancer Res 61:1781–1785

232. Tempel-Brami C, Neeman M (2002) Non-invasive analysis of rat ovarian angiogenesis by MRI. Mol Cell Endocrinol 187:19–22

233. Verhoye M et al (2002) Assessment of the neovascular permeability in glioma xenografts by dynamic T1 MRI with Gadomer-17. Magn Reson Med 47:305–313

234. Goertz DE, Yu JL, Kerbel RS, Burns PN, Foster FS (2002) High-frequency doppler ultrasound monitors the effects of antivascular therapy on tumor blood flow. Cancer Res 62:6371–6375

235. Jorgensen SM, Demirkaya O, Ritman EL (1998) Three-dimensional imaging of vasculature and parenchyma in intact rodent organs with X-ray micro-CT. Am J Physiol Heart Circ Physiol 275:H1103–H1114

236. Blankenberg FG et al (1999) Imaging of apoptosis (programmed cell death) with 99mtc annexin V. J Nucl Med 40:184–191

237. Franklin KBJ, Paxinos G (2008) The Mouse Brain in Stereotaxic Coordinates, 3rd edn. Academic, San Diego

238. Mouse Brain Library. http://www.mbl.org/

239. Ahrens ET, Narasimhan PT, Nakada T, Jacobs RE (2002) Small animal neuroimaging using magnetic resonance microscopy. Prog Nucl Magn Reson Spectrosc 40:275–306

240. Johansson BB (2000) Brain plasticity and stroke rehabilitation: the Willis lecture. Stroke 31:223–230

241. Dijkhuizen RM et al (2001) Functional magnetic resonance imaging of reorganization in rat brain after stroke. Proc Natl Acad Sci USA 98:12766–12771

242. Silva AC, Bock NA (2008) Manganese-enhanced MRI: an exceptional tool in translational neuroimaging. Schizophr Bull 34:595–604

243. Bilgen M, Dancause N, Al-Hafez B, He Y-Y, Malone TM (2005) Manganese-enhanced MRI of rat spinal cord injury. Magn Reson Imaging 23:829–832

244. Acton P et al (2002) Occupancy of dopamine D2 receptors in the mouse brain measured using ultra-high-resolution single-photon emission tomography and [123]IBF. Eur J Nucl Med 29:1507–1515

245. Hume SP et al (1997) In vivo saturation kinetics of two dopamine transporter probes measured using a small animal positron emission tomography scanner. J Neurosci Meth 76:45–51

246. Jongen C, de Bruin K, Beekman F, Booij J (2008) SPECT imaging of D2 dopamine receptors and endogenous dopamine release in mice. Eur J Nucl Med Mol Imaging 35:1692–1698

247. Brownell A-L, Livni E, Galpern W, Isacson O (1998) In vivo PET imaging in rat of dopamine terminals reveals functional neural transplants. Ann Neurol 43:387–390

248. Torres EM et al (1995) Assessment of striatal graft viability in the rat in vivo using a small diameter PET scanner. NeuroReport 6:2017–2021

249. Lewis JS, Achilefu S, Garbow JR, Laforest R, Welch MJ (2002) Small animal imaging: current technology and perspectives for oncological imaging. Eur J Cancer 38:2173–2188

250. Shields AF et al (1998) Imaging proliferation in vivo with [F-18]FLT and positron emission tomography. Nat Med 4:1334–1336

251. Herschman HR (2003) Micro-PET imaging and small animal models of disease. Curr Opin Immunol 15:378–384

252. Czernin J, Weber WA, Herschman HR (2006) Molecular imaging in the development of cancer therapeutics. Annu Rev Med 57:99–118

253. Radu CG et al (2008) Molecular imaging of lymphoid organs and immune activation by positron emission tomography with a new [18F]-labeled 2[prime]-deoxycytidine analog. Nat Med 14:783–788

254. Lapointe D et al (1999) High-resolution PET imaging for in vivo monitoring of tumor response after photodynamic therapy in mice. J Nucl Med 40:876–882

255. Sundaresan G et al (2003) 124I-Labeled engineered anti-CEA minibodies and diabodies allow high-contrast, antigen-specific small-animal PET imaging of xenografts in athymic mice. J Nucl Med 44:1962–1969

256. Koutcher JA et al (2002) MRI of mouse models for gliomas shows similarities to humans and can be used to identify mice for preclinical trials. Neoplasia 4:480–485

257. Pulkkanen K et al (2000) Characterization of a new animal model for human renal cell carcinoma. In Vivo 14:393–400

258. Abdulkadir SA et al (2001) Impaired prostate tumorigenesis in Egr1-deficient mice. Nat Med 7:101–107

259. Ross BD et al (2003) Evaluation of cancer therapy using diffusion magnetic resonance imaging. Molecular Cancer Therapy 2:581–587

260. Jain RK (2005) Normalization of tumor vasculature: an emerging concept in antiangiogenic therapy. Science 307:58–62

261. Gross DJ et al (1999) The antiangiogenic agent linomide inhibits the growth rate of von hippel-lindau paraganglioma xenografts to mice. Clin Cancer Res 5:3669–3675

262. Badruddoja MA et al (2003) Antiangiogenic effects of dexamethasone in 9L gliosarcoma assessed by MRI cerebral blood volume maps. Neuro-Oncol 5:235–243

263. Tiefenauer LX, Tschirky A, Kuhne G, Andres RY (1996) In vivo evaluation of magnetite nanoparticles for use as a tumor contrast agent in MRI. Magn Reson Imaging 14:391–402

264. Cha S et al (2003) Dynamic, contrast-enhanced perfusion MRI in mouse gliomas: correlation with histopathology. Magn Reson Med 49:848–855

265. Sun Y et al (2004) Perfusion MRI of U87 brain tumors in a mouse model. Magn Reson Med 51:893–899

266. Cody DD et al (2005) Murine lung tumor measurement using respiratory-gated micro-computed tomography. Investig Radiol 40:263–269

267. De Clerck NM et al (2004) High-resolution X-ray micro-tomography for the detection of lung tumors in living mice. Neoplasia 6:374–379

268. Edinger M et al (1999) Noninvasive assessment of tumor cell proliferation in animal models. Neoplasia 1:303–310

269. Rehemtulla A et al (2000) Rapid and quantitative assessment of cancer treatment response using in vivo biolumi-nescence imaging. Neoplasia 2:491–495

270. Contag CH, Jenkins D, Contag PR, Negrin RS (2000) Use of reporter genes for optical measurements of neoplastic disease in vivo. Neoplasia 2:41–52

271. Weissleder R, Tung C-H, Mahmood U, Bogdanov A (1999) In vivo imaging of tumors with protease-activated near-infrared fluorescent probes. Nat Biotechnol 17:375–378

272. Becker A et al (2001) Receptor-targeted optical imaging of tumors with near-infrared fluorescent ligands. Nat Bio-technol 19:327–331

273. Whitesides GM (2006) The origins and the future of microfluidics. Nature 442:368–373

274. Lee C-C et al (2005) Multistep synthesis of a radiolabeled imaging probe using integrated microfluidics. Science 310:1793–1796

275. Cho, JS et al (2006) in Nuclear Science Symposium Con-ference Record, 2006. IEEE. 1977–1981. http://ieeexplore.ieee.org/xpl/freeabs_all.jsp?arnumber=4179415

276. Vu NT et al (2006) in Nuclear Science Symposium Confer-ence Record, 2006. IEEE. 3536–3539. http://ieeexplore.ieee.org/xpl/freeabs_all.jsp?arnumber=4179804

277. Judenhofer MS et al (2008) Simultaneous PET-MRI: a new approach for functional and morphological imaging. Nat Med 14:459–465

278. Catana C et al (2008) Simultaneous in vivo positron emis-sion tomography and magnetic resonance imaging. Proc Natl Acad Sci 105:3705–3710

279. Esenaliev RO et al (2002) Optoacoustic technique for noninvasive monitoring of blood oxygenation: a feasibility study. Appl Opt 41:4722–4731

280. Eghtedari M, Liopo AV, Copland JA, Oraevsky AA, Motamedi M (2008) Engineering of hetero-functional gold nanorods for the in vivo molecular targeting of breast cancer cells. Nano Lett 9(1): 287–291, http://pubs.acs.org/doi/abs/10.1021/nl802915q

281. Kruger RA, Kiser WL, Reinecke DR, Kruger GA, Miller KD (2003) Thermoacoustic molecular imaging of small animals. Mol Imaging 2:113–123

282. Chaudhari AJ et al (2005) Hyperspectral and multispectral bioluminescence optical tomography for small animal imaging. Phys Med Biol 50:5421–5441

283. Zavattini G et al (2006) A hyperspectral fluorescence system for 3D in vivo optical imaging. Phys Med Biol 51:2029–2043

Index

Printing and Binding: Stürtz GmbH, Würzburg